THE SOFT TISSUES

Trauma and Sports Injuries

Edited by

G. R. McLatchie FRCS
Consultant in General and Peripheral Vascular Surgery, The General Hospital, Hartlepool, UK; Director of the National Sports Medicine Institute, London, UK; and Visiting Professor in Sports Medicine, University of Sunderland, UK

and

C. M. E. Lennox FRCS (Orth) (Ed)
Consultant Orthopaedic Surgeon, The General Hospital, Hartlepool, UK

Assistant Editors

E. C. Percy BSc, MD CM, MSc, Dip Surg (McGill), FACS, FRCS(C)
Associate Professor, Department of Surgery and Adjunct Associate Professor, Department of Exercise and Sport Sciences, University of Arizona, USA (Retired)

and

J. Davies LRCS, LRCP, DPhys Med
Consultant in Rehabilitation and Sports Medicine, Devonshire Hospital, London, and Guy's Hospital, London, UK

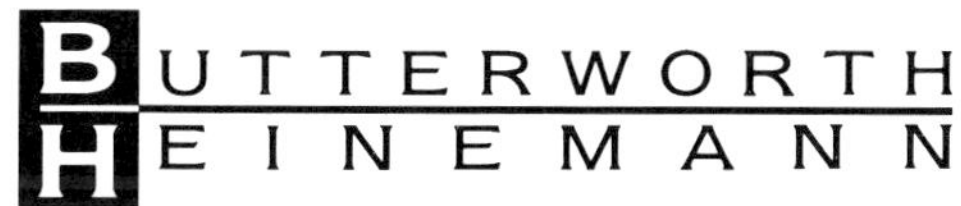

Butterworth-Heinemann
Linacre House, Jordan Hill, Oxford OX2 8DP
A division of Reed Educational and Professional Publishing Ltd

A member of the Reed Elsevier plc group

OXFORD BOSTON JOHANNESBURG
MELBOURNE NEW DELHI SINGAPORE

First published 1993
Paperback edition 1996
Reprinted 1996

British Library Cataloguing in Publication Data
A catalogue for this book is available from the British Library

ISBN 0 7506 3065 5

Phototypeset by Wilmaset Ltd, Birkenhead, Wirral
Printed and bound in Great Britain

Contents

Part III – Sports Injuries

Contributors

Adewale Adebajo MB, BS, FACP, is Arthritis and Rheumatism Council of Great Britain Research Fellow at the Department of Rheumatology, Addenbrooke's Hospital, Cambridge. In addition to managing sports injuries, his research interests include new diagnostic and therapeutic measures for sports injuries.

Malcolm B Bottomley MB, ChB, is the Medical Officer to the University of Bath. He is also an Honorary Medical Officer to the British Athletics Federation and is Medical Director of the Distance Learning Course in Sports Medicine for doctors offered by the University of Bath. His experience in sports medicine includes previous posts as an Honorary Medical Officer to the Football Association of Wales and to Bath Rugby Football Club. He attended the 1988 Olympic Games as Medical Officer to the Great Britain track and field athletics team.

Hugh C Burry MB, ChB, FRACP, FRCP (Lond), D Phys Med, FACRM, FACSP, lately Professor and Director of Rehabilitation Medicine, Melbourne University and Royal Melbourne and Essendon Hospitals, Australia. Previous posts include Director of the Department of Rheumatology, Guy's Hospital, London; Consultant Physician to the Sports Council of Great Britain; and Associate Professor of Rheumatology, Wellington Clinical School of Medicine, Australia.

Tony Butlin MA, Adv Dip Phys Ed, MIHE, is Principal Lecturer in the School of Health Sciences at the University of Sunderland. His lecturing and research commitments are in the field of exercise physiology, from which he has gained a vast amount of experience in the fitness assessment of both the élitist in sport and in members of the community. He is a fitness consultant to many sports clubs and community leisure centres on methods of training and their assessment.

Kenneth S Carnine MD, Chief of the Department of Surgery, Head of Orthopedic Division, Affiliated Health Services Hositals, Skagit County, Washington, USA. Member of 15 medical societies. Multiple previous pubications. Current Medical Director of Pacific Coast Rugby Football Union and Co-Medical Director of USA Rugby Football Union.

John L Chase MD, FACS, Fellow, American Academy of Orthopedic Surgery, President of Benchmark Medical Group, Orthopedic Consultant to the United States Air Force Reserve, Honorary Medical Advisor to the United States Rugby Football Union, Chief Physician for the US Eagles Rugby Team, Founding Member International College of Rugby Medicine. He maintains active practice in orthopedics, trauma and sports injuries in Oakland, CA and Sacramento, CA, USA.

Mary Dyson BSc, PhD, is Director of the Tissue Repair Research Unit, Division of Anatomy and Cell Biology, United Medical and Dental Schools of Guy's and St. Thomas's Hospitals, London, UK, and Reader in Tissue Repair Biology of the University of London. She is an Honorary Fellow of the American Institute of Ultrasound in Medicine, and of the Chartered Society of Physiotherapy.

Roger Evans MB, BS, FRCP, is Consultant in Emergency Medicine at the Cardiff Royal Infirmary. He was previously Consultant in Emergency Medicine at the Royal Devon and Exeter Hospital.

Shirley Hancock ONC, MCSP, SRP, is Physiotherapy Manager at the RDC Physiotherapy Clinic, London, the Royal Ballet Schools and the Royal Academy of Dancing.

Brian Hazleman MA, FRCP, is Consultant Rheumatologist at Addenbrooke's Hospital, Director of the Rheumatology Research Unit and Fellow at Corpus Christi College in Cambridge. He is interested in many aspects of the rheumatic diseases and, in particular, assessing the treatment of soft tissue rheumatism. In addition he carries out research studies into the causation and treatment of soft tissue rheumatism.

Justin Howse MB, BS, FRCS, is Consultant Orthopaedic Surgeon, Medical Director of St. Vincent's Orthopaedic Hospital, Director of the RDC Physiotherapy Clinic, London. Orthopaedic Consultant to the Royal Ballet Schools, the Royal Academy of Dancing and the Royal Society of Musicians. Trustee and Council Member of the British Performing Arts Medicine Trust.

Simon L Knight MB, FRCS, is a Consultant in Plastic Surgery and Hand Surgery, at the Plastic Surgery Unit, St James's University Hospital, Leeds.

Michael Kody MD, is currently in private practice as an orthopaedic surgeon in Spokane, Washington, USA, and has completed a 1-year fellowship at the Orthopedic Specialty Hospital.

Catherine M E Lennox MB, ChB, FRCS (Orth) (Ed) began her orthopaedic career in her native Scotland and subsequently in Newcastle upon Tyne, spending several years training on a part-time basis while being mother of two. She is now a full-time Consultant Orthopaedic Surgeon in Hartlepool General Hospital, Hartlepool, Cleveland. She is currently involved in establishing a 'knee injury clinic' and arthroscopy service to complement the sports medicine clinic in Hartlepool.

Evan Llewelyn Lloyd MB, ChB, FRCS (Ed), FCAnaes, is a Consultant Anaesthetist at Princess Margaret Rose Orthopaedic Hospital in Edinburgh. Previous posts include Medical Officer, Bamdah Mission Hospital in India, posts in geriatrics and general medicine in Scotland, and Staff Anaesthetist, Toronto General Hospital, Canada.

John Lloyd Parry MA, MB, BChir, is Medical Adviser to the Fédération Equestre Internationale and to the Governing Body of the British Horse Society Horse Trials (Eventing). He is also a Member of the Committee of the Medical Commission on Accident Prevention (Sports).

Caroline J MacEwen MB, ChB, FRCS (Ed), FC, Ophth, is a Consultant Ophthalmologist at Ninewells Hospital and Medical School, Dundee.

Donald A D Macleod FRCS, is a Consultant General Surgeon, St John's Hospital, Livingston, West Lothian, UK. Honorary Medical Advisor to the Scottish Rugby Union and Chairman of the Scottish Sports Council Consultative Group on Sports Medicine and Sports Science.

Greg R McLatchie FRCS, is Consultant in General and Peripheral Vascular Surgery, The General Hospital, Hartlepool. He is also Director of the National Sports Medicine Institute, London, and Visiting Professor in Sports Medicine, University of Sunderland.

Ian McLean BSc (Hons) MB, ChB, FRCS (Glas), is a Registrar in Orthopaedic Surgery in Falkirk. A member of the Scientific Group of the International Orienteering Federation, he is also assistant medical officer to the British Orienteering Squad and part of the medical team of the Royal and Ancient Golf Club.

M O'Brien is Professor of Anatomy, Trinity College, Dublin, where she is also Director of the Human Performance Laboratory.

Lonnie Paulos MD, is currently in private practice in Salt Lake City, Utah, USA. He is Co-Director of the Orthopedic Specialty Hospital and Medical Director of the Orthopedic Biomechanics Institute. He is an Associate Clinical Professor at the Division of Orthopedic Surgery, University of Utah Medical School. Previously, he was the Co-Director of Cincinnati Sports Medicine Institute.

Edward C Percy BSc, MD CM, MSc, Dip Surg (McGill), FACS, FRCS(C), is Associate Professor, Department of Surgery and Adjunct Associate Professor, Department of Exercise and Sport Sciences, University of Arizona, USA (retired).

Arup K Ray MB, BS, MS (Gen. Surg.), FRCS (Ed) is Senior Registrar in Plastic Surgery at the West of Scotland Regional Plastic and Maxillofacial Surgery Unit, Canniesburn Hospital, Glasgow, Scotland.

David A Sherlock BM, BCh, MA, DPhil, FRCS, is a consultant at both the Royal Hospital for Sick Children and the Southern General Hospital in Glasgow. His previous posts include Oxford, Reading and Swindon.

Roger Soames BSc, PhD, is a Senior Lecturer in Anatomy at King's College London. His previous publications include *Anatomy and Human Movement: Structure and Function*.

David S Soutar ChM, FRCS (Ed), FRCS (Glas), MB, ChB, is Consultant Plastic Surgeon at the West of Scotland Regional Plastic and Maxillofacial Surgery Unit, Glasgow and Honorary Clinical Senior Lecturer at the University of Glasgow. His previous posts include Senior Registrar in Plastic Surgery, Canniesburn Hospital and Registrar in General Surgery, Grampian Health Board.

Ian G Stother MA, MB, BChir, FRCS (Ed) FRCS (Glas) is a Consultant Orthopaedic Surgeon at Glasgow Royal Infirmary, Glasgow, Scotland. He is also an Honorary Clinical Senior Lecturer in Orthopaedic and Accident Surgery at the University of Glasgow and an Honorary Lecturer in Bioengineering at the University of Strathclyde. He has been Orthopaedic Advisor to the Scottish Ballet and the Dance School for Scotland.

Jonathan Vafidis MA, FRCS, is a Consultant Neurosurgeon working at the University Hospital of Wales, Cardiff. His specialist training was undertaken at Cardiff, and subsequently the Radcliffe Infirmary, Oxford and Manchester Royal Infirmary.

Michael Whittle BSc, MB, BS, MSc, PhD, occupies the Cline Chair of Rehabilitation Technology at the University of Tennessee at Chattanooga. His previous posts include Acting Director of the Oxford Orthopaedic Engineering Centre at the University of Oxford, where he ran the gait analysis laboratory, and principal coordinating scientist for NASA's Skylab Medical Experiments. His previous publications include *Gait Analysis: an introduction*.

Foreword

It was with a great deal of pleasure that I accepted the invitation to provide the foreword to this book in view of the friendship and association with the editor, which I have enjoyed over many years.

He continually reminds me that I was one of his teachers during his undergraduate years in Glasgow, but even in those early formative years I became aware of his interest in injuries sustained during sporting activities. Himself no mean sporting performer he found time within his busy workload as a junior hospital doctor to publish reports on surveys of injuries in different sports.

From this beginning his interest expanded to encompass many aspects of sports medicine, including its teaching, to the extent that he was an ideal appointment to the Directorship of the National Sports Medicine Institute.

Over many years our knowledge of the nature and healing of injuries of the soft tissues has grown very slowly, although steadily, based largely on empiricism but it has been with the application of modern technology that methods of diagnosis, treatment and rehabilitation have significantly advanced more recently.

These advances are reflected in the various chapters of this book extending from the modern imaging techniques which have proved so useful in diagnosis through logical treatment both conservative and surgical to rehabilitation based on a better knowledge of the behaviour of the soft tissues.

Professor McLatchie is to be congratulated on persuading such experts in their field to participate then compiling their contributions into such a single important volume on soft tissue injuries which has been sorely needed.

James Graham MB, ChB, FRCS(Ed), FRCS(Glas)
Department of Orthopaedics
Western Infirmary
Glasgow

Preface

The diagnosis, treatment and rehabilitation of patients with problems relating to the soft tissues constitute a significant part of the workload of doctors in many disiplines. All age groups can be affected but the pathologies are often ill-understood and the management based on empirical methods. The fact that many soft tissue lesions will settle spontaneously further compounds the issue but should serve as positive reassurance for many patients who are losing time from work (for the economic implications are considerable), sport or play. So extensive is the problem that it has been described as the 'unthwarted epidemic' by some authorities in the USA.

Against this background we have invited specialists in specific areas of soft tissue management worldwide to crystallize their experience, our aim being to increase the general understanding of this complex clinical minefield in the hope that it will lead to a more structured approach to dealing effectively with our patients. We are grateful to all the contributors for addressing their task so comprehensively and enthusiastically. They have fulfilled their part of this commitment. We hope, in drawing together these disparate subjects, that we have fulfilled ours.

G R McLatchie
C M E Lennox
Hartlepool, UK, 1993

Acknowledgements

We are grateful to all who have been involved:

- our contributors for meeting such high standards and their deadlines
- our secretaries for their hard work and surprisingly happy dispositions
- all who have contributed photographs and line drawings
- the staff at Butterworth-Heinemann committed to this project
- and James Graham, FRCS, who gave us the idea in the first place!

The photographs on pages 83, 90, 351, 371, 383, 389, 395, 415, 467, 468 and 469 are courtesy of Dirk van der Werff and Tom Collins of the Hartlepool Mail.

The publishers would like to thank Paul Elliott and Corydon Lowde of the Oxford City Ryobukai Karate Club for the photograph appearing on page 443.

Part I

General Principles

1

Incidence, nature and economic effects of soft tissue injury

A. O. Adebajo
B. L. Hazelman

Introduction

Soft tissue injuries, although commonly overlooked in the planning and provision of health care, are disorders of major and increasing importance. Fortunately there has been an increase in interest with regard to these lesions concomitant with an increase in our understanding of these disorders.

Soft tissue rheumatism includes lesions of tendons and the tenoperiosteal junction, and the development of the unifying concept of the local enthesopathies is a recent finding marking progress in the field of soft tissue rheumatism. The primary forms of these conditions are unassociated with arthritis or connective tissue diseases. Some of these disorders are regional, including sports-related and occupational soft tissue rheumatism problems, whereas others are generalized such as the fibromyalgia syndrome. In general laboratory and roentgenographic examination findings are normal.

Whilst soft tissue problems are rarely associated with mortality there is a high morbidity from these lesions. Since these patients seldom come to surgery, the opportunity to study their pathology has hitherto been infrequent and consequently poorly understood. Recently however much attention is being focused on the histology and biochemistry of tendon (Chard *et al.*, 1985, 1987; Webster and Burry, 1982). A large proportion of local causes of soft tissue rheumatism are related to chronic repetitive low-grade trauma and excessive and unaccustomed use (both at work and at play). These factors may also cause partial interruption of the blood supply resulting in incomplete attempts at healing and degeneration, which render these tissues more vulnerable in the middle-aged and the elderly in whom these lesions predominate. Since the vascular supply to adult tendon is poor, healing of these lesions is slow. Poor tendon repair and degeneration would appear to explain the chronicity of tendon lesions. *In vivo* work has suggested that tendon healing after damage involves the reaction of surrounding tissue and adhesion without participation of the tendon tissue itself (Moushe *et al.*, 1984). Other studies have revealed that tendons are capable of responding to injury, although it does appear that most actively dividing cells are derived from the superficial part of the tendon. Chard *et al.* (1987) have shown that the majority of cells obtained from tendon that are capable of replication *in vitro* are derived from the superficial layer of tendon (epithelium).

Growth characteristics of the cell lines have been established by investigating DNA synthesis using thymidine incorporation in response to stimulation by fetal calf serum. No significant reduction in growth response with increasing age was found.

Initial light microscopy analysis of normal

rotator cuff tendons (Chard *et al.*, 1989) suggests a general thickening of blood vessels, fewer tendon fibroblasts, increased mucopolysaccharide and increased calcification with increasing age. Attention has been drawn to the unifying concept of the enthesopathies, suggesting that local ischaemia is the common denominator in their causation. The enthesis is always at risk because the working muscle takes up most of the blood at the expense of the tendon and insertion. Other contributory factors include overstressing, microtraumatization, muscular hypertonus and excessive cooling. Endogenous factors such as impaired vascularization, metabolic disorders, endocrine disorders, trophic disorders, toxic damage and even psychological factors may also influence damage to the enthesis. Those tendons without sheaths are better supplied with blood than tendons in sheaths and studies of dynamic *in vivo* blood flow in these regions may yield valuable information.

Collagen is the basic framework of all soft tissues. Once a tear occurs within the collagen bundles, the defect is replaced by haphazard, loose connective tissue formed in the blood clot which initially fills the torn area. Thus the intrinsic structural strength may be reduced significantly, leading to impaired power, mobility, skill and eventually to further damage.

Recent interest has centred on the role of prostaglandin synthesis and release in response to soft tissue injury due to either trauma or overuse. After injury a prostaglandin 'cascade' occurs as a secondary event. Prostaglandins may act synergistically with other inflammatory mediators such as histamine, serotonin and bradykinin to potentiate both swelling and pain. Muscle injuries are associated with bleeding to a greater or lesser degree and interstitial haematomas produce marked pain and loss of function. Muscle regeneration is a slow process. Strains affect muscles; with minor strains, only fibre damage occurs and the muscle sheath is left intact. With more severe strains a partial or complete rupture of fibres and sheath is present. A sprain is an overstretch injury of a ligament. It may affect only a few fibres, or complete or partial tears of tendons may occur. Each tendon is surrounded by a paratenor and, in sites where movement occurs around bone, is further enclosed in a fibrous sheath. Most tendon injuries are due to overuse. In tendinitis and peritendinitis, either the tendon or its sheath becomes inflamed and swollen. Tendovaginitis occurs in sites where there is no synovial sheath such as the anterior tibial tendons as they traverse the front of the ankle joint. The sheath becomes inflamed and there is crepitus and pain on movement (tendovaginitis crepitans). Bursae are found where tendons or muscles move over bony prominences. They may also be subcutaneous and can become acutely inflamed.

Soft tissue injuries due to sport are in essence acute or severe forms of the soft tissue disorders seen in non-sportsmen. The increasing popularity of sport is evidenced by the sight of joggers in the streets and the increasing popularity of marathon runs, gymnasia and fitness training. The last General Household Survey conducted in the UK in 1985 showed that the highest involvement in at least one outdoor sport, excluding rambling, was by full-time students (41%), falling off after this generally young age group, with a continuing greater involvement by professional (27%) than unskilled manual workers (9%). The last decade has seen a dramatic increase in the number of participants in sport. Folsom *et al.* (1985) state that the proportion of Americans taking regular exercise has more than doubled since 1961. As in the UK, the professional groups participate more and this more vocal group is likely to insist on proper health provision for their sports injuries.

This increase in participation has occurred for several reasons. Firstly there is a general awareness that regular exercise is related to good health. Secondly there is broader acceptance of the 'sport for all' concept promoted by successive governments, especially in the USA and Germany but also in the UK, with regular aerobic exercise being advocated as a major component of health promotion and disease prevention for all age groups, from children to the elderly. Unfortunately there is a high level of neuroticism amongst some people with injuries. Even Hippocrates recognized this problem and stated that 'all parts of the body which have a function, if used in moderation and exercised in labours in which each is accustomed, become thereby healthy, well-developed and age more slowly, but if unused and left idle they become liable to disease, defective in growth and age quickly'. The overstepping of Hippocrates's suggestion of moderation in exercise, and thus sports appropriate to the individual, leads not to health but to injury, most frequently involving the soft tissues.

Reliable information about sports injuries is scarce. There is a suggestion that the incidence of sports-related symptoms is increasing (Newman *et al.*, 1969). It is however impossible to know whether such data represent real demand, changing demography or improved clinical services. Body contact sports are the most likely to cause injury and endurance sports are those most likely to induce overuse problems. In one sports clinic, overuse injuries accounted for 32% of the total injuries, and of these 64% were found in track and field athletes (Sperryn, 1972). Application of broad epidemiological considerations to a range of sporting activities in the community is yet to be performed. Much less arduous are those epidemiological surveys conducted by questionnaire. This approach has the advantage of allowing manageable access to large populations. One British study questioned 1700 injured joggers and marathan runners to determine the distribution of injuries (Temple, 1983). Problems affecting the knee had the highest frequency (25%), followed by Achilles tendon symptoms (17%). An American investigation of 2500 runners concluded that more than one-third of the runners had musculoskeletal problems attributable to running over 1 year (Koplan *et al.*, 1982). Only one-seventh had sought medical attention, indicating how unrepresentative clinic-based surveys may be. In sports participants the relationship of symptoms to overuse, inadequate training or repeated minor trauma is often easy to establish. The same mechanisms are also usually responsible for similar conditions in non-sportsmen, requiring the same prompt treatment and advice to avoid exacerbation by altering work patterns. Occupational repetitive strain injuries have in particular become a significant source of disability at work in recent years.

An accurate diagnosis of soft tissue rheumatism can be made by taking a careful history considering possible trauma or overuse, and carrying out a systematic examination. For most local lesions, further investigation is unnecessary and X-rays which reveal the expected age-related degenerative changes can often confuse. It is usually apparent if there is a more generalized condition which needs appropriate investigation. One feature common to all soft tissue syndromes is a tendency to spontaneous remission. Many of the lesions take weeks to improve and only few persist with significant symptoms beyond 6 months. A clear diagnosis consequently evokes a doctor to reassure the patient that the prognosis is good and that failure to resolve is often due to further injury. Few of the conditions require complete rest, but most respond to selective rest of the involved region. Modalities of treatment, where required, include the use of splints, exercises and forms of physiotherapy including such measures as ultrasound and megapulse. The short-term use of non-steroidal anti-inflammatory drugs may be necessary. Their immediate use is beneficial in limiting the pain and swelling of soft tissue trauma. Many soft tissue lesions respond to a local well-placed injection with steroid and anaesthetic.

Recent advances in the diagnosis and management of the more common syndromes has helped in a better understanding and care for patients with these varied problems. As knowledge of the anatomical, biochemical, physical, emotional and behavioural mechanisms contributing to these syndromes improves, their management will become better standardized and more effective.

Epidemiology

Statistics on the incidence of soft tissue injuries are sadly inadequate as the much needed epidemiological studies have hitherto only infrequently been performed. Indeed Dixon (1979) has described soft tisssue rheumatism as the great outback of rheumatology, a vast frontier land, ill-defined and little explained, its features poorly categorized and far from internationally agreed. The fact that any or all of these soft tissue lesions may be associated with overt systemic disease makes classification and interpretation of data difficult. The lack of universally acceptable defined criteria for these injuries has been a major obstacle to conducting epidemiological studies.

The absence of specific diagnostic tests for the soft tissue syndromes highlights the importance of developing diagnostic criteria based on combinations of the predominant clinical features that are sensitive enough to exclude those without the syndrome. Most of these syndromes will be covered by the inclusion criteria of pain at a specific site or sites, local tenderness, limitation of movement and pain on specific restricted movement or movements. There is a need for rigorous diagnostic criteria taking into account the lack of a 'gold standard' reference test, the continuous distribution pattern of the symptoms and signs, the variation in disease expression and different time points and the inter- and intraobserver variation in eliciting these clinical signs. Such diagnostic criteria are required for defining occurrence, measuring outcome and assessing the effect of intervention, for example in recruitment to clinical trials.

Lawrence (1977) gives a review based on the occurrence of pain in various parts of the body, without attempting to determine the scope and incidence of soft tissue lesions *per se*. A population survey by the Swedish National Central Bureau of statistics indicates a prevalence of all forms of soft tissue rheumatism of 1.6% in men and 3.6% in women (Bjelle *et al.*, 1980). Chronic complaints attributed to non-articular rheumatism as well as miscellaneous back disorders were estimated to occur in about 3% of the adult (18–70 years) US population in the 1976 National Health Interview survey (National Center for Health Statistics, 1976). This compared with a frequency of about 3% of symptoms attributed to rheumatoid arthritis and 8% to degenerative joint disease. Together soft tissue lesions represent one-third of all rheumatic diseases seen by family physicians and represent 3–4% of all ambulatory medical care visits (Wood *et al.*, 1979).

There is considerable confusion in diagnostic terminology and a wide variation in reported incidence between countries, probably reflecting the contrasting as well as legal attitudes to these conditions. In general the increased incidence of these disorders appears to be due to new technology lending to advanced automation and mechanization. With most other rheumatic diseases, however, one is uncertain whether there is an apparent increase in risk in certain industries, or whether there is an absolute increase in risk or an increase in the rate of developing these lesions. Occupational disorders are of interest because, theoretically at least, it should be possible to devise methods of working that could prevent their development. Certainly sufferers are at present in considerable hazard of repeated attendances, as indicated by recrudescence rates reported for 'beat' knee (12%), 'beat' elbow (7%) and tenosynovitis of the wrist (6%) by Wood and McLeish (1974).

It would be of interest to learn why only a proportion of individuals exposed to particular methods of working develop soft tissue injuries. Automation and mechanization have led to the need for reptitive movements often limited to the upper limbs or even the hands and wrists alone. Although actual physical work loads may be lighter, it is this increased rate of work concentrated locally on an individual's musculoskeletal system that results in repetition strain injuries and associated overuse syndromes. This has been a focus of recent attention (Editorial, 1987; Barton, 1989; Brooks, 1989). The role of occupation and how we use or overuse parts of our body is striking and suggests that if alternative ways of accomplishing various activities can be developed then at least a part of the problem could be controlled. In this regard, ergonomic and behavioural studies have much to offer (Elland, 1985).

The crude differences in age patterns may be discerned between traumatic and non-traumatic forms of soft tissue rheumatism. The frequency of spells of strains and sprains tends to reduce after the 30s, whereas non-traumatic conditions show a less marked decline and this does not appear until after the 40s. Rates in women tend in general to be less than in men. The most recent population study available which includes specific concern with certain forms of soft tissue rheumatism is that by Allander (1974). Unfortunately age and sex-specific prevalence ratios were quoted only for four quinquennial groups between the ages of 30 and 75 years, so that an overall population frequency cannot be determined. Nevertheless, the data suggest surprisingly high rates – the unweighted mean prevalence in the groups was 16% for the painful shoulder and 3% for tennis elbow.

Of localized problems, the painful shoulder ranks highest in frequency and consequently has been better documented than most other soft tissue lesions. Regional shoulder complaints rank fifth among the regional rheumatic diseases as a course of incapacity or of visiting a physician. This contrasts with one in 30 for back pain. Nearly one million cases were recorded in the USA in 1976 by the National Center for Statistics (Kelsey, 1982). Data from UK general practices (Department of Health and Social Security, 1986) suggest that approximately one in 170 of the adult population will present to their general practitioner with a new episode of shoulder pain each year. This contrasts with one in 30 for back pain.

The elderly frequently have considerable functional impairment and Chard and Hazleman (1989a) found that over 20% of the elderly hospital population have shoulder disorders: less than one-fifth of these had sought medical attention. Community-based studies also indicate that there is a large reservoir of elderly people with soft tissue shoulder disability (Chard and Hazelman, 1989b; Chakravarty and Webley, 1990).

The association between shoulder pain and occupation was highlighted in a study of the medical outpatient departments of six heavy industries by Bjelle *et al.* (1979). Approximately one-third of the visits were for non-traumatic musculoskeletal complaints, of which 30–50% were neck–shoulder complaints. In Allander's study (Allander, 1974) a significantly higher prevalence of painful shoulder was found in males than in females in the age groups 56–60 (27 and 20% respectively) and 70–74 years (21 and 16% respectively). The prevalence of painful shoulder was similar in males and females in two younger age groups – 31–35 (7–8%) and 42–44 years (15%) – and lower than in the age groups 50–60 and 70–74 years. The annual incidence peaked significantly in the age group 42–46 years (2.5 and 2.2% in males and females, respectively), compared to around 1% in both sexes in age groups 31–35 and 56–60 years, and 0.9% (females) and 1.6% (males) in the oldest age group of 70–74 years. In the USA, the Health and Nutrition Examination Survey 1971–1975 (Miller, 1973) studied the adult population aged 25–74 years. They found that 4.2% had suffered from shoulder complaints and physician-observed abnormalities were present in 1.2% (Cunningham and Kelsey, 1984). Almost 40% had associated neck complaints. In over 80%, the complaints had occurred during the year before the study. However, only a few of the other 6000 probands reported that these shoulder complaints had caused absence from work. Physician-observed abormalities in the shoulder were found in 3%.

An interview survey from Finland carried out in 1973–1974 (Takala *et al.* 1982) studied the prevalence of shoulder pain occurring fairly often, often, or continuously during the year preceding the interview. In women an annual prevalence of right-sided shoulder/upper arm region pain was found in 11% under the age of 50 and in 25% over the age of 50 years. On the left side, the prevalence was somewhat lower, at 9 and 20% respectively. In men, the prevalence was 11% under 50 and 22% over 50 years of age, with a similar prevalence for left and right sides. An interview survey in a Philippine village (Manahan *et al.*, 1985) found a prevalence of reported shoulder pain of 1.7% in males and 2.8% in females in the population over 15 years of age. Trapezius and neck pain was significantly more frequent in farmers than in non-farmers, suggesting an association between working conditions and pain in the neck–trapezius area. A study of past shoulder complaints in the inhabitants of an Indonesian village reported that 10% of the population over 15 years of age was affected (Darmanan, 1988). Similar figures have been found in an indigenous African population (Adebajo and Hazleman, 1990).

In a study of the elderly in Sweden (Bergstrom *et al.*, 1985a), shoulder complaints were reported by 16% of women and 15% of men in a representative population sample of 79-year-olds. At physical examination, rotator cuff tenderness on palpation was noted on the dorsal aspect in 6%, on the anterior aspect in 10%, and on the upper part of the right shoulder in 12% of the females and in 0, 0 and 8% respectively of the males. Similar figures were obtained on examination of the left shoulder. The range of motion was normal in 61%. Active internal rotation was decreased in one-third of the individuals, passive internal rotation in only 16%. The frequency of restricted range of motion in individuals reporting shoulder complaints was 50% (Bergstrom *et al.*, 1985b). There was no difference in the frequency of complaints in individuals with either active or passive restricted range of motion. Active as well as passive restriction of movement was significantly associated with difficulty in entering public transport.

Age, sex and occupation appear to be definite risk factors for shoulder lesions. Health care (Kvarnstrom 1983; Dimberg, 1985) and insurance data (Kivi, 1984) support the role of age in shoulder complaints amongst workers in the production industry. The influence of age may partly be due to the frequent finding of degenerative changes of the rotator cuff (Post, 1978; Chard and Hazleman, 1989a), making this tissue highly vulnerable to trauma after the fifth decade. Similarly, regardless of the study design, there seems to be overwhelming evidence that females run a higher risk than males of developing shoulder complaints when working in production industries. Health care data (Kvarnstrom, 1983), insurance registers (Kivi, 1984) and cross-sectional studies (Dimberg, 1985) all point in the same direction. In the Finnish study (Kivi, 1984) on reports on occupational disorders in which repetitive tasks were mentioned as an associated factor, periarthritis of the shoulder accounted for 9% of all cases. It was more frequent in females than in males and correlated with age. Butchers and workers in the food-processing industry were at highest risk of developing painful shoulders. For the entity referred to as frozen shoulder or adhesive capsulitis, the peak incidence is between 50 and 70 years (Hazleman, 1972). The condition is encountered slightly more commonly in women than in men. The left (non-dominant) shoulder is more frequently involved and, although rarely recurring, the contralateral shoulder may become affected more commonly than would be expected by chance (Kessel *et al.*, 1981).

Further studies are required to determine whether the age, sex and occupation pattern seen with shoulder lesions is equally applicable to other specific soft tissue injuries. Data available for tenosynovitis of the wrist show an apparent similarity in a predominant sex incidence (Muckart, 1986). Tennis elbow or lateral epicondylitis affects 1–3% of the population (Allander, 1974). It occurs mostly between 40 and 60 years of age and usually affects the dominant arm. Interestingly, while some 40–50% of tennis players suffer with it, and it is more frequent and severe in older players (Nirschl and Pettrone, 1973; Gruchow and Pelletier, 1979), less than 5% of cases are related to the game (Conrad and Hooper, 1973) and it is found more often in non-athletes. The majority are not manual workers and many cannot describe any precipitating factors (Binder and Hazleman, 1983). As previously mentioned, occupation repetitive strain injury is obtaining increasing prominence. The apparent increase in its incidence in recent times may be due to an increased acceptance and recognition of the condition among doctors. Thus its true incidence remains unknown.

Various statistics are available to indicate the burden that back pain causes to the community. These show clearly that back pain resulting from soft tissue back injury is an important component of the morbidity from soft tissue problems. Unfortunately semantic difficulties over what is meant by back pain results in different criteria being used by different workers. Furthermore the symptoms are often intermittent, such that less than half of those with back problems can be detected by a cross-sectional study. There is also a high spontaneous recovery rate. Dixon (1980) has suggested that 92% of those who sought medical advice for back pain recovered within 2 months. On the other hand, Quinet and Hadler (1979) estimated that about 70% of the population will be affected by backache at some time in their lives. They also claimed that 90% of those who have to seek medical advice will have a recurrence and that

10% will have prolonged disability. Of a cross-sectional study of 2684 men from a range of occupations (Anderson, 1983), 17.8% had back pain for which no obvious bony cause was found.

Within the UK there are regional variations to the burden that back pain presents to the community. In our region, East Anglia, back pain accounts for the highest percentage of total sickness absence in the region (Office of Population Censuses and Surveys, 1974) and this is nearly double that of the South-East region. These regional differences may be due to attitudes towards sickness absence and the sick rate, in addition to any environment and occupational practices. In industry, back pain is an important cause of absence from work with consequences to industry, society and the individual. It has been estimated that out of the 22 900 000 episodes of ill health experienced in the UK in one year, approximately 10% will consult their general practitioners with back pain. Of these, 330 000 will be referred to hospital, 63 000 will be admitted, and of all those hospitalized, 60% bear the diagnosis of non-specific back pain (Office of Health Economics, 1985). Insufficient information is available on ethnic, socioeconomic, racial or genetic predisposition of various forms of soft tissue rheumatism and further epidemiological studies are keenly awaited.

Economic effects and burden on health care service

Soft tissue rheumatism is a major cause of morbidity and of loss of productive hours at work, and a heavy burden on medical resources. Judged by certification of sickness incapacity and of those who attend medical, rheumatological and orthopaedic outpatients in hospitals or by the burden of consultation with general practitioners and private specialists, soft tissue rheumatism is a conspicuous feature of the scenery of ill health. Among younger and middle-aged adults in particular, problems caused by soft tissue rheumatism collectively may be expected to be the most common rheumatic disorder – possibly the main cause of absenteeism and decreased productivity. Almost everyone experiences transient signs of soft tissue rheumatism due to the periodic excesses of normal living. The inconvenience and discomfort of sports injuries are personal measures of importance; however, there are other dimensions which are relevant to society as a whole. There is an increasing demand for medical attention for both acute and chronic injuries. A significant portion of this burden falls on hospital orthopaedic and rheumatology services with a consequent strain on health resources. Orthopaedic and accident departments, for example, are now accustomed to the Saturday influx of acute trauma from the playing fields. Sportspeople in particular are unusually demanding and often have unrealistic expectations of treatment. It is sadly not uncommon for such patients to seek multiple hospital opinions, especially where professed treatment has failed, thus compounding the final burden of such injuries on the community.

Data from the UK general practices for five common conditions are shown in Figures 1.1–1.5 (Royal College of General Practitioners, 1979, 1986), indicating the workload on primary care of these conditions. These studies from the Royal College of General Practitioners highlight the very low rate of referral for soft tissue problems to hospital and thus the outcome from hospital series does not, in this area of medicine in particular, reflect the outcome from the syndrome as a whole. There is also considerable variation between hos-

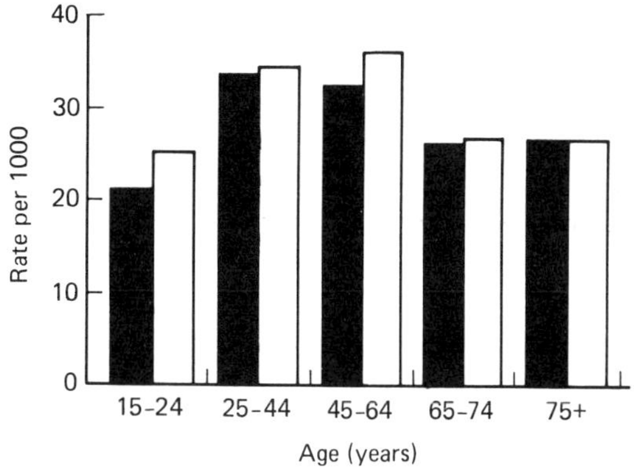

Fig. 1.1. Incidence of back pain (no sciatica). ■ = Male; □ = Female.

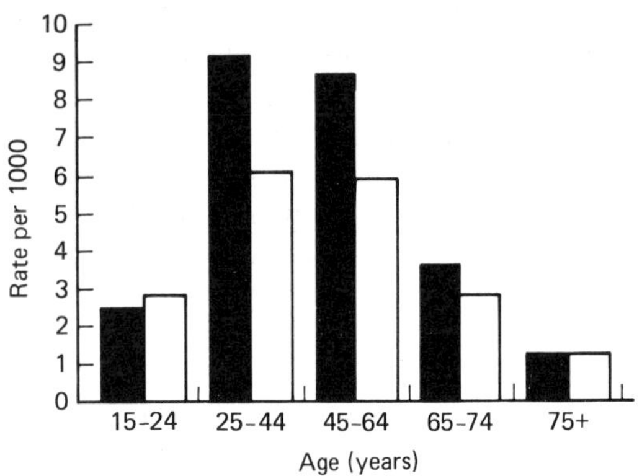

Fig. 1.2. Incidence of prolapsed intervertebral disc. ■ = Male; □ = Female.

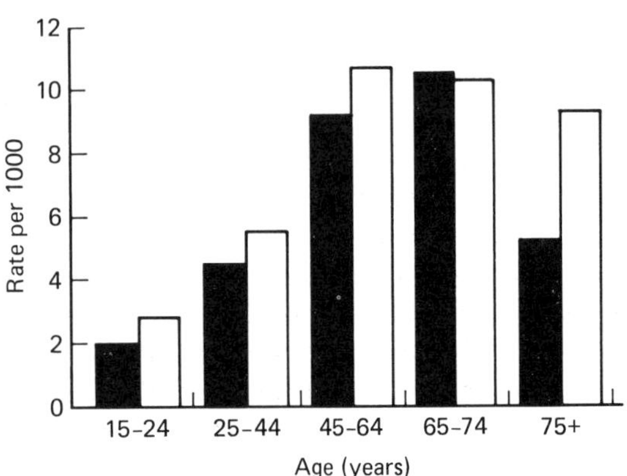

Fig. 1.3. Incidence of all shoulder syndromes. ■ = Male; □ = Female.

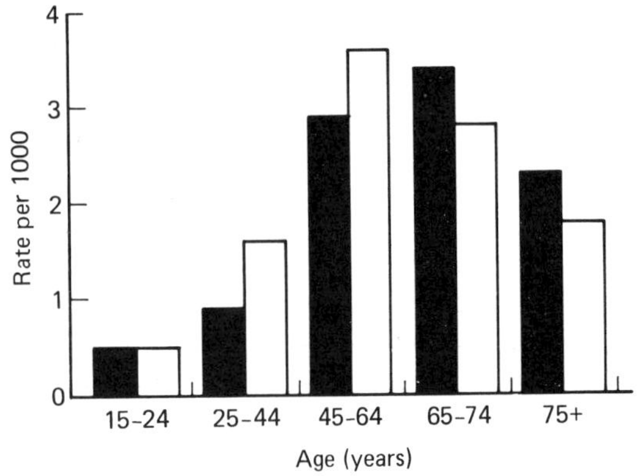

Fig. 1.4. Incidence of frozen shoulder. ■ = Male; □ = Female.

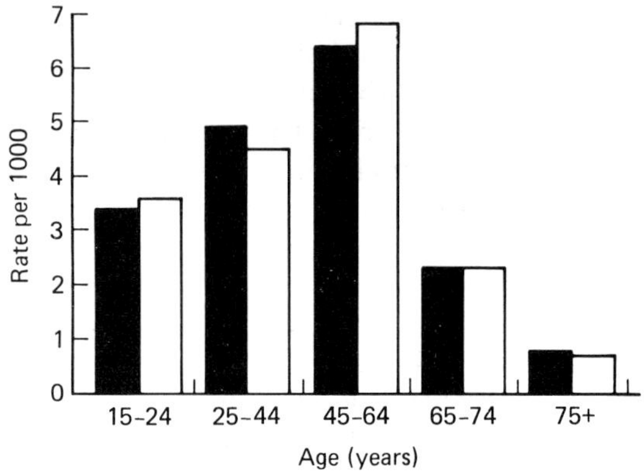

Fig. 1.5. Incidence of tenosynovitis. ■ = Male; □ = Female.

pital units in case severity of new attenders. Such variation is a function of waiting list time, and both general practitioner and hospital clinicians declared interests, with some general practitioners referring very few patients (Barker, 1977). There is, therefore, a need to amalgamate the diagnostic expertise of hospital units with the case mix in general practice, to investigate the true natural history of most of these disorders.

In general, rheumatic disorders account for approximately 10% of all consultations in general practice, one-third of all rheumatic consultations in primary care being due to soft tissue rheumatism. This amounts to 3–4% of the overall workload. Experience in females generally tends to resemble that in males, although consultation rates are proportionately slightly lower for bursitis and rather more or non-articular rheumatism other than frozen shoulder, for tenosynovitis and for less well-defined complaints (Wood *et al.*, 1979). Of those who do go to a general practitioner, most experience only a single episode during the course of a year. When divided according to geographical location the samples were not really large enough to permit any conclusions to be drawn about variation between regions.

Soft tissue rheumatism represents the most commonly encountered rheumatic cause of sickness absences from work, accounting for 44% of certified rheumatic spells and 6% of all incapacity spells. As is known from their natural history however, the volume of time lost from work is comparatively less impressive. Thus the average duration of incapacity of 21 days when aggregated amounts to 2.5% of rheumatic days or 3.5% of all days lost from work. These figures include absences on industrial injury as well as sickness benefit, the former making up about one-fifth of the total. There is an age relationship in days lost. Traumatic disorders show no very marked trend, but the non-traumatic complaints are associated with an increase in days lost that is progressive with age – the rate is at least six times greater in the oldest as compared with the youngest quinquennium. This pattern reflects the fact that the average duration of incapacity spells grows longer with age, those occurring in the oldest group being more than twice as long as those in younger people.

The overall pattern of incapacity spells is generally similar in most of the diagnostic categories, but muscle tendon and fascia lesions are unusual for the undue length of some incapacity spells. Wood (1970) indicates that both incapacity spells and days lost from non-articular rheumatism showed little change between 1961 and 1967. However, Woods's later report (Wood *et al.*, 1979) indicated that this period may have been somewhat unusual with rates diminishing slightly since then. Thus between the two periods 1968–1970 and 1972–1974, both rheumatic incapacity spells and days lost fell by 8%, although strains and sprains increased by a similar proportion. Underlying these changes was some indication that the new length of incapacity spell reduced frequently in older people.

Within the UK there is a marked regional variation in sickness absence from soft tissue lesions. This is up to 50% above the average for the country as a whole in Wales and the Northern and Yorkshire–Humberside regions and the excess is only slightly less marked in the North-West and Scotland. By comparison, it is 40% below average in East Anglia and the South-East, while the deficit in the South-West and the West Midlands is somewhat less. In Wales, it is lost days that are disproportionately greater, the mean incapacity spell duration being 50% above the average, and this is most noticeable with non-articular rheumatism. Sickness incapacity data on differences between industrial groups in the UK are available but incomplete. Workers involved in gas, coke and chemical production have high rates for non-articular rheumatism.

As would be anticipated from the nature of soft tissue lesions, less than a quarter of all rheumatic admissions are due to these disorders, and back pain makes up a considerable proportion of these. This total accounts for only 1.3% of all non-psychiatric admissions (Wood *et al.*, 1979). In women, all these proportions tend to be marginally lower than in men. For all except traumatic and ill-defined complaints the admission rates are highest in the 45–64-year age group. For every 27 men who have a period off work for soft tissue rheumatism during the course of a year, there is probably one who is chronically disabled by these complaints.

In the UK alone, the resultant loss of working days from soft tissue lesions is likely to cost the country almost a billion pounds in lost productivity, apart from the value of social security payments, lost tax revenue and health and social services applied to this problem. Behind these huge sums is a great deal of pain and misery and much disruption to family life and work arrangements. The economic effects, loss of time from work and the load that such patients present to both general practitioners and hospital doctors are clearly immense. Greater attention needs to be focused on these diseases.

Nature of soft tissue lesions

Soft tissue shoulder lesions

Terminology is a problem in defining shoulder lesions but most attention has been directed towards disease of the rotator cuff. This is because both mechanical and electromyographic studies indicate that the rotator cuff is the main stabilizer of the glenohumeral joint and is also important in monitoring nutrition of the cartilage. Rotator cuff tendinitis appears to be due to a combination of mechanical factors as well as tendon degeneration associated with vascular impairment. Impingement may occur on the anterior edge and undersurface or the anterior third of the acromion, the coracoacromial ligament and the acromioclavicular joint. The mechanical impingement of the rotator cuff may be influenced by variations in the shape and slope of the acromion. Pathophysiologically, there is an initial inflammatory tendinitis with oedema and haemorrhage which then progresses to tendon fibrosis, degeneration, and finally tears develop. This is reflected by increasing clinical features of shoulder pain, restriction of movements and weakness. With progression of the disease, wearing and attrition result in a full-thickness rotator cuff tear. Such tears also occur as a result of direct trauma, traction injury or recurrent shoulder instability.

With rotator cuff lesions, full painless passive elevation is possible. A painful arc is frequently present and may suggest a subacromial bursitis or tendon inflammation. Chronic bursitis is characterized by the gradual onset of persistent pain, often referred to the deltoid insertion. There is a painful arc on passive elevation and particularly pain on passive rotation of the abducted humerus. Active movements are painful and active abduction is less than that of the passive range. When impingement is present, there will often be point tenderness over the greater tuberosity and anterior acromion and the shoulder pain can be reproduced when the arm in neutral position is forcibly flexed by the examiner, jarring the greater tuberosity against the anterior inferior surface of the acromion (Neer and Welsh, 1977). With the elbow and shoulder flexed by 90°, the examiner forcibly internally rotates the arm, driving the greater tuberosity against the coracoacromial ligament (Hawkins and Kennedy, 1980). Relief of pain by injections of 1% lignocaine under the anterior acromion helps confirm the diagnosis (Brown, 1949). There are many athletic patients who put excessive demands on their shoulders, resulting in very abnormal stresses on the rotator cuff which in turn can produce tendinitis and a painful shoulder. In a select high-profile athletic population, excessive overload may be the cause.

A plain x-ray is helpful when arthritis is suspected. In patients with shoulder pain three routine views are obtained – an anteroposterior view at right angles to the scapula, an axillary view and a lateral scapular view with the beam tilted 10° caudally (Bigliani *et al.*, 1986). The anteroposterior view provides analysis of the undersurface of the acromion, acromioclavicular joint, the greater tuberosity, and clearly visualizes the glenohumeral joint. It allows an estimation of the distance between the undersurface of the acromion and the superior surface of the humeral head. If this space is less than 6 mm, a rotator cuff tear is probably present. Norwood and colleagues (1989) have suggested that certain radiographic features are useful in distinguishing between symptomatic patients with or without rotator cuff tears. These include the concavity of the acromion and the presence of cysts at the greater tuberosity. Computed tomography of the shoulder is rarely used as an initial investigation and is not particularly useful for imaging of soft tissue lesions but may serve to exclude a fracture or assess the thickness of the cartilage or of the labrum. Arthrography remains the most widely used shoulder imaging procedure, especially for the demonstration of rotator cuff tears. This technique can be performed using single or double contrast and can be combined with computed tomography to enhance interpretation. In addition to evaluating problems of the rotator cuff, arthrography is useful in evaluating the glenoid labrum and shoulder capsule. Single positive contrast bursography can be used as a complementary procedure to arthrography. Tears may however be demonstrated at surgery or post-mortem when arthrograms have been normal, particularly when the bursa has sealed off a small full-thickness tear.

Sonographic evaluation of the rotator cuff is a non-invasive, safe, rapid and inexpensive procedure with satisfactory accuracy (Mack *et al.*, 1988). The major disadvantage is that sonography is highly operator-dependent and a significant learning curve is required. The normal rotator cuff tissues are seen as a band of low echogenicity between the deltoid muscle and bone of the humeral head. Inflammatory change and small tears are seen as areas of increased echogenicity within this band. Magnetic resonance imaging (MRI) appears of potential benefit in depicting small rotator cuff tears. The absence of an intact

Table 1.1. Features of various diagnostic methods when used to detect rotator cuff tears

	Arthrography	Sonography	Magnetic resonance imaging	Thermography	Arthroscopy
Invasive	+	−	−	−	+++
Technical requirements	+	+++	++	+	+
Cost in money	+	+	+++	+	+++
Cost in time	++	+	+++	+	+++
Accuracy	+++	+/++	++	+	+++

subdeltoid fat line is associated with a cuff tear (Zlatkin *et al.*, 1988). MRI can detect subdeltoid bursitis and may even be able to identify cuff tendinitis (Kieft *et al.*, 1988). The high cost currently prohibits its wide usage and MRI involves a long examination time as well as technical difficulties.

Scintigraphy of the shoulder may be useful in excluding glenohumeral disease. We have found thermography useful in the diagnosis of rotator cuff tendinitis but not for identifying cuff tears. The arthroscope is becoming a useful investment in the differential diagnosis of a patient who has confusing shoulder pain, particularly in the younger athletic population in whom there is a variety of causes for shoulder tendinitis. Arthroscopy allows a simultaneous assessment under anaesthesia, identifies partial articular or bursal surface tears of the cuff, estimates the size of tears, identifies intra-articular bicipital or labral lesions and evaluates the articular surfaces (Table 1.1).

Various treatment modalities have been suggested for rotator cuff lesions. For rotator cuff tendinitis the offending activity, such as an occupation involving repetitive overhead arm movement, should be avoided whenever possible. In the early stages a short course of a non-steroidal anti-inflammatory drug should be tried. This is combined with home exercises. These exercises initially consist of pendulum-type exercises and then wall-climbing exercises. Where a non-steroidal anti-inflammatory drug proves unhelpful then a subacromial local corticosteroid injection either preceded by or mixed with a local anaesthetic should be administered. A second injection may be administered a few weeks later if the first injection has provided incomplete relief. We do not advocate giving more than two injections and certainly no more than three as there is some evidence that this is deleterious to the tendons. Furthermore Bjorkenheim and co-workers (1988) found that the administration of more than three local corticosteroid injections preoperatively was associated with a poorer surgical outcome. Various other therapies have been suggested (Table 1.2) with varying success. We have found pulsed electromagnetic field therapy to be of benefit (Binder *et al.*, 1984). Surgery can be helpful when conservative measures fail (Hawkins and Brock, 1979; Whipple and Goldner, 1979). Subacromial decompression serves to eliminate or diminish friction between the humeral head and the undersurface of the acromion, thus allowing free movement (Neer, 1972). Acromioplasty, acromioclavicular excision arthroplasty and excision of the coracoacromial ligament are effective procedures (Watson, 1989).

Opinion is divided over the management of small cuff tears. Whilst conservative treatment clearly provides relief in many patients with cuff tears, there are those who believe that such tears are almost certain to enlarge with time. Constant

Table 1.2. Suggested therapies for rotator cuff tendinitis

Analgesics
Non-steroidal anti-inflammatories (oral and topical)
Heat and ultrasound
Physiotherapy and graded exercises
Corticosteroids (oral and intra-articular)
Laser therapy
Pulsed electromagnetic field therapy
Surgery

and Welsh (1985) suggest that surgical decompression and repair are both safe and effective, particularly in early lesions, and that conservative treatment for such tears simply delays surgery which then becomes a more difficult procedure. For patients with a full-thickness rotator cuff tear surgical repair is usually required. Older patients with chronic rotator cuff tears frequently choose to accept their disability, contributing further to the level of disability from shoulder problems in the community (Chard and Hazleman, 1989a, 1989b; Chakravarty and Webley, 1990).

Some orthopaedic surgeons believe that surgery should be offered more widely than is currently the practice (Barrett, 1990). There will however always be patients who have other problems precluding surgery, such as severe myocardial disease. We are currently looking at the role of suprascapular nerve block for this type of patient as this procedure has already been proven of value in the treatment of patients with shoulder involvement from rheumatoid arthritis (Emery *et al.*, 1989). In massive rotator cuff tears which are irreparable, subacromial decompression alone occasionally offers pain relief (Rockwood, 1986).

Bicipital tendinitis may occur as an isolated condition affecting the long head of the biceps; however this is less common than in conjunction with rotator cuff pathology. The patient notices an area of discomfort in the anterior and upper region of the bicipital tendon. This area is frequently injected during forced resistance to the flexed elbow while the forearm is supinated. The biceps tendon can be palpated as it runs in the bicipital groove, which is brought to the forefront with the humerus externally rotated approximately 20°. The abducted arm is then rotated through the external rotation and any subluxation of this tendon is noted. With biceps tendinitis, passive movement remains normal. Rupture of the biceps tendon results in visible swelling of the biceps muscle belly in the distal third of the arm, and weakness of elbow flexion is apparent. Surgical repair is rarely required but is usually successful. Bicipital tendinitis improves with rest and ultrasound.

Subacromial and subcoracoid bursitis may occur primarily rather than being secondary to adjacent tendon injury. The onset may be acute or chronic. Pain is usually present and worsened by active abduction of the arm. Calcification of rotator cuff tendons is a common cause of shoulder pain; however, it may occur in asymptomatic individuals and is not necessarily the cause of shoulder problems when present. Ruttimann (1959) reported a high incidence of 20% in 100 individuals without symptoms. According to Bosworth (1941), 35–45% of individuals with radiologically visible calcification in their shoulders develop symptoms. It has been argued that a primary degeneration of the tendon tissues is responsible for the subsequent deposition of calcium. The sequence of events is suggested as degeneration, necrosis and calcification (Macnab, 1973). Uhthoff and colleagues (1976) however, emphasize that the self-healing nature of calcifying tendinitis is not indicative of a degenerative disease.

In the early part of the condition during the formative phase of calcification the patient typically complains of varying degrees of chronic pain that does not seriously impair the movement of the arm. A painful arc of motion between 70 and 100° has been described by Kessel and Watson (1977). In contrast to the chronic symptoms, acute symptoms during the resorptive phase incapacitate the arm almost completely. The acute symptoms tend to subside in 1–2 weeks even in the absence of treatment. Chronic pain may also persist during the period of repair (post-calcific stage), probably before the newly synthesized collagen fibres align along the axis of the tendon. Conservative treatment comprises a daily programme of exercises to maintain glenohumeral mobility, especially in the formative stage of calcification. When symptoms are acute a non-steroidal anti-inflammatory drug or subacromial cortocosteroid injection is administered. Analgesics as adjunctive treatment may be required during the formative, resorptive or post-resorptive phase. Where conservative measures fail, surgical excision of the calcium deposit is performed under general anaesthesia. Copious lavage and physiotherapy for improving the range of rotation and strengthening exercises are required. Seldom does a frozen shoulder result.

Frozen shoulders are commonly idiopathic. As with soft tissue lesions generally, nomenclature can often be confusing. The label used however is less important than a clear notion of what is meant by the term when applied. We recognize a frozen shoulder as referring to a soft tissue shoulder lesion in which there is restriction of both passive and active movement characterized by prominent reduction in the glenohumeral range of movement and external rotation. Reduction in external rotation is accepted as being a reduction of 50% or more when compared with the normal shoulder. There are three phases: painful, adhesive and resolving. A secondary frozen shoulder is one which occurs in conjunction with an identifiable disorder such as diabetes mellitus, ischaemic heart disease, thyroid disease, pulmonary disease (e.g. tuberculosis), antituberculosis drugs, a readily recognizable precipitating event such as recent cardiac surgery or shoulder trauma, or neurological disorders associated with impaired consciousness or hemiplegia.

The annual cumulative risk for developing a frozen shoulder is under 2% (Lundberg, 1969). Women may be more commonly affected than men and although the evidence is conflicting, the consensus favours involvement of the non-dominant shoulder (Lundberg, 1969; Rizk and Pinals, 1982). No well documented case of recurrence of the condition in the same shoulder has been described.

The aetiopathogenesis of the condition is not known (Bulgen *et al.*, 1976). Diseases such as diabetes mellitus which are associated with a secondary frozen shoulder indicate that microvascular disease may be involved. Various studies have looked at the natural history of this condition (Hazleman, 1972; Clark *et al.*, 1975; Binder *et al.*, 1984). Reeves (1976) has demonstrated that the painful phase lasts 10–36 weeks, the adhesive phase 4–12 months and the resolution phase 12–42 months (with a mean disease duration of 30.1 months). Arthrography shows limitation of joint capacity, a small or non-existent dependent axillary fold and irregularity of the capsular insertion on the anatomical neck of the humerus. Normal arthrograms are seen in the resolution phase when shoulder range has recovered (Reeves, 1966).

Bone densitometric studies of the affected humeral head show on average 50% reduction in bone mineral content compared to the unaffected side. An increased uptake in the affected shoulder region is found with bone scintigraphy. Scintigraphy does not however appear to be useful in predicting outcome (Binder *et al.*, 1984). Our preliminary work with thermography indicates that this may be a useful diagnostic procedure. It shows a localized region of coolness in the affected shoulder which may relate to the involvement of vascular factors pathogenetically.

Various therapies have been suggested for the treatment of the frozen shoulder (Table 1.3). Shoulder mobilization through shoulder exercises should be encouraged, although physiotherapy is frequently unhelpful during the painful phase, when control of pain is a major priority as further shoulder mobilization is precluded by pain. Simple analgesia and non-steroidal anti-inflammatory drugs are used but are frequently inadequate to control symptoms. Oral corticosteroids in two blinded and, controlled studies (Blockley *et al.*, 1954; Binder *et al.*, 1986) have been shown to improve pain, although the rate of recovery may not be improved. Several studies (Murnaghan and MacIntosh, 1955; Lee *et al.*, 1974; Bulgen *et al.*, 1984) have shown that local corticosteroid injections result in improvement of pain and range of movement. We favour injecting both the subacromial space and glenohumeral joint. In controlled studies, cervical sympathetic ganglion blockade has not been shown to give more than temporary relief (Turek, 1967; Callicet, 1986).

Table 1.3. Suggested therapies for frozen shoulder

Analgesics
Non-steroidal anti-inflammatory drugs
Heat and ultrasound
Physiotherapy and graded exercises
Corticosteroids (oral and intra-articular)
Stellate ganglion blockade
Magnetic necklace
Dimethyl sulphoxide (topical)
Arthrographic distension
Joint irradiation
Manipulation under anaesthetic (early/late)

For the adhesive stages graded exercises are the mainstay of management. We would only advocate the use of manipulation under the anaesthesia for those cases in which restriction of shoulder movement is abnormally prolonged. Good controlled studies are lacking but improvements in pain and range of movement are claimed (Kessel *et al.*, 1981). In general, frozen shoulder is a protracted painful illness with some patients having residual, clinically detectable limitation of shoulder movement. A smaller number have residual impairment of function.

Soft tissue elbow lesions

Soft tissue elbow lesions encompass several entities. Tennis elbow, golfer's elbow, olecranon bursitis and javelin thrower's elbow are the commonest. Nerve entrapment is often important in the differential diagnosis.

Tennis elbow is a common condition affecting the arm and characterized by pain over the lateral aspect of the elbow aggravated by gripping. There is some confusion as to whether Renton (1830) or Runge (1873) was the first to describe the condition. The name itself originates from Morris's description of the lawn tennis arm in the *Lancet* (1982). It affects 1–3% of the population and the peak age incidence is 40–60 years of age (Allander, 1974; Kivi, 1982). Forty to fifty per cent of tennis players are affected by the condition (Nirschl and Petrone, 1973; Gruchow and Pelletier, 1979) although only 5% of patients seen with this condition are tennis players (Conrad and Hooper, 1973). This is because non-athletes are more commonly seen. Many patients cannot identify a precipitating event. Tennis elbow rarely occurs before the age of 30 years and this may relate to its pathogenesis.

The heterogeneity of disorders grouped together as tennis elbow makes it difficult to unravel its definitive aetiology. Almost 30 different conditions have been cited as causes of tennis elbow in the literature (Cyriax, 1936; Roles and Maudsley, 1972; Newman and Goodfellow, 1975). These include tendon ruptures, radiohumeral synovitis, periostitis, neuritis, aseptic necrosis and displacement of the orbicular ligament (Goldie, 1964). The vast majority of cases are believed to be musculotendinous in origin with a lesion at or near the attachment of the common extensor tendon to the epicondyle, particularly that part derived from extensor carporadialis brevis (Bosworth, 1955; Cyriax, 1982), and consequently lateral epicodylitis is used as an alternative term. There is evidence that at least relative overuse of wrist and finger extensor muscles may cause the onset of symptoms as the condition is much more common in the dominant arm, and the incidence is influenced by occupation and sport (Kivi, 1982). In a few cases tennis elbow is bilateral, and this may be due to increased stress placed on the unaffected arm. The higher than expected prevalence of other soft tissue lesions in patients with tennis elbow may provide further evidence for the unifying concept of the enthesopathy (Neipal and Sitaj, 1979). Tennis players, particularly novices, suffer tennis elbow often as a result of pressure grip strain during backhand shots. Tennis elbow may also be more common in loose-jointed individuals (Berhang *et al.*, 1975).

Pain is localized to the lateral epicondyle but may spread up and down the upper limb to the shoulder and hand respectively. Pain occurs on gripping objects and the patient may remark that he or she has inadvertently dropped a few things. Grip strength may be severely disabled by limited arm function. Examination reveals tenderness located to the lateral epicondyle. Although most commonly tenderness is maximal over the epicondyle, sometimes it is above on the supracondylar ridge (at the site of insertion of extensor carpi radialis longus) or more distal towards the head of the radius or even occasionally elsewhere (Bosworth, 1955). Pain on resisted wrist dorsiflexion with the elbow in extension is the other cardinal sign. An X-ray of the elbow is usually normal in tennis elbow, although flecks of calcification have been reported on rare occasions (Hughes, 1950).

Approaches to management have varied over the years, depending on the perception of pathology and of anticipated prognosis (Table 1.4). Over 40 consecutive therapies have been attempted for tennis elbow at one time or another.

Table 1.4. Conservative treatment of tennis elbow

Prolonged observation	*Physiotherapy*
Rest and imobilization	*Ultrasound*
Sling	Diathermy
Wrist splint	Massage
Backslab	Ice packs
Elastic bandage/strapping	Hot soaks or hot air
Pressure pad	Paraffin baths
Brace	Faradism
Systemic medications	Galvanic acupuncture
Corticosteroids	Microthermy
Non-steroidal anti-inflammatories	Ultraviolet
Thyroid extract	Infrared
Vitamin D	*Local procedures*
Local injection	Analgesic ointment
Steroids	Painting with iodine
Local anaesthesia	Ichthymol ointment
Alcohol	Blistering
Histamine	Cauterization
Carbolic acid	*X-ray therapy*
Oxygen or air	*Miscellaneous*
Acupuncture	Special diet
	Sedatives
	Digital rupture of bursa
	Change of occupation

These have ranged from prolonged observation (Cyriax, 1936) to X-ray therapy (Meheim and Cooper, 1950). Properly conducted controlled clinical trials have seldom been performed. In early cases rest and immobilization together with elimination of the underlying cause are simple and effective. Use of a tennis elbow splint or sling may be tried in assisting immobilization. Non-steroidal anti-inflammatory drugs are seldom effective. Topical anti-inflammatory agents are currently being evaluated. Ultrasound, by its ability to cross myofascial planes and concentrate near bone, has theoretical advantages (Binder *et al.*, 1985). Acupuncture has also been used in treatment (Brattberg, 1983). We have looked at a novel physical treatment using pulsed electromagnetic field therapy for patients with chronic tennis elbow unresponsive to the more usual conservative therapies. Although results consistently favoured the treatment group, the differences were not significant (Devereaux *et al.*, 1985). Local corticosteroid injections have been used since the early 1950s and are widely used. The superiority of local corticosteroid injection over local saline injection has been shown (Day *et al.*, 1978), and there remains no overall agreement in the literature as to the best steroid preparation, correct dosage or best form of administration (single spot or multiple punctures). If there is no response to two injections then further attempts are unlikely to be effective (Calvert *et al.*, 1985).

Up to 10% of patients have been reported as being resistant to the simple measures or injections (Wadsworth, 1987); however, less than 5% are considered for surgery. Options other than surgery for those who fail to respond to conservative treatment are limited.

The Mills manipulation (Mills, 1982) has been advocated by some (Marlun, 1930; Cyriax, 1936) but its efficacy remains unproven (Meheim and Cooper, 1950). Wadsworth (1987) has suggested a combination of anaesthetizing the patient, injecting steroid locally and manipulation, envisaging that the manipulation frees adhesions.

The suggested surgical management, like that of conservative treatments, has over the years been influenced by perceptions with regards to pathology. Lateral release has been successful in 90% of cases and is as effective as that for more extensive procedures (Gerberich and Priest, 1985); it is probably the surgical procedure of choice. We think infrared thermography is a useful tool in monitoring progress. Thermography of the lateral elbow in tennis elbow revealed a localized hot spot over the epicondyle 1–3°C higher than the background isotherm in 98% of affected elbows and analysis of the gradient across the abnormal area showed correlation with clinical severity (Binder *et al.*, 1983). Cyriax (1982) indicated that tennis elbow is a self-limiting soft tissue lesion, with most patients recovering within 1 year and recurrence occurring in 0–38%. Other workers report relapse rates of between 18 and 50% 6 months after conservative treatment (Clarke and Woodland, 1975; Nevelos, 1980).

Many of the comments with regards to tennis elbow are also applicable to golfer's elbow, a medial epicondylitis. This condition is about 15 times less common than tennis elbow (Conrad and Hooper, 1973) although both conditions can coexist. Thus a golf player may develop tennis elbow in the leading arm and a golfer's elbow in the following arm. The condition can also result during a snatch lift in weightlifting. Golfer's elbow is generally milder than tennis elbow. Tenderness in this condition is more diffuse and may occur distal to the common flexor origin at the medial epicondyle.

Repeated forced extension produces pain over the triceps insertion, causing tricipital tendinitis. Treatment involves rest, anti-inflammatory treatment and light exercises within the limits of pain. Occasionally a local injection into the joint of tenderness is needed. Surgical repair is however required if a suspected tear is present (McLatchie *et al.*, 1980). Bicipital tendinitis at the elbow presents as antecubital fossa pain which is aggravated by resisted elbow flexion and forearm supination.

Stenosing tenosynovitis of the abductor pollicis longus or extensor pollicis brevis may result from repetitive activity or direct injury. Tenderness is maximal in the anatomical snuffbox. The Finkelstein test (Finkelstein, 1930) is positive and is carried out by clenching the fist with the fingers of the involved hand folded over the thumb. The involved tendons are stretched by ulnar deviation of the hand. This results in exacerbation of pain. Crepitus on thumb movements may be present. Tenography, although available (Engel *et al.*, 1981), is not widely used but may assist in determining those patients requiring surgery. Ultrasound examination is of similar value (Fornage and Rifkin, 1988). MRI may also prove to be useful (Herman *et al.*, 1987).

Rest and avoidance of the causative activity may provide relief and indeed the condition may resolve spontaneously. Wrist splints may assist immobilization. Ultrasound treatment may also be of value (Lanfear and Clarke, 1972). Where the condition recurs or persists, however, local corticosteroid and the injection of local anaesthesia may be required. If the condition becomes chronic, marked thickening of the fibrous sheath with accompanying radiological changes may occur (Rhoades *et al.*, 1984). If conservative measures have failed the surgical tendon release should be carried out (Reed and Harcourt, 1943; Potenza, 1963), taking care to avoid the adjacent sensory branches of the radial nerve.

Tenosynovitis of the wrist

Acute frictional tenosynovitis of the extensor tendons at the wrist occurs as a result of repetitive use. There is pain over the dorsum of the wrist. Tenderness, boggy swelling and crepitus with pain on extension during applied pressure may occur. The condition is treated by splinting in slight dorsiflexion. Anti-inflammatory drugs may be required.

Flexor tenosynovitis occurs with palm and/or trigger pain which is worse on tight grip. Trigger finger results from an incomplete obstruction to the movement of a finger flexor tendon in its sheath, most commonly affecting the middle finger of the dominant hand of middle-aged females. For both trigger thumb and trigger finger the usual treatment is a local corticosteroid injection into the tendon sheath. If this fails then surgery is required.

The commonest site for a tenoperiosteal strain in the hand is in the insertion of flexor carpi ulnaris (Yates, 1977). This gives rise to localized tenderness both proximal and distal to the pisiform. Murray and Jacobson (1977) describe calcific tendinitis affecting the insertion of flexor carpi radialis in a violinist and extensor pollicis brevis in a radiologist who had for many years operated the on–off button of his dictaphone with the affected thumb. Calcific tendinitis of the insertion of abductor pollicis has also occurred in a young woman who had subjected her right thumb to excessive use while working as a filing clerk (Evans, 1985). These lesions generally improve after a period of splintage with spontaneous resolution of the calcific mass. If this fails, the material can be aspirated, combined with local injection of steroid, or evacuated surgically.

Soft tissue lesions of the hip and knee

No single entity stands out as a major cause for low pelvic, hip and thigh regional pain. Trochanteric bursitis present with lateral hip pain which is often acute and usually more severe at night, particularly if the patient lies on the affected side. The trochanteric bursa lies between the tendon of the gluteus maximus and the posterior prominence of the great trochanter and the ileotibial tract (Swezey and Spiegel, 1979). Physical examination reveals point tenderness over the bursa in the region of the greater trochanter. Conservative measures includes treatment with cold packs, anti-inflammatory drugs and rest. In chronic cases, local cortocosteroid injection is effective, although a spinal needle may sometimes be required.

The iliopectineal bursa lies between the iliopsoas muscle and the iliopectineal eminence. Bursitis causes pain in the anterior pelvis, groin and thigh region. Local corticosteroid treatment is the treatment of choice. 'Weaver's bottom' or 'tailor's bottom' arises from pain in a bursa overlying the ischial prominence (Swartout and Compere, 1974).

Fascia lata fasciitis causes discomfort over the low back and lateral hip and thigh region. Treatment includes injecting the tender points with a local corticosteroid injection, stretching exercises and conditioning exercises before engaging in sporting activities.

Adductor longus tendoperiostitis is an injury frequently associated with adductor longus muscle strain. An iliopsoas strain gives rise to pain on the medial aspect of the thigh over the insertion of the tendon into the lesser trochanter.

The rectus femoris muscle can be strained as a result of repetitive movements. Conservative measures are adequate for incomplete tears; however, surgery is required for complete tears. Hamstring tears are common injuries which tend to be recurrent. The muscles may be avulsed from their origins, torn completely or strained. Early treatment is important. Minor pulls can be treated conservatively. Causative activity must be avoided until healing is complete and this may take several weeks. Controlled stretching exercises enable maintenance of muscle length. Avulsion of the origin and complete ruptures require surgical management.

Rupture of the quadriceps tendon or muscle is relatively common. In young athletes rupture generally involves the muscle mass whilst in older persons rupture usually occurs at the tendinous portion. Such patients are treated by immobilization of the limb in extension followed by gradual mobilization. With complete rupture however immediate surgical repair is recommended.

Pain in the region of the suprapatellar pouch may occur as a result of calcific quadriceps tendinitis. Such calcification at the upper or lower pole of the patella can occur with 'jumper's knee' or Sinding–Larsen–Johansson disease. Otherwise well children or adolescents present with pain, swelling, tenderness and crepitus (Sinding–Larsen, 1921; Johansson, 1922). Treatment is by avoidance of precipitating activity whilst occasionally a period of rest in a plaster of Paris cylinder is required. Some patients obtain relief with ultrasound and a local corticosteroid injection into the tender area may also be attempted; however, injection into the tendon may cause rupture. Surgical decompression is rarely required.

Numerous bursae occur near the knee in relation to the attachments of the various muscles and ligaments (Bywaters, 1979). They may communicate constantly or occasionally with the knee joint. The suprapatellar, prepatellar, infrapatellar and an adventitious cutaneous bursa lie in the anterior knee region. The sartorius and anserine bursae lie medially whilst three bursae lie adjacent to the fibular collateral ligament and the popliteus tendon in the lateral region of the knee (Stuttle, 1959; Henderson, 1946) isolated at the front edge of the anterior fibres of the medial collateral ligament.

Prepatellar bursitis is a chronic condition associated with occupations requiring repetitive kneeling and hence is also referred to as housemaid's knee. Pain is usually slight unless there is direct pressure on the swollen area found on inspection. Treatment is by rest, aspiration and corticosteroid injection. Anserine bursitis is to be suspected when pain occurs in the medial knee region. There is point tenderness over the medial tibial collateral ligament. Treatment is by local cortocosteroid injection.

Baker (1877) was one of the first to draw

attention to popliteal cysts. These cysts may be formed either by enlargement of the semimembranous or gastrocnemius bursae or direct herniation from the back of the knee joint. Surgery is rarely indicated (Dinham, 1975). The patient frequently presents with aching discomfort in the popliteal region, leg and calf. The discomfort is aggravated by walking and often relieved by rest. The patient may report the presence of a swelling behind the knee. Treatment includes aspiration of the cyst and/or the knee joint, followed by injection of a corticosteroid agent. Isometric quadriceps exercises are helpful. Surgical excision should be considered for recurrent cysts.

Popliteus tendinitis may give rise to posterolateral knee pain and may be produced by hyperpronation of the foot. Tenosynovitis of the tendons of insertion of the other hamstring muscles and their associated bursae may cause pain in the back of the knee and palpation during straight leg raising reveals marked tightness of involved muscles (Halperin and Axer, 1980). Local corticosteroid injections into areas of tenderness and short-wave diathermy are helpful whilst hamstring stretching exercises should be performed. Non-steroidal anti-inflammatory drugs and cooling are useful for acute episodes.

Pellegrini–Stieda disease consists of calcification in the region of the medial tibial collateral ligament. Local corticosteroid injection may be helpful, otherwise treatment is by muscle-strengthening exercises and gradual mobilization within the limits of pain.

Ligamentous injuries occur most usually when the knee is bent, as this permits relaxation of the collateral ligaments together with knee rotation. The medial collateral ligament is most frequently involved. Valgus or varus forces produce partial or complete rupture of these ligaments. A complete tear is painful. Swelling and localized tenderness are present above the joint line. Most importantly there is no abnormal movement on stressing the ligament. By contrast, complete tears may be relatively painless, with minimal swelling. Confirmation is by stress radiography, arthroscopy and arthrotomy. Partial tears can be treated in a plaster of Paris cylinder. Complete tears of the lateral and medial ligament are repaired surgically. After collateral ligament repair, a plaster of Paris cylinder is worn for 6 weeks. Early operation within 2 weeks of injury gives the best results.

The cruciates can be torn either alone or in conjunction with a collateral ligament tear. Isolated tears of the anterior cruciate are not common and associated damage to the collateral ligaments and posterior cruciate are often found. When there is anterior cruciate insufficiency, an anterior drawer sign with the knee at 90° flexion or the more sensitive Ritchie–Lachmann test with the knee at 0–20° flexion is positive (Ritchie, 1960; Hughston *et al.*, 1976; Frank, 1986). Time can in some measure compensate for anterior cruciate weakness but in the presence of marked laxity a direct repair or a late reconstruction operation using the semitendinosus tendon can be performed.

Posterior cruciate damage is more serious and although direct or reconstructive surgery can be employed, the end results are frequently poor (Muckle, 1983). Although menisceal tears are a common cause of knee pain, they may be asymptomatic. Pain, if present, is usually located at the affected joint margin. Intermittent catching, locking or clicking may be reported, leading to sudden changes in muscle tone in the leg such that the knee 'gives way'. On physical examination quadriceps wasting may be present. If the joint locks, it is held flexed to about 10° or 20° and extension is painful. Lateral or medial rotation may be painful and extension is painful.

Meniscal tears may be partial or complete and are characteristically produced when weight is taken on a semiflexed knee and there is a superimposed twisting sprain. If partial, it is the posterior horn that is most commonly affected. Complete tears create 'bucket-handle' lesions on the meniscus. A plain radiograph should be taken to exclude loose bodies or avulsion fractures. An arthrogram will demonstrate about 90% of tears. Arthroscopy, although invasive, directly confirms the diagnosis. MRI is being increasingly used for diagnosis. Some patients in whom meniscus tears are diagnosed settle without any treatment. When the patient complains of recurring episodes or has a locked joint, surgery is required. Whenever possible, partial meniscectomy is performed to reduce the risk of post-meniscectomy osteoarthritis (Pettrone, 1982).

Achilles tendinitis is often associated with training errors. Achilles tendinitis may present with heel pain and tenderness over the insertion of the tendon. Pain may appear early during exercise, later subsiding, only to reappear to a severer degree after activity is stopped. Gentle progressive heel cord stretching exercises are helpful. Both acute and chronic cases respond to cryotherapy. Heel raises are used to place the foot in slight equinus and to relieve the strain on the tendon. Anti-inflammatory drugs are useful in acute cases and both ice packs and ultrasound treatment may be beneficial. In resistant cases however surgical intervention is required. Local steroid injections are to be avoided because of the risk of rupture.

A complete or partial tear of the Achilles tendon is often a sudden event which may occur after a burst of physical activity, usually involving a sudden plantar flexion force of the foot. The best results are obtained by surgical repair. A plaster of Paris full-length cast is applied with the foot in slight equinus or in a neutral position for 6 weeks. Calcification may be present in the Achilles tendon (Fisher and Woods, 1970). Visible firm swellings or 'bump pumps' may be present at the lower end of the Achilles tendon, especially in those who wear closely contoured heel counters. The ill-fitting shoes may also cause another adventitial bursitis, 'last bursitis', located lateral to the heel (Layfer, 1980).

Treatment consists in removing the source of pressure. Anti-inflammatory drugs and surgery may also be required if symptoms persist or if the bursae become acutely swollen.

With ankle ligament injury there are three grades of severity. Grade 1 is a ligament sprain without instability; grade 2 is an incomplete tear with mild instability and grade 3 a complete tear with marked instability. Prognosis is good for grades 1 and 2. Non-steroidal anti-inflammatory drugs, elevation, ice packs, compression dressing, local corticosteroids, strapping and rest may be used in the acute phase, when there is much pain and swelling. Movements within the limitations of pain are subsequently encouraged (McLatchie *et al.*, 1985). With grade 3 tears, a below-knee plaster of Paris cast may be applied for 6 weeks, after which mobilization is commenced. Cast braces may also be used and can be worn for a shorter period (3 weeks). In general, patients who have inversion ankle injuries should be actively exercised as soon as they have relief from pain. This prevents proprioceptive loss in the joint and recurrent injury. A wobble board is frequently useful (Leach *et al.*, 1981). Other exercises include a gentle full range of ankle movements within the limits of pain. As recovery progresses, heel raises, hopping and progressive resistance exercises with weights can be introduced.

Injury to the medial ligament is less common (Glick, 1978) and more usually results in an avulsion fracture. A sprain of this ligament can however occur and pain is accentuated by eversion. Treatment is as for the lateral ligaments.

Plantar fasciitis is a frequent cause of pain over the plantar and medial aspects of the heel (Moskowitz, 1975). A minority are associated with plantar ligament enthesopathies found in seronegative arthropathies (Gerster *et al.*, 1977). Heel spurs often coexist (Campbell and Inman, 1974) and may represent a secondary response to an inflammatory reaction. In one study (Furey, 1975) over half of the patients had calcaneal spurs but their presence did not affect outcome. Plantar fasciitis is commonly related to abnormal stresses applied to the foot, particularly conditions resulting in unusual torsion or tension on the plantar fascia (Lester and Buchanan, 1984). Such forces are magnified in the foot with an inherent tendency to evert. This is the flexible flat foot and is associated with excessive motion at the talonavicular and naviculocuneiform joints (Scranton *et al.*, 1982).

Treatment in the early stage (within 6 months) may include the use of pressure-relieving heelpads (Eggers, 1957) made up of sponge, rubber, orthopaedic felt or plasterzote with or without a cut-out area. Thick-cushioned-sole training shoes may be more comfortable. Shortening of the Achilles tendon complex may aggravate symptoms and stretching exercises may help to reduce the tension placed on the proximal origin of the plantar fascia. A short course of an oral non-steroidal anti-inflammatory drug may also prove beneficial in the early stages (Snider *et al.*, 1983). Physiotherapy and ultrasound treatment have little effect but if symptoms persist then an injection of hydrocortisone and local anaethetic into the calcaneal tubercle area at the point of maximal tenderness should be performed. Proper shoes or sandals, particularly with rubber soles for working on concrete, may be helpful. Excessive heel strike, as in jogging, should be curtailed and obesity should be controlled. Treatment of flat feet and systemic inflammation are also undertaken when present. Local strapping of the plantar arch and midfoot may also be helpful (Mann and Duvries, 1978). A soft mouldable flexible insert that can be shaped to the foot while it is held in the position of correction may be helpful (Lester and Buchanan, 1984) and a modified valgus convex heel insole, the Taylor–Rose orthosis, has been shown to be effective if worn long-term (Campbell and Inman, 1974; Rose, 1979).

Plantar fascial fibromatosis or Dupuytren's contracture of the foot is a diffuse, localized or multiple nodular hyperplasia of the plantar aponeurosis. It is similar to Dupuytren's palmar contracture in the hand (Pentland and Anderson, 1985) but uncommonly involves the toes (Stoyler, 1964). Although a small number result from direct trauma or lacerations to the palmar or plantar fascia, studies have shown the majority have no association and the pathogenesis is different, suggesting that this is an autoimmune phenomenon (Buren, 1966). The nodules only give pain when excessive pressure develops. Contoured insoles and pads may alleviate the problems; however, exercise may be required to give long-term relief. Wide exposure of the plantar fusion is necessary with wide clearance of the lesions to present recurrence (Peterson and Day, 1954).

Disorders of the arch of the foot result in pes planus, when the arch collapses, or pes cavus, when it is too high. Of patients with flat feet, 70% have an inherited predisposition to flat feet (Dothie and Ferguson, 1973). Spasmodic flat foot results from spasm of the peroneal muscles often associated with a bony bar arising from the calcaneus articulating with the navicular or talus (Outland and Murphy, 1960). There is a consequent eversion deformity of the foot. Oblique tarsal radiographs may reveal a bony bridge but occasionally the bar is a synchrondrosis, when the appearance is of incomplete bony bridging.

Flat feet may be symptomless (Mann and Du Vries, 1978) and even when painful, the degree of flatness bears no correlation to future foot pain (Giannestras, 1978). Symptoms, when present, include foot pain, excessive muscular fatigue and aching and intolerance to prolonged walking or standing. In some patients walking improves symptoms (Dothie and Ferguson, 1973). The anterior and posterior tibial tendons and plantar muscles are found to be stretched and the Achilles tendon may become shortened (Turek, 1977). The flat foot can be either flexible or rigid depending on whether or not it can be inverted (Giannestras, 1978).

Treatment depends on strengthening the foot inner soles to help them restore the arch. Grasping exercises for intrinsic foot muscles and mobilizing exercises that plantiflex the foot and invert the ankle are helpful. Failing this, the foot has to be shod in a surgical shoe with a deeply cushioned insole. If there is hyperpronation a medial wedge is indicated. A Thomas heel may be useful in providing a varus tilt and can extend to the mid-part of the navicula so that it intersects the longitudinal axis of the fibula (Mann and DuVries, 1978). An attempt should be made to identify any precipitating or aggravating factors and these should be eliminated where possible. In severe cases, talonavicular, naviculocuneiform or talocalcaneal arthrodeses may be necessary.

Pes cavus with a high longitudinal arch results from contracture of the plantar aponeurosis and deep plantar ligaments, leading in the majority of cases to loss of fibrosis of the intrinsic muscles and overextension of the extrinsic muscles. Approximately one-third of these deformities are idiopathic or a normal variant, whereas two-thirds are secondary to a neuromuscular disorder (Brewerton *et al.*, 1962). Many cases require no treatment. Special shoes may be worn to accommodate the altered foot shape. Surgical correction of the claw toes reduces the disability arising from corns and calluses and makes the choice of footwear easier. Severe cases may merit more radical bone and tendon surgery.

In general, the foot is frequently affected by overuse. A tendon attachment strain may result. Oral anti-inflammatory drugs and the use of an orthotic device combined with reduction in activity are standard methods which produce good results. Strapping or splints can also be used to prevent excessive movement.

Back pain

Back pain, as previously stated, is a major cause of rheumatic disability throughout the western world. The causes of low back pain are numerous, ranging from a wide variety of congenital disorders to traumatic states, inflammatory and osteoarthritic processes, infectious diseases, metabolic abnormalities, and primary and metastatic neoplastic diseases. We are only concerned here with soft tissue causes but it has been suggested that most cases of back pain (estimated at 22.9 million episodes per annum in 1980 in the UK) are due to soft tissue lesions (Office of Health Economics, 1985). Frequently the natural history of the disorder is benign and self-limiting. Recurrences occur but these tend to disappear in later life. Very occasionally an incapacitating back condition results (Sternback *et al.*, 1973). Myofascial back pain syndromes constitute part of a series of localized disorders in which focal pain is associated with an irritable focus within the muscle, termed a trigger spot, which on palpation produces referred pain (Simons and Travell, 1980). Back pain may also be present as part of the more generalized fibromyalgia syndrome. Tender points are found on palpation in association with other features such as sleep disturbance, excessive fatigability, headiness, paraesthesiae and morning stiffness (Wolfe, 1986). The patient is typically a middle-aged female. Back pain was present in 94% of patients with this syndrome in one series (Wolfe, 1986) and 66% in another (Yunus and Masi, 1985). Investigations such as radiographs are normal but serve to exclude other causes of back pain. The injection of a myofascial trigger point with local anaesthetic and corticosteroid may be diagnostic as well as therapeutic in myofascial back pain.

Management in the main is largely preventive with the emphasis on avoiding aggravating factors through lifestyle modification both at work and in leisure activities in an attempt to avoid injury or overuse of the spinal tissues. Muscle-strengthening exercises may also prove helpful in rehabilitating patients. Exercises that strengthen abdominal muscles are of established value (Nachemson, 1969). A range of other therapeutic exercises for back protection may be performed. Steindler and Luck (1938) claimed lasting relief with the injection of trigger points in myofascial back pain. Oral analgesics may be useful in those with acute symptoms. Non-steroidal anti-inflammatory drugs may be helpful in some patients with chronic back pain. The use of antidepressants for nocturnal sedation as well as depression may be helpful in those with chronic back pain, particularly in those in whom the back pain is in association with the fibromyalgia syndrome. Outcome may be influenced by the motivation of the patient and good communication between all involved parties, including the patient, patient's family, physician and even the insurer and lawyer (Mooney and Cairns, 1978). The patient with chronic back pain must want to recover.

General measures

In general the specific exercise programme must be individualized, based on a prior appropriate evaluation of the musculoskeletal system. Therapists should determine the potential response capabilities of the patient based on an assessment of strength, range of movement and functional ability. Specific exercises and number of repetitions should be stated. An exercise schedule should include weight-training for the unaffected muscle groups, stretching exercises, specific exercises in a pool where weight-bearing is eliminated and use of an exercise cycle. Most of the exercises for soft tissue injuries involve mobilization and stretching exercises. Exercise in some form will psychologically assist an athlete who will feel that he or she is still training, maintaining fitness and losing the minimum amount of time in returning to full function. This can prevent an undesirable early return to competition. Therapeutic exercise can, however, be overdone. Pain may result from improper performance, inaccurate diagnosis or too vigorous a programme.

In order to improve blood flow and to provide optimum healing conditions and reduce pain so that normal movement can be resumed, various treatment techniques can be used as adjuncts. Hot water baths, gelpacks, infrared lamps, short-wave and microwave diathermy all increase tissue temperature. Infrared heat is of value in inducing relaxation and reducing muscle spasm and heat packs have similar effects. Short-wave diathermy is used for treating subacute or chronic soft tissue lesions as well as for injury to more deeply placed soft tissue structures. Microwave diathermy differs in that microwaves tend to concentrate in tissues with a high fluid content, such as muscle. Thus microwave diathermy has a greater healing effect on muscle than short-wave diathermy. Microwaves are particularly useful for the treatment of small localized lesions.

Ultrasound, which is also a heat modality, may facilitate the extensibility of soft tissues (Gestern, 1955). The biological effects of therapeutic ultrasound aid tissue repair. Reduction of chronic inflammatory processes and stimulation of protein synthesis associated with an increase in lysosomal permeability have been observed (Harvey *et al.*, 1975). Deep friction breaks down adhesion in muscle, tendons and ligaments and is especially useful in chronic lesions. Strapping of the affected part may provide physical support for the injured part, limiting pain, assisting or resisting specific movements and allowing an injured area to come into graduated use. It allows normal movement distal and proximal to the lesion and prevents atrophy and abnormal postures.

Ice application for soft tissue injuries may act via local anaesthesia produced by a reduction in the rate of conduction of sensory nerves, decrease in metabolic rate in the area treated and changes in local circulation. The system of applying ice to numb the part, moving it actively, then repeating the procedure three to four times is known as cryotherapy or cryokinetics (Grant, 1964; Hayden, 1964). Compression, applied by tubular or elastic bandage or by an air splint applied from below to above the lesion (avoid constriction) decreases inflammatory exudate. Elevation allows for draining of oedema by gravity. This in turn produces pain relief. More recently, laser therapy has been used for soft tissue lesions and its role is currently under investigation.

In summary, in the first 24 hours of a soft tissue injury, treatment aims to reduce inflammatory exudate and subsequent secondary damage. Relative rest is indicated: movement should be within limits since activity may further aggravate the lesion. After the first 24–48 hours gentle non-weight-bearing exercises should be initiated. Such early contraction is thought to influence the direction in which collagen fibres are laid down. To avoid shortening, stretching exercises are required. Prompt treatment prevents the risk of secondary damage and may accelerate primary healing. Where symptoms persist due to continued overstretching of scar tissue, strapping may limit movement within a painfree range. If pain persists splinting may be required. Heating may also be beneficial and may be applied in a form dependent on the nature and extent of the lesion. Transverse friction often proves beneficial in specific conditions such as chronic tenosynovitis. When the problem begins to resolve, rehabilitation follows the same guidelines as in the acute stage, with emphasis on regaining length by static stretching exercises.

In the main, preventive measures involve a common sense attitude towards thc usc of such tissue structures. Individualized and appropriate training for an athlete is an obvious example. A skilled coach will include certain training activities which, whilst not enhancing performance, reduce the chance of injury. Such activities may vary depending on the time of year, the athlete and the sport. Training benefits are specific to the training activities that produce them. When dealing with a beginner athlete, tolerance for the training process needs to be developed. Thus training frequency is increased first, later duration of training is increased and finally intensity is increased. Too rapid training leads to soft tissue injury. When injuries are prevented, standards are improved without spoiling enjoyment (McLatchie and Morris, 1977).

Medical practitioners, physiotherapists, nurses

and others who come into contact with soft tissue lesions need to be educated as regards their diagnosis and management. Close liaison with physiologists, biochemists, pathologists, bioengineers and others involved in research into soft tissue lesions is important. The current state of teaching in medical schools with regard to the soft tissue problems is grossly inadequate. Deans of clinical schools should ensure that more attention is paid to these problems. Even rheumatologists and orthopaedic surgeons often surprisingly lack knowledge about these lesions. It will bode well in the future if more sports and soft tissue lesion clinics are established. We can only ignore these important disorders at our peril.

References

Adebajo AO, Hazleman BL (1990) Painful stiff shoulder in Africans – a combined hospital and community study. *British Journal of Rheumatism* **29** (suppl 1), 32.

Allander E (1974) Prevalence, incidence and remission rates of some common rheumatic diseases and syndromes. *Scandinavian Journal of Rheumatology* **3**, 145–53.

Anderson JAD (1983) Occupational factors in arthritis and rheumatism. In: Hawkins L, Currey HLF (eds) *Collected Reports on Rheumatic Diseases 1959–1983*. London: Arthritis and Rheumatism Council for Research, p. 28.

Baker WM (1877) On the formation of synovial cysts in the leg in connection with disease of the knee joint. *St Bartholomew's Hospital Reports* **13**, 245–61.

Barker ME (1977) Pain in the back and leg. A general practice survey. *Rheumatology and Rehabilitation* **16**, 37–45.

Barrett D (1990) Disorders of the shoulder. *British Medical Journal* **300**, 1141.

Barton N (1989) Repetitive strain disorder. *British Medical Journal* **299**, 405–6.

Bergstrom G, Bjelle A, Sorensen LB, Sundh V, Svanborg A (1985a) Prevalence of symptoms and signs of joint impairment at age 79. *Scandinavian Journal of Rehabilitation Medicine* **17**, 173–82.

Bergstrom G, Aniunsson A, Bjelle A, Grimby G, Lundgren-Lindquist B, Svanborg A (1985b) Functional consequences of joint impairment at age 79. *Scandinavian Journal of Rehabilitation Medicine* **17**, 183–90.

Berhang AM, Dehner W, Fogarty C (1975) A scientific approach to tennis elbow. *Orthopaedic Review* **4**, 35–41.

Bigliani LU, Morrison DS, Arpil EW (1986) The morphology of the acromion and its relationship to rotator cuff tears. *Orthopaedic Transactions* **10**, 228.

Binder AI, Hazleman BL (1983) Lateral humeral epicondylitis – a study of natural history and the effect of conservative therapy. *British Journal of Rheumatology* **22**, 73–6.

Binder A, Parr G, Page Thomas P, Hazleman BL (1983) A clinical and thermographic study of lateral epicondylitis. *British Journal of Rheumatism* **22**, 77–81.

Binder A, Bulgen D, Hazleman B, Robert S (1984) Frozen shoulder: a long-term prospective study. *Annals of Rheumatic Disease* **43**, 361–4.

Binder A, Hodge G, Greenwood AM, Hazleman BL, Page Thomas DP (1985) Is therapeutic ultrasound effective in treating soft tissue lesions? *British Medical Journal* **1**, 512–14.

Binder A, Hazleman B, Parr G, Roberts S (1986) A controlled study of oral prednisolone in frozen shoulder. *British Journal of Rheumatism* **25**, 288–92.

Bjelle A, Hagberg M, Michaelson G (1979) Clinical and ergonomic factors in prolonged shoulder pain among industrial workers. *Scandinavian Journal of Work and Environmental Health*, **5**, 205–10.

Bjelle A, Allander E, Magi M (1980) Rheumatic disorders in the Swedish population and health care system. *Journal of Rheumatology* **7**, 877–85.

Bjorkenheim JP, Paavolainen P, Ahoto J, Slatis P (1988) Surgical repair of the rotator cuff and surrounding tissues: factors influencing results. *Clinics in Orthopaedics and Related Research* **236**, 148–53.

Blockley N, Wright J, Kellgren J (1954) Oral cortisone therapy in periarthritis of the shoulder. *British Medical Journal* **1**, 1455–7.

Bosworth BM (1941) Calcium deposits in the shoulder and subacromial bursitis: a survey of 12 122 shoulders. *Journal of the American Medical Assocation* **116**, 2477–82.

Bosworth DM (1955) The role of the orbicular ligament in tennis elbow. *Journal of Bone and Joint Surgery (America)* **37**, 527–33.

Brattberg G (1983) Acupuncture therapy for tennis elbow. *Pain* **16**, 285–8.

Brewerton DA, Sandifer P, Sweetnam R (1962) Pes cavus. *Journal of Bone and Joint Surgery* **44B**, 741.

Brooks P (1989) RSI – regional pain syndrome. The importance of nomenclature. *British Journal of Rheumatology* **28**, 180–2.

Brown JT (1949) Early assessment of supraspinatus tears: procaine infiltration as a guide to treatment. *Journal of Bone and Joint Surgery* **318**, 423–6.

Bulgen DY, Hazleman BL, Voak D (1976) HLA B27 and frozen shoulder. *Lancet* **1**, 1042–4.

Bulgen D, Binder A, Hazleman B (1984) Frozen shoulder: prospective clinical study with an evaluation of three treatment regimens. *Annals of Rheumatic Disease* **43**, 353–60.

Buren PRJ (1966) Duputryen's contracture and autoimmune disease. *Journal of Bone and Joint Surgery* **48B**, 312.

Bywaters EGL (1979) Lesions of bursae, tendons and tendon sheaths. *Clinics in Rheumatic Disease* **5**, 893–926.

Callicet R (1966) *Shoulder Pain*. Philadelphia: FA Davis.

Calvert PT, Macpherson IS, Allum RL, Bentley G (1985) Simple lateral release in treatment of tennis elbow. *Journal of the Royal Society of Medicine* **78**, 912–15.

Campbell JW, Inman VT (1974) Treatment of plantar fasciitis and calcaneal spurs with the UC-BL shoe insert. *Clinics in Orthopaedics* **103**, 57–62.

Chakravarty KK, Webley M (1990) Disorders of the shoulder: an often unrecognised cause of disability in elderly people. *British Medical Journal* **300**, 849–50.

Chard MD, Hazleman BL (1989a) Shoulder disorders in the elderly (a hospital study). *Annals of Rheumatic Disease* **46**, 684–7.

Chard MD, Hazleman BL (1989b) Shoulder disorders in the elderly (a community survey). *British Journal of Rheumatism* **28** (suppl 2), 21.

Chard MD, Wright JK, Cawston TE, Hazleman BL (1985) The production of latent collagenase and the tissue inhibitor of metalloproteinase by adult human tendon fibroblasts. *British Journal of Rheumatism* **25**, 52.

Chard MD, Wright JK, Hazleman BL (1987) The isolation and culture of adult human tendon fibroblasts. *Annals of Rheumatic Disease* **46**, 385–90.

Chard MD, Gresham A, Hazleman BL (1989) Age related changes in the rotator cuff. *British Journal of Rheumatology* **18**, 19.

Clark E, Willis L, Fish W *et al.* (1975) Preliminary studies in measuring range of motion in normal and painful stiff shoulder. *Rheumatology and Re-habilitation* **14**, 39–46.

Clarke AK, Woodland J (1975) Comparison of two steroid preparations used to treat tennis elbow, using hypospray. *Rheumatic Rehabilitation* **14**, 47–9.

Conrad RW, Hooper WR (1973) Tennis elbow: course natural history, conservative and surgical management. *Journal of Bone and Joint Surgery (America)* **55**, 1177–87.

Constant CR, Welsh RP (1985) *Shoulder Replacement*. Berlin: Springer.

Cunningham LS, Kelsey JL (1984) Epidemiology of musculoskeletal impairments and associated disability. *American Journal of Public Health* **74**, 574–9.

Cyriax JH (1936) The pathology and treatment of tennis elbow. *Journal of Bone and Joint Surgery* **18**, 921–40.

Cyriax J (1982) Diagnosis of soft tissue lesions. In: *Textbook of Orthopaedic Medicine*. London: Bailliere Tindall.

Darmawan J (1988) Rheumatic conditions in the northern part of central Java. An epidemiological survey. Thesis, Erasmus University, Rotterdam.

Day BH, Gordinasamay N, Patnaik R (1978) Corticosteroid injections in the treatment of tennis elbow. *Practitioner* **200**, 459–62.

Department of Health and Social Security (1986) *Morbidity Statistics from General Practice. Third National Study 1981–1982*. London: HMSO.

Devereaux MD, Hazleman BL, Page Thomas P (1985) Chronic lateral humeral epicondylitis – a double blind controlled assessment of pulsed electromagnetic field therapy. *Clinics in Experimental Rheumatism* **3**, 333–6.

Dimberg L (ed) (1985) Symptoms from the neck and upper extremities – an epidemiological, clinical and ergonomic study. Gothenburg: Volvo.

Dinham JM (1975) Popliteal cysts in children. *Journal of Bone and Joint Surgery* **57B**, 69–71.

Dixon A St J (1979) Soft tissue rheumatism. Concept and classification. *Clinics in Rheumatic Diseases* **5**, 739–42.

Dixon A (1980) Diagnosis of low back pain – sorting the complainers. In: Jayson MIV (ed) *The Lumbar Spine and Back Pain* 2nd edn. Kent: Pitman Medical, pp 135–55.

Dothie RB, Ferguson AB (1973) *Mercer's Orthopaedic Surgery*. Baltimore: Williams & Wilkins.

Editorial (1987) Repetition strain injury. *Lancet* **ii**, 316.

Eggers GWN (1957) Shoe pad for treatment of calcaneal spur. *Journal of Bone and Joint Surgery* **39A**, 219–20.

Ellard J (1985) Compensation neurosis. *Medical Journal of Australia* **142**, 535.

Emery P, Bowman S, Wedderburn L, Grahame R (1989) Suprascapular nerve block for chronic shoulder pain in rheumatoid arthritis. *British Medical Journal* **299**, 1079–80.

Engel J, Luboshit ZS, Israeli A, Ganel A (1981) Tenography in De Quervain's disease. *Hand* **13**, 142–6.

Evans G (1985) Calcific tendinitis of the insertion of abductor pollicis. *Clinical Notes On-line* **1**, 6.

Finkelstein H (1930) Stenosing tenovaginitis at the radial styloid process. *Journal of Bone and Joint Surgery* **12**, 509–40.

Fisher TR, Woods CG (1970) Partial rupture of the tendocalcaneus with heterotopic ossification. Repeat of a case. *Journal of Bone and Joint Surgery* **52**, 334–6.

Folsom AR, Casperson CJ, Taylor HL *et al.* (1985) Leisure time, physical activity and its relationship to coronary risk factors in a population based sample.

The Minnesota Heart Survey. *American Journal of Epidemiology* **121**, 570–0.
Fornage BD, Rifkin MD (1988) Ultrasound examination of the tendons. *Radiologic Clinics of North America* **26**, 87.
General Household Survey (1985) London: HMSO, pp 186–207.
Gerberich SG, Priest JD (1985) Treatment of lateral epicondylitis: variables related to recovery. *British Journal of Sports Medicine* **19**, 224–7.
Gerster JC, Vischer TL, Benani A, Fallet GH (1977) The painful heel. *Annals of Rheumatic Disease* **36**, 343–8.
Gersten JW (1985) Effect of ultrasound on tendon extensibility. *American Journal of Physical Medicine* **34**, 362–9.
Giannestras NJ (1978) *Foot Disorders.* In: *Duties' Surgery of the Foot.* Mann RA (ed) St Louis: CV Mosby.
Glick JM (1978) Traumatic injuries to the soft tissues of the foot and ankle. In: Mann RA (ed) *DuVries' Surgery of the Foot.* St Louis: CV Mosby.
Goldie I (1964) Epicondylitis lateralis humeri (epicondylalgia or tennis elbow). A pathogenetic study. *Acta Chirurgica Scandinavica. Supplementum* **339**, 1.
Grant AE (1964) Massage with ice (cryokinetics) in the treatment of painful conditions of the musculoskeletal system. *Archives of Physical Medicine and Rehabilitation* **45**, 233–8.
Gruchow HW, Pelletier BS (1979) An epidemiologic study of tennis elbow. *American Journal of Sports Medicine* **7**, 234–8.
Halpern N, Axer A (1980) Simple reconstruction of anteromedial rotational knee stability. *Injury* **12**, 53–8.
Harvey W, Dyson M, Pond JB, Grahame R (1975) The in vitro stimulation of protein synthesis in human fibroblasts by therapeutic levels of ultrasound. In: *Proceedings of the 2nd European Congress on Ultrasonics in Medicine.* Excerpta Medica: International Congress series 363; pp. 10–21.
Hawkins RJ, Brock RM (1979) Early results for impingement with intact rotator cuffs. *Orthopaedic Transactions* **3**, 274.
Hawkins RJ, Kennedy JC (1980) The impingement syndrome in athletes. *American Journal of Sports Medicine* **8**, 151–8.
Hayden C (1964) Cryokinetics in an early treatment programme. *Journal of the American Physiotherapy and Therapeutics Association* **44**, 990–93.
Hazleman BL (1972) The painful stiff shoulder. *Rheumatology and Physical Medicine* **11**, 413–21.
Hendryson IE (1946) Bursitis in the region of the fibular collateral ligament. *Journal of Bone and Joint Surgery* **28**, 446–50.
Herman A, Levin DN, Beek RN (1987) Oscillating intensity display of soft tissue lesions in MRI. *Medical Imaging* **6**, 370–3.
Hughes ESR (1950) Acute deposition of calcium near the elbow. *Journal of Bone and Joint Surgery* **32B**, 30–5.
Johansson S (1922) A previously undescribed lesion of the patella. *Hygiea* **84**, 161–6.
Kelsey JL (1982) *Epidemiology of Musculoskeletal Disorders.* New York: Oxford University Press, p 194.
Kessel L. Bayley I, Young A (1981) The frozen shoulder. *British Journal of Hospital Medicine* **25**, 334–8.
Kessel L, Watson M (1977) The painful arc syndrome. *Journal of Bone and Joint Surgery* **59B**, 166–72.
Kieft GJ, Bloem JL, Rozing PM, Oberman WR (1988) Rotator cuff impingement syndrome: MR imaging. *Radiology* **166**, 211–4.
Kivi P (1982) The aetiology and conservative treatment of humeral epicondylitis. *Scandinavian Journal of Rehabilitation Medicine* **15**, 37–41.
Kivi P (1984) Rheumatic disorders of the upper limbs associated with repetitive occupational tasks in Finland 1975–1979. *Scandinavian Journal of Rheumatology* **13**, 101–7.
Koplan JP, Powell KE, Sikes RK, Shirley RW, Campbell CC (1982) An epidemiological study of the benefits and risks of running. *Journal of the American Medical Association* **248**, 3118–21.
Kvarnstrom S (1983) Occurrence of musculoskeletal disorders in a manufacturing industry with special attention to occupational shoulder disorders. *Scandinavian Journal of Rehabilitation Medicine* **8** (suppl 8), 1–114.
Lanfear RT, Clarke WB (1972) The treatment of tenosynovitis in industry. *Physiotherapy* **58**, 128–9.
Lanzetta A, Meani E, Tinti G (1981) Injuries of the Achilles tendon in athletes: their causes and the indication for their treatment. *Italian Journal of Sports Traumatology* **3**, 113–21.
Lawrence JS (1977) *Rheumatism in Populations.* London: Heinemann.
Leach RE, Osamu N, Richard PG, Stockel J (1981) Secondary reconstruction of the lateral ligaments of the ankle. *Clinical Orthopaedics and Related Research* **160**, 201–11.
Lee P, Lee M, Haq A (1974) Periarthritis of the shoulder – trial of treatments investigated by multivariate analysis. *Annals of Rheumatic Disease* **33**, 116–19.
Lester DK, Buchanan JR (1984) Surgical treatment of plantar fasciitis. *Clinics in Orthopaedics* **186**, 202–4.
Lundberg B (1969) The frozen shoulder. *Acta Orthopaedica Scandinavica* (suppl) 119.
Mack LA, Cannon MK, Kikoyne RF, Matsen III FA (1988) Sonographic evaluation of the rotator cuff. Accuracy in patients without prior surgery. *Clinics in Orthopaedics Related Research* **234**, 21–7.
McLatchie GR, Morris EW (1977) Prevention of karate injuries – a progress report. *British Journal of Sports Medicine* **11**, 78–82.

McLatchie GR, Fitzgerald B, Davies JE (1980) The medical implications of weight training and weight lifting. *Medisport* **2**, 69–72.

McLatchie GR, Allister C, Hamilton G *et al.* (1985) Variable schedules of ibuprofen for ankle sprains. British Journal of Sports Medicine 19.

Macnab I (1973) Rotator cuff tendinitis. *Annals of the Royal College of Surgeons of England* **53**, 271–87.

Manahan L, Caragay R, Muirden KD, Allander E, Valkenburg HA, Wigley RD (1985) Rheumatic pain in a Philippine Village. A WHO-ILAR COPCORD study. *Rheumatology International* **5**, 149–53.

Mann RA, DuVries HL (1978) Acquired non-traumatic deformities of the foot. In: Mann RA (ed) *DuVries' Surgery of the Foot*. St Louis: CV Mosby.

Marlun T (1930) Treatment of tennis elbow with some observations of joint manipulation. *Lancet* **i**, 509–11.

Meheim JM, Cooper CE (1950) Tennis elbow. *American Journal of Surgery* **80**, 622–5.

Miller HW (1973) *Plan and Operation of the Health and Nutrition Examination Survey: United States 1971–3*. Vital and Health Statistics series 1, no. 10. Washington: Public Health Service, US Department of Health.

Mills GP (1982) The treatment of tennis elbow. *British Medical Journal* **i**, 12–13.

Mooney V, Cairns D (1978) Management in the patient with chronic low back pain. *Orthopaedics of North America* **9**, 543–57.

Morris H (1822) Riders sprain. *Lancet* **ii**, 557.

Moskowitz RW (1975) *Clinical Rheumatology*. Philadelphia: Lea & Febiger.

Moushe PR, Gilberman RH, Vande-Berg JS, Lesker PA (1984) Intrinsic flexor-tendon repair. A morphological in vitro study. *Journal of Bone and Joint Surgery* **66A**, 685–96.

Muckart RD (1986) Stenosing tenovaginitis of abductor pollicis longus and extensor pollicis brevis at the radial styloid (de Quervain's disease). *Clinical Orthopaedics* **33**, 201–8.

Murnaghan G, MacIntosh D (1955) Hydrocortisone in the painful shoulder – a controlled trial. *Lancet* **ii**, 798.

Murray RD, Jacobson HG (1977) *Acute Calcific Tendinitis. Radiology of Skeletal Disorders*. Edinburgh: Churchill Livingstone, 876.

Nachemson A (1969) Physiotherapy for low back pain. A critical look. *Scandinavian Journal of Rehabilitation Medicine*.

National Center for Health Statistics (1976) National Health Interview Survey. Public Health Service publication no. 79–1552, series 10, no. 124. Washington DC: US Government Printing Office.

Neer CS (1972) Anterior acromioplasto for the chronic impingement syndrome in the shoulder. A preliminary report. *Journal of Bone and Joint Surgery* **54A**, 41–50.

Neer CS, Welsh RP (1977) The shoulder in sports. *Orthopaedic Clinics of North America* **8**, 583–90.

Neipal GA, Sitaj S (1979) Enthesopathy. *Clinics in Rheumatic Disease* **5**, 857–72.

Nevelos AB (1980) The treatment of tennis elbow with triamcinolone acetonide. *Current Medical Research Opinion* **6**, 507–9.

Newman JH, Goodfellow JW (1975) Fibrillation of the radial head as one cause for tennis elbow. *British Medical Journal* **ii**, 328–30.

Newman PH, Thompson JPU, Barnes JM, Moore TM (1969) A clinic for athletic injuries. *Proceedings of the Royal Society of Medicine* **62**; 939–41.

Nirchl RP, Pettrone FA (1973) Tennis elbow. *Journal of Bone and Joint Surgery* **61A**, 832–9.

Norwood LA, Barrack R, Jacobson KE (1989) A surgical viewpoint of clinical features predictive of rotator cuff tears. *Journal of Bone and Joint Surgery* **71A**, 499–505.

Office of Health Economics (1985) *Back Pain*. London: Office of Health Economics.

Office of Population Censuses and Surveys (OPCS) (1985) *Mortality Statistics for 1984 by Cause*. Series DH2, no. 11. HMSO: London.

Outland T, Murphy ID (1960) Peroneal flat foot. *Clinical Orthopaedics* **16**, 64–73.

Pentland AP, Anderson TF (1985) Plantar fibromatosis responds to intralesional steroids. *Journal of the American Academy of Dermatology* **12**, 212–4.

Peterson HE, Day AJ (1954) Dupuytren's disease of the foot. *Journal of the American Medical Association* **154**, 33.

Pettrone FA (1982) Menisectomy: arthrotomy versus arthroscopy. *American Journal of Sports Medicine* **10**, 355–9.

Post M (1978) *The Shoulder, Surgical and Non-Surgical Management*. Philadelphia: Lea & Febiger, pp 306–10.

Potenza AD (1963) Clinical evaluation of flexor tendon healing and adhesion formation with artificial digital sheaths. *Journal of Bone and Joint Surgery* **41A**, 1217–33.

Quinet R, Hadler N (1979) Diagnosis and treatment of backache. *Seminars in Arthritis and Rheumatism* **8**, 261–87.

Reed JV, Harcourt AK (1943) Tenosynovitis. *American Journal of Surgery* **62**, 392–6.

Reeves B (1966) Arthrographic changes in frozen and post traumatic stiff shoulders. *Proceedings of the Royal Society of Medicine* **59**, 827–30.

Reeves B (1976) The natural history of the frozen shoulder syndrome. *Scandinavian Journal of Rheumatology* **4**, 193–6.

Renton J (1830) Observations in acupuncturation. *Edinburgh Medical Journal* **34**, 100.

Rhoades CE, Gelberman RH, Manjamis JF (1984) Stenosing tenosynovitis of the fingers and thumb. *Clinics in Orthopaedics* **190**, 236–8.

Ritchey SJ (1960) Ligamentous disruption of the knee. A review with analysis of 28 cases. *US Armed Forces Medical Journal* **11**, 167–76.

Rizk TE, Pinals RS (1982) Frozen shoulder. *Seminars in Arthritis and Rheumatism* **11**, 440–52.

Rockwood CA (1986) The management of patients with massive rotator cuff defects by acromioplasty and rotator cuff debridement. *Orthopaedic Transactions* **10**, 622.

Roles NC, Maudsley RH (1972) Radial tunnel syndrome: resistant tennis elbow as a nerve entrapment. *Journal of Bone and Joint Surgery* **54B**, 499–508.

Rose GK (1979) Soft tissue and bony operations for cavus and planus. In: Rob C, Smith R (eds) *Operative Surgery* 3rd edn. London: Butterworths, pp 894–900.

Royal College of General Practitioners (1979) Office of Population Censuses and Surveys, Department of Health and Social Security. *Morbidity Statistics from General Practice. Second National Study 1971–2*. London: HMSO.

Royal College of General Practitioners (1986) Office of Population Censuses and Surveys, Department of Health and Social Security. *Morbidity Statistics from General Practice. Third National Study*. London: HMSO.

Runge F (1873) Zur Genese und Behandlung des Schreiberkrumpfes. *Berliner Klinische Wochenschrift* **10**, 245–8.

Rurek S (ed.) (1967) The shoulder. In: *Orthopaedics: Principles and Applications*. Philadelphia: JB Lippincott.

Ruttimann G (1959) Uber die Haufigkeit rontgenologischer Verunderungen bei Patienten mit typischer periarthritis humeroscapularis und schultegesunden. Inaugural dissertation University of Zurich.

Scranton PE, Pedeganon LR, Whitesel JP (1982) Gait analysis: alterations in support phase forces using supportive devices. *American Journal of Sports Medicine* **10**, 6–10.

Simons DG, Travell JG (1980) Myofascial origins of low back pain. 3. Pelvic and lower extremities. *Postgraduate Medicine* **73**, 99–108.

Sinding-Larsen MF (1921) A hitherto unknown affection of the patella. *Acta Radiologica* **1**, 171–3.

Snider MP, Clancy WG, McBenth AA (1983) Plantar fascia releases for chronic plantar fasciitis in runners. *American Journal of Sports Medicine* **11**, 215–9.

Sperryn PN (1972) Athletic injuries. *Rheumatology and Rehabilitation* **11**, 246–9.

Steindler A, Luck JV (1938) Differential diagnosis of pain low in the back: allocation of the source of pain by the procainamide hydrochloride method. *Journal of the American Medical Association* **110**, 106–13.

Sternback RA, Murphy RW, Akeson WH, Wolf Sr (1973) Chronic low back pain: the 'low back laser'. *Postgraduate Medicine* **53**, 135–8.

Stoyler TF (1964) Duputyren's contracture in the foot. *Journal of Bone and Joint Surgery* **46B**, 218.

Stuttle FL (1959) The no-name and no-fame bursa. *Clinics in Orthopaedics* **15**, 197–9.

Swartout R, Compere EL (1974) Ischio-gluteal bursitis. *Journal of the American Medical Association* **227**, 551–2.

Swezey RL, Spiegel TM (1979) Evaluation and treatment of local musculoskeletal disorders in elderly patients. *Geriatrics* **34**, 56–75.

Takala J, Sievers K, Klaukka T (1982) Rheumatic symptoms in the middle aged population in South Western Finland. *Scandinavian Journal of Rheumatology* **47** (suppl), 15–29.

Temple C (1983) Sports injuries. Hazards of jogging and marathon running. *British Journal of Hospital Medicine* **29**, 237–9.

Turek SL (1977) *Orthopaedics; Principles and their application*. Philadelphia: JB Lippincott.

Uhthoff HK, Sarkar K. Maynard JA (1976) Calcifying tendinitis. *Clinics in Orthopaedics* **118**, 164–8.

Wadsworth TG (1987) Tennis elbow conservative, surgical and manipulative treatment. *British Medical Journal* **294**, 621–14.

Watson M (1989) Rotator cuff function in the impingement syndrome. *Journal of Bone and Joint Surgery (Am)* **3**, 361–6.

Webster DF, Burry HC (1982) The effects of hypoxia on human skin, lung and tendon cells in vitro. *British Journal of Experimental Pathology* **63**, 50–5.

Whipple TL, Goldner JL (1979) A consideration in patient selection and operative technique. *Orthopaedic Transactions* **3**, 40.

Wolfe F (1986) The clinical syndrome of fibrositis. *American Journal of Medicine* **81**, 7–14.

Wood PHN (1970) Statistical appendix – Digest of data on the rheumatic diseases: Recent trends in sickness, absence and mortality. *Annals of Rheumatic Disease* **29**, 324–9.

Wood PHN, McLeish CL (1974) Statistical appendix. Digest of data on the rheumatic diseases: 5. Morbidity in industry, and rheumatology in general practice. *Annals of Rheumatic Disease* **33**, 93–105.

Wood PHN, Sturrock AW, Badley EM (1979) Soft tissue rheumatism in the community. *Clinics in Rheumatic Disease* **5**, 743–54.

Yates DA (1977) Non-articular rheumatism. *Physiotherapy* **63**, 393–5.

Yunus MB, Masi AT (1985) Juvenile primary fibromyalgi syndrome. *Arthritis and Rheumatism*, **28**, 138–44.

Zlatkin MB, Reicher MA, Kellerhouse LE, McDade W, Vetter L, Resnick D (1988) The painful shoulder: MR imaging of the glenohumeral joint. *Journal of Computer Assisted Tomography* **12**, 995–1001.

2

Anatomy of the soft tissues

R. W. Soames

The skin

Introduction

The skin is a tough, pliable waterproof covering which is continuous with the more delicate membranes lining the various openings of the body. Indeed it lines the terminal parts of many duct systems that open externally and are liable to trauma, e.g. the anal canal, vagina and ear. Skin, however, is more than a mere covering – it protects the deeper tissues, controls body temperature, prevents fluid loss, absorbs certain drugs, vitamins and hormones, excretes certain crystalloids, and is the largest single sensory organ in the body. In addition to these various functions the skin plays an important role in general medical diagnosis and surgery, as well as being liable to many diseases of its own.

The surface area of the skin is between 1.8 and 2.0 m^2, and is some seven times greater in the adult than at birth. Its thickness varies from 0.5 to over 3 mm; however, for the most part it is between 1 and 2 mm thick, and generally thicker over extensor than flexor surfaces. It is thinner in infancy and in old age. Total thickness of the skin depends on the thickness of both the epidermis and the dermis. In areas of great wear and tear (e.g. the palm of the hand and the sole of the foot) the epidermis is primarily responsible for the thickness of the skin; the dermis is relatively thin.

The skin is generally loosely applied to the underlying tissues so that it is easily displaced. In some areas, however, it is firmly attached to the underlying structures, e.g. the subcutaneous periosteal surface of the tibia. In other places it must be firmly bound down to allow freedom of movement without interference from subcutaneous fat and otherwise highly mobile skin, e.g. to the deep fascia surrounding joints.

In young individuals the skin is extremely elastic, returning to its original shape and position after distortion. This elasticity is increasingly lost with age so than unless it firmly attaches to the underlying tissues it stretches. Stretching tends to occur in one direction due to the orientation of the collagen in the deeper layers; this tends to run predominantly at right angles to the direction of stretch. In adjusting to allow movement the skin follows the contours of the body. Although this is enabled by its intrinsic elasticity it is nevertheless subject to internal stresses which vary from region to region. These stress lines are referred to as Langer's lines or cleavage lines (Fig. 2.1). Langer's lines do not always correspond with the stress lines of life; they merely reflect the stresses within the skin at rest. They are important because surgical incisions along these lines tend to heal with a minimum of scar, whereas wounds across them lead to thicker scar formation with the possibility of scar contraction, due to the edges of the wound being pulled apart by the internal stresses within the skin.

Structure

The skin consists of two distinct layers, each of different embryological origin. The epidermis is

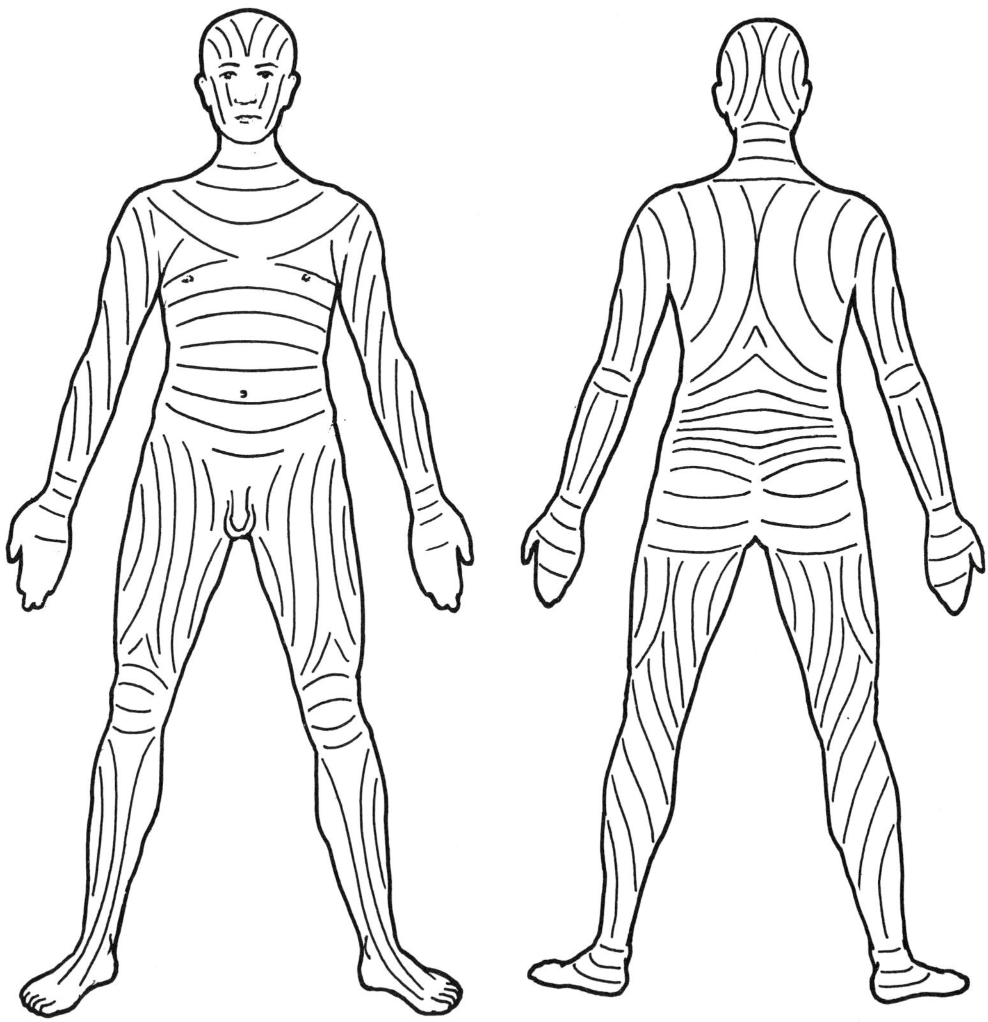

Fig. 2.1 The orientation of the natural lines of cleavage of the skin, known as Langer's lines.

the superficial layer and is of ectodermal origin, while the underlying dermis is a mesodermally derived layer. Beneath the dermis is a layer of loose connective tissue which varies from areolar to adipose in character. This layer is sometimes referred to as the hypodermis and is essentially the superficial fascia of the body: it is not considered to be part of the skin.

Epidermis

The epidermis is an avascular but richly innervated layer of stratified squamous epithelium of varying thickness (0.3–1.0 mm), consisting of several distinct layers of cells, which are more easily visible in thick skin, i.e. on the palms and soles. The deeper cells are living and actively proliferating, with the cells produced gradually passing towards the surface, becoming progressively keratinized as they do so. Keratin eventually replaces the majority of the cytoplasm, the cell dies and is finally shed from the surface. The deep surface of the epidermis is firmly locked on to the underlying dermis by projections into it known as epidermal pegs, while the reciprocal dermal projections are known as dermal papillae (Fig. 2.2).

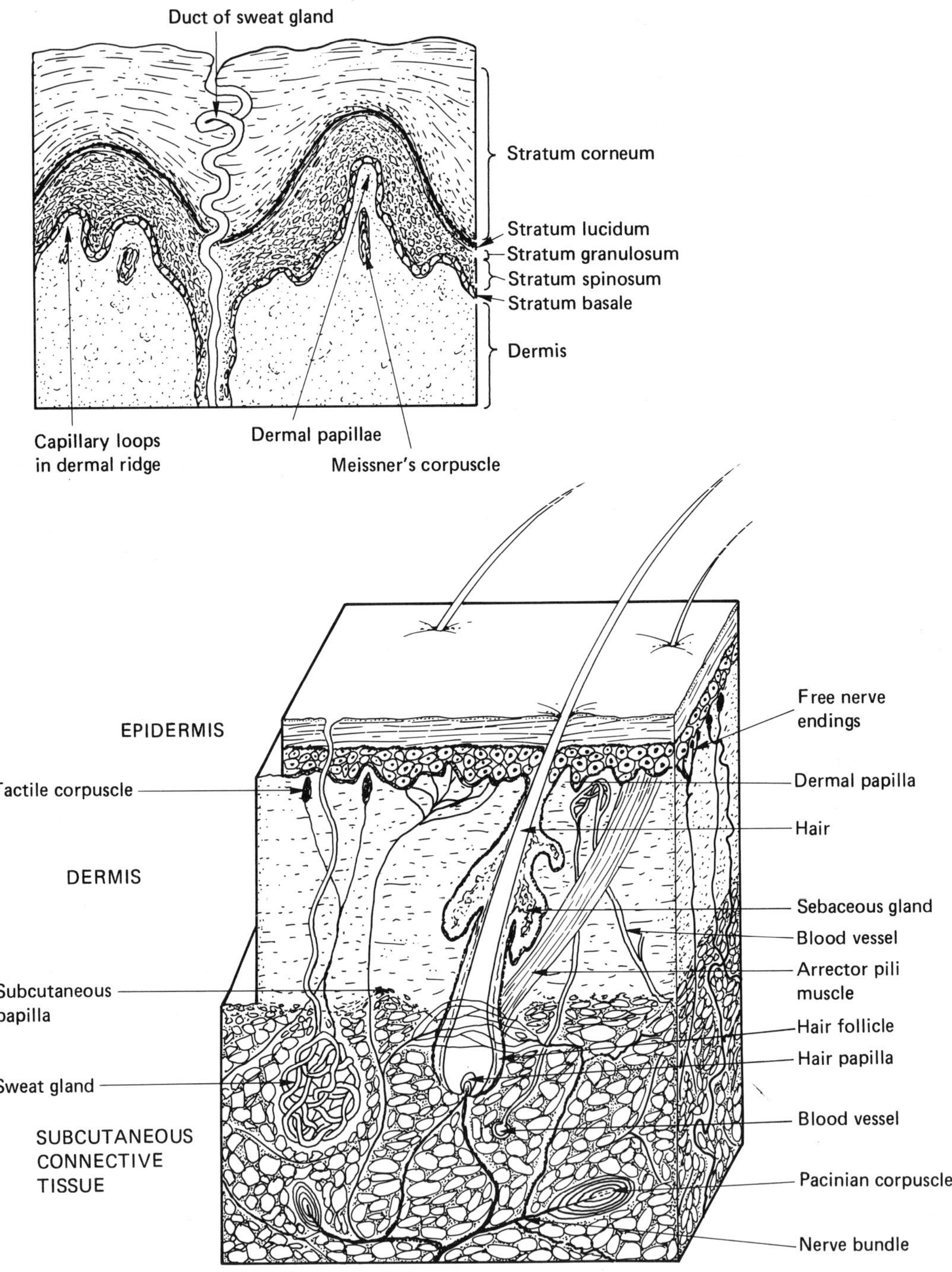

Fig. 2.2 The structure of skin.

Where the epidermis is thick it presents as five distinct layers, with the outer three sometimes being referred to as the horny layer, and the deeper two as the Malpighian layer (stratum

Malpighii). The layers are, from deep to superficial, the stratum basale (or germinativum), stratum spinosum, stratum granulosum, stratum lucidum and stratum corneum. The stratum basale consists of a single layer of columnar cells with short thin cytoplasmic processes on their basal surface which fit into pockets of the basal lamina and appear to anchor the epithelium to the underlying dermis. New cells are produced in this layer and displaced upwards. The stratum spinosum is several layers thick and consists of irregular polyhedral cells which become flattened towards the surface. The cytoplasm contains many bundles of filaments which form the tonofilaments, which in turn are the principal precursor of keratin. The stratum granulosum consists of three to five layers of flattened cells whose long axes lie parallel to the skin surface. It is in this layer that the cells of the epidermis die. The stratum lucidum is a clear translucent layer, again three to five cells deep, with the cells not being clearly distinguishable as separate entities: they are flattened and closely packed together. The final layer, the stratum corneum, consists of clear, dead scale-like cells which become progressively flattened and fused. The most superficial layers of the stratum corneum are flat horny plates which are continually lost from the skin surface.

The epidermis over the remainder of the body is thinner and simpler than the palms or soles. All the layers are reduced, and the stratum lucidum is often absent. The reduction in thickness of the so-called 'thin' skin is probably due to the fact that keratinization is less marked and is not a continuous process. Even so, keratin is present throughout the epidermis and is readily hydrated, hence the swelling of skin when immersed in water; dryness of the skin is due mainly to a lack of water.

Skin colour is dependent on three factors: (1) the presence of carotene which gives the skin a yellow appearance; (2) blood showing through from the underlying dermis; and (3) the presence of varying amounts of melanin pigment giving various shades of brown. The melanin is present mainly in the stratum basale and deeper layers of the stratum spinosum, with the pigment being in specialized cells, called melanocytes, derived from the neural crest.

Human epidermis shows a rhythmic mitotic cycle, with mitosis being more active at night. It is stimulated by loss of the horny layer. Part or all of the dermis may be raised in the form of blisters, due to the accumulation of underlying plasma, when the skin is damaged. In addition prolonged pressure and friction produce callosities and corns.

When an area of epidermis, with or without any underlying dermis, is destroyed, new epidermis is formed from hair follicles as well as from sudoriferous and sebaceous glands when present. If the injury is deep and involves the whole thickness of the dermis, repair can only take place by a growing over of the surrounding edge of the epidermis or alternatively by the use of an autograft. Free skin grafts of the epidermis, together with part or all of the thickness of the dermis can be applied; vascularization takes place between the subcutaneous vessels and those in the graft.

Dermis

The dermis, also known as the corium, is the deeper interlacing mesh of collagen and elastic fibres which constitutes the greater part of total skin thickness. The exact limits of the dermis are difficult to define since it merges into the underlying subcutaneous layer; however it has an average thickness of 0.5–3.0 mm. The undersurface of the dermis is invaginated by tufts of subcutaneous tissue similar to but larger and more dispersed than the dermal papillae. The larger spacing of these invaginations is a guide to the proper plane of separation between the dermis and the subcutaneous tissues. The tufts also serve for the entrance into the dermis of blood vessels and nerves.

The dermis can be subdivided into superficial and deep layers. The superficial layer is a finely textured layer of thin collagenous, reticular and elastic fibres arranged in an extensive network, together with fibroblasts, mast cells and macrophages. Just beneath the epidermis the reticular fibres of the dermis form a close feltwork into which the basal processes of the stratum basale of the epidermis are anchored: this is the basal lamina. The superficial layer of the dermis includes the ridges and papillae, which may number 100 per mm^2, that project into the epidermis. The papillae tend to occur in double rows and are often branched. Some contain special nerve terminations (nervous papillae), while others possess capillary loops (vascular papillae).

The thicker deeper reticular layer is the main fibrous bed of the dermis. It consists of coarse, dense interlacing collagenous fibres together with a few reticular and numerous elastic fibres. Most fibres lie parallel to the skin surface, giving rise to lines of skin tension known as Langer's lines (see earlier). Some of the fibres in this layer enter the subcutaneous tissue where they form bundles between lobules of fat. The main cellular elements in this layer of the dermis are fibroblasts and macrophages, with some fat cells either singly or in groups. As well as the connective tissue cells, pigmented, branched cells called chromatophores may be present. They tend, however, to occur only in areas where the overlying epidermis is heavily pigmented, and probably obtain their pigment from melanocytes. True dermal melanocytes tend to be rare.

Smooth muscle fibres are also present in the dermis. These are arranged in bundles in connection with hair follicles, the arrectores pilorum muscles, and also scattered throughout the dermis in considerable numbers in some areas (areola and nipple, scrotum and penis), giving the skin in these regions a wrinkled appearance. In the neck and face fibres of some skeletal muscles terminate in the delicate elastic fibre networks of the dermis.

Hypodermis

Although not part of the skin, this subcutaneous layer appears as an extension of the dermis. It is the density and arrangement of this subcutaneous layer which determines the mobility of the skin. Depending on the region of the body and the nutritional status of the individual, varying amounts of fat cells are found in the hypodermis. This fatty layer overlies the more densely fibrous fascia (the superficial fascia). The superficial part of the hypodermis contains part of the hair follicles and sweat glands.

Derivatives of skin

Several structures are derived from the epidermis – sebaceous, sweat and mammary glands, nails and hair.

Sebaceous glands

These are associated with all hairs and hair follicles; between one and four being associated with each hair. Where they are independent of hairs their ducts open directly on to the skin surface, e.g. the tarsal (meibomium) glands of the eyelids. Sebaceous glands are absent on the palms and soles.

They are simple alveolar glands forming lobes in the dermis, usually in the angle between the hair follicle and the arrectores pilorum. The epithelial cells of the gland are continuously destroyed in the production of their oily secretion (sebum) into the lumen of the hair follicle – holocrine secretion. The sebum keeps the stratum corneum pliable and aids the conservation of body heat by hindering evaporation. Discharge of the secretion is aided by contraction of the arrectores pili muscles.

An excessive secretion of sebum (seborrhoea) may collect on the skin surface as scales known as dandruff. Chronic inflammation and accumulation of secretion within the gland itself give rise to acne. If the duct is blocked a blackhead (comedo) results; however, if the blockage is permanent a sebaceous cyst (wen) may form in the duct and follicle.

Sweat glands

Sweat glands develop in the fetus as epidermal downgrowths which become canalized. They are simple, unbranched tubular glands with a coiled secretory unit situated in the dermis or subcutaneous tissue, with a long winding duct extending through the epidermis to open on the skin surface by a minute pit. The glands produce sweat, a clear fluid without any cellular elements (eccrine secretion), and are important in temperature regulation as its evaporation from the skin surface promotes heat loss. The eccrine sweat glands are innervated by sympathetic fibres. Consequently any disturbance in the sympathetic system may result in a warm, dry skin (anhydrosis) either locally or extensively.

Sweat glands have a wide distribution throughout the body, being more numerous on its exposed parts, particularly the soles, palms and flexor surfaces of the digits. Here their ducts open on to the summit of the epidermal ridges.

In certain areas (axilla, areola and around the anus) larger sweat glands are found. The secretory portion lies deeply in the subcutaneous layer, while the ducts may be associated with a hair follicle or open directly on to the skin surface. The secretions from these glands include some disintegration products of the gland cells (apocrine secretion). These apocrine glands vary with sexual development, enlarging at puberty. In females they show changes associated with the menstrual cycle. The glands in the external auditory meatus (ceruminous glands) and those which open at the margins of the eyelids (ciliary glands) are modified uncoiled sweat glands.

Mammary glands

These are specialized localized glands situated in the subcutaneous tissue. They develop from the nipples during fetal life. The mammary glands are modified sweat glands with apocrine secretions. Each gland consists of 15–20 lobes, each of which is an independent gland, with a duct opening at the apex of the nipple. Mammary glands are present in both sexes, but in children prior to puberty and adult males they remain rudimentary while in post-pubescent females they enlarge, principally as a result of the development of adipose and other connective tissue. Even in females the glands remain incompletely developed until pregnancy when there is rapid proliferation of the glandular tissue and a decrease in interlobar fat and connective tissue.

Nails

These are hardened plates formed from the horny layer of the epidermis and are situated over the dorsal aspect of the distal phalanges. They develop as epidermal thickenings that undercut the skin to form folds from which the horny substance of the nail grows. The horny part consists of hard keratin and has an exposed distal part, the body, and a hidden proximal part, the root (Fig. 2.3). The root is covered by an extension of the stratum corneum, consisting of soft keratin, forming the eponychium. Deep to the distal part of the nail the horny layer of the fingertip is thickened – the hyponychium. The epidermis beneath the nail forms the nail bed, with the proximal part (or matrix) producing hard keratin. However, the most superficial layer of the nail may be produced by the epithelium between the nail root and the eponychium.

The nail plate itself is translucent and transmits the pink of the highly vascular nail bed. Nail growth, which averages 0.5 and 1.00 mm per week (quicker in the finger nails than in the toe nails), is affected by nutrition, hormones and disease. It involves considerable protein synthesis, consequently non-specific changes occur in the nails in response to various local and systemic disturbances. If a nail is removed a new nail will grow providing that the matrix is not destroyed.

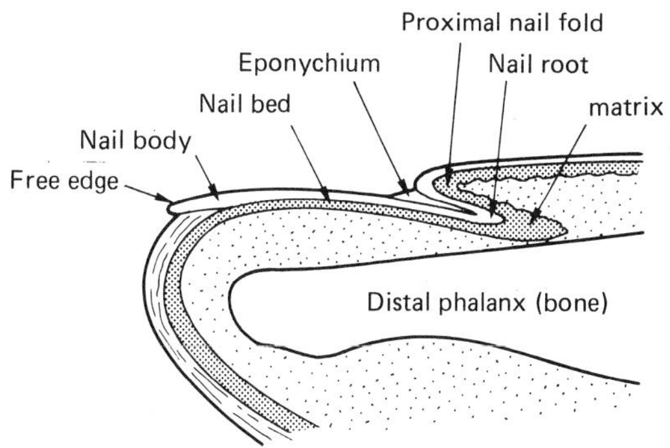

Fig. 2.3 The relationship of nail to the skin.

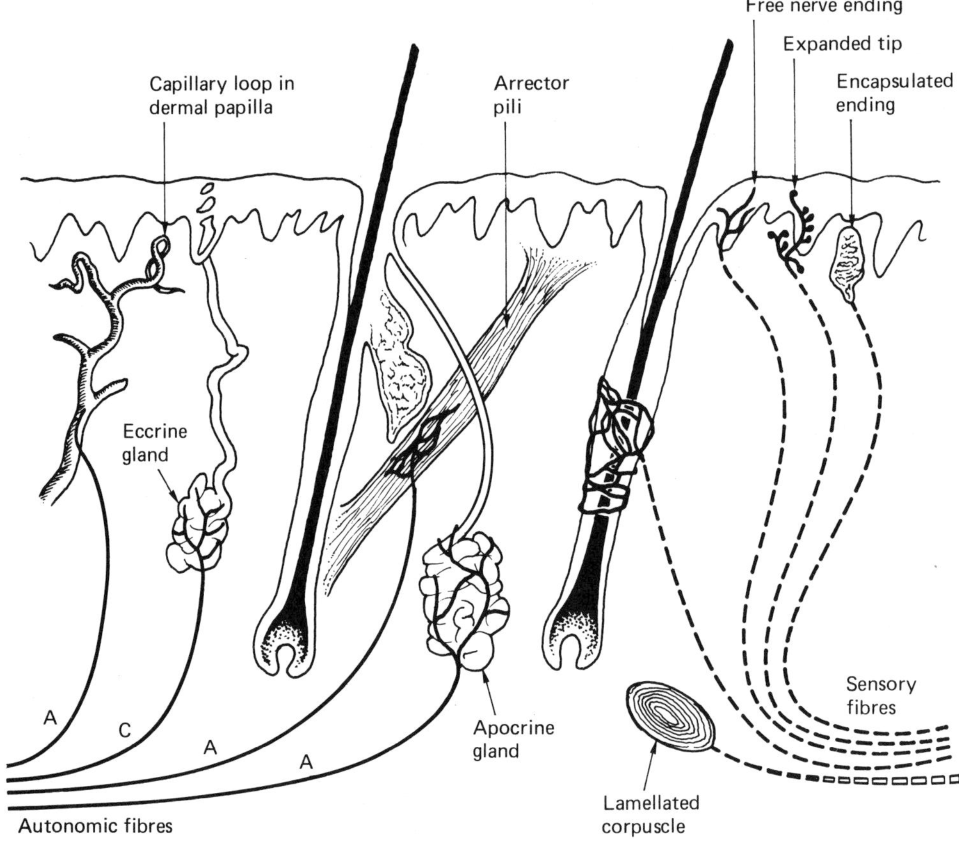

Fig. 2.4 Schematic representation of the innervation of the skin. A = Adrenergic nerve fibres; C = cholinergic nerve fibres.

Hairs

Hair is widely distributed over the body surface, notable exceptions being on the palm of the hand, the sole of the foot, the dorsal surfaces of the distal phalanges, the red portions of the lips and the nipples. The functions of hair include protection, regulation of body temperature and sensory perception. Hairs develop as epidermal downgrowths in the fetus that invade the underlying dermis. Each downgrowth terminates in an expansion that becomes invaginated by a mesodermal papilla. The central cells of the downgrowth become keratinized forming the hair, which then grows upwards to reach the surface. The initial hair (lanugo) is shed shortly before birth and finer hair subsequently develops (the vellus). Some of this latter hair is replaced by terminal hair, particularly on the scalp, eyebrows and eyelids, and after puberty over the pubes, in the axilla, and in males on the face. Although hairs on many parts of the body are inconspicuous their actual number per unit area is large.

Hairs are elastic keratinized threads, varying from 1 mm to over 1 m in length, and from 0.05 to 0.5 mm in thickness. Each has a free shaft and a root embedded in the skin. Surrounding the root is the tubular hair follicle, which extends deep into the dermis (Fig. 2.4). The lower end of the follicle is dilated forming the hair bulb. A connective tissue papilla projects into the bottom of the bulb conveying blood vessels into it.

Hair consists of epidermal cells arranged in three concentric layers: the medulla, the cortex and the cuticle. The medulla forms the loose central part of the hair and consists of two or three layers of shrunken cells, containing soft keratin and often pigment, separated by air spaces. The medulla is absent from vellous hair, some scalp hair and from blonde hair. The main bulk of the hair consists of the cortex which is composed of several layers of long flattened cornified cells containing hard keratin; pigment cells are found in and between the cells (oxidized pigment gives rise to black hair). Air accumulates in the intercellular spaces of cortical cells modifying hair colour. The outermost layer of hair is a single layer of thin clear cells forming the cuticle. They overlap like tiles on a roof, but with the free edges directed upwards.

The shaft of straight hair is circular in cross-section, while that of curly hair is oval. Hair lasts for definite periods from 2–4 years on the head to only 3–5 months in the eyelashes. When growth ceases the root of the hair becomes detached from the matrix and falls out. After a resting phase the remaining epithelial cells of the follicle undergo a period of growth and establish contact with a papilla, either the old one or a new one. A new matrix develops and the new hair begins to grow up from the reforming follicles.

Blood supply and lymphatic drainage

The skin has a profuse blood supply which is from large arteries in the subcutaneous connective tissue. From this subcutaneous network, at the junction between the dermis and hypodermis, branches pass to one side to supply the subcutaneous tissues, including sweat glands and the deeper parts of the hair follicles, and on the other side to form a subpapillary plexus in the dermis. This latter plexus gives rise to capillary loops which pass into the dermal papillae, supplying the papillae, sebaceous glands and the intermediate parts of the hair follicles. The avascular epidermis is bathed in tissue fluid derived from these capillary loops.

A network of veins immediately beneath the papillae collects blood from the area supplied by the subpapillary plexus. It is this network which gives the skin its pink appearance; the vessels become dilated when the skin is heated, giving a red glow. This venous network communicates with a second network immediately beneath it, and via this with a third at the junction of the dermis with the hypodermis. Into this third plexus pass most of the veins from the fat lobules and sweat glands. From this deeper (third) plexus veins pass to a network of vessels in the subcutaneous tissues, which in turn drain into larger veins. Arteriovenous anastomoses are common within the deeper layers of the dermis.

The lymphatics of the skin begin in the papillae as endothelial-lined clefts which pass to a mesh of lymphatic capillaries in the papillary layer. This mesh communicates with a network of larger capillaries in the subcutaneous tissue, which also receives lymph from plexuses surrounding sebaceous and sweat glands and hair follicles.

Innervation

The skin has a rich innervation. Nerves are of two types: afferent somatic fibres mediating pain, touch, pressure, heat and cold (general sensory), and efferent autonomic (sympathetic) fibres supplying blood vessels, glands and arrectores pilorum.

The cutaneous fibres pierce the fascia and form plexuses in the subcutaneous tissue and in the dermis. The sensory (afferent) nerve endings have several forms. Fine free nerve endings pass between the deeper cells of the epidermis and also pass to terminate around and adjacent to hair follicles. They are receptive to general tactile sensations as well as painful stimuli. Enclosed tactile corpuscles lie in the dermal papillae and are sensitive to touch. Pacinian corpuscles exist in the subcutaneous tissue, and are particularly plentiful along the sides of the digits, and act as pressure receptors. Specific endings for heat and cold have been described, although general agreement as to their identity has yet to be reached.

Trauma to the skin

Burns

Burns are a common trauma to skin. They are classified by severity, i.e. the degree of the burn, and by extent, i.e. the percentage body surface area affected. A burn is an excess energy transfer to the skin and other tissues; its severity is determined by the factors responsible. Partial-thickness burns involve only the epidermis and are referred to as first-degree burns. Mixed-thickness burns (second-degree burns) involve the dermis, while full-thickness burns (third-degree burns) include the hypodermis. First-degree burns always heal as they involve loss of the epidermis only. Second-degree burns may heal, depending on the depth of the burn, or they may progress to a full-thickness burn. Third-degree burns do not heal as the tissue is unable to regenerate itself. It is in these cases that skin grafts must be applied to the affected area. If the extent of the burn is small skin may be grafted from another region of the body such as the buttock or thigh. However, if the affected area is large skin may be cultured to replace that lost.

Burns affecting less than 10% of the total body surface area are considered to be minor in nature, and generally do not require formal resuscitation of the tissue, although this will be influenced by the patient's age. If the burn affects more than 10% of the surface area it is considered to be major, while if more than 30% of the surface area is affected it is classified as a serious burn. In both of the latter cases formal resuscitation is required, involving fluids etc.

The extent of the surface area affected can be quickly ascertained by applying the rule of nine (the head and neck together, and each upper limb are each approximately 9% of the total surface area; each lower limb, the front of the trunk, and the back of the trunk are each approximately 18% of the total surface area). However, the approximation is not so accurate in children because of the larger head size with respect to the body. Nevertheless, it provides a valuable first-hand guide.

Skin grafts

Skin grafts are often used to repair or replace an area of damaged skin. Various thicknesses of skin graft (Fig. 2.5) can be used depending on the severity of the initial injury. A superficial (Thiersch) graft involves the epidermis and the immediately underlying dermis; a split-thickness graft includes one-quarter to one-third of the dermis; a full-thickness (Wolfe) graft takes the majority of the dermis with the epidermis.

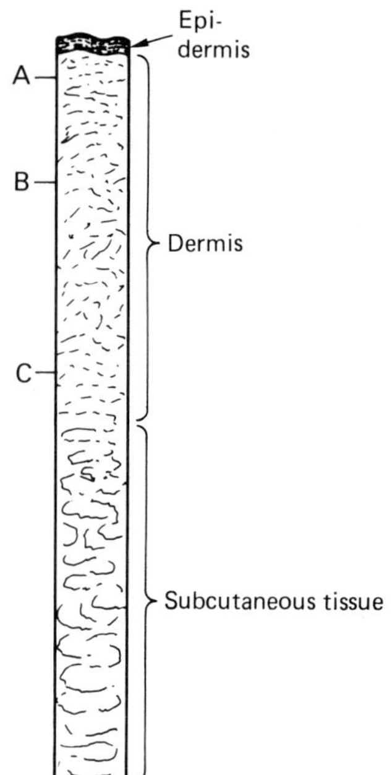

Fig. 2.5 Thicknesses of skin grafts. A = level of a superficial graft; B = level of a split-thickness graft; C = level of a full-thickness graft.

Muscle

Introduction

Muscle tissue is a specialized form of connective tissue having contractile properties, and as such enables movement of the many parts of the body with respect to one another, and of the body as a whole. Because of its contractile function the individual cells in muscle tissue are elongated in the direction of the axis of contraction. Consequently the cells are usually referred to as fibres.

There are three well-defined types of muscle as well as the myoepithelial cells of sweat and mammary glands. The main types are smooth muscle (also known as non-striated, involuntary or visceral muscle), cardiac muscle and skeletal muscle (also referred to as somatic, striated or voluntary muscle). The different types can be distinguished from each other on both a structural (Fig. 2.6) and a functional basis. Because muscle tissue performs mechanical work it requires a rich network of blood capillaries to provide nutrients and oxygen, as well as to eliminate the toxic waste products associated with contraction. The blood vessels, together with nerve fibres, are conveyed in fibroconnective tissue which also serves to bind the individual fibres together.

Smooth muscle typically forms the walls of hollow organs and blood vessels, as well as being present in the dermis. The cells are fusiform, elongated and closely associated with connective tissue. Each cell contains only a single nucleus which is centrally placed or slightly eccentric in position. Smooth muscle contracts relatively slowly and less powerfully than skeletal muscle, but is able to maintain its contraction longer. Its contraction is not under voluntary control since it is innervated by the autonomic nervous system. It does, however, have the ability to contract automatically, spontaneously and often rhythmically without the stimulus of a nervous impulse. Smooth muscle fibres are differentiated from splanchnic mesenchyme surrounding the endoderm of the primitive gut and its derivatives. That in the walls of many blood and lymphatic vessels arises from somatic mesoderm (Moore, 1988).

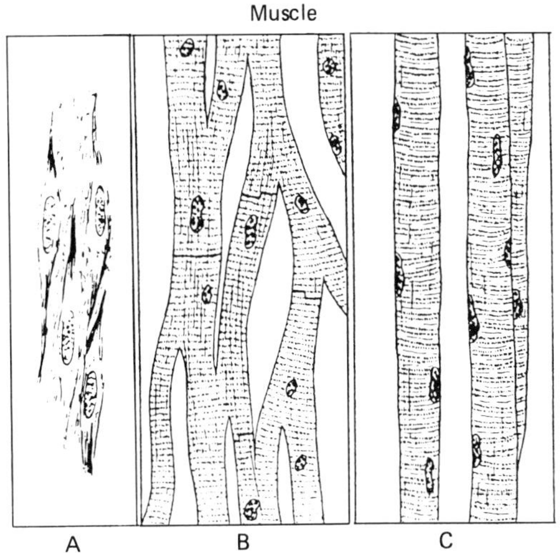

Fig. 2.6 Varieties of muscle. A = Smooth; B = cardiac; C = skeletal muscle.

In many of its structural features cardiac muscle is intermediate between smooth and skeletal muscle. It is found only in the myocardium and walls of the great vessels joining the heart. Cardiac muscle contracts automatically and rhythmically, i.e. it is myogenic; although not initiated by nervous impulses the rate of contraction can be modified by the autonomic nervous system. Cross-striations are visible in cardiac muscle; however, the structural arrangement of the fibres is different from that in skeletal muscle: the fibres branch and anastomose with other fibres. Muscle cells which make up an individual cardiac muscle fibre are joined end to end at specialized junctional zones known as intercalated discs. The nuclei are elongated and situated centrally in the fibre, usually between diverging myofibrils. Cardiac muscle develops from splanchnic mesenchyme surrounding the endocardial heart tube. Cardiac myoblasts are differentiated from the myoepicardial mantle and form the myocardium (Moore, 1988).

Skeletal muscle accounts for some 40% of total body mass in humans. It has various forms (flat, thick, long or short) and may attach directly to bone or be connected by an intermediate tendon. The length of a muscle, excluding its associated tendon, is closely related to the distance through which it is required to contract. The muscle fibres have been shown to have the ability to shorten to almost half (57%) of their relaxed length. An important aspect of movement produced by muscle action is that it is the result of muscle shortening, i.e. by contraction. The action is usually exerted across a joint pulling the two bones together.

Skeletal muscle

Skeletal muscle consists of many individual, unbranched muscle fibres, each of which is a long, cylindrical, multinucleated cell (Fig. 2.6), the ends of which taper to a point or are rounded or notched at the myotendon junction. Individual fibres may vary in length from a few millimetres to over 30 cm, and in diameter from 10 to 100 μ. However, in many muscles the fibres are shorter than the overall length of the muscle; one end is attached to tendon and the other to a connective tissue septum within the muscle. The many nuclei (approximately 35 per mm length) are ovoid, situated at the periphery and oriented lengthwise: no cell boundaries exist between the nuclei.

Structure

Skeletal muscle fibres show both a longitudinal striation and a characteristic transverse arrangement of light and dark bands. The sarcoplasm (cytoplasm of the fibre) is surrounded by the sarcolemma (cell membrane), which has the typical three-layered structure characteristic of boundary membranes.

The sarcoplasm is occupied mainly by longitudinal, parallel columns of myofibrils of about 1 μ diameter. The myofibrils extend the whole length of the muscle fibre. They are unbranched and vary in diameter from 1 to 3 μ. Each myofibril exhibits alternate discs or bands of light and dark material; the bands are in step with each other across myofibrils, thus producing the characteristic cross-striations (Fig. 2.7). The lighter bands are the I bands (isotropic), while the darker ones are the A bands (anisotropic). [The terms anisotropic (birefringent) and isotropic refer to the appearance of the myofibrils when seen with polarized light.] In the centre of the I band is a thin dark line known as the Z disc. A pale thin H band bisects the A band, and within this a very dark M stripe is present. The segment of the fibril that extends between two Z discs is the sarcomere. In relaxed muscle the major crossbandings (i.e. A and I) are distinct. However, in contracting muscle the fibrils are thicker and the sarcomeres shorter: the distance between Z discs becomes progressively smaller due to the shortening of the I bands. Consequently the A bands approach the Z disc so that eventually the I and A bands are indistinguishable: the length of the A band, however, remains constant.

The myofibrils consist of bundles of smaller units called myofilaments, which are of two kinds (thick and thin), each being of different chemical composition. Each myofibril contains upwards of 1000 myofilaments, of which some two-thirds are of the thin type. The thicker filaments, which consist of the protein myosin, are about 1.5 μ long and 10 nm in diameter. Each filament has short lateral projections arranged in six helical rows along its length. Each myosin filament, which lies in the A band (Fig. 2.8a), is formed by light and heavy meromyosin. The core of the myosin filament consists of light meromyosin, while heavy meromyosin forms the lateral projections.

The thinner filaments, which are composed of the protein actin, are about 1 μ in length and 5 nm in diameter: they constitute the I band (Fig. 2.8a). One end of each actin filament is attached to the Z disc while the other is free, interdigitating with the myosin filaments. The degree of overlap between the actin and myosin filaments varies with the state of contraction. Actin filaments consist of two longitudinal strands coiled around each other in the open helix, with each strand formed by globular subunits (G actin) lying end to end. Tropomyosin is a slender protein lying between the two actin strands, while troponin is found at regular intervals along the length of the filament. Alpha-actin, a third protein, is also associated with the actin filament and forms part of the Z disc complex.

In cross-section the actin and myosin filaments in the outer portion of the A band form a hexagonal pattern (Fig. 2.8b), with six actin filaments lying around each myosin filament.

Non-fibrillar areas occur in the sarcoplasm between the myofibrils and also close to the nuclei. They contain numerous large sarcosomes (mitochondria), which are concentrated near the poles of the nuclei and in parallel rows between the myofibrils. Small Golgi apparatuses are also found in a paranuclear position, together with ribosomes, a few lysosomes, numerous glycogen particles (concentrated between the myofibrils at the I band) and some lipid droplets (which tend to increase with age).

The sarcoplasmic reticulum is a continuous system of membrane-limited sarcotubules enclosing each myofibril. In the region of the A band the sarcotubules are arranged longitudinally with

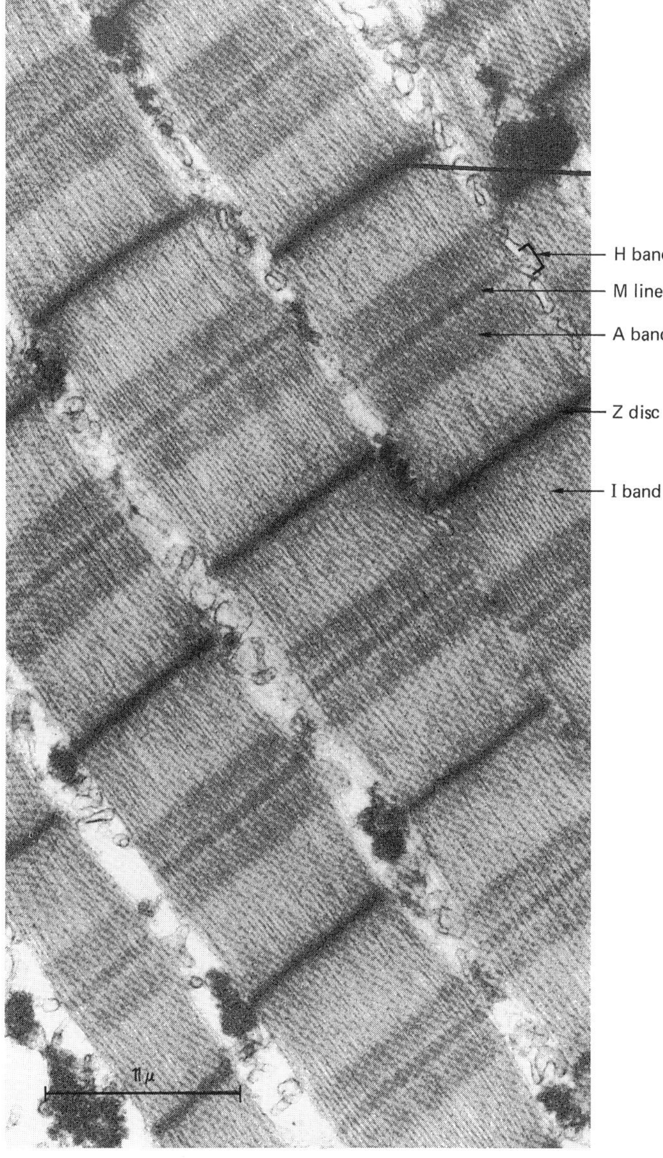

Fig. 2.7 Light microscopy appearance of skeletal muscle, the organization of the different bands and their relationship to the sarcomere.

many cross-connections near the H band. Close to the A–I junction the tubules from each side are connected to dilated transverse cisternae (terminal cisternae). The two terminal cisternae of a pair are separated by a small, central, transverse tubule (the T tubule) situated at the A–I junction. This arrangement is known as a triad, and there are two triads to each sarcomere. The T tubule is not part of the sarcoplasmic reticulum; it is an invagination from the surface sarcolemma. Its lumen is therefore continuous with the extracellular space and not with that of the reticulum. Collectively the T tubules are known as the T system.

Outside the sarcolemma of each muscle fibre is the delicate endomysium which serves to separate

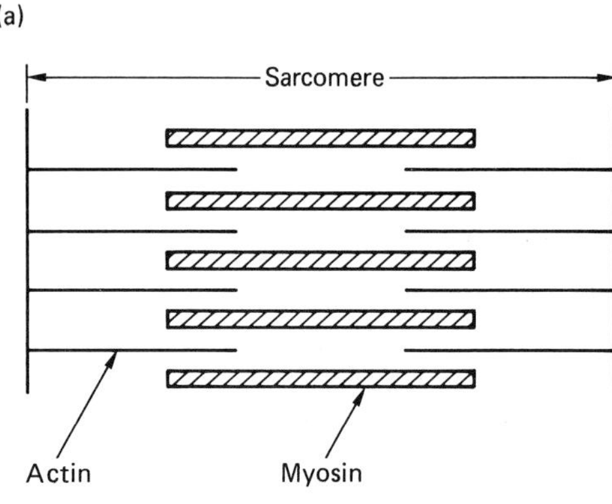

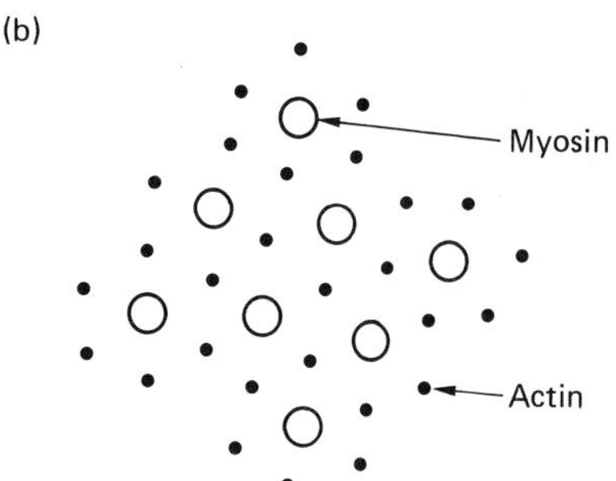

Fig. 2.8 Schematic representation of (a) the longitudinal arrangement of the actin and myosin filaments, and (b) transverse section through a myofibril.

each fibre from its neighbour yet connect them together. Individual fibres are arranged in parallel bundles (fasciculi) which are bound together by the denser perimysium. Fasciculi are enclosed within the fibrous epimysium (Fig. 2.9), which may be thick and strong or thin and almost transparent. It is through these connective tissue elements that skeletal muscle is able to produce traction on bones and hence movement. The collagenous bundles of the endomysium and perimysium pass directly over into those of the tendon, which in turn become continuous with those of the periosteum, penetrate the bone, or blend with the fibres of joint capsules or other connective tissue structures.

The total amount of fibroconnective tissue present varies between muscles; some have large amounts and others very little. However, the amount of connective tissue tends to increase with age. Fine slips of elastic tissue are also present between adjacent muscle fibres, with the amount again varying from muscle to muscle. Elastic tissue tends to be prominent in the extraocular and facial muscles.

Fibre types

Within skeletal muscle two different types of muscle fibre can be identified on the basis of their structural appearance and speed of contraction. Red muscle fibres contain a large amount of myoglobin and have a rich capillary network. They tend to be slender, have poorly defined myofibrils of varying diameter, numerous sarcosomes and contract more slowly than white fibres. The red fibres are designed for a relatively slow but repetitive contraction over long periods of time, as in postural muscles. White fibres are of larger diameter, have more myofibrils, a more extensive sarcoplasmic reticulum and fewer sarcosomes. They are present in greater numbers in muscles used for rapid contraction and, in contrast to red fibres, fatigue more easily. 'Fast' muscle can sustain more intense activity but only on an intermittent basis, since it derives the majority of its energy anaerobically. Both types of fibre are present within an individual muscle, as well as fibres intermediate between red and white.

Muscle fibres do not normally act individually but in groups (motor units) innervated by the branches of a single motor axon. All of the fibres of a single motor unit are of the same histochemical type, with different motor units distributed with overlapping territories. The motor units of slow muscle fibres tend to be innervated by motor neurons which have a low threshold for firing, whereas motor units of fast muscle fibres are innervated by motor units with higher thresholds. Consequently when movement is initiated the motor units tend to be recruited in a fixed order corresponding to the hierarchy of thresholds of the motor neurons. In this way the slow fibres receive continuous levels of activity (postural activity), while the fast fibres are involved in brief bursts of more intense activity (purposeful or protective movements). Experiments have suggested that it

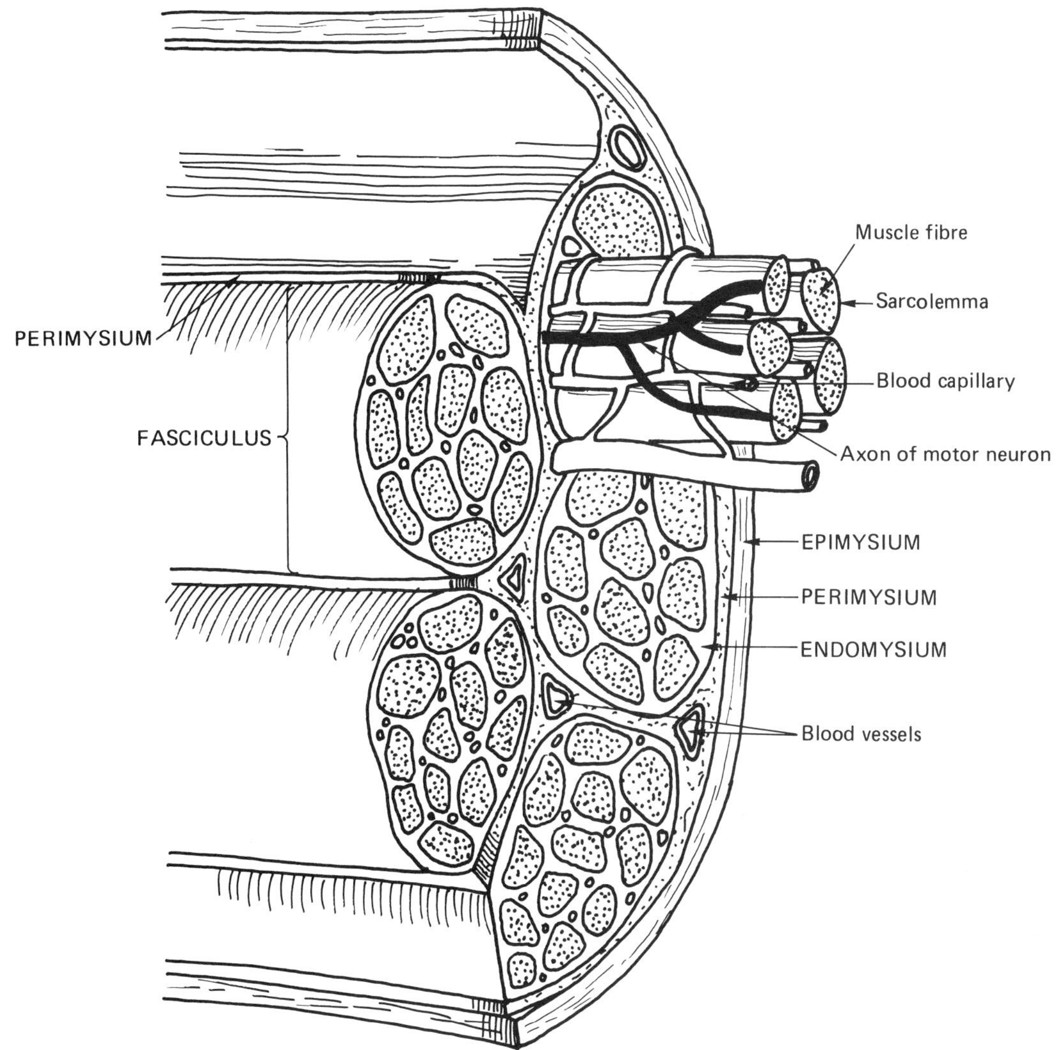

Fig. 2.9 The gross organization of muscle from bundles of fibres, together with the investing connective tissue layers.

is the impulse activity which brings about matching of the neural and muscular elements. Salmons (1980) has shown that under conditions of continuous electrical stimulation a 'fast' muscle gradually acquires all the physiological, biochemical, histochemical and ultrastructural properties of a 'slow' muscle, including a shift from a predominantly anaerobic to a predominantly aerobic metabolism. The evidence from such studies suggests that the process of fibre-type transformation occurs within individual muscle fibres without alteration to the motor unit organization, and that it is completely reversible.

Endurance training, although a less continuous stimulus, also evokes adaptations similar to the early stages of the response to electrical stimulation. Luthi *et al.* (1986), however, found no change in fibre-type distribution patterns of exercised muscles following 6 weeks of heavy-resistance exercise. Nor did they observe any significant change in capillary-to-fibre ratio or the capillary density.

Mechanical properties

The same motor command to a muscle, whether reflexly or voluntarily generated, can result in different forces being developed within it, depending on the state of the muscle. These differences are primarily due to the length of the muscle, its velocity of shortening or lengthening,

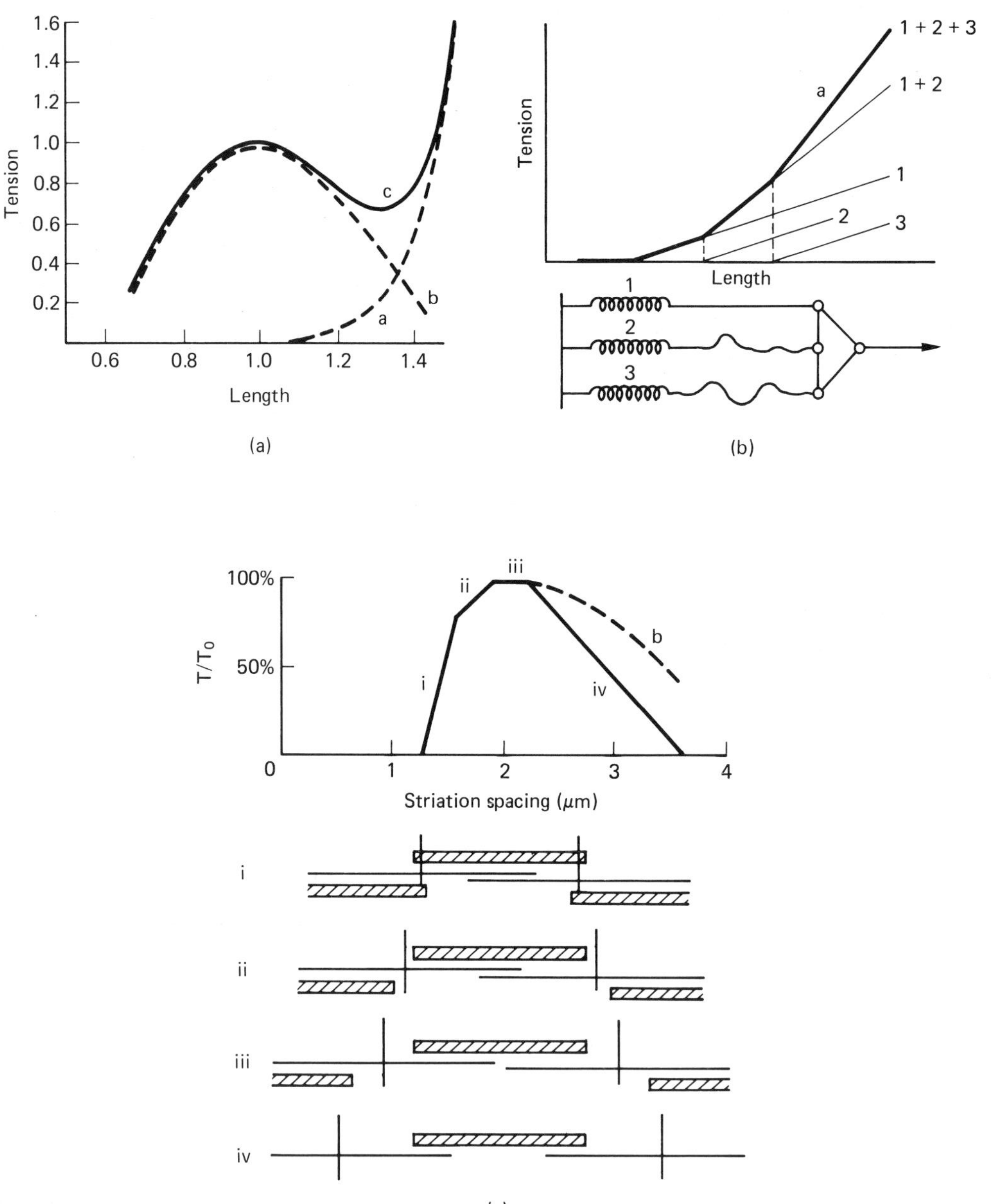

Fig. 2.10 (a) Characteristic length–tension diagram for skeletal muscle (1.0 = resting muscle length); (b) the contribution of the connective tissue elements (see text for details); (c) the length–tension diagram of a single sarcomere, also showing the relationship between the actin and myosin at each part of the curve. [Curve b in (a) is smoother due to the summation effects of many sarcomeres.]

its state of activation prior to receiving the stimulus, and to some degree its temperature.

The relationship between the length of the muscle and the tension it can develop is shown by curve c in Figure 2.10a: curve c is obtained by adding together curves a and b. Curve a represents the tension developed by the non-contractile elements of the muscle. Many of these elements lie parallel to the muscle fibres while others lie in series with them. Those lying parallel will have different 'slack' lengths such that as the muscle is progressively stretched the tension contributions of the individual elements are added together (Fig. 2.10b). (In Figure 2.10b the parallel components are represented by individual springs.) The series elastic elements modify the characteristics of the muscle by increasing its stiffness when the muscle is stretched (Lensel and Goubel, 1988). Curve b in Figure 2.10a represents the summated effects of the length–tension relationships of many individual sarcomeres; the tension at different parts of the curve is determined by the degree of overlap of the actin and myosin filaments (Fig. 2.10c).

The force–velocity relationship of skeletal muscle at its resting length is shown in Figure 2.11. For shortening, the curve resembles a rectangular hyperbola, while for lengthening the muscle is able to develop a force greater than isometric tension if it is forcibly extended at a moderate speed. Because the force–velocity curve will be modified by the length of the muscle, the contractility of a muscle is therefore a complex relationship between its length, the tension developed and the velocity of shortening or lengthening (Fig. 2.12), to which can be added the relatively small effects of its temperature.

Passive tension is important in embryonic and neonatal muscle development, where rapid changes in bone length place the attached muscle fibres under continuous tension (Stewart, 1972), resulting in increases in myofibril length and the addition of further myofibrils in series (Williams and Goldspink, 1971). In young animals passive muscle stretching and the resulting increase in muscle tension play a major role in stimulating muscle growth (Goldspink, 1977) by increased protein accumulation. Vandenburgh (1987) has shown that the changes observed *in vivo* also occur *in vitro*.

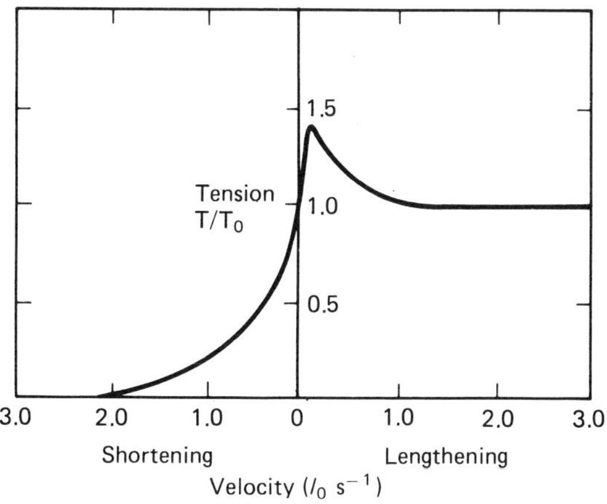

Fig. 2.11 Force–velocity curve for tetanized muscle. T_0 = tension developed at resting length; T = tension; l_0 = resting length.

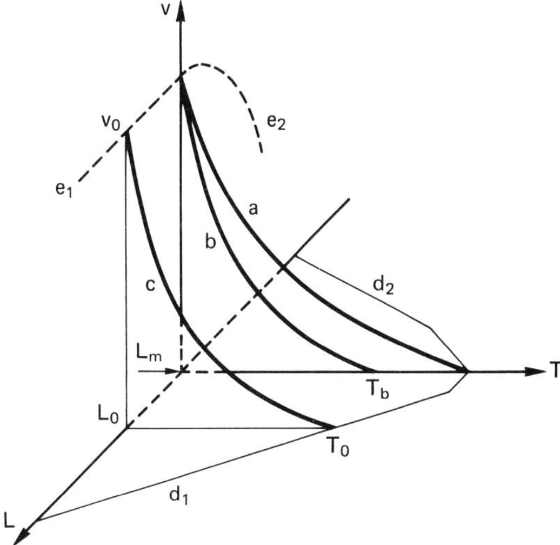

Fig. 2.12 The three-dimensional relationship of muscle contractility. L = muscle length; T = developed tension; v = velocity of shortening; a,b, and c represent three force–velocity curves at different tensions; d_1, d_2 = tension–length curve; e_1, e_2 = maximum velocity–length curve. Adapted from Mashima (1984).

The Tendon

Introduction

Tendon is a regularly arranged form of connective tissue, consisting principally of type I collagen together with some elastin and reticular fibres. It is in apparent continuity with muscle fibres, serving to attach the muscle to bone. Tendons generally serve to concentrate the pull of a muscle on to a small area. They enable muscles to act from a distance, e.g. the digitorum tendons of the fingers and toes, as well as to change the direction of pull and so increase the velocity ratio of the muscle at the expense of its leverage power. The length of a tendon is determined by the length of the fleshy fascicules of muscles fibres, which in turn are related to the range of movement required.

Tendon consists of bundles of collagen fibres arranged parallel to each other. The bundles are surrounded by a woven mesh of loose connective tissue, the endotenon, containing elastic fibres that tend to draw the bundle into a wavy formation (crimp) when relaxed. The whole tendon is surrounded by a sheath, the epitenon, around which is a loose, fatty areolar tissue, the paratenon. The paratenon allows the tendon to glide freely against the surrounding tissues. When the tendon passes over a structure that might harm it, e.g. bone, a synovial sheath or bursa is formed.

Tendons, and ligaments, are among the most static structures in the body with regard to their metabolism. Once collagen is mature its turnover is very slow. Because the growth rate of intercellular substances exceeds that of the cells, the number of cells per unit volume decreases rapidly after birth. The endo- and epitenon constitute approximately 25% of the tendon area in the newborn, but only some 12% in the adult. Tendon tissue from older individuals contains more collagen but the water content decreases independently of the functional state of the tissue.

The stimulus to the initial development of tendon is probably a tensile stress imposed by a muscle on undifferentiated mesenchyme, leading to a proliferation and axial orientation of fibroblasts and the deposition of parallel bundles of collagen fibres. Nevertheless, fibroblasts cultured in a Petri dish on an appropriate substrate have been shown to aggregate themselves in one direction. Such action is presumably in response to the chemical transmission of information initiated by autonomous cells.

Structure

Tendon

The only cell types present in tendon are fibroblasts, which are aligned in rows between the collagen fibres. Each fibre is composed of a large number of fibrils; individual collagen fibrils, consisting of intertwining molecules of tropocollagen, are suspended in a mucopolysaccharide gel.

The essential feature of all collagen molecules is their stiff, triple-stranded structure. Three collagen polypeptide chains (the alpha-chains) are wound around each other in a regular helix forming a rope-like collagen molecule about 300 nm long and 1.4 nm in diameter (Grodzinsky, 1983), which is conventionally referred to as tropocollagen. After being secreted into the extracellular space, type I (and for that matter, types II and III) collagen molecules assemble into ordered polymers known as collagen fibrils, which are long (up to many μm), thin (10–300 nm) strands. Isolated collagen fibrils show cross-striations every 67 nm, reflecting the arrangement of the individual collagen molecules within the fibril. These fibrils are grouped together into larger bundles several μm in diameter.

Special properties of the particular amino acid sequences in the collagen chains favour interchain hydrogen bonding. This greatly affects the structural rigidity of the resting molecule, enabling a stable helix to exist at 37°C. In addition special covalent bonds (unique to collagen and elastin) and crosslinks exist between the three chains (intramolecular crosslinks) and between the molecules of a fibril (intermolecular crosslinks). The high degree of crosslinking of collagen in tendon is presumably in response to the requirement for great tensile strength, and is therefore an important determinant of fibril function.

Bundles of fibrils lying between fibroblasts and often surrounded by their processes make up tendon fibres. These are grouped into secondary bundles (or fascicules), which are in turn combined into larger bundles. Within the fasciculi the individual fibres are interwoven with one another. Secondary and tertiary bundles are arranged in three-dimensional networks, probably as helices with cross-branching between loops (Proske and Morgan, 1987).

A tendon within a digital sheath is a unique collagenous tissue that differs in terms of its nutrient pathways and vascularity from tendons in other areas. The mixture of cellular and matrix components varies considerably along the length of such a tendon from the myotendinous junction to its bony insertion, particularly along long flexor or extensor tendons. The differences appear to correlate with nutritional and mechanical factors. Where such tendons bear large compressive forces on their concave surfaces areas of fibrocartilaginous metaplasia develop within the digital sheath (Okuda *et al.*, 1987). It has been observed that mesenchymal cells cultured under conditions of compressive stress and low oxygen concentration produce cartilage, while cells subjected *in vitro* to tensile stress and high oxygen concentration produce fibrous tissue (Bassett and Herrmann, 1961). A knowledge of this diversity may help explain differences observed in tendon healing, as well as provide an insight into the cellular mechanisms of matrix modulation in response to external mechanical and nutritional factors (Okuda *et al.*, 1987).

The myotendon junction

The myotendon junction is the region where the tendon attaches to the muscle. It is also the site where muscle fibres grow in length by the addition of sarcomeres. At this junction there is an intimate relationship between the muscle fibres and the collagen fibril bundles, although there is no direct continuation between them. The sarcolemma is intact at the myotendon junction, with the tendon bundles invaginated into the ends of muscle fibres in the many terminal indentations of the outer layer of the sarcolemma (Viidik, 1966). Consequently a considerable contact area between the muscle fibre and the collagen fibril is achieved.

In the mature myotendon junction densely packed sarcoplasmic organelles, including high concentrations of mitochondria, and satellite cells are present at the ends of the muscle fibres. The organelles are associated with the high level of metabolic activity at this site, while the functional significance of the satellite cells is uncertain (Ovalle, 1987). However, the presence of the latter suggests that the potential for maintenance, repair and remodelling is retained after normal growth has ceased and, subsequently, throughout life.

In neonatal and adolescent myotendon junctions leptomeric organelles are present in subsarcolemmal regions. They resemble the cross-striated structures seen at the myotendon junction in the fetus. Their presence at the ends of growing muscle fibres is consistent with them being involved in the formation of new myofibrils by the splitting of existing sarcomeres. It is possible that they also function as anchoring sites for myofibrils to the terminal sarcolemmal membrane (Ovalle, 1987).

Regardless of age fibroblasts at the myotendon junction show a regular spatial orientation with respect to the prevailing direction of the surrounding collagen fibres. At birth and during adolescence tendon fibroblasts are plentiful and their morphological features are consistent with high metabolic and secretory activity. Attachments between fibroblasts in growing myotendon may serve to anchor the cells together, forming a structural syncytium to counteract the repetitive changes in stretch and contraction that normally occur at this interface. Alternatively, groups of fibroblasts in rapidly growing tendon may need to be coupled, either metabolically or electrically, in order to synchronize their secretory activity.

Attachment of the tendon to bone

The collagen fibres of tendon pass directly into bone where they intermingle with the perforating fibres of Sharpey: thus they are firmly anchored.

However, because of the tensile strength of the collagen fibres it is not uncommon, under certain circumstances, for the bone tendon interface, or indeed the myotendon junction, to give way in preference to the tendon itself.

Blood and nerve supply

Tendons tend to be comparatively poorly supplied with blood vessels. Those that are present enter at both ends, from the muscle and from the periosteum at the site of its attachment to the bone. In long tendons, e.g. those of the fingers, an additional supply reaches them along their course via reflections from the lining of the tendon sheath, i.e. by the vinculae tendinae.

The sensory supply to tendons is relatively abundant, with nerve fibres terminating either as Golgi tendon organs or as Pacinian corpuscles. The Golgi tendon organs are found within the substance of the tendon itself close to the myotendon junction, while the Pacinian corpuscles are found in the tendon sheath. Both of these nerve endings provide an important mechanism whereby changes in tension in the tendon are conveyed to the central nervous system. Also surrounding tendons and their sheaths is a plexus of fine nerve fibres similar to those associated with the conduction of painful impulses. This latter plexus probably accounts for the sensitivity of tendons to painful stimuli such as prolonged pressure.

Properties

Tendon properties have to conform with what appears as conflicting requirements. A muscle attached to a very 'stretchy' tendon would delay the reaching of a required level of tension, because of the time taken to stretch the tendon. There are, however, advantages for the muscle in having a compliant tendon. If, for example, the muscle and tendon are shortening under conditions where the overall tension level was decreasing, a significant amount of shortening can be taken up by recoil of the previously stretched tendon (Proske and Morgan, 1987). Tendon recoil is also energy-efficient in that it allows recovery of much of the elastic energy stored during the stretch. A stiff tendon, however, will transmit most of an imposed load change to the muscle fibres, which will subsequently shorten more rapidly and be able to bear less load. On the other hand stiff tendons will transmit rapid tension changes and thus promote accurate movements.

An important role of tendon is that while many movements require active shortening of the muscle, others involve muscle lengthening (eccentric contraction). Eccentric contraction makes severe demands upon the muscle's tendinous attachments as the tension developed can be considerably greater than the maximum reached under isometric (constant-length) conditions.

It should be remembered that tendons lying in series with muscle fibres have to bear the same tension as the muscle; the stretch applied to a muscle is distributed between the muscle fibres and the tendon in proportion to their respective stiffnesses.

A force applied to a tendon elicits a non-linear response (Fig. 2.13). Initially a small load produces a relatively large extension (region 1), but as the load increases the tendon stiffens (region 2) until a linear relationship is attained (region 3), which continues until yield and subsequent rupture of the tendon occurs. The non-linear response of tendon is thought to be due partly to the presence of elastin producing the crimp in relaxed tissue, and partly to the inter- and intramolecular crosslinking within the collagen.

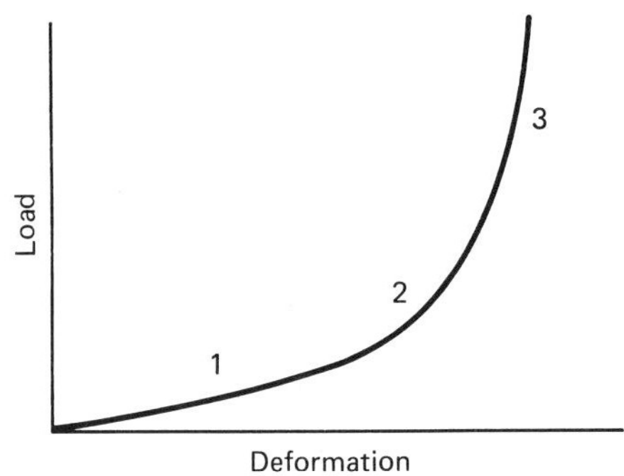

Fig. 2.13 Typical load–extension curve for tendon. 1 represents the 'toe' region; 2 is the limit of the non-linear curve; 3 is the region of linear elastic deformation.

When initially loaded these crosslinkings yield relatively easily and the elastin becomes stretched, straightening the crimp, thus accounting for region 1. In region 2 some fibrils still exhibit crimping while others have straightened. By the time region 3 has been reached all of the fibrils have been straightened. Provided that the yield point is not exceeded the crimp reappears when the load is removed. Both the structural basis of the crimp, and its reversible non-linear mechanical behaviour, and the relationship of molecular bonding to these properties is not fully understood.

If a tendon is loaded beyond region 3 in Fig. 2.13 such that its yield point is exceeded it will be permanently deformed. This is the plastic, as opposed to the elastic, region of the curve. It is in this region that individual fibrils fail, with increasing numbers failing as the load increases. Finally a point is reached when sufficient fibrils have failed that the tendon as a whole ruptures.

Quantitative characterizations of the behaviour of tendon up to the yield point and beyond is important in relation to the design of prostheses. In this context several criteria are commonly used: (1) the toe limit strain; this represents the transition from region 1 to region 3; (2) the modulus of elasticity (E), which is the gradient of region 3; (3) the stress and strain to yield; and (4) the stress and strain to rupture, that is the ultimate tensile stress and strain.

Under physiological loading conditions the yield point is not normally exceeded, so that when the load is removed the tendon returns to its resting state. This is not, however, a purely elastic response as hysteresis is observed between the loading and unloading curves (Fig. 2.14a) representing the storage and loss of energy during the loading cycle. When a tendon is subjected to repeated cyclical loads the hysteresis curve shifts to the right with each cycle (Fig. 2.14b), with a consequent apparent increase in the toe limit strain. This change between successive cycles decreases until a steady state is reached; the tendon is then said to be preconditioned.

Because tendon is a composite material consisting largely of the fibrous protein collagen, a small amount of mucopolysaccharide, mainly hyaluronic acid, and elastic tissue, the role of collagen is primarily mechanical and, like any other polymer, exhibits viscoelastic mechanical behaviour such as stress relaxation and creep. Stress relaxation occurs when a tendon stretched to any point in region 3 (see Fig. 2.13) is held at constant length, the force required to maintain this length decreases exponentially with time (Fig. 2.15a). On the other hand, if a constant force is applied to a tendon in region 3, over time it will progressively increase in length; this is the phenomenon of creep (Fig. 2.15b).

All tendons exhibit a non-linear response to applied load, hysteresis, preconditioning, stress relaxation and creep to a variable extent.

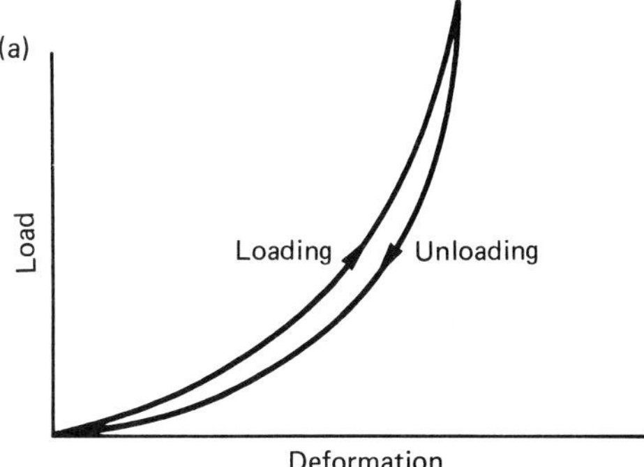

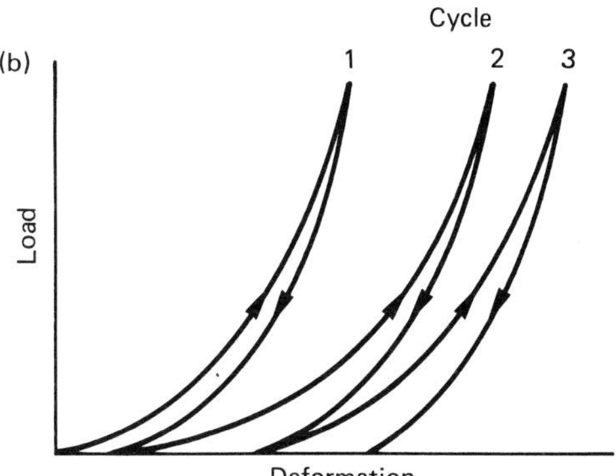

Fig. 2.14 (a) Complete cycle of loading and unloading showing a small degree of hysteresis. (b) Repeated cyclical loading within the linear elastic portion of the load–extension curve showing a gradual movement of the hysteresis curve to the right. Eventually a steady state is reached when the tendon is said to be preconditioned.

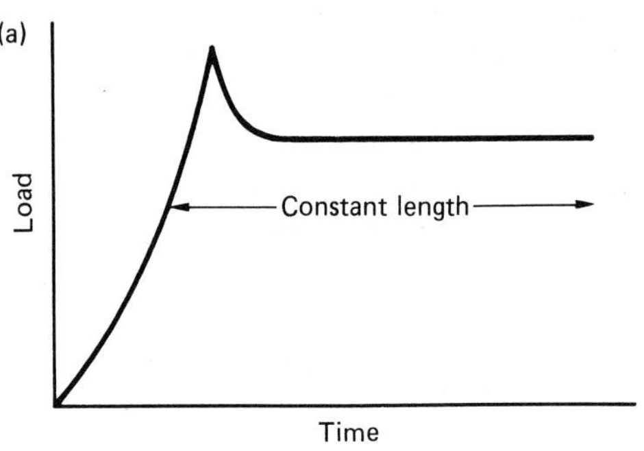

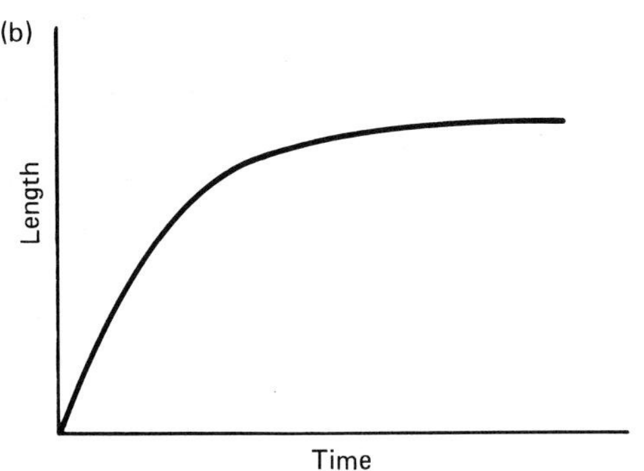

Fig. 2.15 (a) Stress–relaxation curve showing that a reduced load is required to maintain a constant deformation over time. (b) Creep – a constant load produces an increasing deformation.

Tendon healing

The physical, mechanical and chemical properties of collagenous tissue are an inherent part of its structural organization. In wound healing architectural changes in the collagen matrix occur as a result of the intricate process of remodelling.

Approximately 5 days after the beginning of wound healing the connective tissues begin to increase both their collagen content and tensile strength (Goldin *et al.*, 1980). Histological studies have shown that the collagen content of a healing tendon is constant after 5 weeks; collagen synthesis is at a maximum at 4 weeks and is still elevated at 12 weeks (Birdsell *et al.*, 1966). Presumably these rates reflect collagen turnover secondary to remodelling. Collagen remodelling and maturation have been observed up to 1 year after wounding (Greenlee and Pike, 1971). Two weeks after wounding the repair tissue is highly cellular and distinct from the surrounding areolar tissue. The extracellular matrix is noticeable for its wavy pattern, numerous blood vessels and very fine fibres. At 3 weeks cellularity and vascularity have decreased and collagen fibres are clearly visible: actively mobilizing pump cells are present between the collagen fascicles at the severed stumps of the tendon. By the fourth week both the cellularity and vascularity of the tissue have further decreased; the collagen fibres are longer, wider and show a better longitudinal alignment along the cell axis. At no period during this repair phase is there evidence of cartilage or bone metaplasia (Steiner, 1982).

The phase of fibroplasia appears to be initiated between the second and third week of healing. During this period the extracellular matrix progresses from a reticulin filigree to a distinct collagenous structure. This fundamental change improves all biomechanical parameters except elongation. In the 3–4 week period the strength, elongation and energy-absorbing capacity of the tendon increase, suggesting that function at lower loads is relatively constant once a rudimentary fibrous structure has been established. By the end of the fourth week the healing tendon has recovered 70% of its normal stiffness and 40% of its rupture strength. This relative return of stiffness before strength has also been demonstrated for skin and ligament wounds following immobilization (Zingg, 1975; Noyes, 1977).

During the wound-healing process increased numbers of intermolecular covalent bonds develop between the amino acid polymer chains, giving a stronger anatomical configuration and consequently a change in the mechanical and chemical properties of the collagen fibres. An increase in the amount of crosslinking in collagen fibres is consistent with maturation, leading to increases in tensile strength. Tensile strength has been evaluated as a function of suture method, with the breaking strengths of tendons sutured end-to-end reaching a nadir at the end of the first week of healing. Their strengths double after a further 2–3 weeks of healing, and then double again after a further 4–12 weeks.

Cyclic loading of a damped tendon has been demonstrated to improve significantly the visco-elastic parameters of the tendon after 8 weeks of healing, while significantly improved strength and stiffness are seen after 24 weeks of healing (Hirsch, 1974).

Ligaments

Introduction

An important role of ligaments is the provision of stability at joints, while enabling free movement to occur. This is usually achieved by having the ligament pass obliquely across the joint. In addition the ligament itself may exhibit some degree of spiralling as it passes between its two bony attachments. In this way distruction or dislocation of the joint during its normal range of movement is minimized.

As with tendons, ligaments have a complex internal arrangement which allows for their diverse tensile functions at a wide range of sites. They transmit longitudinal, rotatory and shear stresses, as a consequence of which no single prosthetic ligament can simulate the mechanical characteristics of all ligaments which may require replacement. Not only is there variation in the requirements and properties of different ligaments, both between and within individuals, but the response of a specific ligament is influenced by the individual's age and habitual level of activity.

Structure

The basic structure of ligaments is essentially similar to that of tendons; the only cell-type present being fibroblasts arranged in rows between the collagen fibres (for further details the reader is referred to Chapter 6). Like tendon, 65–70% of the total weight of ligament consists of water. Similarly, 75–80% of the fat-free dry weight is collagen, up to 5% may be elastin in ligament, whereas this is usually only of the order of 3% in tendon. Proteoglycans account for between 1 and 3% of the fat-free dry weight in ligament; the precise amount depends on the site and function of the ligament: for example, the cruciate ligaments contain 2.5–3%, while the collaterals of the knee contain only 1–1.5%.

When a joint is immobilized so that the ligament is relieved of tensile stresses, even in the absence of wound healing resulting from injury or surgical manipulation, it undergoes active contraction (Wilson and Dahners, 1988). Histological studies do not reveal an increased cellularity in contracted ligaments; however there is heavy staining for the contractile protein actin. It is thought that ligament fibroblasts, which have become modified to a form containing increased quantities of actin, play an important active role in the contraction of ligamentous tissue.

At the site of attachment of ligament to bone there is a change in composition of the surrounding medium as the collagen fibres of the ligament (zone 1) pass through fibrocartilage (zone 2), mineralized fibrocartilage (zone 3) and into bone (zone 4).

Blood and nerve supply

Histological studies have shown that the individual fasciculi which make up the ligament are separated from each other by spaces that contain loose connective tissue and tortuous blood vessels supplying the tissues.

Nerve fibres are present in all regions of ligament. The majority are paravascular in position, although some ramify among the connective tissue elements. It has been shown that human cruciate ligaments contain a fusiform mechanoreceptor, axons within the substance of the ligament, and a mechanoreceptor resembling a Golgi tendon organ (Schultz *et al.*, 1984). Although much of the work on innervation has been conducted using the cruciate ligaments, it is highly probable that all ligaments will have a similar pattern of innervation. The concentration of mechanoreceptors appears to be greatest in areas related to the extremes of movement and probably represents the first line of defence in sensing that these extremes are being reached. These afferent discharges are reinforced by those from mechanoreceptors within the joint capsule and also from those in the surrounding muscles. The total afferent output serves to alert the central nervous system of impending injury, which can then be averted through reflex activity (Zimny, 1988).

Growth

Longitudinal growth occurs throughout the length of a ligament, there being no specific region responsible for its enlargement (Muller and Dahners, 1988). The magnitude of ligament growth is proportional to the rate of growth of its associated joint. The rapid changes seen near the attachment sites are for the purposes of moving the ligament insertion with respect to the metaphysis, so as to adjust for bone growth and thus maintain stability at the joint.

Properties

The mechanical behaviour of ligaments depends not only on the material properties of the fibres themselves, but also on the geometrical arrangement of the collagen fibre bundles, the proportions of the different types of fibrous constituents and the relatively unknown effect of the surrounding ground substance. The ligament insertion site and the underlying bone are additional parts of the ligament unit which have to be considered when evaluating ligament strength.

Forces applied to ligament elicit non-linear responses, with a small load producing a relatively large extension. However, as the load increases, the ligament stiffens until little or no further extension is possible (Fig. 2.16). As with tendon, the non-linear response is thought to be due partly to the presence of elastin, which gives the crimp seen in relaxed tissue. Ligaments with a large elastin content will show a more pronounced toe region in Figure 2.16. The more linear portion of the load–deformation curve probably corresponds to the condition where the fibres are fully oriented and under tension. Because of the complex arrangement of ligaments along their length it is also probable that the straightening of the collagen bundles, e.g. unspiralling of the ligament between its bony attachments, will modify the load–deformation curve. Nevertheless, an excessively loaded ligament will tend to rupture.

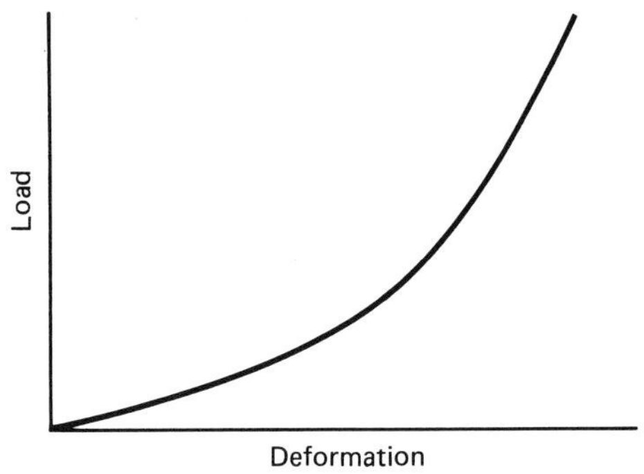

Fig. 2.16 Typical load–deformation curve for ligament.

Being a composite material, ligaments exhibit viscoelastic mechanical behaviour in the same way that tendon does (see Fig. 2.15).

Failure

Under excessive tensile loading conditions, ligaments tend to fail in one of three ways. The first is ligament failure in which the collagen fibres are pulled apart. This tends to occur throughout the body of the ligament and is not restricted to one specific area. It appears that the geometric arrangement of the fibre bundles determines the region of greatest stress, deformation and initial damage, leading to the serial rupture of other fibres (Noyes *et al.*, 1974). This pull-apart type of fracture suggests that there is little cohesion between the major fibre bundles. The second mode of failure is an avulsion fracture, most commonly seen through the cancellous bone immediately beneath the denser cortical bone at the site of ligament attachment. The third, and least common, mode of failure involves cleavage of the ligament–bone interface. Cleavage has been observed throughout the four zones of ligament attachment; there is no prediliction for failure to occur through zone 3 (mineralized fibrocartilage).

Immobilization is often required in the treatment of musculoskeletal trauma. It is generally recognized that immobility can lead to significant changes in bone, joint and soft tissues (see earlier for contraction changes in ligament). Reconditioning exercises following a period of immobilization greatly improve the mechanical behaviour of the ligament, such that there is an almost complete return to normal values.

Failure of ligament after a period of immobilization usually involves one or more of the following: minor or major avulsion fractures at the insertion site; ligamentous failure (the most common); a pulling apart of the fibre bundles, followed by a shear fracture between the fibre bundles; and, rarely, fracture at the bone–ligament interface.

Immobility leads to a weakening of the functional ligament unit, with only partial recovery after 20 weeks of resumed activity. The decrease in strength of this unit can be explained in part by the resorption of haversian bone and the resultant weakening of the cortex beneath the insertion site. Because most ligaments insert into bone via well-defined zones of fibrocartilage, ultimate failure of the ligament unit tends to occur through the underlying cortical bone at the insertion site, through the body of the ligament, or by both modes. This protective effect of the fibrocartilage probably also applies to tendons which have a similar type of attachment. In addition to these mechanical effects the zones impose a barrier to the vascular supply of the ligament from the underlying bone.

The mechanisms by which immobility leads to a decrease in ligament stiffness are unknown. However, a reduction of almost 40% in the concentration of hyaluronic acid and of 32% in the concentration of chondroitin-4 and chondroitin-6 sulphate in the periarticular tissues in animal studies has been observed following 9 weeks' immobilization (Partington and Wood, 1963; Woesner, 1968). This suggests that the surrounding matrix and its interaction with collagen are important in maintaining the strength and integrity of connective tissues. Other mechanisms implicated in changing the properties of connective tissue include: changes in the synthesis and degradation equilibrium of collagen (Peacock, 1963); changes in collagen crosslinks at both the inter- and intramolecular levels (Peacock, 1963); alterations in the water and electrolyte content of the connective tissue itself; and changes in the arrangement, number and thickness of the collagen fibres (Elliott, 1965).

References

Bassett CAL, Herrmann I (1961) Influence of oxygen concentration and mechanical factors on differentiation of connective tissue in vitro. *Nature* **190**, 460–1.

Birdsell DC, Tunstanoff ER, Lindsay WK (1966) Collagen production in regenerating tendon. *Scandinavian Journal of Plastic and Reconstructive Surgery* **23**, 504–11.

Elliott DH (1965) Structure and function of mammalian tendon. *Biological Reviews* **40**, 392–421.

Goldin B, Block WD, Pearson JR (1980) Wound healing in tendons. I. Physical mechanical and metabolic changes. *Journal of Biomechanics* **13**, 241–56.

Goldspink DF (1977) The influence of immobilization and stretch on protein turnover of rat skeletal muscle. *Journal of Physiology* **264**, 267–82.

Greenlee RK, Pike D (1971) Studies of tendon healing in rat. *Scandinavian Journal of Plastic and Reconstructive Surgery* **48**, 260–70.

Grodzinsky AJ (1983) Electromechanical and physicochemical properties of connective tissue. *CRC Critical Reviews in Biomedical Engineering* **9**, 133–99.

Hirsch G (1974) Tensile properties during tendon healing. *Acta Orthopaedica Scandinavica*, suppl. 153.

Lensel G, Goubel F (1988) Series elasticity in contracted muscle during stretching. In: *Biomechanics XIA*. Amsterdam: Free University Press, pp 26–30.

Luthi JM, Howald H, Claasen H, Rosler K, Vock P, Hoppeler H (1986) Structural changes in skeletal muscle tissue with heavy-resistance exercise. *International Journal of Sports Medicine* **7**, 123–7.

Mashima H (1984) Force–velocity relation and contractility in striated muscles. *Japanese Journal of Physiology* **34**, 1–17.

Moore KL (1988) *The Developing Human: Clinically Oriented Embryology* 4th edn. Philadelphia: WB Saunders.

Muller P, Dahners LE (1988) A study of ligamentous growth. *Clinical Orthopaedics and Related Research* **229**, 274–7.

Noyes FR, Delucas JL, Torvik DJ (1974) Biomechanics of anterior cruciate ligament failure: an analysis of strain rate and sensitivity and mechanics of failure in primates. *Journal of Bone and Joint Surgery* **56A**, 236–53.

Noyes FR (1977) Functional properties of knee ligaments and alterations reduced by immobilization. *Clinical Orthopaedics and Related Research* **123**, 210–42.

Okuda Y, Gorski JP, An K-N, Amadio PC (1987) Biochemical, histological, and biomechanical analyses of canine tendon. *Journal of Orthopaedic Research* **5**, 60–8.

Ovalle WK (1987) The human muscle–tendon junction. A morphological study during normal growth and at maturity. *Anatomy and Embryology* **176**, 281–94.

Partington FR, Wood GC (1963) The role of non-collagen components in the mechanical behaviour of tendon fibres. *Biochemica Biophysica Acta* **69**, 485–95.

Peacock EE (1963) Comparison of collagenous tissue surrounding normal and immobilised joints. *Surgical Forum* **14**, 440–1.

Proske U, Morgan DL (1987) Tendon stiffness: methods of measurement and significance for the control of movement. A review. *Journal of Biomechanics* **20**, 75–82.

Salmons S (1980) Functional adaptations in skeletal muscle. *Trends in Neuroscience* **3**, 134–7.

Schultz RA, Miller DC, Kerr CS, Micheli L (1984) Mechanoreceptors in human cruciate ligaments. *Journal of Bone and Joint Surgery* **66A**, 1072–6.

Steiner M (1982) Biomechanics of tendon healing. *Journal of Biomechanics* **15**, 951–8.

Stewart DM (1972) The role of tension in muscle growth. In: Goss RJ (ed) *Regulation of Organ and Tissue Growth*. New York: Academic Press, pp 77–100.

Vandenburgh HH (1987) Motion into mass: how does tension stimulate muscle growth? *Medicine and Science in Sports and Exercise* **19**, S142–9.

Viidik A (1966) Biomechanics and functional adaption of tendons and joint ligaments. In Evans F (ed) *Bone and Joints*. Chicago: CC Thomas, pp 17–39.

Williams PE, Goldspink G (1971) Longitudinal growth of striated muscle fibers. *Journal of Cell Science* **9**, 751–67.

Wilson CJ, Dahners LE (1988) An examination of the mechanism of ligament contracture. *Clinical Orthopaedics and Related Research* **227**, 286–91.

Woesner JF (1968) Biological mechanisms of collagen resorption. In: Gould BS (ed) *Treatise on Collagen* vol 2, Part B Biology of Collagen. New York: Academic Press, pp 253–330.

Zimny ML (1988) Mechanoreceptors in articular tissues. *American Journal of Anatomy* **182**, 16–32.

Zingg W (1975) Bioengineering analysis of healing tissue. *Journal of Sports Medicine* **3**, 61–70.

3

Skin injuries and wound healing

A. K. Ray
D. S. Soutar

Principles

A fundamental requisite for the survival of a living organism must be its ability to repair the site of traumatic disruption of its tissues, especially a breach in its protective integument.

In the more primitive orders of organisms this mechanism of repair is often by a process of rapid regeneration. In the more evolved species of living creatures such as humans, the full regenerative abilities of the integument appear to be limited to the cells of the epidermis and the lining cells of the respiratory, alimentary and genitourinary tracts.

The process of healing of a skin wound in mammals is a combination of epidermal regeneration and wound contraction (Fig. 3.1). Epidermal continuity is re-established initially by a process of sliding out of the cells at the periphery of the wound, accompanied by brisk cell regeneration. The damaged dermal and deeper elements of the wound are replaced by scar tissue, which is initially laid down in a random and disorganized fashion in order to bridge the wound gap but has poor breaking strength. This is reorganized over a period of several months to produce a stronger mature scar with considerably greater breaking strength (Fig. 3.2).

Epidermal regeneration, wound contraction and the production and final maturation of scar tissue are ill-understood processes and the topic of considerable scientific debate. Local production of hormone-like substances which regulate the healing process have been implicated but none have been convincingly demonstrated. Hypertrophic scarring and the formation of keloids (see later in this chapter) are of special interest as they appear to represent a form of failure of a local regulatory mechanism.

However certain general and local factors which influence wound healing are well established (Table 3.1).

Table 3.1 Factors affecting wound healing

General factors
Age
Race
Nutrition
Disease
Iatrogenic
Local factors
Site
Orientation
Type of trauma
Blood supply
Sepsis

General factors

Age

Healing is a rapid and vigorous process in children and the incidence of hypertrophic scarring is

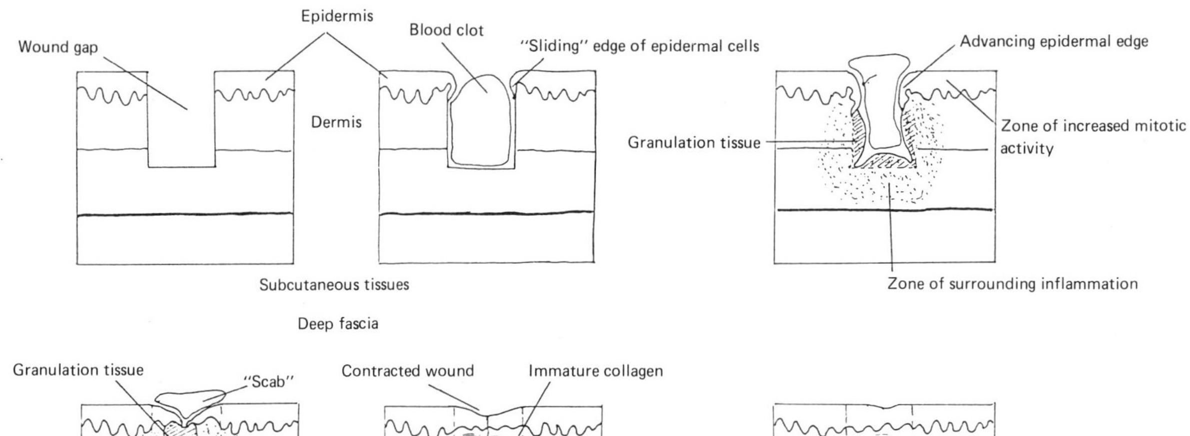

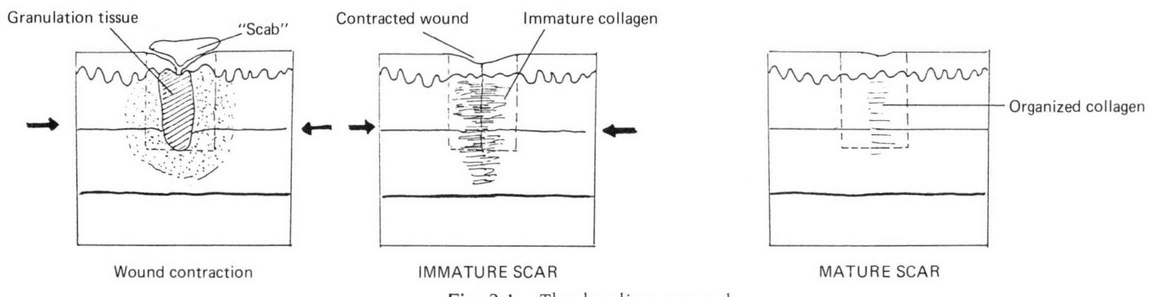

Fig. 3.1 The healing wound.

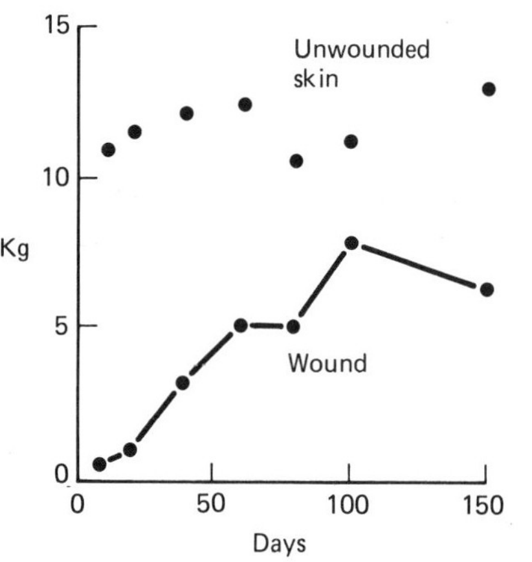

Fig. 3.2 Wound strength. Graph showing the mean tensile strength of sutured skin incision from 10 to 150 days compared with the strength of unwounded skin. (Redrawn from Sundell, 1979.)

certainly higher than in the elderly who often heal slowly but with remarkably little visible scars. Considerable interest has been aroused in the field of fetal surgery where the primitive ability to repair wounds almost completely by local regeneration of tissues results in healing with virtually no replacement by scar.

Race

The predilection for hypertrophic scarring and especially the formation of keloids in people of Afro-Carribean origin can pose a serious problem even with minimal trauma such as a pierced ear lobule.

Nutrition

Wound healing is impaired in protein deficiency states, though considerable hypoproteinaemia and a loss of more than 10% of the body weight has to occur before this is manifest. Rapid protein depletion and severe catabolic states following extensive injuries such as burns may result in impaired wound healing. In chronic malnutrition, malignant cachexia or protein depletion from large decubitus ulcers, wound dehiscence is a well-known risk.

Several vitamin deficiency states are known to affect wound healing adversely. Ascorbic acid plays an essential role in collagen synthesis and poorer wound healing in scorbutic patients has been noted following surgery.

Depletion of vitamin A appears to interfere with epithelial integrity and results in unstable epithelial lining, manifest readily as ulceration of the delicate epithelial lining of the cornea. Thiamine and riboflavine have also been implicated in wound healing.

Trace metals such as zinc also play a vital role in collagen synthesis and the administration of zinc in burns patients with zinc depletion appears to promote wound healing. The topical application of zinc or the boosting of normal zinc levels does not appear to have any beneficial effect. Abnormal wound healing has also been recorded in copper and magnesium deficiency states.

Disease

Wound healing is adversely affected in the presence of a variety of diseases, the most prominent of which are diabetes mellitus, jaundice, uraemia and advanced malignancy. In conditions such as diabetes mellitus and Cushing's disease, multiple factors may be responsible for the impairment of wound healing.

Iatrogenic

Administration of drugs or agents which interfere with collagen maturation and cell multiplication affects healing. Steriods, cytotoxic drugs, immunosuppression, or radiation therapy and their adverse effects on the healing of wounds are well-documented in clinical practice.

Local factors

Local factors which influence the quality of wound healing are often most amenable to manipulation by the surgeon and contribute to the fundamental principles of wound surgery.

Site

Certain sites especially overlying the sternum, shoulder and on the chin have a propensity for forming hypertrophic scars or keloids.

Orientation

The final appearance of a scar resulting from a healed wound is dependent on the orientation of the wound relative to the lines of tension in the region where it lies. In the face, these lines are dictated by the attachment of the underlying muscles of facial animation. At other sites, the orientation of the collagen fibres closely parallels the lines of tension. A linear wound produced at an angle or perpendicular to the lines of tension will tend to stretch, resulting in a cosmetically unacceptable scar. (Fig. 3.3 and 3.4).

Blood supply

The repair of wounds is an active metabolic process which utilizes energy. Wound healing is faster and results in a mature, stable scar much earlier in tissues which are well-perfused, such as the face, when compared to regions such as the pretibial skin. The delivery of oxygen and other nutrients and the removal of metabolic waste products are also impaired in the presence of non-viable tissues, foreign bodies, infection or peripheral vascular disease.

Sepsis

Sepsis remains the single most important cause for poor wound healing. The multiplication of Gram-positive, Gram-negative and/or anaerobic organisms at the site of injury results in a virtual arrest of the healing process as a result of the production of local toxins, and tissue damage. The inflammatory response mounted at the site of injury is diverted to the control of the local sepsis by the production of a temporary granulation tissue barrier and the activity of the inflammatory exudate. The form-

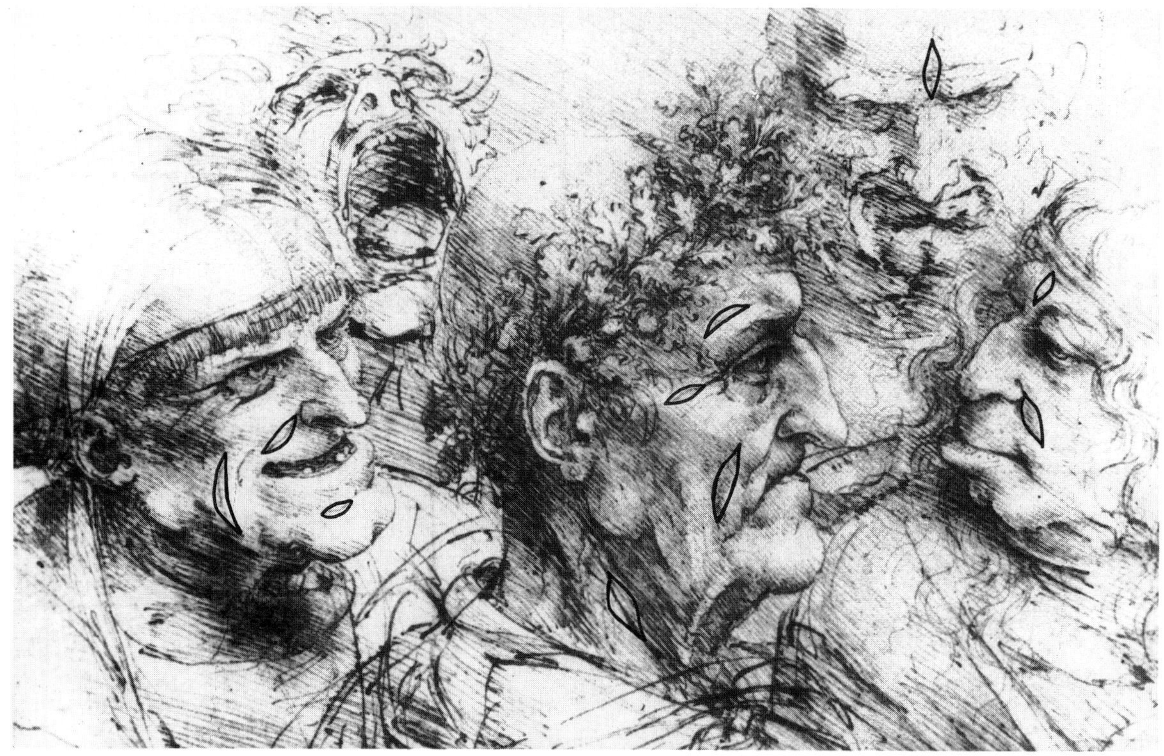

Fig. 3.3 Lines of election of the face. From Devane (1988), with permission.

ation of scar tissue is grossly altered under these circumstances, resulting in an initial failure of deposition and organization of collagen, followed by an overproduction and delayed maturation of scar tissues, resulting in hypertrophic scars or keloids.

The nature of injury

The mechanisms of tissue injury may be:

1. Mechanical.
2. Thermal.
   (a) Hot.
   (b) Cold.
3. Chemical.
4. Electrical.
5. Radiation.

These forces which produce injury may result in the following variable effects depending on the nature and intensity of the injuring force and the site to which it is applied.

Ecchymoses

Minimal to moderate blunt trauma may produce the disruption of small blood vessels at the site of injury resulting in localized ecchymoses or bruising with no breach of the epithelium.

Haematoma

Rupture of larger blood vessels or the presence of a bleeding diathesis may result in a large collection of blood in the subcutaneous tissues producing a haematoma, the size of which will be governed by the vascularity of the tissues, the size of vessels affected and the laxity of the tissues.

Ecchymoses and small haematomata require no treatment but larger haematomata may warrant

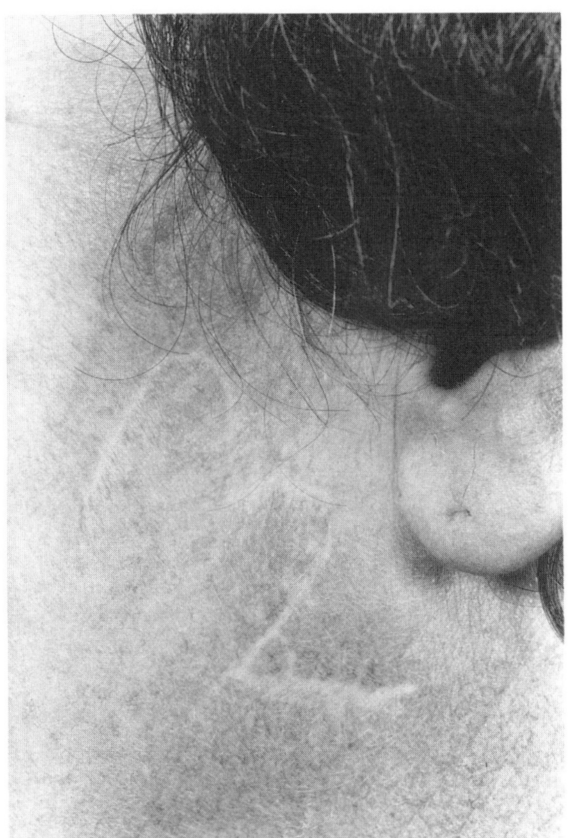

Fig. 3.4 Bilobed flap on the face. Note the minimum stretching of the scar in areas parallel to the lines of election and the unacceptable stretching of scar in the area transversing these lines.

surgical evacuation. Occasionally such surgical intervention may require to be performed urgently if the perfusion of tissues is at risk. Notable examples of such situations are retrobulbar haemorrhages, scrotal haematomata, haematoceles and degloving injuries.

Blisters

Blisters are produced by a cleavage at the dermal epidermal interface resulting in a space which rapidly fills and distends with fluid. This may be produced by chronic repetitive trauma as with ill-fitting shoes, thermal or chemical injury resulting in superficial or partial-thickness burns, or in certain disease states (e.g epidermolysis bullosa) and adverse drug reactions. Small blisters do not warrant any active treatment and will resolve spontaneously if the cause is appropriately treated.

Larger areas of blistering are best treated by careful deroofing of the blisters and the application of a sterile emollient dressing or a mild topical antiseptic. The basis for such intervention is that in extensive injuries the blisters are uncomfortable, are unlikely to persist without rupture and are prone to colonization of the blister fluid by the resident flora. It is therefore preferable to drain the blisters and eliminate all dead skin under controlled aseptic conditions to obtain optimum healing.

Abrasions

Abrasions of skin are produced by subjecting the surface to a tangential injury by an abrasive surface resulting in multiple partial-thickness lacerations. In its simplest form of a 'graze', abraded skin appears as a red somewhat raw surface which may be very painful. Such an injury will heal spontaneously by rapid re-epithelialization from all remaining dermal and epidermal elements.

Abrasions may however be complicated by ingrained tattooing of the skin produced by embedded particles of the abrasive surface or dirt. This ingrained material, if left in the wound, may be covered over by granulation tissue and subsequently epithelium, resulting in a scarred surface with obviously visible and irregular tattoo marks. The embedded material also represents an extensive contamination load with a potential for gross wound infection and delayed healing, and the formation of hypertrophic scar.

Such wounds must be treated aggressively as early as possible after injury and the surface vigorously scrubbed with a stiff nail brush and some foaming antiseptic preparation such as Hibiscrub to eliminate as much as possible of the embedded dirt. Any material which is deeper must then be thoroughly and individually debrided. If sufficient dermal elements remain after such a procedure – as is usually the case – the wound should be dressed with an emollient or a topical antiseptic and spontaneous healing will occur with surprisingly little final scar.

Abrasions may also be noted as an associated finding in more complicated cutaneous injuries produced by tangential forces due to rapidly spinning objects such as industrial rollers. These may produce extensive and full-thickness friction burns due to the rapid generation of heat at the contact surfaces. Such injuries however will not heal spontaneously as the underlying cutaneous elements are not perfused or viable. They may be recognized quite easily by their pale or light brown stained appearance and the lack of bleeding, pain or sensory perception.

Degloving injuries

Tangential forces which impart a sudden and severe shearing force to skin may produce extensive rupture of the blood vessels in the subcutaneous fat and fascia as they cross this region from relatively fixed points in the deep fascia to the dermis. Such an injury, which may or may not be associated with overlying abrasions, may result in effective devascularization of the skin with no obvious breach in the skin (Fig. 3.5). In both deep burns and degloving injuries, the affected skin is not viable and will require excision and resurfacing by one of the techniques described later in this chapter.

Lacerations

A force of sufficient intensity, if produced by a blunt object, may result in a 'fracture' of the skin, especially if it overlies a bony structure. Lacerations of skin produced by blunt trauma tend to be irregular with marked contusion of the skin edges and attenuation of the collagen, producing a soft pulpy feel with a lack of firm elastic recoil. The dissipation of the injuring force also produces a considerably greater amount of deeper tissue damage than is immediately apparent. Such wounds often require radical debridement (Fig. 3.6).

Penetrating injuries

Sharp objects tend to produce linear lacerations with very localized tissue damage (Fig. 3.7). It is often difficult however to determine the depth or the extent of the deeper tissue injury from the overlying laceration, especially in oblique penetration, and surprisingly small lacerations may be associated with extensive deeper tissue damage. In all lacerations therefore it is certainly rewarding to have a high index of suspicion.

A careful clinical history is invaluable in estimating the likely amount of underlying damage.

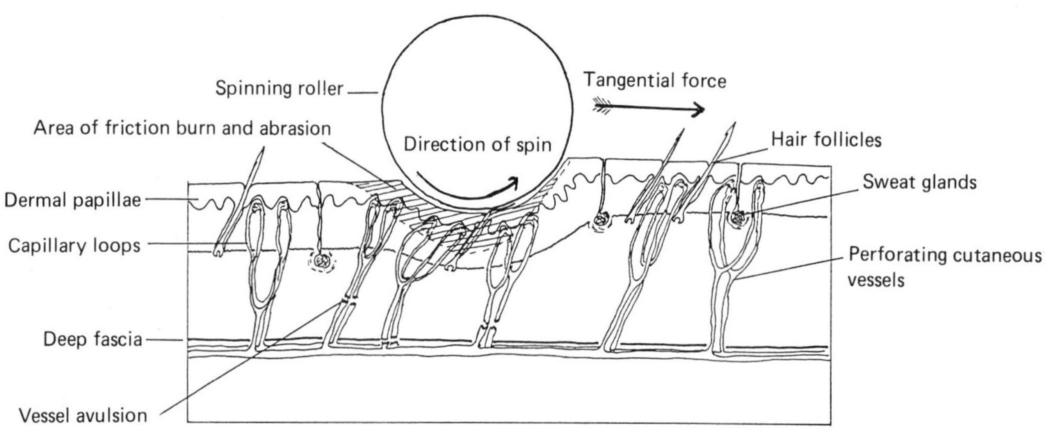

Fig. 3.5 Degloving injury.

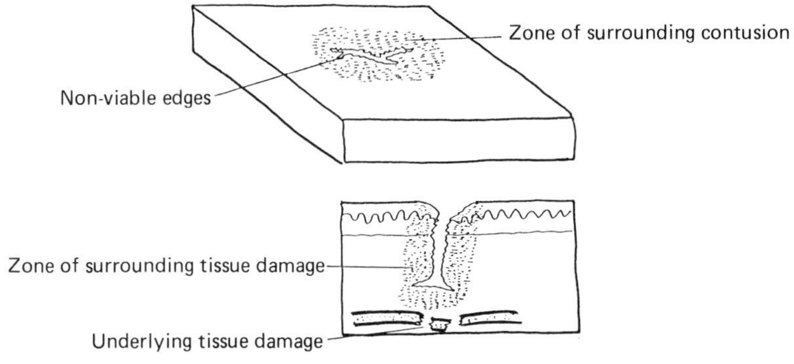

Fig. 3.6 Blunt penetrating injury.

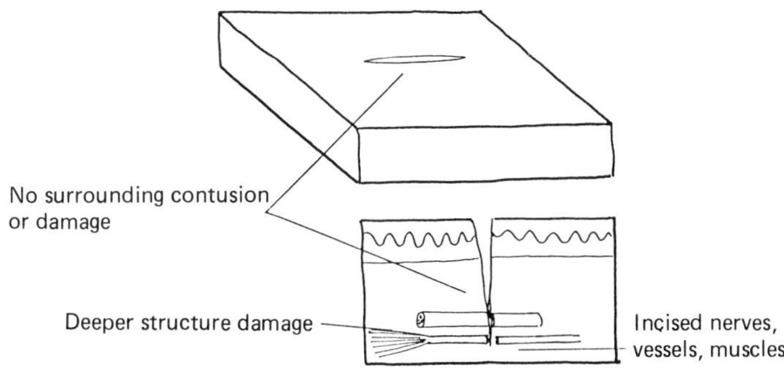

Fig. 3.7 Sharp penetrating injury.

In the course of the physical examination of all such injuries, a knowledge of anatomy is crucial to identify the structures adjacent to the injury which may have been damaged in order to apply the relevant clinical tests to examine their function (e.g. nerve, tendon, joints etc.). The possibility of retained foreign bodies such as shards of glass or pieces of metal must be considered and radiological examination used to exclude their presence. Where there is definitive evidence of deeper structure injury, exploration and repair are mandatory. In cases where the clinical history and the physical findings do not tally or the results of any tests are equivocal, formal exploration of the wound should be performed. This is especially relevant in injuries produced by glass.

Formal wound exploration should ideally be performed in a well-lit operating theatre with appropriate anaesthetic facilities to ensure adequate exposure and facilitate the meticulous examination of the injured tissues.

Burns

Thermal, chemical and electrical or radiation injury produces coagulation of proteins and cell death, commonly expressed as burn injury.

The severity of the injury is related to:

1. *The site of injury*: Burns of the eyelids, though small in area, are potentially serious. Circumferential burns of digits or limbs can result in peripheral ischaemia.
2. *The depth of the burn*: Deep burns may result in damage to vital structures such as blood vessels or nerves.
3. *The type of burn*: Chemical injury (e.g. with caustic soda) may continue for a considerable period of time after contact has ceased.

Electrical burn injury may be associated with extensive systemic tissue damage and the area of burn injury is often greater than is immediately apparent. The entry and exit points for the electric current are the areas of maximum injury and must be identified. A patient presenting with hand burns may have associated and unrecognized deep burns of the feet through which the injuring current may have exited to the earth.

4. *The area of burn*: This may be expressed as a percentage of the total body surface area.

The management of burn injuries is complex but is crucial and may be defined as follows:

At the site

1. Isolate the patient from any further contact with the burning agent.
2. Douse all flames or smouldering clothing and in the case of chemical agents, wash liberally to remove any residual contact with the skin. It is generally recommended that neutralizing agents such as alkalis for acid contact are not used since the neutralizing reactions are often exothermic and may produce further damage.
3. Observe all first-aid manoeuvres to ensure an adequate airway, breathing and circulation.
4. Administer an analgesic if available early. Absorption of intramuscular or subcutaneously injected drugs is erratic once shock has set in.
5. If the area of burn is more than 5% in a child or 10% in an adult, an attempt should be made to start a secure peripheral infusion as soon as possible, to maintain fluid replacement during transfer.

Shock phase

The patient should then be transferred to the nearest hospital equipped to deal with such emergencies.

The management of the fluid and metabolic disturbances produced by an extensive burn injury is a complicated and highly specialized subject and should be dealt with only in a designated unit with an appropriate burns team with rapid access to all major specialties.

The mortality and morbidity of patients with burn injury are significant, especially in the very young and the very old. Survival and the decision to practise triage in situations where the predicted mortality is extremely high is only possible with considerable experience in the field.

The post-shock phase

The capacity for spontaneous healing of a burn of the skin is largely dependent on the depth of the burn and consequently the quantity of remaining cutaneous appendages. Burns may be conveniently classified as follows (Fig, 3.8):

1. Superficial.
2. Partial-thickness.
   (a) Superficial.
   (b) Deep (deep dermal).
3. Full-thickness.

Superficial burns such as sunburn or light scalds will heal rapidly because the underlying dermis is intact. Superficial partial-thickness burns will also heal from the remaining dermis within 5 – 6 days.

Deep partial-thickness burns or deep dermal burns heal slowly by epithelial outgrowth from the remaining cutaneous appendages such as hair follicles, sweat glands and sebaceous glands and any remaining dermal papillae. The management of these burns is controversial as they tend to heal with considerable hypertrophic scarring and are difficult to distinguish from full-thickness burns.

Full-thickness burns leave no residual cutaneous appendage or skin alive and will heal only by separation of the eschar and wound contraction if left untreated.

The management may therefore be outlined as follows:

1. *Conservative*: If the burn is likely to heal spontaneously within a few days, the wounds should be cleaned and all blisters deroofed. The burn areas should then be dressed with non-adherent dressings. Appropriate topical agents such as nitrofurazone (Furacin) or silver sulphadiazine (Flamazine) may be used. *Note*: Flamazine should not be used on the face as the silver salts are capable of producing an intense chemical conjunctivitis.
2. *Surgical excision and skin cover*: If the burn is full-thickness in nature or does not show promising signs of healing with conservative management of about a week, surgical debridement

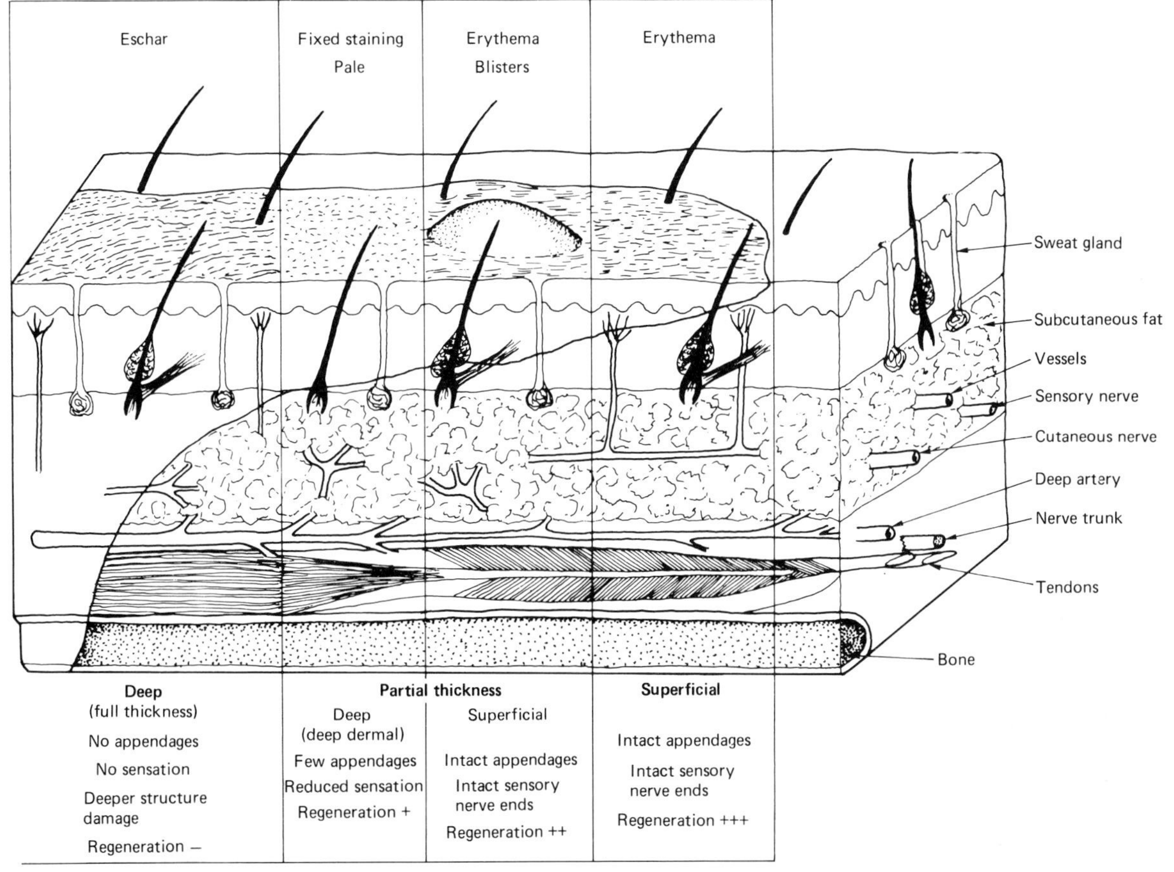

Fig. 3.8 Depth of burn injury.

should be undertaken and the defect skin grafted (see below).

Rehabilitation and secondary management

The overall management of burn injury must include, in the early stages, physiotherapy to encourage full mobilization, nutritional support, psychiatric and psychological evaluation and social support and rehabilitation.

Extensive or severe burns will require multiple operations for secondary cosmetic and functional deformities. Occupational therapeutic help may be necessary to encourage the patient to resume a normal life.

Skin infections

Exogenous

Exogenous invasion of the skin by pathogenic organisms results in infection. The skin is a potent barrier to infection and is able in most instances to resist penetration. The surface of the skin and the depths of the cutaneous appendages such as the sweat and sebaceous glands are normally inhabited by commensal organisms such as *Staphylococcus albus*.

In situations where the continuity of the integument is breached, a localized colonization by organisms such as streptococcus or staphylococcus may occur. In conditions where the patient's immunity may be compromised, this infection may rapidly spread and become generalized, if not treated in time.

Endogenous

Wound infection following trauma or surgery is also commonly recognized to occur from the patient's own respiratory tract and nasal passages and may be proven by typing of the offending organism. Endogenous infection by pathogenic strains of *Staphylococcus aureus* following surgery is a common manifestation of this route.

Systemic diseases

Cutaneous eruptions may also be a manifestation of systemic disease e.g. septicaemia, varicella. Secondary infection of such eruptions should be avoided as far as possible and treated appropriately with dressings and suitable antibiotics if indicated.

The management of cutaneous infection is at three levels – prevention, early recognition and treatment.

Prevention

Isolation – for communicable diseases. Strict codes of practice for barrier nursing must be applied in specialized units designed for this purpose to contain the infection.

Aseptic technique – Bacterial colonization of wounds and the transfer of nosocomial infective agents can be minimized by employing careful aseptic techniques in the peri- and postoperative phase.

Immunization – Resistance to several infective agents can be significantly enhanced by the use of the appropriate immunizations, e.g. tetanus toxoid, measles vaccine, hepatitis B serum.

Passive immunization may be employed in situations where host defences are compromised or the patient is at risk, e.g. antitetanus globulin, anti-gas gangrene serum, immunoglobulin.

Early recognition

A high index of suspicion and awareness of the predilection for specific infections at certain sites or clinical situations are crucial. The risk of gas gangrene in crushed and devitalized tissues or fulminating infections after human bites (see below) are examples.

It is often possible to identify the infecting organism by its clinical behaviour, e.g. streptococcus – rapidly spreading cellulitis with lymphangitis and toxaemia; staphylococcus – folliculitis, abscesses, impetigo; *Pseudomonas* – greenish pus with extensive necrosis (Table 3.2).

Table 3.2 The progression of cutaneous infection

Early inflammation
Erythema
Increased temperature
Pain
Cellulitis
Increasing erythema
Persistent local hyperthermia
Pain
Induration and oedema
Subcutaneous gangrene or abscess formation
Generalized infection
Septicaemia
Toxaemia
Pyaemia
Metastatic abscesses
Osteomyelitis
Death

Treatment

Identification – Microbiological culture and antibiotic sensitivity patterns of the infecting organism should be carried out. Identification of the particular strain or type of the organism is useful in the study of nosocomial infections, to locate the source.

Appropriate antibiotic therapy.

Surgery – If warranted, surgery should be carried

out for the drainage of abscesses, excision of necrotic tissue and mechanical toiletting of a wound to reduce the bacterial load.

Wound management

The primary objective of all skin wound healing is to achieve a rapid re-establishment of continuity in the integument.

Until the breach in the external defences has been sealed, the repair of exposed structures in the deeper tissues such as tendons, nerves, bones and blood vessels will not proceed. Hence skin cover following injury is of primary importance and must be achieved, sometimes at the expense of delayed repair of other damaged structures.

Principles of wound management

1. Early assessment and treatment.
2. Debridement.
3. Haemostasis.
4. Meticulous repair.

Early assessment and treatment

Wounds should be assessed and treated as early as possible to minimize bacterial contamination, inflammation and oedema. The timing of wound repair was an important consideration in the pre-antibiotic era and formed the basis of:

Primary repair – within 6–12 hours.
Delayed primary repair – within 4–6 days.
Secondary repair – 2–3 weeks.

Rigid adherence to such a time schedule is no longer considered necessary and the protocol for management is based more on the nature of the injury.

Debridement

All non-viable or doubtfully viable tissues should be excised as far as possible till healthy, well-perfused tissues are reached. In situations where extensive areas of doubtful viability exist, there may be a need to cover the wound with sterile dressings and reassess the tissues in 24–48 hours, by which time the demarcation between non-viable and viable tissues should be evident. Rarely, in the hands of the inexperienced, a third or fourth-look operation may be necessary. The dictum for debridement is thoroughness and if any doubt about the viability of tissues exists, no attempt should be made to close the wound.

All potential sources of contamination should be eliminated as far as possible and the wound must be explored for buried foreign materials and debris. The efficiency of pulsed saline irrigation has been well-established in cleaning most surface contamination. Deep-seated and more extensive debris will require thorough debridement. To this end, the surgeon should lose no opportunity to extend a smaller wound to permit a detailed exploration wherever indicated.

Haemostasis

Adequate haemostasis must be achieved before attempting wound closure to prevent the formation of a haematoma, which is a potent nidus for bacterial contamination and is also locally disruptive by mechanically separating the wound edges and tissue planes and interfering with tissue perfusion due to pressure.

The adoption of these three principles should result in a surgically clean, healthy and viable wound. In some instances, due to delayed presentation, extensive contamination or infection and tissue damage or oedema, attempting wound closure may not be a feasible proposition. It may be necessary to await spontaneous separation of necrotic tissues and resolution of the cellulitis before attempting repair as a secondary procedure.

Meticulous repair

Skin cover may be achieved surgically by one of three means:

1. Direct closure.
2. Skin graft.
   (a) Split-thickness.
   (b) Full-thickness.
   (c) Pinch.
3. Flap cover.

Direct closure

This is the method of choice in wounds with no skin loss or minimal skin loss where the edges of the wound can be apposed with minimal tension. It is obviously easier to obtain closure if the surrounding skin is lax as in elderly people or in sites such as the abdominal wall, breasts, neck or genitalia. The skin over the mastoid or the scalp, by comparison, may be very difficult to approximate.

Great care should be exercised however in attempting direct closure of wounds in areas where the mobility of adjacent structures can create the illusion of skin laxity. This is applicable in the vicinity of the eyelids, the mouth or the

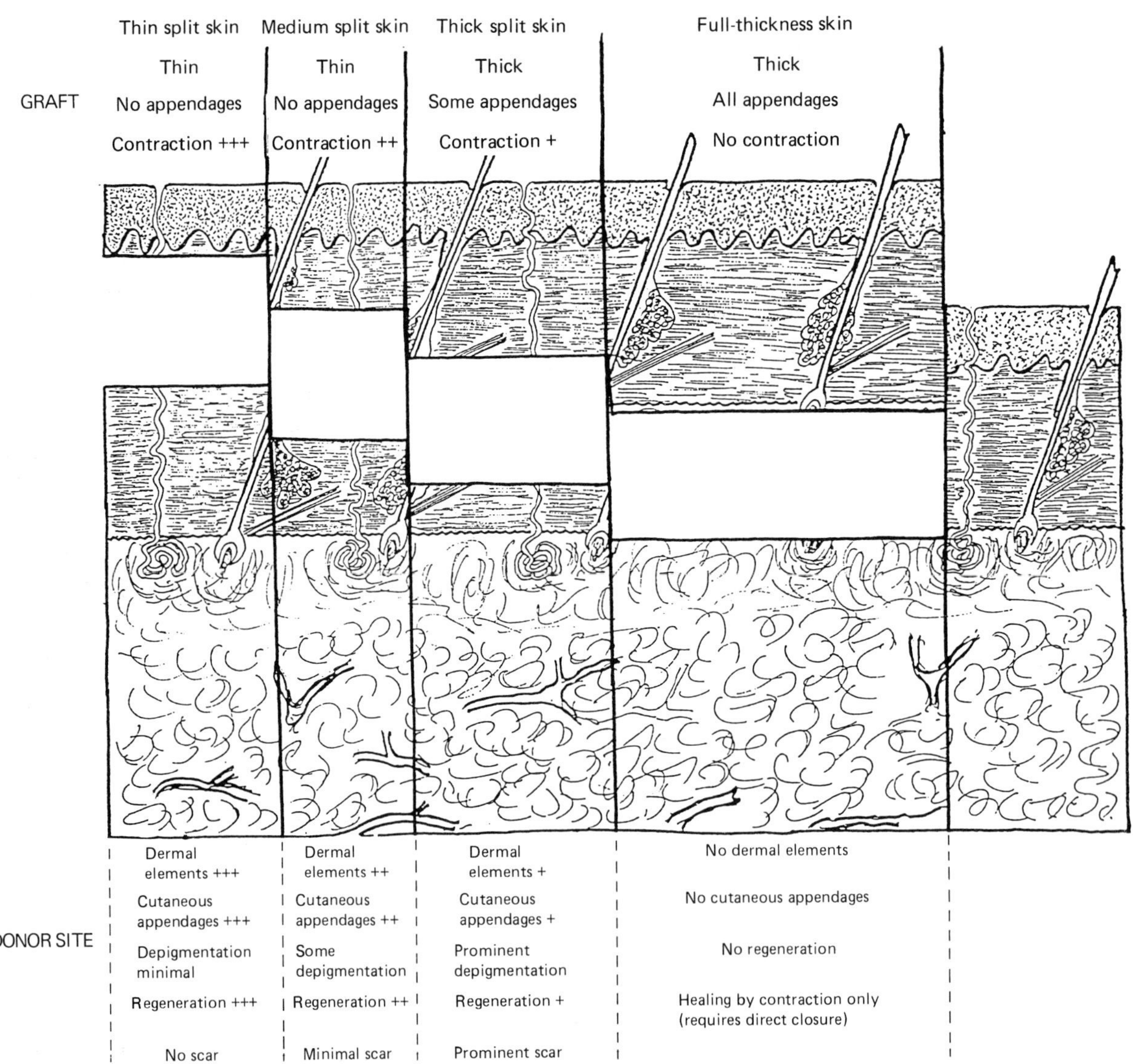

Fig. 3.9 Different types of skin grafts.

Table 3.3 Advantages and disadvantages of various types of skin graft

Type of graft	Donor site		Recipient site		Uses
	Advantages	Disadvantages	Advantages	Disadvantages	Uses
Thin split-thickness graft	Minimal cosmetic deformity Rapid re-epithelialization Repeated harvesting from the same donor site at 2–3-week intervals	Painful Difficult to harvest without experience	Higher 'take' rate Easy to apply Large thin sheets	Cosmetic appearance is often unsatisfactory Graft contains no dermal appendages Prone to shrinkage Pigmentation unpredictable Graft often unstable	Extensive areas of skin loss or for temporary skin cover Inadvisable for the face
Thick split-thickness graft	Easier to harvest	Prolonged healing time Hypertrophic scarring Mature scars are visible Hypopigmentation	Better cosmesis Less prone to contracture More supple and more stable	Reduced 'take' rate May contain unwanted hair follicles Difficult to resurface large areas	Resurfacing of areas where contracture is undesirable, e.g. joints, hands
Full-thickness graft	Harvested from flexural creases and inconspicuous sites Defect closed as a linear scar	Limited number of appropriate donor sites Size of graft may be small Graft behaviour is identical to donor site skin	Good-quality skin with all dermal appendages and hair follicles Pliable, soft and stable Not prone to contracture	Only possible to resurface small areas 'Take' may be precarious compared to split-skin grafts Application must be meticulous Unwanted hair	For cosmesis, e.g. face Avoidance of contractures, e.g. joints, digits Transfer of hair-bearing skin, e.g. eyebrow reconstruction
Pinch grafts	Easy to harvest	Unacceptable cosmetic deformity if visible Scars may be concealed by hair	Useful for transferring hair follicles	Unsightly patchy appearance, irregular pigmentation, scarring and uneven texture	Only used for transfer of hair follicles on the scalp for treatment of alopecia

flexor surfaces of joints. Direct closure of wounds with skin loss or subsequent scar contracture will result in marked tethering, retraction, ectropion or flexion contractures in joints.

The elastic recoil of the collagen in the dermis can convey the false impression of skin loss, especially with V or C-shaped lacerations. Careful apposition and matching of the wound edges will reveal that direct closure is possible with no tension.

Skin grafts

Skin grafts are a simple solution in situations where skin loss cannot be rectified by direct closure.

Skin grafts however are only suitable in those circumstances where the bed or surface which requires to be covered is adequately vascularized. As the graft derives its nutritional and vascular support from the underlying bed, it will fail to survive in the presence of relatively avascular surfaces such as bare bone devoid of periosteum, bare tendon devoid of paratenon or exposed ligaments and joints, or in the presence of dead tissue, exposed foreign bodies or any sepsis.

A split-thickness skin graft is a shaving of skin taken from a suitable donor site at a depth which will allow rapid re-epithelialization of the donor surface from the dermal elements and cutaneous appendages left behind (Fig. 3.9). The properties of the various types of grafts are summarized in Table 3.3.

Flap cover

Flaps of skin and soft tissues are distinct from grafts in that their viability is maintained by their own independent blood supply and therefore they are not to any great extent dependent on the vascularity of the wound bed (Fig. 3.10).

They are therefore suitable for use in almost all instances where skin grafts are precluded and also in instances when it may be desirable to transfer a vascular zone into an area of poor vascularity, such as the pretibial area.

In regions such as the face, local flaps have a special role in situations where direct wound closure may not be possible, by mobilizing adjacent tissues with a good colour and surface texture match from a suitable donor site, which may be successfully concealed in a natural skin crease or anatomical area, into the wound defect (Fig. 3.11).

A local skin flap can be transposed to alter the axis of tension of wound closure in order to minimize the resultant cosmetic deformity or traction on adjacent structures.

The commonest application of this principle is the Z-plasty where the axis of the wound can be altered to fit a natural skin crease (Fig. 3.12).

Sutures and suturing techniques
(Figs 3.13 and 3.14)

The purpose of all sutures or other approximating devices such as staples or steristrips is to bring wound edges into apposition to facilitate the bridging of the wound gap by regenerating epidermis and scar tissue while conferring some mechanical resistance to separation of the wound by any distracting forces.

A delicate balance however has to be achieved as each suture effectively increases the foreign material load in the wound, which potentially

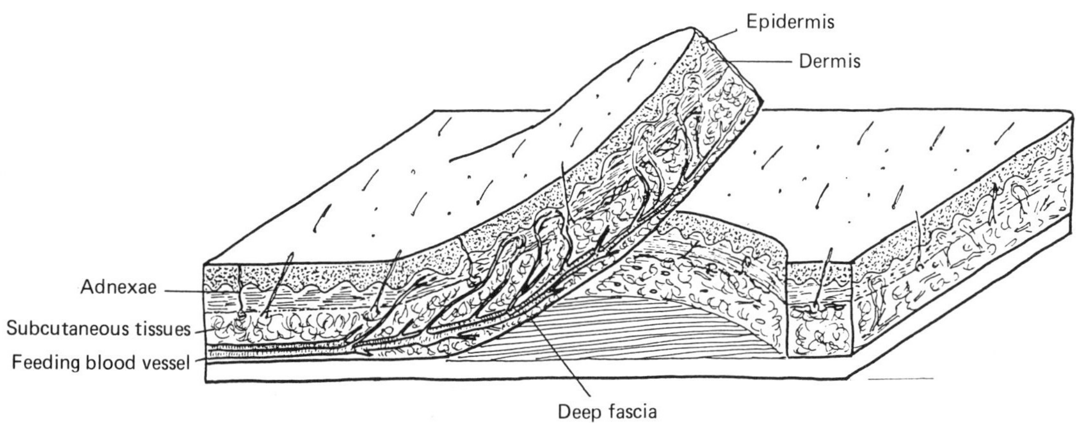

Fig. 3.10 Skin flap showing an independent vascular pedicle which maintains its nutrition.

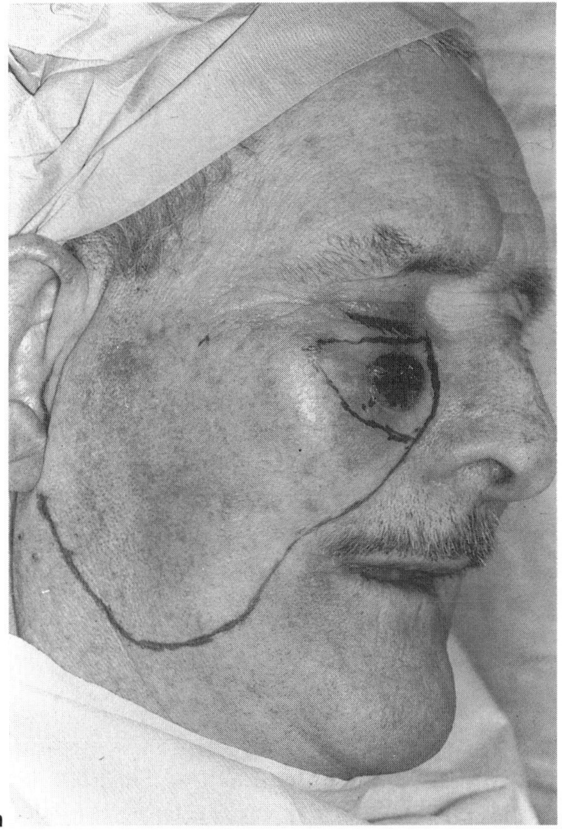

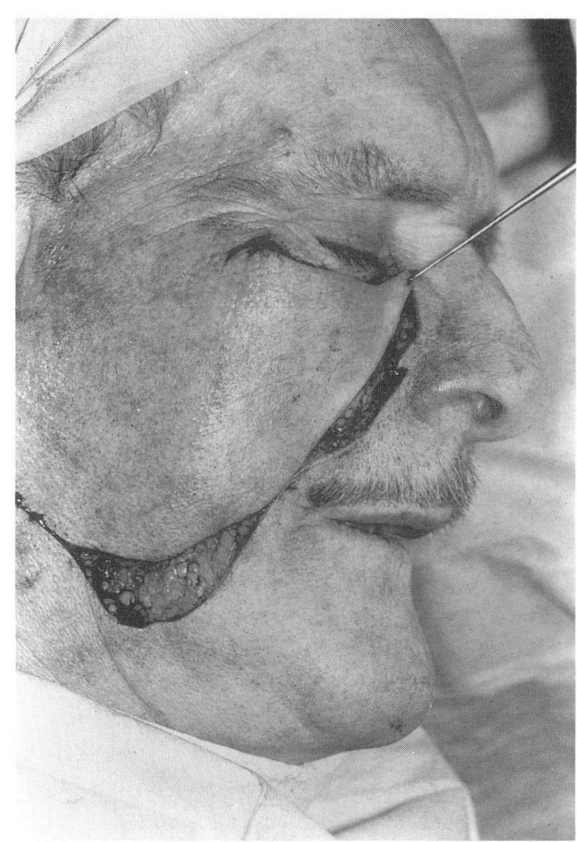

a b

Fig. 3.11 (a–b) Cervicofacial flap used to resurface a defect on the cheek, (a) The skin incisions are carefully positioned along the perimeter of the flap to ensure their orientation along the lines of election. (b) The flap is rotated and advanced; the original defect is transposed into the lax tissues of the neck.

inhibits wound healing and promotes bacterial colonization or ingress of organisms along the suture tracks.

The wide choice of suture materials available today often makes selection of the appropriate suture difficult and the choice of material is often based on personal preference.

The general principles on which suture selection is based are summarized in Tables 3.4 and 3.5.

Facial injury

Nowhere else should the principles of plastic surgery be applied more meticulously than in the management of facial injury. Fortunately facial tissues are also extremely vascular and capable of tolerating a greater degree of insult in terms of injury and contamination than tissues elsewhere.

Accurate assessment of the extent of injury and meticulous repair are the essential features of facial trauma management.

Assessment

History

A detailed history of the mechanism of injury is invaluable in determining the extent of the underlying damage. A tearing injury and the laceration produced by a direct blunt blow may appear superficially similar but the latter may be associated with considerable underlying bony damage.

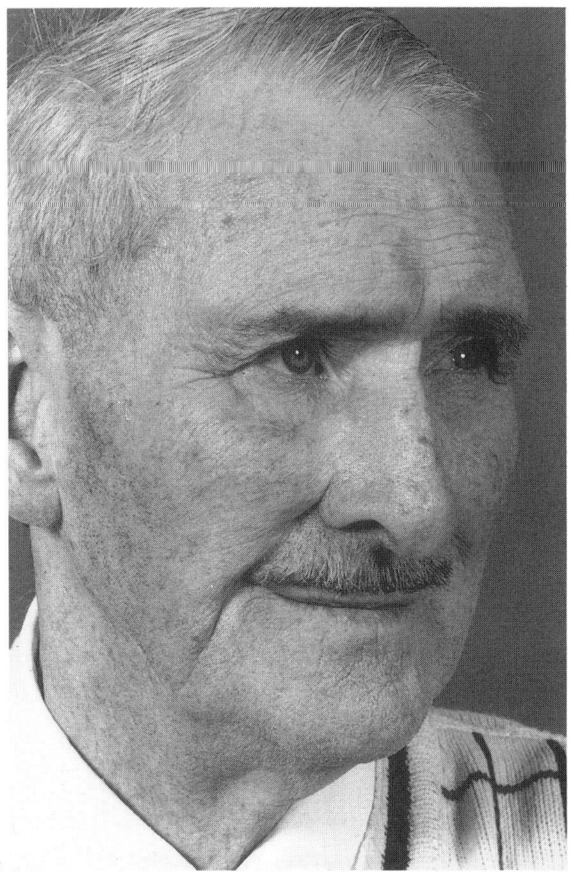

c

Fig. 3.11 (c) The final result.

In the unconscious patient, it is important to obtain information from witnesses as far as possible.

Associated symptoms following the injury may be useful indicators of underlying tissue damage. Numbness of the lower lip and chin may suggest a fractured mandible with injury to the inferior alveolar nerve. Facial asymmetry or motor weakness indicates facial nerve injury. Constant watery discharge from the nose could be cerebrospinal fluid rhinorrhoea.

Examination

Facial injuries must be carefully examined within a few hours of the injury. The laxity of facial skin and its relatively greater vascularity result in the rapid onset and development of tissue oedema and/or extravasation of blood, which distorts facial contours and makes the assessment of the extent of injury difficult if not impossible.

The possibility of damage to the underlying and adjacent structures must always be borne in mind and excluded. The results of early recognition and repair of nerve injuries and bony displacement are certainly gratifying and the consequences of missed penetrating injuries such as those involving the eyeballs or periorbita could be disastrous.

Investigation

Any suspicion of underlying injury must be investigated thoroughly using the appropriate radiography, computed tomography scans, ultrasound or other imaging techniques which may be relevant.

Management

The management of facial injuries will depend on several factors, the most important of which are:

1. The nature of the injury.
2. The extent of the injury.
3. The site.
4. The degree of potential or actual contamination.

Only the simplest facial injuries such as contusions or haematomata with no underlying injury, superficial abrasions with no embedded foreign material or small clean lacerations which lie along the lines of minimum tension or in relatively inconspicuous sites should be managed conservatively.

Contusions or subcutaneous extravasation of blood are usually self-limiting and warrant only the use of analgesia and possibly cold compresses or ice packs to minimize the extent of oedema. Active drainage or needle aspiration of a haematoma may be indicated in the vicinity of cartilaginous structures such as the nasal septum or external ear which, if left untreated, may produce a

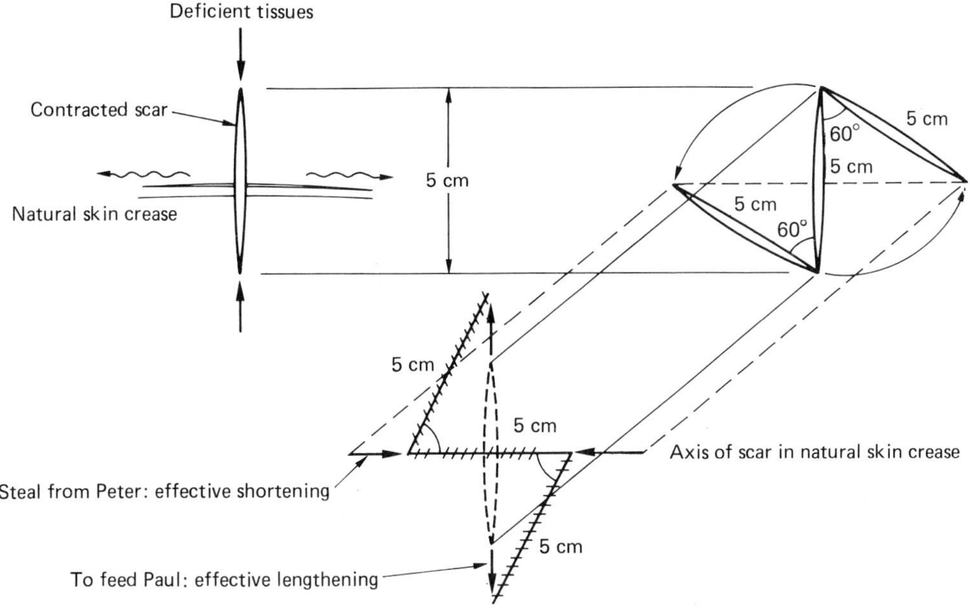

Fig. 3.12 The principle of Z-plasty, demonstrating the effective lengthening of a contracted scar by tissue transposition and the realignment of a scar along the lines of tension to achieve an optimum cosmetic result.

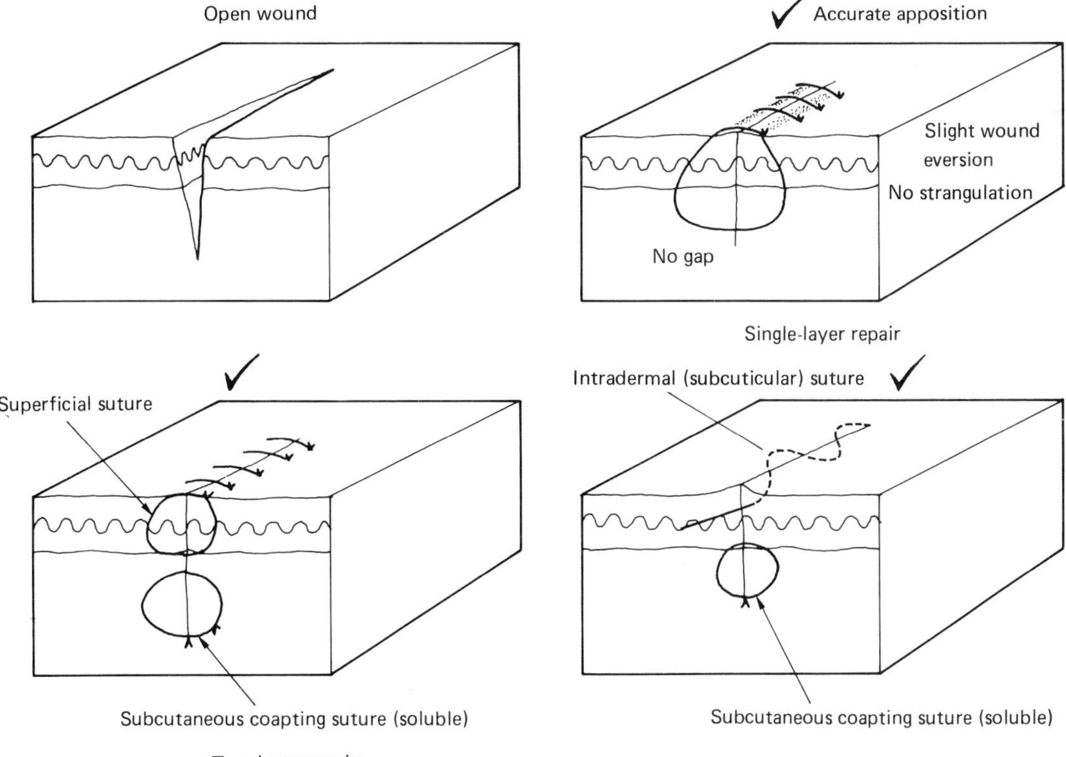

Fig. 3.13 Correct suturing technique.

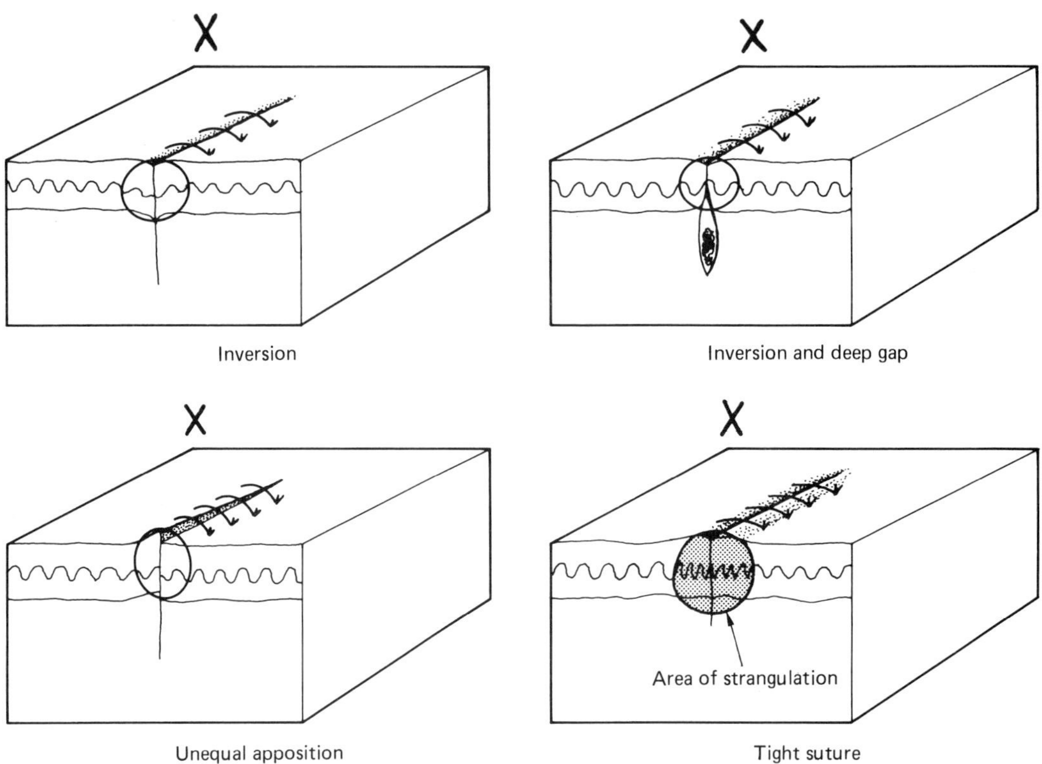

Fig. 3.14 Incorrect suturing technique.

pressure necrosis and subsequent distortion of the cartilage. Simple abrasions require gentle cleaning and topical application of an emollient and or non-adherent dressing.

Very small, clean, incised lacerations may be dealt with by steristrip apposition of the wound edges.

Local anaesthesia may be appropriate for small uncomplicated injuries in patients who are co-operative. Lignocaine 0.5–1% with 1:200 000 adrenaline is usually adequate for simple procedures and local distortion of tissues or the obliteration of vital landmarks such as the vermilion border can be avoided by using regional nerve block techniques.

Any injuries which are more extensive or complicated, and wounds in children, should be explored, preferably under a general anaesthetic.

The general principles of wound management outlined earlier should be applied meticulously and all contamination and obviously non-viable tissues excised carefully, followed by the apposition of wound edges under optimum conditions. Accurate replacement of tissues is crucial in areas such as the eyebrows, the eyelids, the nose and the lips. Failure to note anatomical landmarks such as the vermilion border of the lips or the eyebrow margins can produce gross cosmetic deformity for which only the surgeon may be held responsible. Landmarks should be carefully marked and eyebrows should *never* be shaved to facilitate repair (Fig. 3.15).

The principle of wound excision to eliminate ragged and partially devitalized, contaminated wound edges and surgically produce clean, incised and relatively uncontaminated, well-vascularized wound edges which are oriented as far as possible along the lines of minimum tension should be applied only as long as excision does not compromise closure. Facial skin is remarkably well-vascularized and even relatively long and narrow flaps of skin in ragged, tearing injuries, multiple lacerations or stellate injuries will survive and should be replaced as accurately as possible, if there is a

Table 3.4 Advantages and disadvantages of soluble and insoluble sutures

Advantages	Disadvantages
Soluble sutures	
Appropriate when suture removal is difficult or impossible, e.g. deeper tissues, unco-operative patients, children No foreign material remains after dissolution May be used intradermally and left *in situ* to prolong wound support	Dissolution time is unpredictable Tensile strength falls rapidly during dissolution Process of dissolution produces an inflammatory response which may adversely affect the resultant scar Unsuitable for surface use unless removed
Insoluble sutures	
Mechanically more reliable than soluble sutures Confer predictable resistance to disruption Induce a smaller inflammatory response Suitable for prolonged wound support, e.g. tendon repair	Some synthetic sutures are difficult to handle If used in deeper tissues, they persist as foreign bodies and may cause problems of stitch abscesses or extrusion

Table 3.5 Advantages and disadvantages of monofilament and braided sutures

Advantages	Disadvantages
Monofilament	
Smooth glide Suitable for use in potentially contaminated tissues and in vascular repairs Wide variety of materials Finer grades of sutures available (down to 13 μ)	Tend to have poor knot capacity and security Tendency to fracture and stretch
Braided sutures	
Easier to knot with better knot-holding capacity and security Often softer and more pliable No problems with 'memory' No stretch	Poor glide More thrombogenic if used in vascular repairs Prone to bacterial colonization within the braids Higher incidence of granulomata and stitch abcesses Unsuitable for use in infected or potentially infected environments Tendency to fragment

reasonable chance of viability. Secondary revision of unsightly scars in these circumstances is justified since the extent of revision is often much less than the original injury.

Complex injuries of the face with a potential for serious cosmetic deformity should be referred to an appropriate plastic surgical unit. Injuries which warrant such referral for primary management in a specialized unit may be summarized as follows:

1. Injuries in difficult sites such as the eyelids, the nose and irregular tearing injuries of the lips.
2. Complicated injuries with underlying bony or nerve injury or tissue loss.
3. Damage to deeper structures such as salivary glands, jaws and teeth.
4. Amputation injuries of the nose and ears. Replantation of the amputated segment using microvascular surgical techniques is often possible if the patient and the amputated tissue are managed correctly and transferred quickly to the nearest unit capable of dealing with such an emergency. The amputated segment should be preserved *dry*, after gentle cleaning with saline if severely contaminated, in a clean (not necessarily sterile) polythene bag which should be surrounded loosely with ice. On no account should the part be directly immersed in an iced solution or frozen. The patient should be kept warm and transferred with the amputated segment as soon as possible, with a reliable peripheral infusion to correct hypovolaemia and prevent peripheral shutdown.

Hand injuries

Injuries involving the hands are the source of considerable disability and loss of work hours. The management of even simple injuries of the hand in order to minimize functional disability is suffi-

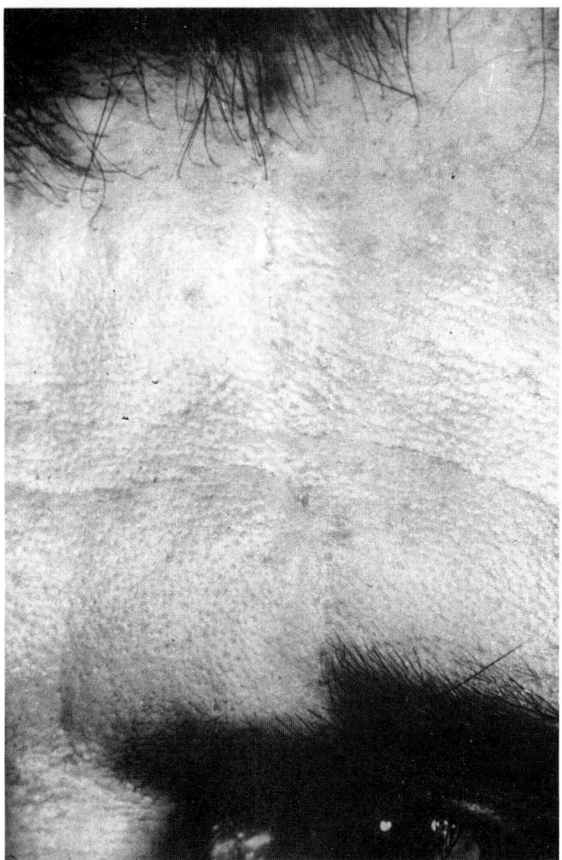

Fig. 3.15 Inaccurate apposition of the eyebrow resulting in a prominent step (see text).

ciently complex to justify the referral of virtually all hand injuries to a specialized unit with appropriate ancillary facilities such as physiotherapists, occupational therapists and orthotists.

The logical progression in the management of injuries of the hand is aimed at defining the extent and nature of injury, which may often be more serious than is immediately apparent. A systematic examination of motor, sensory and circulatory function is crucial to identify any damage to underlying structures before undertaking an exploration under an anaesthetic. Such examination may not be possible in the very young or the unco-operative patient and in such situations formal exploration is mandatory.

The repair of injured structures such as tendons, nerves, blood vessels, bones and joints is a sufficiently delicate and specialized procedure to merit the attention of a hand surgeon.

The management of hand injuries consists of

1. Early exploration and repair.
2. Elevation.
3. Mobilization.

Early exploration and repair

It is preferable to undertake the repair of all hand injuries within a few hours of the injury before the onset of oedema and sepsis. Virtually all surgical procedures on the hand should be performed in an operating theatre with suitable lighting and under tourniquet control. Field magnification using binocular loupes is desirable. Regional anaesthetic block, digital nerve block for finger injuries or the administration of a general anaesthetic may be necessary. Local infiltration of an anaesthetic agent is rarely satisfactory if any form of exploration is indicated and is justifiable in only the simplest of lacerations where direct closure is the only procedure required. Local anaesthetic agents containing adrenaline or any other vasoconstrictor must never be used for digital or ring blocks, which may jeopardize the circulation to the relevant digit.

Clean wounds should be repaired primarily with minimal or no tissue excision. If formal exploration is warranted there should be no hesitation in extending the wound to obtain a better exposure and carry the limits beyond the zone of injury. The planning of the surgical incisions to extend the wound must take into account the vascularity of the resultant flaps and the risk to underlying structures or contractures across joint lines.

Untidy injuries should be thoroughly debrided and all non-viable tissue excised. Skin cover may then be achieved by direct closure, grafts or the use of flaps.

Indeterminate injuries warrant careful and meticulous exploration and debridement to eliminate as far as possible all contamination and non-viable tissues. In difficult cases, it may be necessary to cover the hand in moist dressings and re-explore the hand in 24 hours for further debridement. The management of such injuries is often complex and skin cover may only be achieved by the use of pedicled or free flaps.

Elevation

The enemies of the hand surgeon are infection, oedema and stiffness. Even trivial trauma of the hand can often produce impressive oedema of the entire hand, which is more evident on the relatively lax skin of the dorsum. Hand oedema interferes with wound healing and predisposes to joint stiffness, especially in the elderly. The severity of oedema can be minimized by a combination of high elevation and early mobilization. All postoperative hands should be elevated in slings as high as is comfortably possible. Care should be taken to ensure that dressings or plaster casts do not impede venous return and the periphery should be monitored regularly for signs of ischaemia. The hand should be immobilized initially in a comfortable position with all the joints partially flexed over soft padding. If the risk of subsequent stiffness is high, as in complicated injuries or the elderly patient, or if early mobilization is contraindicated, it is preferable to splint the fingers and thumb in a more functional position.

Mobilization

Early mobilization under the supervision of a trained hand physiotherapist is vital in the management of the injured hand. Mobilization should be commenced as early as possible in the postoperative phase. Simple lacerations or fingertip injuries may be mobilized within a few hours of surgery. More extensive injuries or wounds which have required grafting or flaps may need immobilization for a few days. During this period, every effort should be made to maintain a full range of movement in the uninvolved digits and hand. The crucial role of early mobilization cannot be stressed enough for the consequences may be irreversible.

Stiffness and consequent loss of function in the injured hand are unusual in the young and common in the elderly. The formation of inflammatory adhesions and subsequent scar will result in stiffness. Early mobilization encourages the dissipation of oedema and limits the formation of dense adhesions which interfere with the smooth gliding and movement of tendons and joints.

The role of antibiotics in the management of hand injuries is controversial. They do not appear to confer any additional advantage over mechanical cleansing in most instances. They do have a role in grossly contaminated wounds such as human or animal bites and in delayed treatment, or in the presence of obvious sepsis.

Fingertip injuries

The commonest form of hand injuries are crush, avulsion or amputations of the fingertips. Though the size of the injury is often small, the functional magnitude is considerable as the fingertips represent the organs of tactile perception. An insensate or, worse, painful scar on the fingertip can render a digit unusable and compromise hand function.

Injuries of the pulp alone with no exposure or loss of bone may be treated conservatively if only a small area is involved. Larger areas may be resurfaced with a split-skin graft. There is however evidence to suggest that grafting of pulp defects does not confer any special advantage over conservative management with dressings and mobilization. Crushing or burst injuries are best treated conservatively to determine tissue viability.

Avulsed finger nails should always be carefully replaced under the eponychium to prevent synechiae which will result in subsequent dystrophic nail growth. If the avulsed finger nail is not available, a nail splint can be designed using aluminium foil or soft plastic.

Pulp loss with exposure of bone may warrant soft tissue flap cover, if sufficient distal phalangeal length is retained, to be of functional use. If however the remaining stump is too short, it is preferable to terminalize the digit by resecting the distal phalangeal bone and using the soft tissues to close the defect.

The manual worker who is not particularly concerned about cosmesis but requires to return to work as quickly as possible may prefer to have a digit terminalized rather than undergo a procedure which may involve a more protracted recovery. A society hostess may desire however to preserve the cosmetic appearance of the finger at all costs.

Flaps from adjacent digits or the thenar eminence may be inadvisable in the elderly due to the risk of permanent stiffness in the affected digit.

The obliquity of the amputation and the digit involved are important in deciding the course of action. The thumb pulp or the radial aspect of the index finger pulp should be reconstructed with sensate tissue if possible in order to preserve tactile pinch function.

Terminalization of a digit is often the easiest option but the procedure must be executed with care.

The bony stump should be smoothed and shaped to eliminate any sharp spurs or projections. If the phalangeal stump requires to be disarticulated, the exposed articular cartilage should be excised and the tip fashioned to produce a tapering surface. The skin flaps should be designed to obtain maximum volar sensate skin cover with the underlying padding over the tip to minimize the problem of a painful scar at the tip. The digital nerve stumps should be buried deeply into the soft tissues or preferably into drill holes in the phalangeal bone to prevent painful neuromas.

Physiotherapy, mobilization and restoration of hand function under supervision are vitally important, even with fingertip injuries, in order to avoid a stiff and useless or painful finger.

Bites

Human and animal bites represent a special category of injury due to penetration which embeds a considerable load of pathogenic organisms deep into the soft tissues, associated with a crushing or devitalizing injury of the surrounding tissues. The resident organisms in the human mouth appear far more virulent than those in animals and are often responsible for florid infections with extensive soft tissue damage after relatively trivial injuries. A common site for such injuries is overlying the dorsal aspect of the metacarpophalangeal joints following a punch to the mouth. If indequately treated this may result in gross destruction of the underlying joint, delayed rupture of extensor tendons, florid sepsis of the hand and marked stiffness of the joints.

Early exploration, debridement and vigorous cleansing of bites with mechanical irrigation are essential. Intravenous administration of antibiotics such as a combination of penicillin and metronidazole is necessary to ensure adequate and sustained serum levels.

Lower limb injuries

Lower limb injuries are common in sports and constitute a large proportion of all injuries. Simple abrasions and lacerations of the lower limb are treated as described earlier in this chapter.

Pretibial injuries

Pretibial injuries of the skin merit special attention due to the peculiarly precarious blood supply of the skin which often results in poor wound healing, especially in the elderly. Shearing forces such as a kick or accidental blunt trauma to the pretibial region result in a flap of skin, often V-shaped, which may be partially avulsed from the underlying periosteum or deep fascia. These flaps may be distally or proximally based. The viability of such skin flaps following a pretibial injury is often borderline and attempting to replace the flap and suture the skin edges is likely to result in failure due to necrosis.

The treatment should therefore be aimed at early excision of all non-viable tissues and split-skin grafting of the deficit. In borderline cases, fluorescein injection studies have been used to determine the extent of perfusion in the skin flap. In the postoperative period, the patient should be nursed with the leg elevated for 4–5 days. In elderly, obese or female patients, prophylactic subcutaneous injections of Minihep 5000 units b.d. is recommended to minimize the risk of deep vein thrombosis during the period of immobilization. Gradual mobilization is then commenced with the injured leg supported in a compression stocking or bandage.

Some success has been reported with the technique of careful defatting of the skin flap and its replacement as a full-thickness graft with multiple stab incisions to facilitate drainage and permit some expansion of the residual skin. If successful, this obviates the need to harvest a skin graft from a distant site.

Support stockings should be used for 4–6 weeks to minimize the formation of oedema and graft loss.

Grafts in the pretibial region are also often unstable and small areas of graft loss may be expected when mobilization is commenced. These will usually heal spontaneously with regular dressings. Persistent instability of a graft may warrant the use of local flap cover, for which the patient should be referred to a specialist unit.

Degloving injuries (see Fig. 3.5)

The shearing forces required to avulse the attachments and blood supply of the skin and subcutaneous tissues from the deeper tissues are a common feature in industrial and road traffic accidents.

The mechanism of injury should alert the examining doctor to the possibility of degloving, for the initial appearance of the skin on a cursory examination may be unimpressive. The clinical signs to look for are:

1. Extensive bruising or pallor of the skin.
2. Excessive mobility of the skin.
3. Poor or absent blanching and refill on digital pressure or poor bleeding on pinprick.
4. Loss of sensation over the injured skin.
5. Drop in skin temperature.

The area of degloving may be mapped using fluorescein injection. These injuries are often part of more complicated injuries with underlying damage and the risk of compartment syndromes or peripheral ischaemia.

Surgery in degloving injuries is a matter of urgency. Under an appropriate anaesthetic, the degloved limb should be explored and all the underlying haematoma evacuated. Extensive fasciotomies may be required to minimize the risk of compartment syndromes. Any bony, joint or soft tissue injuries are dealt with at this time. The degloved skin is then examined carefully and all the potentially non-viable skin excised. The subcutaneous tissues attached to the excised skin can be shaved using a Gibson–Tough dermatome designed especially for this purpose, or with any available skin graft knife. This skin is then stored under refrigeration in a sterile container.

The injured limb is wrapped up in moist dressings and elevated. It is re-explored in 24 hours and any further areas of non-viable skin and tissue excised and discarded. The previously defatted stored skin may now be applied as a graft to the exposed soft tissues. Multiple punctures should be made in the grafted skin to facilitate drainage of any underlying seroma or haematoma. If no suitable skin is available for storing, split-skin grafts harvested from other areas may be used.

The limb is redressed and elevated and the graft inspected 4–5 days later.

Mobilization should be commenced as soon as the grafts are stable and/or underlying tissue damage will allow. Compression support using stockings or bandages is essential for upper and lower limb injuries. Circumferential degloving injuries will be associated with long-term problems of peripheral venous and lymphatic drainage and custom-made gradient-pressure garments may have to be worn for several years.

Tattoos

Tattoos are produced by embedding insoluble pigments into the dermis. Tattoos produced by professional tattoo artists may use several colours and the depth of the dye is uniform.

Amateur tattoos are produced by manual

embedding of India ink into the dermis and are therefore often made with variable depth and density of dye penetration.

Traumatic tattoos produced by impregnation of dirt or grit following accidental injury should be avoided by definitive primary treatment, as outlined earlier.

None of the methods that are currently available for the removal of tattoos is entirely satisfactory. The simplest method of treatment in suitable cases is excision and direct closure. The other surgical methods available are:

1. Split-thickness tangential excision and extrusion of dye using a variety of substances such as tannic acid, salt etc.
2. Dermabrasion.
3. Full-thickness excision and skin graft.

In all these techniques it is important to impress upon the patient that the degree of scarring is prominent and often disfiguring, and the best that can be achieved is trading the tattoo for a scar.

Laser obliteration of tattoos is eminently suitable for carbon-based tattoos such as those produced with India ink and produces good results with minimal scarring in suitable cases.

The disadvantage of laser therapy is that its use is limited, expensive, and restricted to a few specialized centres.

Decubitus ulcers

Prolonged cutaneous ischaemia due to unrelieved pressure especially against underlying bony prominences such as the sacrum or ischial tuberosities can result in a breakdown of the skin and a subsequent pressure sore. They are commonest in debilitated patients who are unable to move themselves or in paraplegic or quadriplegic patients with sensory loss.

The exact mechanism which contributes to the formation of pressure sores is not fully understood. Prevention however is certainly better than cure and a constant awareness of the risk of decubitus ischaemia is essential. Diligent nursing care and awareness have contributed to a significant fall in the incidence of pressure sores.

The localized changes which herald an impending decubitus ulcer are persistent erythema and induration with slight oedema of the affected area which usually overlies a bony prominence. This subsequently progresses through the stages of superficial skin loss, full-thickness necrosis with or without osteomyelitis and, in long-standing cases, the formation of an extensive bursa-like cavity.

If recognized in the very early stages before the onset of full-thickness necrosis, decubitus ulcers will heal with conservative management as follows:

1. Relieve pressure from the affected area and ensure that the patient's position is changed frequently to avoid problems at other sites.
2. Keep the area dry and clean to minimize maceration and breakdown.
3. Apply zinc oxide paste or mild antiseptics topically.
4. Use special mattresses or beds designed to relieve decubitus problems.

Deep or long-standing sores with underlying bursae will not heal with conservative management.

The management of the established decubitus ulcer relies on the principle of excision of all diseased tissues and their replacement by healthy well-vascularized tissues. Excision and direct closure of a decubitus ulcer are rarely successful except in very simple cases. A large proportion of decubitus ulcers at this stage will require local flaps to replace the excised necrotic tissue and a reduction or excision of the underlying bony prominence to minimize the risk of recurrence.

In neglected or resistant cases which do not appear to respond to long-term conservative therapy, excision and the use of large local flaps such as myocutaneous flaps are required. The patient should be referred to a specialist unit for such treatment.

Non-accidental injury (NAI)

The entity of NAI is a difficult one to confront and establish. Injuries may be deliberately inflicted on children and infants and the possibility of any injury being non-accidental in nature must always be borne in mind. Suspicions should be aroused if the history and alleged mechanism of injury do not correspond to their clinical extent and distribution. Associated observations such as the appearance of a neglected or malnourished child may contribute to an increased index of suspicion but by no means is this true of all children who have suffered NAI. NAI does not appear to be necessarily related to socioeconomic background, race, size of family or age of the parents. The appearance of love and affection between the parent or involved adult and child or the natural concern of the responsible adult for the injured child may also be misleading. The individual who inflicts such injury is often genuinely concerned for the child at the time of presentation and terrified of his or her own failure to control his or her emotions. The act of bringing the injured child to a hospital or a practitioner for treatment is a 'cry for help'. A repeatedly injured or abused child may also show normal affection and attachment for his or her parents, and he or she is unable to recognize the deliberate nature of the inflicted injury.

In any case where NAI is suspected, a careful examination should be conducted for evidence of previous injuries. Healed scars or bony deformities should be carefully documented. Radiological skeletal survey may be necessary to identify previous fractures. The presenting injury should be meticulously documented and photographed. Examples of common presentations for NAI are perithoracic bruises which correspond with fingerprints carved by tight squeezing of the chest, circumscribed burns produced by lighted cigarette ends, scalds of the feet or buttocks produced by lowering the child into hot water or fractures of the ribs, skull or extremities.

Before the suspicion of NAI is substantiated, it is important to eliminate possible disease entities which may mimic NAI:

- Bleeding or clotting disorders may produce excessive bruising with minimal trauma.
- Multiple fractures may occur due to trivial trauma in conditions such as osteogenesis imperfecta.
- Burns or other injuries may occur in children with peripheral anaesthesia. Epidermolysis bullosa may mimic scalded skin.

The management of children with NAI is complex and should not be attempted by inexperienced practitioners. However, it is vital that the diagnosis is established without delay, for the return of the child to the home environment may be potentially fatal. The parents of the affected child must be confronted and will require the evaluation and help of social services, psychiatrists and, if necessary, marriage counsellors. The child may have to be made a ward of court and fostered if necessary to avoid a recurrence of injury. The advice and guidance of paediatricians experienced in the management of NAI are essential and an opinion should be sought as early as possible.

Dermatitis artefacta

An unstable wound following an operative procedure or injury which fails to heal satisfactorily in spite of all the surgeon's endeavours may be a manifestation of self-inflicted injury, if all other factors can be reasonably excluded. The patient who presents with this problem may often be difficult to identify in the initial stages. The diagnosis should be considered if:

1. On hospital admission and treatment, the wound appears to show signs of healing, only to relapse prior to or on discharge.
2. The dressings applied on the wound appear to have been disturbed.
3. The patient expresses little concern or annoyance at the chronic non-healing and is readily prepared to attend the hospital for regular follow-up or admission.
4. Histological examination of an excised part of

the chronic wound reveals unusual debris or foreign bodies.

The treatment of this condition is difficult and it is necessary to identify the underlying social or psychological cause for such behaviour. The patient's circumstances warrant investigation and the help of a psychiatrist is essential. The patient is often simply lonely or has a very low self-image and thrives on the attention and feeling of importance generated from being a clinical conundrum.

Hypertrophic scars and keloids

In some individuals, the mechanism of wound healing appears to vary, resulting in scars which are unacceptable. The pathogenesis of hypertrophic scars and keloids is not clearly understood.

All healing wounds appear to go through an initial hypertrophic phase with an excessive and disorganized deposition of collagen which is later reorganized as the scar matures. In the initial stages the distinction between hypertrophic scars and keloids may be difficult to identify.

Hypertrophic scars

Such scars remain red, raised, itchy and often unstable for several years but never extend beyond the confines of the original injury. They ultimately regress, often leaving pale stretched or irregular, mature scar tissue behind.

Keloids

Keloids are a special type of hypertrophic scar which occurs commonly in the presternal area in all races but is unusually common at all sites in individuals of negroid origin.

They are distinguished by their clinical behaviour. They often extend well beyond the confines of the original wound and continue to enlarge, reaching impressive proportions after even trivial injuries such as shaving cuts or piercing of the ear lobule. They may grow relentlessly, showing little signs of regression, and remain persistently itchy and unstable (Fig. 3.16).

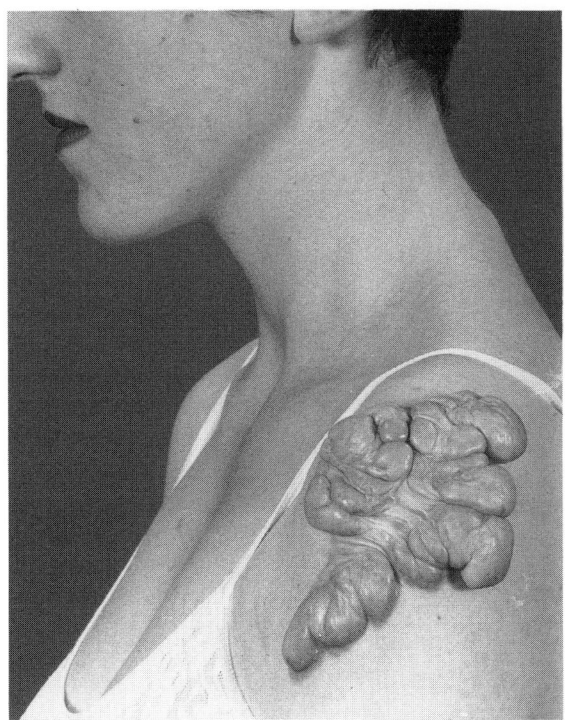

Fig. 3.16 Large keloid on the deltoid area. The keloid did not respond to conventional therapy and was exacerbated by attempted re-excision.

The management of hypertrophic scars and keloids is at best a compromise and should be considered with care. It is important to impress upon the patient that no treatment can guarantee a cure or avoid a recurrence and the general aim of all treatment is to achieve a flat, pale and mature scar.

Variation in the rate of wound healing and scar hypertrophy in individuals is considerable and the initial management of all such scars is conservative. The patient should be reassured and simply advised gently to massage the scar with moisturizing cream once daily. A large proportion of scars will resolve within a year, leaving pale mature and acceptable scars.

In situations where considerable hypertrophy is expected, such as in individuals prone to hypertrophic scarring or following a burn injury or wound infection, more aggressive measures may be adopted to minimize the degree of hypertrophy and effect faster resolution.

The means currently available are:

1. Pressure.
2. Steroids.
3. Radiation.
4. Surgical excision or revision.
5. Silicone gel.

Pressure

The application of pressure to a hypertrophic scar appears to accelerate resolution and produce more acceptable scars.

The use of pressure garments which are custom-designed for patients with hypertrophic scars following burns is widely accepted. The disadvantage of this procedure is that it requires a considerable amount of patient compliance as the garments have to be worn for up to 23 hours a day. Hypertrophic scars and keloids of the ears and lobules have been similarly treated using acrylic oyster splints to maintain constant and uniform pressure. Pressure garments or devices are unsuitable for use on sites such as the neck, shoulder or axilla for obvious reasons.

Steroids

Patients with Cushing's syndrome have atrophic scars. The intralesion injection of steroids such as triamcinolone or the topical application of steroid cream also facilitates scar resolution. Excellent results have been obtained with 4–6-weekly injections or Dermojet instillation of triamcinolone into scars and keloids.

Radiation

In extreme cases, radiation has been used to control the formation of keloids. Its use may be difficult to justify on the grounds of its carcinogenic potential and unpredictable results.

Surgical excision or revision

This procedure is to be approached with caution for the risk of recurrence is high. It is always advisable to allow a hypertrophic scar to mature before contemplating any revision surgery. Surgery in hypertrophic scars is justified only if the predisposing cause for the hypertrophy can be identified, such as burns, infection, wound necrosis or breakdown. Care should be taken to ensure that the wound is located in a suitable site and the individual is not otherwise prone to hypertrophic scarring, as manifested by the appearance of other scars.

Surgical excision of keloids is even more problematic since the risk of producing a greater keloid is considerable. Intrakeloidal excision, leaving the perimeter of the original keloid undisturbed, is advisable to avoid the risk of further extension. Intrakeloid instillation of triamcinolone and/or the application of sustained pressure using custom-made pressure garments is mandatory within a week of the excision and should be continued till final scar maturity has been achieved. The risk of recurrence, however, is high.

Silicone gel

The exact mechanism of action of silicone gel and its effects on hypertrophic scars and keloids is a subject of current study and debate. Its use is controversial.

Conclusions

The role of the surgeon involved in the management of all tissue trauma must depend on the recognition of the nature of the injuring agent and the pattern of injury it is liable to produce, coupled with an indepth knowledge of the factors which would influence the outcome of healing and recovery.

The judicious application of this knowledge to forestall or modify the course of a potentially unfavourable outcome by the 'stitch in time saves

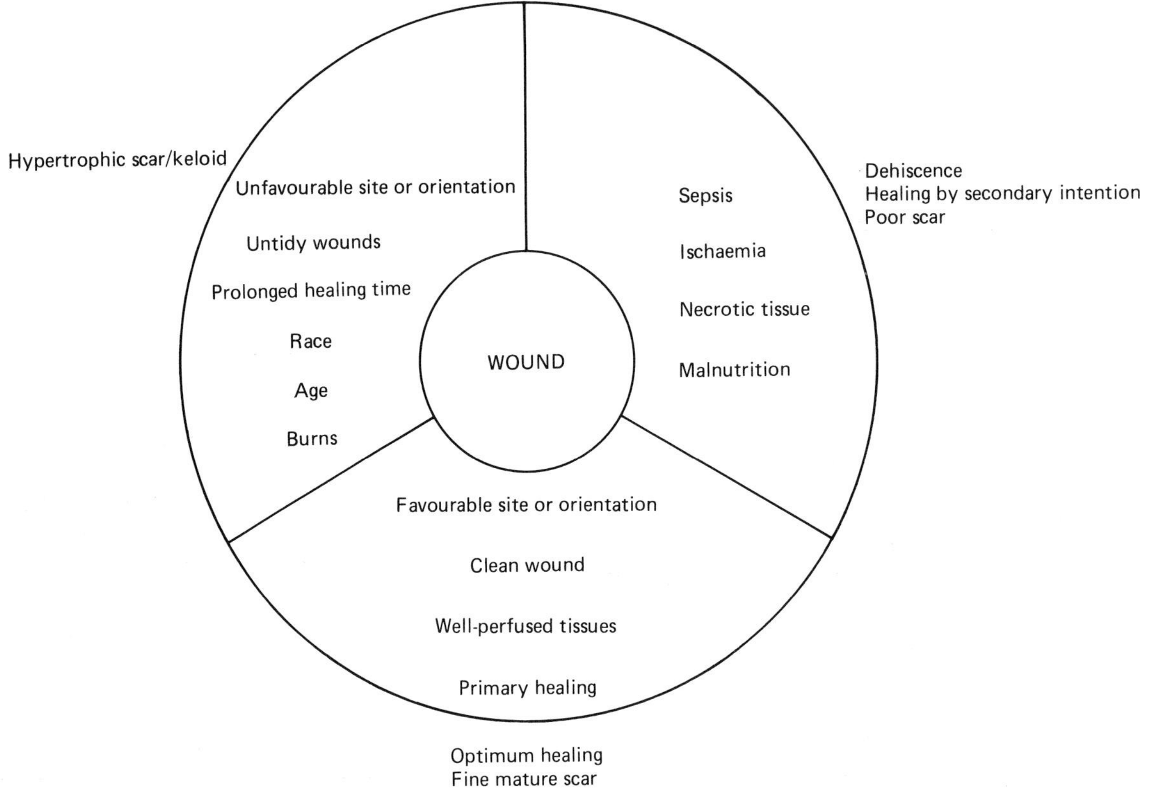

Fig. 3.17 Factors affecting the outcome of scar formation.

nine' principle comprises the net skills of the plastic surgeon who attempts to achieve optimum healing of the surgically induced or traumatic wound (Fig. 3.17).

These skills and objectives are not the sole preserve of the plastic surgeon and are universally applicable to all disciplines. The timely application of these basic principles contributes greatly towards minimizing the suffering and potential disability and disfigurement of the injured patient.

References

Devane J (1988) *Drawing and Painting the Portrait*. London: Tiger Books International.

Sundell B (ed.) (1979) *Symposium on Wound Healing*. Oslo: A/S Apothekernes Laboratorium.

Further reading

Grabb WC, Smith JW *Plastic Surgery: A Concise Guide to Clinical Practice* (2nd edn). Boston: Little, Brown.

Green DP (ed.) (1988) *Operative Hand Surgery* vols 1–3. Edinburgh: Churchill Livingstone.

Ledingham I McA, MacKay C (1978) *Textbook of Surgical Physiology* 3rd edn. Churchill Livingstone.

McCarthy JG (ed.) (1990) *Plastic Surgery* vols 1–8. Philadelphia: W. B. Saunders.

McGregor IA (1972) *Fundamental Techniques of Plastic Surgery and their Surgical Applications*. Edinburgh: Churchill Livingstone.

Schwartz SI, Lillehei RC, Shires T *et al.* (eds) *Principles of Surgery*. New York: McGraw Hill.

4

Muscle injuries

C. M. E. Lennox

Introduction

The spectrum of injury to muscle is immense, from the minor sprain which is so familiar to all, to the dramatic rupture often captured on camera at sports events (Fig. 4.1), to the chronic pattern preventing full rehabilitation and return to work or sport. Equally important are limb-threatening acute ischaemic syndromes and even life-threatening systemic phenomena, e.g. crush syndrome.

An equivalent injuring force may cause very different patterns of damage depending on the quality of muscle, and that same quality influences significantly the speed and completeness of recovery from trauma. By quality is meant the mechanical efficiency and resilience of muscle, both of which are greatly improved by training. It is therefore important to understand the physiology of healing and the physiological adaptations which occur in muscle after different types of training, and to compare the response to injury of trained and untrained muscle.

Physiology of muscle healing

Controversy has long existed regarding the capacity of skeletal muscle to regenerate after injury.

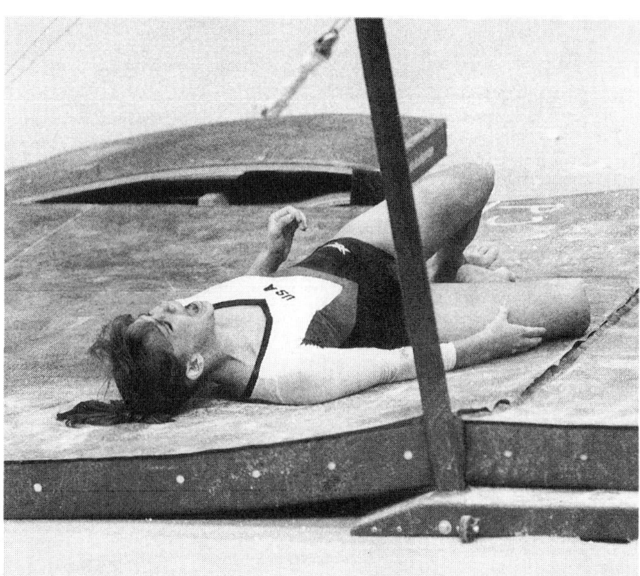

Fig. 4.1 Acute muscle tear.

That skeletal muscle is highly adaptable is without doubt. The phenomenon of disuse atrophy and subsequent reuse hypertrophy demonstrates this adaptability. The efficiency of recovery of muscle function after injury depends on the different healing processes occurring after various types of injury.

Sequence of histological events

Traumatized muscle has the ability to heal either completely with normal muscle tissue, or with more or less scarring, the extent depending on several factors. It is the observation of scarring in injured muscle which has led in the past to some authors declaring that muscle would always heal with scar tissue and not by regeneration.

The best healing is seen to occur after a single incisive injury – if the cut surfaces remain in apposition, as for example after a surgical closure of such a wound, surviving sarcolemmal tissue on either side may unite and encourage immediate bridging of the gap by ingrowth of muscle fibres along the sarcolemmal tube. This situation is not usual however, and in sports injuries to muscle, whether due to direct blow, complete or incomplete tear, there will always be separation of the torn ends of muscle fibres. The sequence of events after this injury (Allbrook *et al.*, 1966) begins with the damage to myofibrils, and the interstitial space surrounding the muscle fibres becoming distended with oedema and haemorrhage, which is later invaded by phagocytic polymorphonuclear neutrophils. These cells act as scavengers so that after a few days the sarcolemmal tubes are free of cellular debris. This surviving basement membrane then acts as a scaffolding for regeneration of muscle tissue by myoblasts. There have been several theories as to the origin of these cells. They probably originate from satellite cells which exist in all normal striated muscle, and are normally dormant, lying under the sarcolemma of the muscle fibre. They have the potential to multiply (in fact they are the only muscle cells which can do so).

Myoblasts multiply and form an elongated syncytium, on either side of which myofilaments are rapidly laid down developing into myotubes – the tube consists of the central core of nuclei and sarcoplasm, with surrounding myofibrils. The myotubes grow forward through the injured area, reconstituting normal muscle.

There are several factors which determine the success or otherwise of this process. Simultaneously with the process of myotube formation, the oedema and haemorrhage are further organized by the appearance of fibroblasts which invade the tissue spaces and deposit connective tissue in a randomly oriented pattern. Plasma fibronectin is a globulin which can be detected in the organizing process even before fibroblasts appear – it is distributed along strands of fibrin in the haematoma and this linkage seems to promote the adhesion of fibrinoblasts to the clot, hence platelet aggregation etc. (Lehto *et al.*, 1985). The presence of fibroblasts is closely linked to the appearance of type III collagen and later type I collagen. This deposition, if unimpeded, will continue and result in a scar which will obstruct further ingrowth of myotubes. Therefore repair of a muscle defect consists of a 'race' between myoblasts laying down muscle fibres and fibroblasts laying down collagen.

There is a complex interaction of factors which determines the winner of the race!

Factors influencing muscle regeneration

Firstly, myotube formation will not continue if a nerve supply does not develop simultaneously by regenerating axons, meeting up with the myotubes and reconstituting neuromuscular units. The new muscle fibre will otherwise undergo denervation atrophy and be replaced by fibrous tissue. The axon regrowth, as with the myotube, may be impeded by the mass of collagenous reticulum in the scar tissue. This obstructive process may be influenced by early activity of the injured muscle, since early intermittent contraction of the muscle will tend to disperse the interstitial oedema and haemorrhage, reducing the amount of scar tissue formation. If the muscle is allowed to contract immediately after injury, the gap will tend to widen, increasing the tendency to scar formation. However, it seems probable that the collagen granulation tissue matrix laid down in the gap acts as a tether, so that after a few days, gentle activity of the muscle is unlikely to cause retraction of the damaged end, because by that time tensile strength of the matrix is sufficient to withstand contraction.

The role of collagen

Also the initiation of contractions has a physical influence on the orientation of the collagen fibres which then line up in the direction of pull (Carlson, 1973). Muscle fibres themselves appear to have an ability to orientate themselves parallel to the line of tension, as has been shown in experiments where a block of muscle is removed and replaced at 90° to the axis of the muscle belly – regenerating fibres grow out of the cut end and turn through 90° (Allbrook, 1973). Likewise, in experiments with minced muscle the fibres regenerate in correct orientation but only if intermittent tension is applied through the muscle (Carlson, 1972).

As the myotubes grow forward between the parallel-oriented collagen fibres (the rate has been measured in rabbit experiments as between 1 and 1.5 mm per day) the number of collagen fibres decreases as muscle fibres enlarge. If the defect is too large there will inevitably always be a scar. Obviously, this will result in reduced function of the muscle, as the scar is inelastic, and may in fact shorten with time, causing an overall shortening of the muscle belly.

Mobilization versus immobilization

Jarvinen performed a series of experiments to illustrate the benefits and disadvantages of mobilization and immobilization after a muscle injury, using a standardized injury with the gastrocnemius muscle in rats. He demonstrated that early mobilization increased the edema and inflammation initially and therefore a larger volume of interstitial collagen deposition occurred but with well-oriented fibres and therefore a rapid return to pre-injury tensile strength (Jarvinen, 1975). On the other hand, immobilization caused less inflammatory reaction and therefore less scarring, but with poor orientation of both collagen and muscle fibres. This smaller but weaker scar is more likely to re-rupture when mobilization does occur. He also showed a more rapid and intensive ingrowth of capillaries after early mobilization, especially in the first few days after surgery (Jarvinen, 1976a). The speed and intensity of tissue repair are directly correlated to the rate of vascular ingrowth (Anderson, 1975).

The same author further showed that 'breaking strength' and energy absorption of the muscle returned to normal much sooner after mobilization than after immobilization (Jarvinen, 1976b).

Clinical application

The significance of this work in planning the treatment of muscle injuries is that after a major injury, a period of immobilization is advisable to allow tensile strength to build up, but that thereafter further immobilization will promote poor healing, a decrease in breaking strength and later contraction. Mobilization after the first few days of immobilization ensures optimum return to strength, length and 'breaking strength'.

Other forms of muscle injury

Other forms of muscle damage behave differently. For example, muscle which has been partly damaged due to ischaemia develops a central necrotic zone (Sanderson *et al.*, 1975). Blood vessels may still enter the muscle belly along tendons or from periosteal vessels at the muscle origin from bone. The repair process is therefore from the periphery into the centre. If incomplete, the central area becomes necrotic, densely scarred and causes contracture of the whole muscle belly with resulting shortening and compromise of any nerves or vessels which pass through the muscle.

After muscle damage due to infection, for example Coxsackie viral myositis, there may be complete regeneration of normal muscle, as there has been no break in continuity during the infection. In contrast, in muscular dystrophy there is often an apparent hypertrophy of some muscles, e.g. the calf muscle. In fact, the increase in bulk is due to swelling of the muscle fibres and fat deposition and later fibrous tissue. These changes are irreversible.

Muscle adaptations to training and their influence on healing after trauma

Muscles which have been trained by an appropriate fitness programme respond differently to stress and resist injury better than do untrained muscles.

An awareness of the physiological and anatomical differences between trained and untrained muscle helps in understanding the pattern of injury seen in each.

Muscle can be trained to adapt either to endurance activities or to short, sharp bursts (supramaximal activity).

Fibre types

There is a significant genetically predetermined factor which influences the individual's ability to excel in one form of sport or another, and that is the composition of fibre type in skeletal muscle (Bergh *et al.*, 1978). The two fibre types are known as fast twitch (FT) and slow twitch (ST) fibres. Each differs from the other in terms of usefulness for specific activities. For example, FT fibres have a lower mitochondrial content, capillary density, and higher anaerobic potential and therefore perform well in supramaximal exertion, e.g. sprinting. ST fibres, on the other hand, have a high resistance to fatigue, a larger number of mitochondria, low anaerobic potential and higher capillary density. They are therefore more efficient in continuous energy production and so perform well in endurance events, e.g. distance running.

A weight-lifter's aim is to build up the bulk of his muscle (because, by and large, muscle strength is proportional to size) by developing the FT fibres. He will only achieve that increase in bulk and strength if he has a genetically predetermined high ratio of FT to ST fibres – increase in bulk is due to hypertrophy of the FT fibres, not to hyperplasia (increase in cell numbers).

In contrast, a marathon runner aims to avoid increasing muscle bulk which would increase body weight, and trains to develop the ST fibres to improve endurance.

Interestingly, FT fibres tend to atrophy before ST fibres with age, which is one reason for decreasing ability to sprint as one gets older!

It has also been shown that capillary density is higher in trained than in untrained muscle (Anderson, 1975).

Biochemical adaptations

Endurance activity requires aerobic glycolysis, and appropriate training increases the efficiency of utilization of oxygen (VO_{2max}) and of glycolysis by increasing the concentration of enzymes and cofactors and muscle glycogen stores (Boobis, 1987). On the other hand, high-intensity exercise requires almost instantaneous availability and utilization of energy by muscle – energy provision is almost entirely anaerobic. It is thought that appropriate training allows muscle to adapt to the resulting increase in lactate (Parkhouse and McKenzie, 1984; Sharp *et al.*, 1986) by an improvement in its ability to buffer hydrogen ions, thus allowing an increased rate of adenosine triphosphate resynthesis. Parkhouse *et al.* (1985) performed a study on two groups of sportsmen – sprinters and rowers in the first group, marathon runners and untrained individuals in the second group. Muscle biopsies were performed after standard exercise and analysed biochemically. An increased buffering capacity was demonstrated in the biopsies from the first group, but not in the second, i.e. the first group had an enhanced capacity for muscle to function under conditions requiring high rates of anaerobic glycolytic energy production, presumably due to repetitive high-intensity training.

The effects of disuse

These adaptive changes take months to achieve but interestingly a spell away from training may result in a rapid loss of these adaptations (Booth, 1977). For example, hypertrophied muscle in a weight-lifter will rapidly return to normal size as the FT fibres lose their bulk. It has been shown that this loss occurs in an exponential fashion with half of the total loss occurring within the first 4–6 days and the rate of loss slowing thereafter. Also, endurance-trained muscle, after enforced bedrest, shows a rapid fall in VO_{2max}. The maximum rate of loss is again in the first few days.

Muscle which is experimentally immobilized in tension can be shown to atrophy more slowly than that which is immobilized in a relaxed position. Therefore, any form of splinting which is required to relieve pain immediately after injury should be applied with the appropriate muscles in tension to minimize the harmful effects of immobilization. Since the musculature of the trained individual rapidly loses its 'superfit' status, although only one limb may be out of action after injury, it is important that the individual as a whole continues to exercise to the maximum possible within the limitations of the handicap.

Trained versus untrained performance

Therefore, the response of trained muscle to exertion is rapid metabolism made possible by increased enzyme activity, and the removal of metabolites by increased vascularity. There is probably also an increase in the flexibility of the muscle substance because of hypertrophy of the fibres.

Untrained muscle, on the other hand, when subjected to unaccustomed exertion, suffers from inflexibility, accumulation of metabolites and therefore oedema. It is also thought that numerous microtears of muscle fibres occur, resulting in microhaemorrhages. The combined effect of these occurrences is a generalized swelling of the muscle mass within the confines of its fascial sleeve, such that the individual experiences muscular pain and extreme stiffness, which may indeed worsen during the following 48 hours and then gradually subside as the swelling disperses. Stretching exercises the day after exertion will encourage dispersal of the oedema and metabolites and will help to ameliorate the symptoms of pain and stiffness (de Vries, 1960).

Classification of muscle injuries

Injury to muscle is most commonly the result of trauma. The term 'torn muscle' covers a wide spectrum of types of trauma to muscle of varying severity. Muscle may also be injured by ischaemic events or by infection.

Muscle tears

Torn muscle may be the result of either direct or indirect violence.

Direct injury

A direct blow will cause variable damage to muscle, the extent of which depends largely on the state of contraction of the muscle at the moment of impact. For example, in association football, the flexed knee of an opponent hitting the anterolateral quadriceps during a tackle from the side can cause crippling muscle damage. The quadriceps muscle is contracting strongly at the moment of impact and therefore retracts fiercely as the blunt impact from the knee compresses the muscle against the underlying bone which acts like an anvil. The resulting rent is much larger than would be the case after a direct blow to a relaxed muscle. In the latter case, the direct force may cause local contusion or haemorrhage but without necessarily causing any significant break in continuity of the fibres.

Direct damage to muscle may also be the result of an incisive force, for example a sharp lacerating injury from without, whether it be due to knife, gunshot or the sharp edge of metal or glass as in a road traffic accident or motorbike injury. Direct division of fibres from within may occur after a fracture of a long bone. Fragments of bone can cut muscle substance and of course may even penetrate skin. However incisive damage is caused, the severity of muscle injury depends (as described above) on the state of contraction of the muscle at the moment of injury. Whatever the nature of the direct force causing injury, the resulting tear tends to be localized to the site of impact or laceration.

Indirect injury

In comparison with the above, indirect violence to a particular muscle may result in damage either at one point or along the whole length of that muscle. The indirect force is an extreme sudden contraction of the muscle causing it to rupture. Although the whole muscle is under severe tension at the moment of injury, the tear may in fact occur at one specific site. The weakest point in a muscle complex is the musculotendinous junction which is therefore often the site of rupture, for example the tendo-Achilles as it emerges from the belly of gastrocnemius. Alternatively, the muscle may be torn away from its bony origin with or without an avulsion fracture. The pattern of damage may be more diffuse than described above – there may be multiple small tears throughout the substance of the muscle and if the fascial sleeve around the muscle remains intact, the resulting swelling and haemorrhage are confined within it. It may be possible to elicit tenderness along the whole length of the muscle. For example, after an acute sprain of the extensor carpi radialis longus muscle in a thrower, tenderness may be demonstrable from the lateral epicondyle of the elbow to the carpus. Similarly, indirect violence due to overstretching may cause the same picture, for example, a fall on to the outstretched hand. Hyperextension of the wrist may overstretch the wrist flexors and cause many small tears within their substance as well as at the musculotendinous junction, with resulting symptoms along the full length of the forearm, and pain which may extend along tendons producing the clinical picture of tenosynovitis. The latter is an example of an extrinsic factor contributing significantly to tension within the muscle, causing its damage.

In order to appreciate the degree of tension which may be generated within the muscle it is useful to look at a biomechanical analysis of the forces acting.

Biomechanics of a muscle tear

Control of joint movement is a balanced interaction between agonists and antagonists which behave synergistically to achieve maximum controlled power as well as providing a protection against injury. The study of isokinetics involves the measurement of magnitude and pattern of torque generated by muscle groups across a specific joint. It can be useful to obtain an objective record of any imbalance between agonist and antagonist. Elaborate and expensive equipment has been used to obtain these measurements, and its application to rehabilitation programmes is slowly being eroded.

The biomechanical analysis of, for example, knee motion, allows the calculation of tensile force in the components of the extensor apparatus and its antagonists, as well as the moment of force around the knee joint. This can be achieved using simple equipment, i.e. a cine camera, stroboscope, electromyography and electrogoniometer.

In the action of kicking a ball (Fig. 4.2), electro-

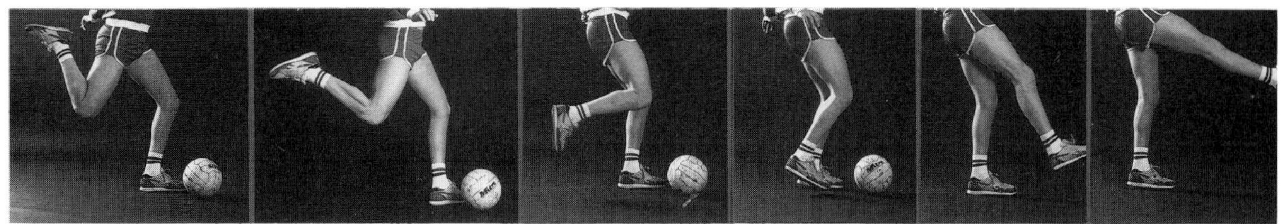

Fig. 4.2 The swing phase from flexion to full extension.

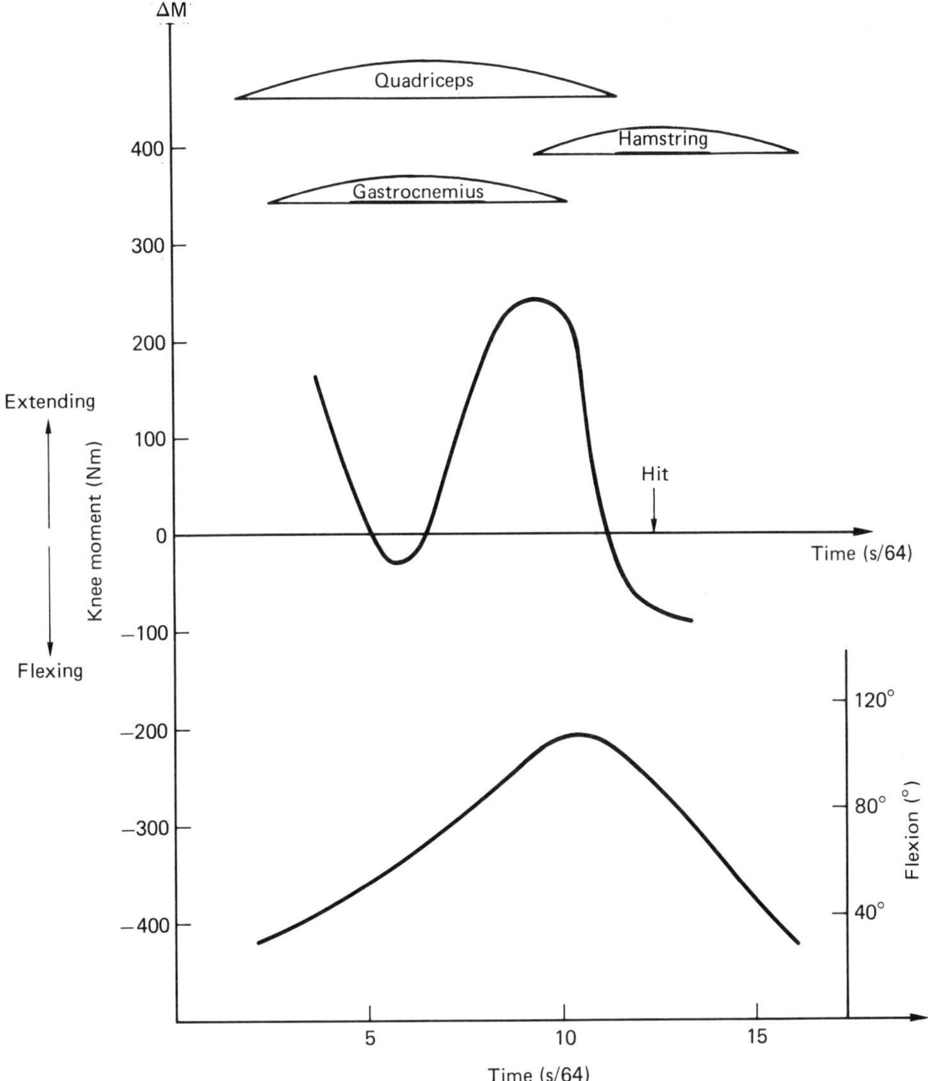

Fig. 4.3 Graph illustrating sequential contraction of agonists and antagonists. Knee moment (M) during the swing phase of kicking in relation to EMG activity (top) and knee angle (bottom). (From Wahrenberg *et al.*, 1978, with permission.)

myography demonstrates that maximum activity in the quadriceps group occurs very early, in the moment when flexion changes into extension, and this peak activity coincides with the calculated maximum moment of force at the knee joint, which occurs just after full flexion (Wahrenberg *et al.*, 1978). Electromyographic activity in the antagonist hamstring group is maximal much later in the swing phase, peaking just before contact with the ball. This muscle group therefore acts as a brake to hyperextension and, without it, much more strain would be put on passive structures, i.e. the ligaments and joint capsule, with increased risk of their rupturing (Fig. 4.3).

When these calculated maximum moments of force at the knee are translated into tensile force across the patellar tendon, and expressed as multiples of body weight, amazing values are obtained. For example, Wahrenberg *et al.* (1978) quote the tension across the patellar tendon occurring early

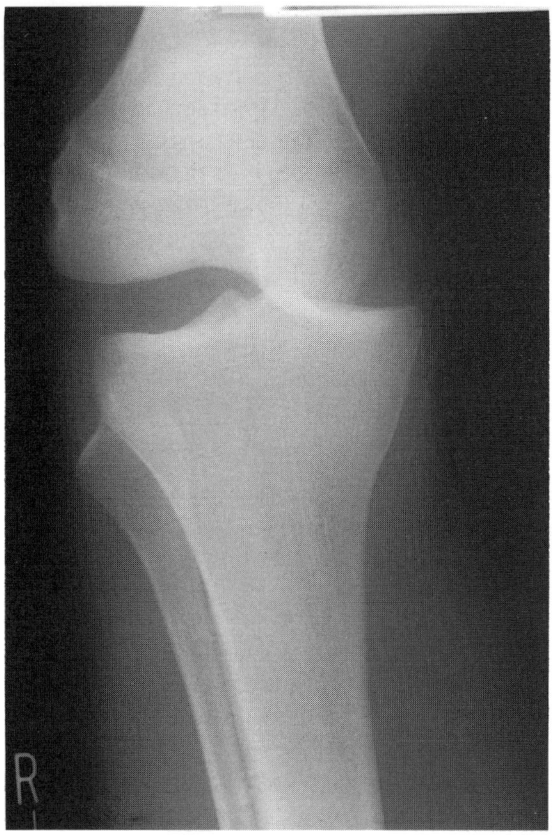

Fig. 4.4 Dislocation of the knee caused by an uneven surface in a long jump pit.

in the swing phase at more than four times body weight. This tensile force is uniform throughout the whole of the extensor apparatus and therefore it is not surprising that if it gives way it does so at the weakest point – the musculotendinous junction or occasionally the muscle belly itself. Any disturbance of the controlled swing of the leg, for example catching the toe in the ground before contacting the ball, will dramatically increase the tension in the extensors and the weakest link is even more likely to give way.

Contact with the ground adds a major extrinsic component to the total force acting across the knee. Obviously, however, under normal circumstances, the knee extensor and flexor mechanism deals more than adequately with the strains imparted during kicking a ball. In circumstances where that synergism between agonist and antagonist is disturbed (Grace *et al.*, 1984) injury is also

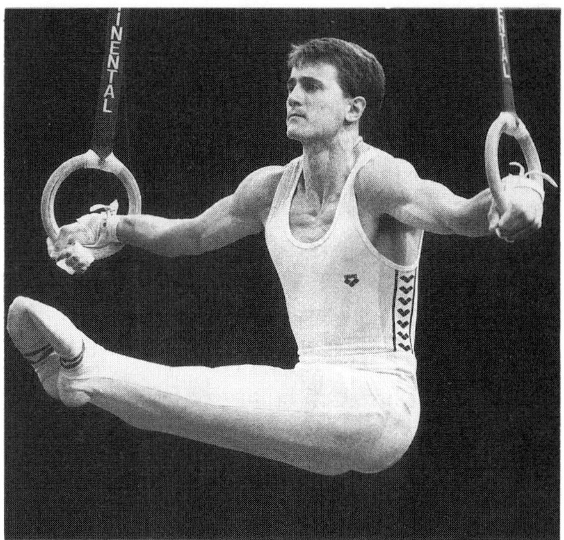

Fig. 4.5 The ultimate in synergism – the 'crucifix'. James May demonstrates.

more likely to occur. For example, there is a very complex interplay between eye–foot co-ordination and the proprioceptive impulses reaching the brain. Figure 4.4 shows an X-ray of a 16-year-old long jumper, who dislocated his knee when his landing foot sank into an unseen depression in the sand. A split second previously that same knee had easily withstood the thrust of take-off. Because he expected to feel a smooth surface under his landing foot, but instead landed in a hollow, the resultant disorganized combination of extensor and flexor contraction failed to protect the knee, which sustained severe damage. This is an extreme example of damage due to momentary loss of co-ordination, but it may be that many serious muscle tears are the result of similar incidents. The ultimate example of co–ordination between agonist and antagonist must be the gymnast's crucifix (Fig. 4.5).

Classification of muscle tears

The anatomical damage resulting from a tear may be classified as complete or partial, and a partial tear may be central or peripheral within the muscle belly.

Complete tear

Complete loss of continuity in a musculotendinous unit will obviously present as loss of function; for example, avulsion of the quadriceps insertion from the proximal pole of the patella presents as a loss of active knee extension. There may also be a palpable, if not visible, defect.

Partial tear

On the other hand, if the loss of continuity is not complete, loss of function will depend more on the severity of associated pain – if the pain is sufficiently intense there may be reflex inhibition of contraction of the muscle, which appears therefore to have lost function.

A central tear deep in the substance of the muscle belly is confined by surrounding intact fibres, therefore oedema and haemorrhage from the injured tissues accumulate under pressure, causing intense pain and secondary loss of function. The haematoma has little opportunity to disperse, therefore rehabilitation is slower.

A peripheral tear, on the other hand, is one in which bleeding from ruptured fibres and vessels disperses rapidly along interstitial planes. Pain is therefore less severe, recovery quicker and dysfunction less. Dramatic bruising may appear distally having tracked down along interstitial planes, for example, bruising around the ankle may appear several days after a rupture of one of the heads of gastrocnemius.

Pain from a muscle tear therefore is largely the result of pressure from the associated haemorrhage. Interestingly, equivalent injury in relatively atrophic elderly muscle tends to be much less painful because of the relatively small blood loss.

As described above, the actual damage to muscle may not be localized and may present as generalized stiffness and tenderness along the length of the muscle due to multiple microtears. These injuries are described rather vaguely as pulled or strained muscle.

Less commonly, if one of the larger veins or arteries is damaged within muscle substance there may be a local accumulation of blood. This may become trapped by surrounding fibrous tissue and an encysted haematoma may result. This will present as persistent local tenderness and loss of function and may be apparent clinically as a palpable cystic swelling and its presence may be confirmed by ultrasonic investigation. This condition will very slowly but gradually regress, but there is a risk of secondary infection causing abscess formation. Once diagnosed, it is wiser to aspirate such a haematoma, or in some instances perhaps even to perform a surgical drainage, and by so doing accelerate return to normal function and eliminate the risk of infection. Such a complication in an otherwise healthy young male would raise the possibility of a bleeding diathesis such as haemophilia and therefore it would be advisable to perform a screen of coagulation studies before embarking on surgical evacuation.

Radiological investigation

The radiological investigation of soft tissue trauma could be regarded as largely superfluous. Adequate clinical examination and a history of the mechanism of injury ought to provide a reliable estimation of the nature and severity of the injury. However, there are a few instances where such investigation might influence treatment, e.g. ultrasound investigation of an intramuscular fluid collection, as mentioned above.

Magnetic resonance imaging will no doubt play an increasing role in the future and some startling images have been published (Bassett and Gold, 1989) (Fig. 4.6).

Vascular injuries of muscle

Vascular compromise of muscle presents in several forms of varying severity.

Cramp

Cramp is an experience with which everyone must be familiar at some time. It consists of an extremely painful, strong muscular spasm, in response either to ischaemia or to metabolic imbalance.

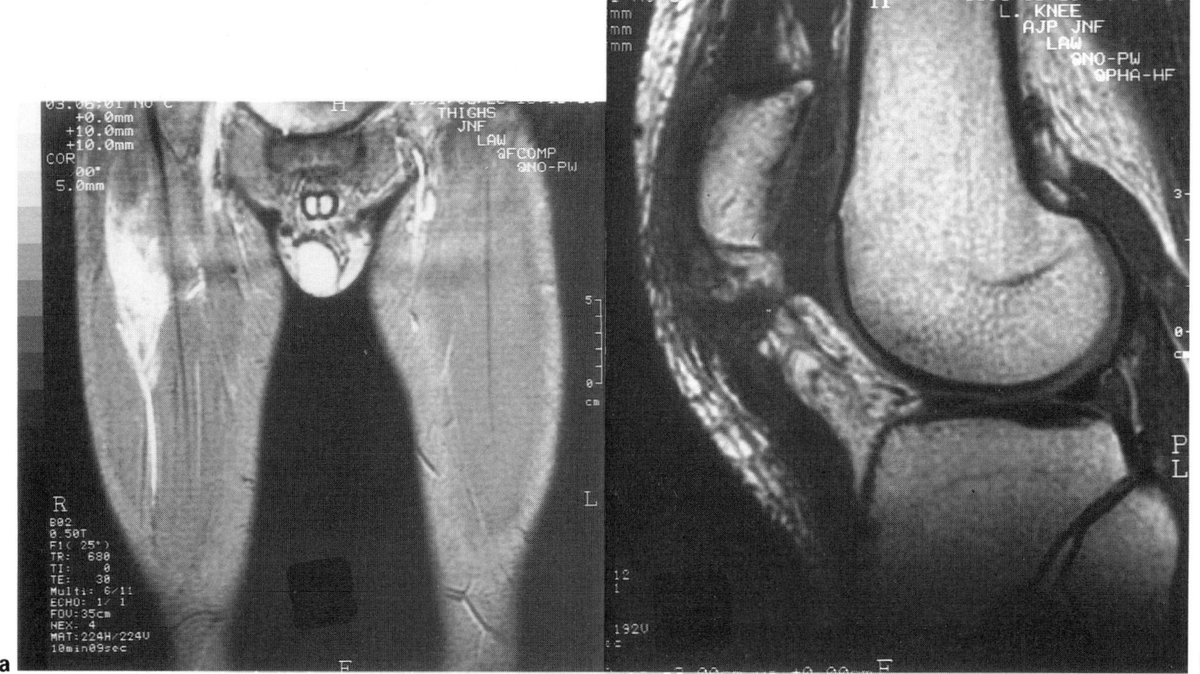

Fig. 4.6 (a) Coronal T2 weighted MRI scan showing a large collection of blood (the white signal) at the site of an acute tear of vastus lateralis muscle. (b) Lateral T1 weighted MRI scan of the knee showing a complete rupture of the patellar tendon – a further example of the excellent imaging of soft tissues available using MRI. (Courtesy of Dr Arnold Williams.)

Ischaemic claudication

Claudication pain in the calves is the hallmark of arteriosclerosis. In these patients, the blood supply to muscles is barely adequate at rest; after muscular work the severely compromised circulation is unable to respond to the demand for increased supply of oxygen, the muscle becomes acutely ischaemic and contracts fiercely in acute painful spasm. This form of cramp usually responds to resting the limb for a few minutes to allow the blood supply to be restored.

Metabolic claudication

The acute cramp experienced in sport has a different aetiology. Prolonged muscular activity and intense competitive exertion lead to excessive loss of fluid by sweating, the purpose of which is, of course, to promote surface cooling by evaporation. Sweat contains a very significant concentration of electrolytes, the most relevant being sodium. Hyponatraemia affects the level of excitability of motor units, hence the development of acute spasm. Controversy exists as to the exact mechanism causing cramp. There may be a superadded element of ischaemic claudication. Since muscle is not perfused during contraction, arterial inflow occurs only between contractions. Prolonged spasm, therefore, will shut off the blood supply encouraging further spasm due to ischaemia.

Treatment

Treatment consists initially of vigorous massage which induces relaxation of spasticity and increased vasodilation, combined with either passive or active stretching of the muscle which is in spasm. Active dorsiflexion of the foot will not only stretch the painful calf muscles but will increase the physiological stretch by contracting the antagonists. Passive dorsiflexion may be instigated by the attending trainer to achieve relief of the acute painful spasm. Prevention consists of avoiding prolonged excessive exertion, especially in hot conditions, and prophylactic extra salt intake.

Trainers often distribute salt tablets to players before a game to reduce the risk of cramp. Even here there is disagreement – some authors consider that oral salt may aggravate the problem because of its osmotic effect, drawing fluid into the lumen of the gut and therefore increasing fluid loss from the circulation (Sperryn, 1983).

It must not be forgotten that any apparently minor obstruction to circulation, for example, a tight garter, may be implicated in the aetiology of cramp.

Cramp in the athlete is most frequently seen in the hamstring group, but also occurs in the calf muscle, adductors, intrinsic muscles of the foot and in segments of the rectus abdominis muscle. The latter may be one cause of 'stitch', another experience with which most of us are very familiar but which is surprisingly poorly understood. The phenomenon of stitch is usually felt on the right-hand side of the abdomen. It often occurs when exercise takes place too soon after a meal, and may be an indication of ischaemic spasm of smooth muscle in the small or large bowel. The splanchnic circulation becomes relatively shut down in deference to the increase in skeletal muscle blood flow which occurs with exercise.

Chronic compartment syndromes

Several muscles and muscle groups are prone to acute and chronic ischaemia because of the nature of the restraining fascial envelope in which they lie (Fig. 4.7).

That which is most frequent is anterior compartment syndrome. Others are lateral compartment (peroneal), deep posterior, tibialis posterior compartment, and common extensor or flexor groups in the forearm. Syndromes included in this group are 'shin splints' and 'medial tibial stress' syndrome.

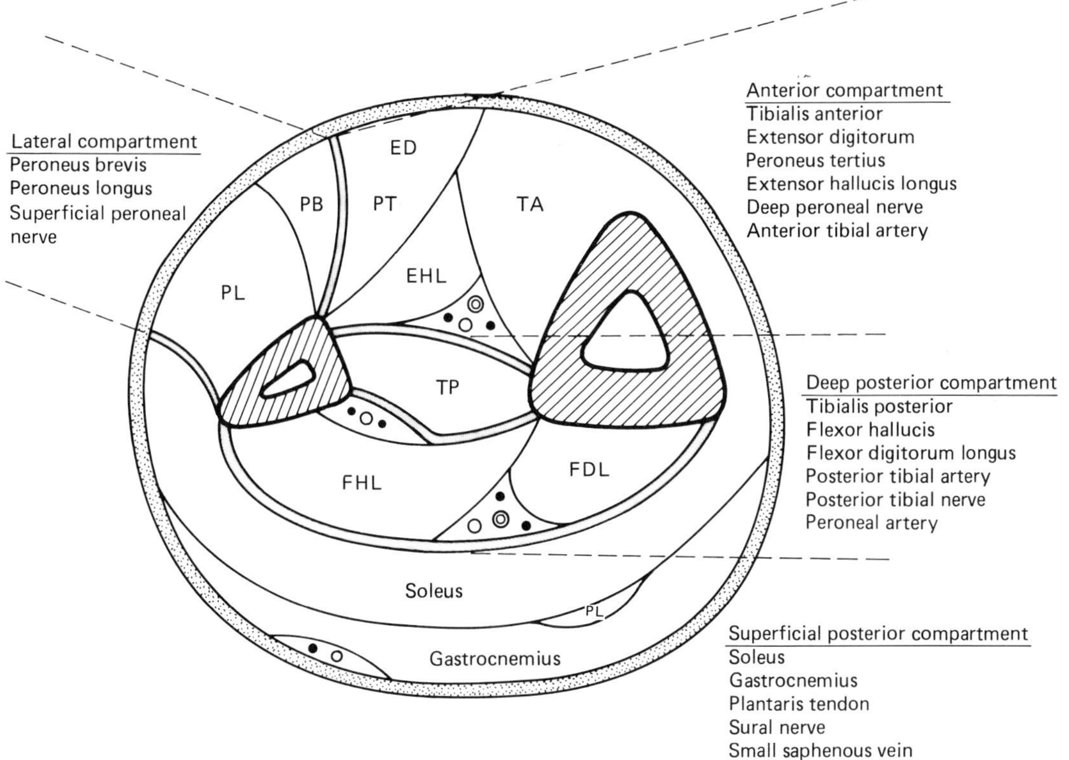

Fig. 4.7 Schematic cross-section of the middle of the lower leg demonstrating five separate compartments. The deep posterior compartment includes the tibialis posterior in its own compartment.

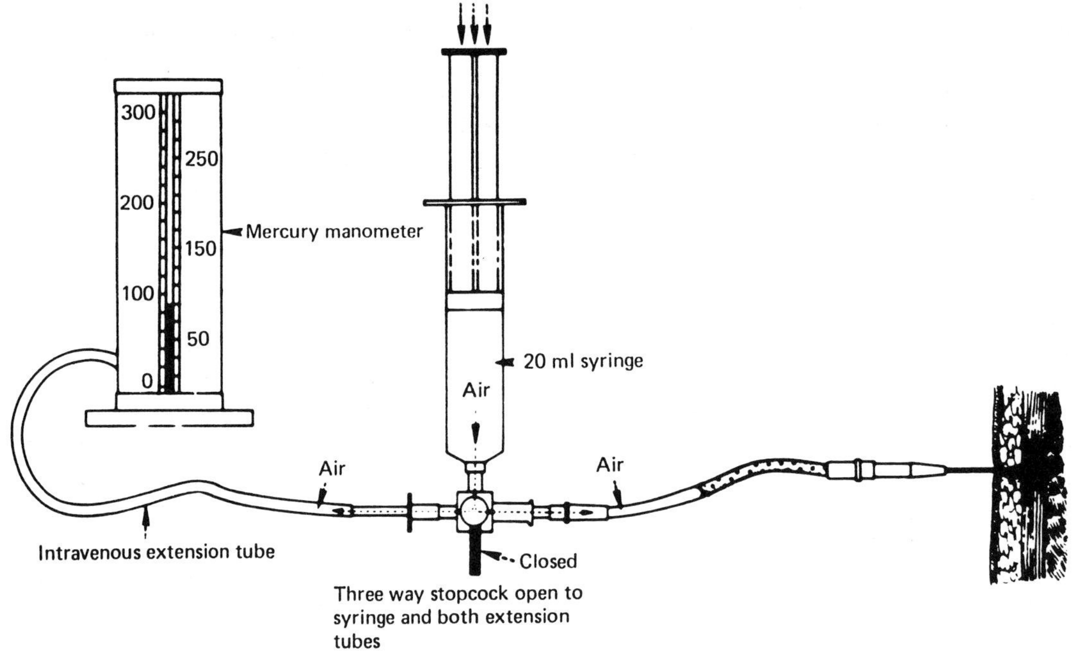

Fig. 4.8 A simple pressure transducer. From Whitesides *et al.* (1975), with permission.

It is possible that the same condition might affect the lumbar extensor muscles. After all, one of the toughest and most confining structures in the body is the lumbar fascia. Recurrent cramp-like lumbar pain with visible and palpable spasm in the erector spinae muscle groups might indicate a form of chronic compartment syndrome.

The criteria for diagnosis of chronic compartment syndromes are based largely on clinical features – signs and symptoms. Cramp-like pains build up on exertion: the longer the history, the earlier the onset of symptoms after the start of exercise. Depending on which muscle group is affected there is often visible and usually palpable and very tender contraction. Objective measurements can be made by various designs of pressure transducer, such as a wick (Mubarak *et al.*, 1976) or slit catheter. Whitesides (1975) described a fairly simple transducer system (Fig. 4.8) which provides reasonably accurate and reproducible readings, and obviously an accurate knowledge of anatomy is required to place the needle in the appropriate muscle for pressure testing. Other means of investigating compartment syndrome are by the xenon-133 clearance technique (Lassen *et al.*, 1964), microtip pressure transducer technique, and the microcapillary infusion technique (Styf and Korner, 1986). The latter provides dynamic measurements during exercise and at rest. Using this technique Styf *et al.* (1987) demonstrated that recording intramuscular pressure during activity was a reliable parameter in diagnosing chronic compartment syndrome. They showed that in muscle affected by the chronic syndrome there was an above-average resting pressure. Since muscle perfusion occurs during relaxation between contractions, the affected muscles become progressively more ischaemic because of the poor inflow during the relaxation phase. Hence the natural history of chronic compartment syndrome is a gradual worsening of symptoms, ischaemic episodes causing damage to a few fibres each time, with resulting scarring and loss of contractile ability.

Chronic anterior compartment syndrome

The anterior muscle compartment contains the muscle bellies of extensor hallucis longus, extensor digitorum, tibialis anterior and peroneus tertius. Overuse of this muscle group is often the result of badly fitting running shoes, or a change from training on soft to hard surfaces, or awkward gait, or constricting garters. An increased incidence was noted when wooden-soled sandals with a single strap were in vogue – the extra dorsiflexion required to keep the sandles on during the swing phase of the gait cycle was probably responsible for the overuse of the dorsiflexors of the foot. Symptoms in this syndrome develop insidiously with exercise and there may be visible and palpable spasm of the muscles in the anterior compartment.

Treatment

Treatment consists in the short term of rest, and a planned reduction in intensity of exercise. Appropriate attention to shoe design may be all that is required.

Sophisticated gait analysis, where available, may identify correctable faults. In the absence of response to these measures, surgery may be indicated, and therefore objective pressure measurements would be useful for reference postoperatively, as well as in identifying which other compartments might also be involved. If the compartment pressure measured with the muscle at rest is more than 35 mmHg the diagnosis is likely.

Surgical decompression of the anterior compartment for the chronic condition is a simple procedure. Through a 2–3-cm incision just lateral to the midpoint of the lateral border of the tibia, the fascia is identified, a small incision made, and then using either a Smillie knife or the slightly opened blades of a pair of dissecting scissors, the fascia is slit subcutaneously as far proximally and distally as possible.

Chronic lateral compartment syndrome

The lateral compartment contains peroneus longus and peroneus brevis muscles. Signs and symptoms are similar to those of the anterior compartment syndrome but the findings are localized to the peroneal compartment. The common peroneal nerve divides just distal to the neck of the fibula into the deep and superficial peroneal nerves. The deep peroneal nerve traverses the peroneal compartment for a short distance before entering the anterior compartment and therefore it may become secondarily affected by pressure necrosis in chronic lateral compartment syndrome. One of the presenting signs of this syndrome may be dysfunction of the deep peroneal nerve causing paralysis of the anterior compartment muscles but in the absence of spasm or pain in that compartment.

Shin splints

This is a term used to describe symptoms of pain along the subcutaneous border of the tibia or just medial to it. The other description of this condition is the medial tibial stress syndrome (Mubarak *et al.*, 1982). The literature is rather muddled regarding the cause – in fact it is likely that the terms cover several diagnoses.

Chronic compartment syndrome of the deep posterior compartment may be the cause; it may involve the whole of the posterior compartment, or be confined to the tibialis posterior muscle which is contained within its own separate fascial envelope and therefore may be affected in isolation (Davey *et al.*, 1984). Needle placement in measuring pressure in the deep peroneal compartment is ideally from a medial approach. The needle is advanced parallel to the posterior surface of the tibia; entrance into the tibialis posterior compartment is relatively easy and considerably safer than the anterior approach, in which injury to the posterior tibial artery or nerve is possible.

Ischaemic change in the posterior tibial and deep posterior compartments is probably more common than is often recognized. It has been reported that there is a significant incidence of contracture of flexor hallucis longus following closed fracture of the tibia, resulting in a degree of clawing of the toes and slight pes cavus, indicating a degree of ischaemia resulting from muscle injury at the time of fracture (Ellis, 1958).

The other possible cause of shin splints is stress fracture of the tibia. This is also a diagnosis which is probably more common than previously appreciated. The classical story is of 'crescendo' pain, i.e. becoming more intense and starting earlier with each training session. Conventional X-rays may be unhelpful in the early stages; the diagnosis may be confirmed either by computerized axial tomography scan or isotope bone scan.

Acute compartment syndrome

Acute compartment syndrome is a major surgical crisis. Fortunately it is not common. It is most usually the result of trauma, for example, fracture of the tibia, or severe crushing injury of a limb where contusion and laceration of muscles cause haemorrhage and swelling; there may also be direct injury to major vessels. Fascial sleeves remain intact, enclosing the damaged tissue and allowing a massive build-up of pressure. If decompression is not accomplished within 6–8 hours, permanent damage may result due to necrosis of muscle and nerve tissue. It has been shown that within 8 hours of acute compartment hypertension, 90% of muscle fibres show evidence of injury. Once necrosis is established there is secondary scar formation which engulfs the remaining normal tissue which is then involved in a generalized contracture. The secondary fibrosis involves any remaining intact nerves and muscle tissue so that there is progressive damage including paralysis, and of course the potential for infection of the dead tissue.

Many authorities in the past have suggested that the presence of a compound wound after fracture prevents the development of an acute compartment syndrome. However, the compound wound may not always act as a pressure-release valve – an understanding of the confining nature of the different facial compartments around the tibia, for example, explains why it is possible that the fractured bone ends may not tear into and decompress every compartment.

A further traumatic version of the syndrome is the ischaemic necrosis occurring in tissues distal to arterial occlusion. For example, a supracondylar fracture of the humerus may result in intimal damage to the brachial artery, acute ischaemia of the forearm muscles and resultant Volkmann's ischaemic contracture. Likewise, in a limb which has been replanted after traumatic amputation, it is vital to do a prophylactic decompression distally because the prolonged ischaemia results in tissue oedema and increased compartment pressure.

A similar disaster may occur without direct trauma however. Acute anterior or lateral compartment syndrome may present without prior warning, after a prolonged spell of strenuous and usually unaccustomed exercise.

Because the condition is not at all common, and in the absence of a history of trauma, it may be undiagnosed until too late, and permanent major damage may result, with resulting necrosis, possibly infection, and certainly late contracture and nerve dysfunction.

Aetiology

The aetiology following acute overuse is thought to be the result of oedema and multiple microhaemorrhages within the muscle fibres with the resulting build-up of pressure. Symptoms increase in the hours after excessive activity, often when the individual is relaxing or trying to sleep. Initially, she or he experiences cramp which fails to settle, but gradually it increases in intensity until the level of pain is excruciating. This is the first pointer to the diagnosis – severity of pain out of proportion to the clinical findings – the patient may even be in neurogenic shock.

Clinical findings

Clinical findings may be misleading, because although the increase in pressure may be enough to shut off arteriolar and capillary circulation and venous return, at least to begin with, major vessels may remain patent and therefore peripheral pulses are palpable. Nerves traversing the tight compartment may lose function at an early stage because of ischaemia and there may be loss of sensation in the toes (loss of sensation in the first web space indicates compromise of the deep personeal nerve). Another diagnostic sign is the dramatic increase in intensity of pain which occurs on passive stretching of the ischaemic muscle, i.e. passive plantarflexion of the foot or even of one toe induces dramatic exacerbation of the pain in anterior compartment compression. As explained above, major vessels are not occluded until late and so colour and temperature of the foot remain normal, which explains why the severity of this condition tends to be underestimated initially.

In the acute syndrome, clinical findings are so dramatic that direct measurement should rarely be necessary, and indeed may encourage procrastination, losing valuable minutes before surgical decompression is achieved. However, if it can be performed expediently, baseline measurement of the pressure in each compartment may help in planning the surgical decompression procedure.

Surgical treatment

Surgical intervention at an early stage will prevent permanent loss of function. High elevation of the limb and the application of ice will reduce damage during preparation for surgery and in transit to theatre.

Several surgical approaches have been described. If only the anterior compartment is affected, and if measurement of compartment pressures in the rest of the leg are within normal limits, then the surgical approach need only be directed to decompressing the anterior compartment. The subcutaneous procedure described under chronic compartment syndrome is usually inadequate in the acute situation, because pressure and swelling may be so great that the skin itself may contribute to the containment of pressure. It is therefore necessary to do a long skin and fascial incision to decompress the compartment adequately and it is usually necessary also to leave the skin open and plan a secondary skin graft. As described above, any fascial compartment may be the site of an acute compartment syndrome and it is therefore considered by many to be expedient to plan a wide decompression of all five compartments in the leg in the acute situation (anterior, peroneal, superficial posterior, deep posterior, and tibialis posterior). This can be achieved either by two separate incisions (posteromedial and anterolateral), or by removing a section of fibula which will decompress four of the five compartments (all except the superficial posterior).

Davey *et al.* (1984) described decompression of all five compartments through a single lateral incision. Of course, in surgery for acute compartment syndrome, it is unwise to use a tourniquet in case of further compromise to the vascular supply. Through a long lateral incision, first of all the skin is reflected anteriorly, allowing a long fasciotomy of the anterior and peroneal compartments. Reflecting the posterior edge allows decompression of the superficial posterior compartment. Thirdly, the incision is deepened between the superficial posterior and the peroneal compartments down to the posterior border of the fibula; periosteum is stripped off the back of the fibula until the tibialis posterior compartment is reached and then a wide fasciotomy is performed of that and of the deep posterior compartment. It may again be necessary to leave the skin incision widely open to maintain the decompression and to plan a split-skin graft at a later date.

Acute compartment syndrome can occur in other sites, for example, the forearm after weightlifting (Bird and McCoy, 1983) or in the thigh after blunt impact, causing muscle damage and bleeding. The syndrome has also been described in the posterior compartment of the thigh.

Crush syndrome

Systemic effects from extensive muscle injury present as crush syndrome. Once established, this condition may be fatal, from acute irreversible renal failure.

Injury of such severity may be the result of burial under masonry, or a mass of bodies, in disasters such as occur only too often and are so vividly and distressingly reported, for example the Hillsborough Football Stadium disaster. Prolonged muscle compression may also be the result of a non-traumatic event, for example prolonged prostration due to unconsciousness or stupor.

Crushed muscle leaks massive volumes of oedema fluid into the interstitial spaces, thus depleting circulating volume. The renal hypoperfusion which results is believed to be a major cause of the renal failure, but there are other possible causes. The full syndrome consists of a metabolic acidosis, myoglobinuria, hyperphosphataemia, hyperkalaemia, hyperuricaemia and, very rarely, coagulation defects. Accumulation of protein debris within the nephron may be one cause of acute renal failure, as may ischaemia, the result of circulatory collapse.

Clinical findings

Clinically, the crushed muscles are paralysed, with absent reflexes and altered overlying skin sensation. Myoglobin is macroscopically evident in urine as a red discoloration. Serum levels of inorganic phosphate, potassium and uric acid are high. The haematocrit is high and there may be a slight fall in platelet count. Urinary pH is low and a 24-hour collection of urine will reveal negative potassium balance; there will also be a raised serum creatine phosphokinase.

Treatment

It has been shown that the condition is reversible if treatment is started at a very early stage. The circulating fluid depletion develops rapidly, and treatment must initially involve rapid intravenous replacement of fluid with electrolyte solution, and the addition of adequate bicarbonate to counteract the acidosis. The infusion and diuresis are monitored carefully by measuring the central venous pressure and mannitol may be added to stimulate further renal flushing.

Ron *et al.* (1982) treated eight patients with major crushing injuries and in none of these cases did the full-blown crush syndrome develop, because they were able to institute immediate intravenous replacement at the site of the accident before transfer to hospital and before even the patients were released from compression. The escape of constituents from damaged muscle begins only after release from compression and continues for a variable length of time up to 60 hours. They therefore advocate an aggressive policy of immediate intravenous volume replacement to avoid the catastrophic renal damage which would otherwise result.

There is some controversy in the literature regarding the advisability of wide fasciotomy after crushing injury, the argument being that it is unlikely that the muscle could be damaged any further by compartment pressure than it had already been by extrinsic pressure. Many patients who initially did well following resuscitation later succumbed to devastating infection which entered via fasciotomy wounds (Reis and Michaelson, 1986).

Myositis ossificans

Myositis ossificans is a dramatic although uncommon sequel of muscle injury. Its incidence may be higher than appreciated since its diagnosis is mainly by radiological means (Fig. 4.9). For example, Jackson and Feagin (1973) reported 65 patients who had moderate to severe quadriceps contusion. In 18 of these cases the contusion was considered to be severe and these patients were X-rayed: 13 of the 18 were found to have myositis ossificans. However, of the remaining 47 patients none was considered to have any more than

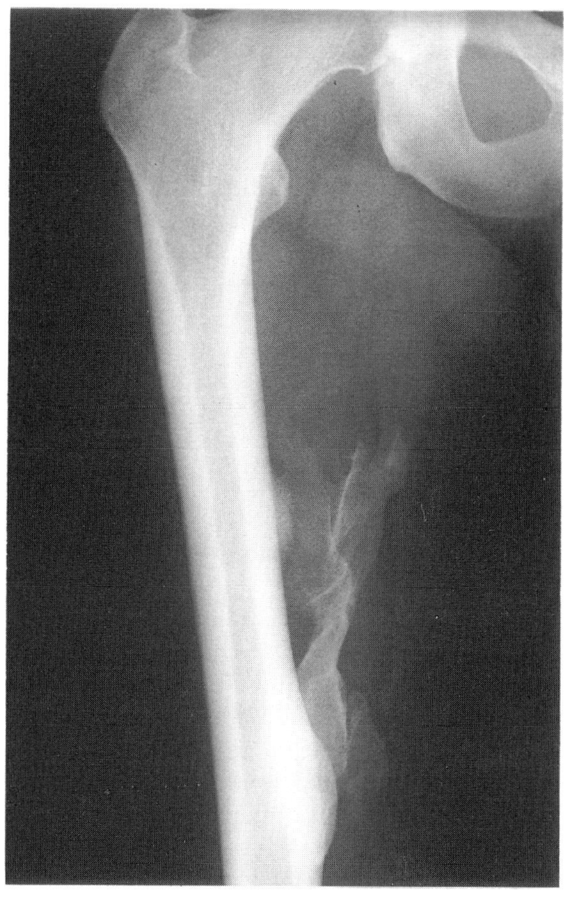

Fig. 4.9 Myositis ossificans of the thigh after quadriceps contusion.

moderate muscle damage and they were not routinely X-rayed, and therefore the true incidence of myositis was not recorded.

The condition is not always the result of trauma – only in 75% or so is there a history of injury. There is a variation reported which is not the result of trauma, and also a very rare progressive form which is eventually fatal. The non-traumatic variant may occur in neurologically deficient patients, for example cerebral palsy, or after a severe head injury; the new bone formation is often periarticular compromising joint function, and may be associated with a systemic febrile illness. In these cases, surgery is occasionally necessary to restore joint function. Interestingly, the incidence of myositis ossificans is higher in cases of traumatic paraplegia than it is in non-traumatic paraplegia – this is thought to be due to gross disturbance of spinal cord reflex activities. Myositis ossificans appears to occur only in those muscles whose nerve supply arises below the level of cord damage.

Aetiology

The aetiology of myositis ossificans is incompletely understood. The post-traumatic type is usually seen around the middle third of the femur although it can occur at other sites, for example the glutei, adductors, or after a supracondylar fracture of the humerus, in which case it appears within the brachialis muscle. Its occurrence at these sites after injury implies that laceration or contusion of muscle substance has a role to play in its aetiology. The main initiating factor is probably interstitial haemorrhage, although muscle necrosis may also play a part. The free blood lying within muscle fibres causes irritation, and oedematous, inflammatory exudate is produced and is invaded by a mass of collagenoblasts. The collagen produced is unusual in that it appears to attract the deposition of mineral i.e. dystrophic calcification. Osteoblasts then appear either invading from neighbouring periosteum, or perhaps by metaplasia of collagenoblasts in response to the heterotopic mineral. Islands of osteoid appear within the collagen until an open network of new bone appears within the muscle belly. Exercise appears to predispose to further proliferation if it is encouraged before the new bone has matured.

Classically, differentiation microscopically between this ectopic bone and osteosarcoma is very difficult. Both conditions show numerous hyperchromatic osteoblasts amid irregular masses of crude osteoid. The differentiating features are that myositis ossificans is usually post-traumatic, as explained above, the cellular components are more organized, cellular activity at the periphery is more like reaction than neoplasia, and the mass is more likely to be well-circumscribed. Also the presence of normal muscle fibres within the osteoid rules out osteosarcoma. Wider examination of myositis ossificans shows a 'zoned' arrangement – central areas are very difficult to differentiate from osteosarcoma but peripherally the tissue is better organized, with muscle fibres included in it. In contrast, osteosarcoma destroys muscle fibres as it advances.

The myositis ossificans may mature into classical cortical bone with cancellous tissue in the middle. It may involve the periosteum and appear on X-ray as cortical thickening or it may grow on a 'stalk'.

Clinical presentation

Post-traumatic myositis ossificans may be suspected if, after injury, the thigh remains swollen, hot and tender for longer than had been anticipated. Knee flexion is persistently very painful and difficult – partly due to the inflammatory nature of the condition and partly to the tethering of the muscle involved in the ossifying process. The erythrocyte sedimentation rate may be raised during the inflammatory phase, and an X-ray taken as early as the second week after trauma shows heterotopic bone.

Treatment

It is well-known that if too much movement is encouraged, the condition tends to progress and involve a larger volume of normal muscle, therefore advice must be to reach a compromise –

resting the affected limb to the extent that the joints above and below should be put through only that range of movement which is painfree. Isometric exercises will maintain some tone in the muscle, since obviously too much enforced inactivity will necessitate very prolonged rehabilitation. Physical modalities such as massage, ultrasound, etc. will result in a delay in maturation and may in fact encourage enlargement of the process. Serial X-rays will demonstrate the process of maturation of the new bone, and once a recognizable lamellar structure is visible, it is unlikely that this condition will progress further.

Prognosis

It is unusual for the established new bone in the quadriceps to compromise muscle action significantly. In Jackson and Feagin's series quoted above, only one patient out of 13 required surgical removal of the lesion to allow return to normal function. The natural history of the condition is that either it becomes so well-circumscribed that it does not obstruct normal muscle and joint function, or it may slowly resolve until it is no longer apparent on X-ray. The lesion affecting brachialis after supracondylar fracture of the humerus is more often removed surgically, because of its proximity to the elbow joint. It may interfere not only with extension of the elbow but, more importantly, it may represent a bony block to flexion. The recommendation is usually to wait until the radiological appearance is of mature bone (usually 6–12 months after injury) before surgical intervention. Dissecting the lesion too early may provoke further myositis. Surgical removal must be followed by 10–14 days of complete immobilization, otherwise a recurrence may appear, even if the lesion seemed mature when removed.

Viral myositis

Some viruses cause muscle damage as part of the overall systemic infective process. Experimentally induced viral myositis in animals has been shown microscopically to consist of a necrotizing myopathy, but this process is usually reversible, for example, in coxsackieviruses, influenza and Bornholm's myalgia. Characteristically, there is generalized malaise associated with muscular pain and stiffness. The muscular symptoms tend to worsen with exercise and therefore rest is a major part of the treatment for these conditions. With recovery the oedema is dispersed and damaged muscle fibres are removed by phagocytosis and usually there is complete recovery.

Rehabilitation and prevention

A structured programme of treatment and rehabilitation after muscle injury is based on a knowledge of the physiology of healing. These principles can be applied immediately after injury, even on the field of play.

Immediate treatment

The mnemonic RICE is well-known.

Rest

As outlined above in the description of the work by Jarvinen and others, after any muscle injury which involves a break in continuity of muscle fibres there is a critical initial period during which the haematoma is becoming organized with deposition of collagen fibres and a gradual increase in tensile strength. Tension through this scar formation too early will result in its disruption, creating a larger scar and more prolonged recovery.

Ice

Any means of cooling the injured area will encourage vasoconstriction and therefore minimize the microhaemorrhages within the injury as well as generally slowing down the rate of metabolism and formation of metabolites.

Compression

Direct pressure over an injury will further restrict local bleeding as well as providing a degree of support of the injured limb, and therefore transport away from the field of play is a degree more comfortable. Of course, it is important that compression is applied correctly; for example, in the thigh muscle injury, there has to be a wide area of compression bandaging including the whole of the thigh and not localized simply to the level of muscle rupture, since the latter may produce a degree of venous obstruction and result in oedema of the lower limb, which in turn may further promote swelling of the actual injury site.

Elevation

By raising the injured limb above the horizontal level, gravity will encourage free drainage away from the injury, thus reducing tissue congestion.

Drug treatment of acute muscle injury

Analgesia

Of course, there will be instances where pain is sufficiently severe to warrant parenteral strong analgesia, even opiates. The judicious use of such drugs in appropriate circumstances may not relieve severe pain but will reduce the associated restlessness, and therefore tend to lessen subsequent damage to the injured limb. There must always be a high index of suspicion, however, that a patient experiencing agonizing pain which seems out of proportion to the injury may be developing an acute compartment syndrome.

Non-steroidal anti-inflammatory drugs

These drugs have a very valuable role to play in the primary treatment of soft tissue injuries, one of the most appropriate being salicylic acid (aspirin) which is not only a very affective analgesic but also has anti-inflammatory properties which are very well-tried and tested. However, the side-effects of aspirin are also well-known and must be respected, and therefore this drug is contraindicated in many patients. The many other non-steroidal anti-inflammatory agents on the market have been appropriately and very effectively used in reducing the inflammatory process in the acute injury.

Local applications

Several preparations are now available of anti-inflammatory agents in a gel form, for example, benzydamine hydrochloride, piroxicam and diclofenac. The efficacy of these preparations probably lies in the transporting agent which carries the active drug through the skin. It is also likely that these preparations are most effective on injuries which are immediately subcutaneous, rather than large-volume muscle injuries such as in the thigh.

There are other well-known preparations in cream form which create a local increase in heat on the skin and therefore act as counterirritants, for example, Wintergreen, or turpentine and camphor preparations. Of course, the massage which is required to apply these ointments is probably also a significant part of the therapeutic effect. Paradoxically, local cooling can also have a counterirritant effect, for example aerosol sprays such as PR, but of course any beneficial effect is very short-lived.

Local anaesthetic

The injection of local anaesthetic into localized sites of pain in acute trauma can only be regarded as foolhardy. Pain is, after all, a protective mechanism to prevent further damage to injured tissue. By abolishing the pain, the inhibitory reflexes are not active and therefore further muscle damage will occur with continued use of the injured part.

Enzymes

Proteolytic enzymes such as trypsin, chymotrypsin, hyaluronidase and streptokinase have been used in both tablet and injectable form, the aim being to disperse the oedema and inflammatory reaction. It is not generally accepted that proteolytic preparations are appropriate in acute trauma.

Steroids

Corticosteroids, for example hydrocortisone and triamcinolone, are widely used in the treatment of soft tissue injuries, but since the effect is catabolic rather than anabolic their use in the acute injury is probably limited. In the chronic injury they can be very effective agents, introduced by injection into the precise area of injury, since they not only suppress the inflammatory process but also encourage resolution of chronic fibrous adhesions.

Anabolic steroids

The effect of anabolic steroids on muscle is to promote the synthesis of protein by increasing nitrogen retention and by an increase of the synthesis of RNA. This, combined with weight-training, increases muscle bulk and therefore strength, especially for events which require explosive power, for example weight-lifting and shot-put. There can be no doubt that anabolic steroids increase muscle bulk but the contention that strength is also increased has never been scientifically proven – clinical trials are not possible because no clinician would consider prescribing steroids in the high doses which athletes administer to themselves (Bergman and Leach, 1985). It may be that the advantageous effects athletes obtain from high-dose steroids are to a larger extent due to the euphoria which they induce (Ryan, 1976).

Rehabilitation programmes

After injury, the ST fibres are found to atrophy first. The FT fibres atrophy secondarily, mainly because pain inhibits their function. Therefore a rehabilitation programme should concentrate initially on building up the ST fibre strength first.

During the initial painful phase in the presence of swelling and irritation, isometric exercises will maintain muscle tone without risking stretching the developing scar formation. At a later stage isotonic exercises are introduced and finally isokinetic work is started in which the speed of working is controlled but the resistance to movement is varied.

Providing this gradual return to function is followed, there should be little risk of re-injury, but often it is the athlete's own overenthusiasm which is the reason for re-injury and delayed return to full sporting activity.

Prevention

The value of a warm-up before competition is the prevention of injury during the more strenuous effort which is to follow. Exercises which encourage suppleness in cold muscle produce an immediate beneficial effect by increasing blood flow and flexibility between individual fibres, so that the muscles are less tight when competition starts. The increase in the muscle circulation and also in the respiration rate and cardiac output conveys more oxygen to muscle cells and speeds up the metabolic process. An efficient warm-up raises the body core temperature by 2–3°C, during which the metabolic efficiency of muscle action increases by 10% or more per 1°C. Consequently, the muscles are better able to withstand sudden sharp contraction and are therefore less likely to be injured.

References

Allbrook DB, Baker W deC, Kirkaldy-Willis WH (1966) Muscle regeneration in experimental animals and in man. *Journal of Bone and Joint Surgery* **488**, 153.

Allbrook DB (1973) Acceleration of muscle regeneration within previously denervated whole muscle autotransplant. Proceedings of the Anatomical Society of Australia and New Zealand.

Anderson P (1975) Capillary density in skeletal muscle of man. *Acta Physiologica Scaninavica* **95**, 203.

Bassett LW, Gold RH (1989) Magnetic resonance imaging of the musculo skeletal system – an overview. *Clincial Orthopaedics and Related Research* **244**, 17.

Bergh U, Thorstensson A, Sjodin B et al. (1978)

Maximal oxygen uptake and muscle fibre types in trained and untrained humans. *Medicine and Science in Sports* **10**, 15.

Bergman R, Leach RE (1985) Uses and abuses of anabolic steroids in Olympic-caliber athlete. *Clinical Orthopaedics and Related Research* **198**, 169.

Bird CB, McCoy JW (1983) Weight-lifting as a cause of compartment syndrome in the forearm – a case report. *Journal of Bone and Joint Surgery* **65A**, 406.

Boobis LH (1987) A study of human muscle metabolism in relation to exercise, training and peripheral vascular disease. MD thesis, University of Leicester, p 262.

Booth FW (1977) Time course of muscular atrophy during immobilisation of hind limbs of rats. *Journal of Applied Physiology* **43**, 656.

Carlson BM (1972) *The Regeneration of Minced Muscles*. London: S Karger.

Carlson BM (1973) The regeneration of skeletal muscle – review. *American Journal of Anatomy* **137**, 119.

Davey JR, Rorabeck CH, Fowler PJ (1984) The tibialis posterior muscle compartment: an unrecognised cause of exertional compartment syndrome. *American Journal of Sports Medicine* **12**, 391.

de Vries HA (1960) Electromyographic observations of the effects of static stretching upon muscular distress. *Research Quarterly* **32**, 468.

Ellis H (1958) Disabilities after tibial shaft fractures with special reference to Volkmann's ischaemic contracture. *Journal of Bone and Joint Surgery* **40B**, 190.

Grace TG, Sweetser ER, Nelson MA et al. (1984) Isokinetic muscle imbalance and knee-joint injuries. *Journal of Bone and Joint Surgery* **66A**, 734.

Jackson DW, Feagin JA (1973) Quadriceps contusion in young athletes. *Journal of Bone and Joint Surgery* **55A**, 95.

Jarvinen M (1975). Healing of a crush injury in rat striated muscle. (A histological study of the effect of early mobilisation and immobilisation on the repair process.) *Acta Pathological et Microbiologica Scandinavica Section A* **83**, 269.

Jarvinen M (1976a) Healing of a crush injury in rat striated muscle. (A micro-angiographical study of the effect of early mobilisation on capillary ingrowth.) *Acta Pathologica et Microbiologica Scandinavica Section A* **84**, 85.

Jarvinen M (1976b) Healing of a crush injury in rat striated muscle. (Effect of early mobilisation and immobilisation on the tensile properties of gastrocnemius muscle.) *Acta Chirurgica Scandinavica* **142**, 47.

Lassen NA, Lindbjerg J, Munck O (1964) Measurement of blood-flow through skeletal muscle by intramuscular injection of Xenon-133. *Lancet* 686.

Lehto M, Duance VC, Restall D (1985) Collagen and fibronectin in a healing skeletal muscle injury. *Journal of Bone and Joint Surgery* **67B**, 820.

Mubarak SJ, Hargens AR, Owen CA et al. (1976) The wick catheter technique for measurement of intramuscular pressure. A new research and clinical tool. *Journal of Bone and Joint Surgery* **58A** 1016.

Mubarah SJ, Gould RN, Lee YF et al. (1982) The medial tibial stress syndrome: a cause of shin splints. *American Journal of Sports Medicine* **10**, 201.

Parkhouse WS, MacKenzie DC (1984) Possible contribution of skeletal muscle buffers to enhanced anaerobic performance: a brief review. *Medicine and Science in Sports and Exercise* **16**, 328.

Parkhouse WS, McKenzie DC, Hochachka PW et al. (1985) Buffering capacity of deproteinised human vastus lateralis muscle. *Journal of Applied Physiology* **58**, 14.

Reis ND, Michaelson M (1986) Crush injury to the lower limbs. *Journal of Bone and Joint Surgery* **68A**, 414.

Ron D, Taitelman U, Michaelson M et al. (1982) Prevention of acute renal failure in traumatic rhabdomyolysis. *Archives of Internal Medicine* **144**, 277.

Ryan AJ (1976) Anabolic and androgenic steroids. In: Kochakian CD (ed.) *Handbook of Experimental Pharmacology* vol. 43, 515. Springer-Verlag.

Sanderson RA, Foley RK, McIvor GWD et al. (1975) Histological response of skeletal muscle to ischaemia. *Clinical Orthopaedics and Related Research* **113**, 27.

Sharp RL, Costill DL, Fink WJ et al. (1986) Effects of eight weeks of bicycle ergometer sprint training on human muscle buffer capacity. *International Journal of Sports Medicine* **7**, 13.

Sperryn PN (1983) *Muscle and Training Adaptations in Sports and Medicine*. London: Butterworths, p. 51.

Styf J, Korner L (1986) Microcapillary infusion technique for measurement of intramuscular pressure during exercise. *Clinical Orthopaedics and Related Research* **207**, 253.

Styf J, Korner L, Suurkula M (1987) Intramuscular pressure and muscle blood flow during exercise in chronic compartment syndrome. *Journal of Bone and Joint Surgery* **69B**, 301.

Wahrenberg H, Lindbeck L, Ekholm J (1978) Knee muscular movement, tendon tension force and e.m.g. during a vigorous movement in man. *Scandinavian Journal of Rehabilitation Medicine* **10**, 99.

Whitesides JE Jr *et al.* (1975) A simple method for tissue pressure determination. *Archives of Surgery* **110**, 1311.

Whitesides JE Jr et al. (1975) Tissue pressure measurements as a determinant of the need for fasciotomy. *Clinical Orthopaedics and Related Research* **113**, 43.

5

Management of the acutely injured joint

L. Paulos
M. Kody

Management of the acutely injured joint is changing as traditional tenets of treatment are gradually replaced with new rules based on scientific advances. In the past, joint injuries were immobilized and diagnosis often postponed until the acute phase of pain and swelling was completed. It is now clear that prolonged immobilization is detrimental and frequently promotes debilitating and irreversible joint stiffness and weakening. Currently, emphasis is on early, accurate diagnosis and treatment.

Treatment of the acute injury

Rest, ice, compression and elevation remain the acute-phase treatments to be instituted as soon after injury as possible. Thereafter, an accurate history with emphasis on the mechanism of injury should be taken. Clinical examination and stress testing usually lead to accurate diagnosis which can then be confirmed or altered in accordance with radiographic evaluation. The examiner categorizes injuries based on the degree of pathological laxity: grade I sprains are categorized as minor injuries; grade II injuries are incomplete ruptures; grade III sprains indicate complete ruptures.

Diagnoses and treatments for the ligamentous and capsular injuries in specific joints are detailed below.

The ankle

Injury to the deltoid ligament

Injury to this ligament occurs with pronation, eversion and external rotation stress to the foot and is manifested by point tenderness and swelling on the medial malleolus. Since the deep and superficial structures of the deltoid are very wide and broad, complete ligamentous disruption is rarely without fracture. Fracture and syndesmotic widening should be verified by radiography following the physical examination (under anaesthesia) for medial instability. Partial injuries are treated with weight-bearing as tolerated, rapid mobilization, and aggressive physical therapy as suggested by Cox (1985). Open repair is mandatory for the rare cases of complete injury where the ligament is interposed in the joint and blocks reduction of the mortise. In all other cases, operative and non-operative therapy seem to offer equivalent results (Colville *et al.*, 1987).

Injury to the lateral complex ligaments

Much more controversy surrounds management of the lateral ligaments, the most commonly injured in the body. This ligament complex consists of the anterior talofibular ligament (ATF), the calcaneofibular ligament (CF) and the posterior talofibular ligament (PTL). Injury

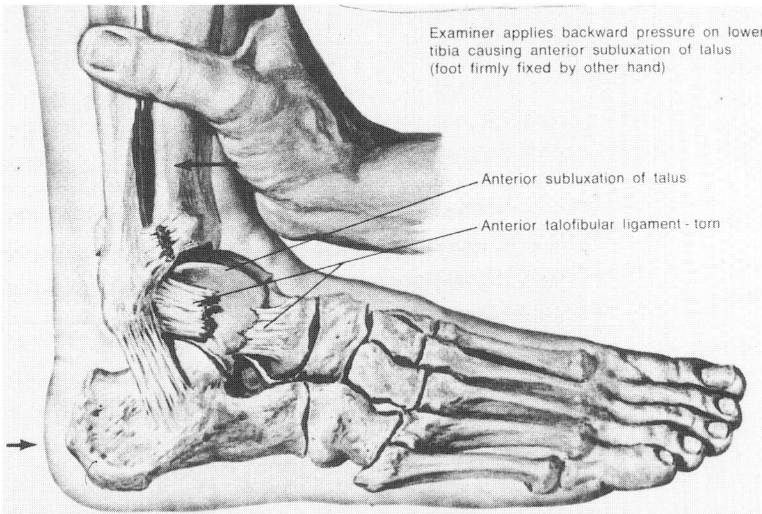

Fig. 5.1 Anterior drawer test for instability of the ankle.

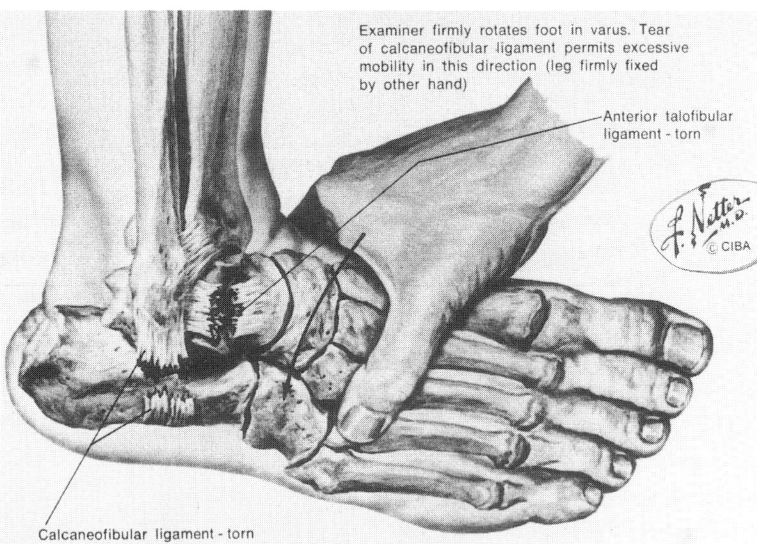

Fig. 5.2 Talar tilt test.

usually results from supination and inversion stress to the foot with external rotation of the tibia and is manifested by lateral pain and swelling.

Proper treatment depends on correctly assessing the magnitude of the injury. Complete rupture of the AFT leads to a positive anterior draw sign when the foot is in the plantigrade (Grace, 1984) position or when the foot is plantiflexed 10° (Larsen, 1986). The rupture can be documented by radiography, which will show a 3 mm difference in the position of the injured ankle with respect to the other (Anderson and Le Coq, 1954; Brostrom, 1966) or a difference of 6 mm in position with stress as described by Grace (1984). Stewart has diagnosed rupture of the calcaneofibular ligament if there is a difference of 8–10° in talar tilt between the two limbs. According to Bonin (1950), less than 15° difference indicates that only the ATF is torn, while a difference greater than 30° shows that all three ligaments are torn (Fig 5.1–5.3).

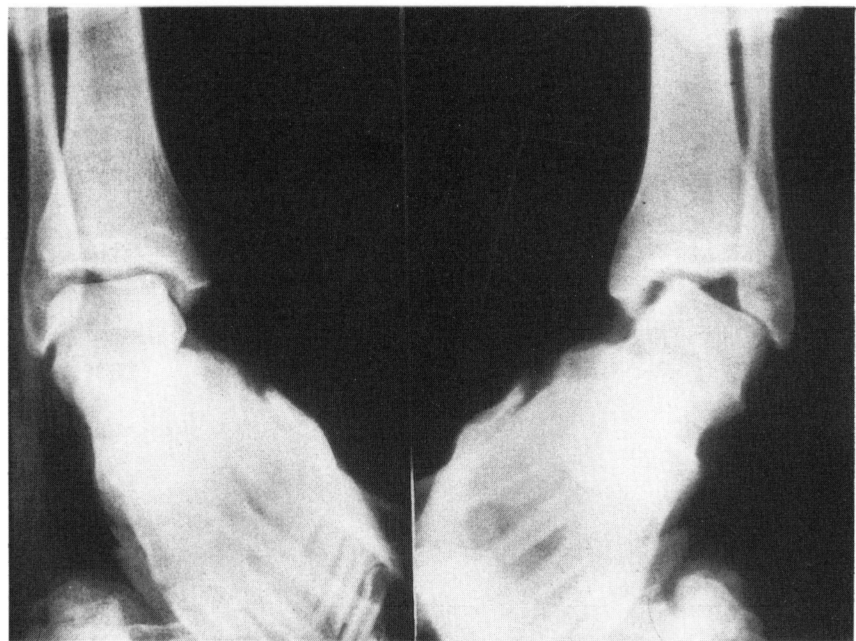

Fig. 5.3 Stress radiograph revealing excessive talar tilt consistent with lateral instability.

Controversy prevails over conservative versus operative therapy. Staples (1975) found that only 58% of patients with rupture of the lateral ligamentous complex were asymptomatic after conservation therapy, whereas early surgical repair yielded much-improved results. Comparing the results of strapping, casting and surgery in patients with arthrogram ligament ruptures, Brostom (1966) found primary surgical repair superior to non-operative treatment; there was 3% residual instability in the operated group and 20% amongst the non-operated. The earliest return to work occurred with strapping, which was as effective as casting. Niedermann *et al.* (1981) compared 107 conservatively treated ankle ruptures to 102 surgically treated ruptures and found good results in 76 and 81% respectively. Evans *et al.* (1984) divided 100 ankle sprains into two groups – those with isolated ATF tears (30 patients) and those with both ATF and CF tears (20 patients). The operative group experienced more complications and delayed return to work; there was no difference in the end-result for the two groups.

We treat ATF tears by muscle strengthening, taping and sometimes use a laced ankle corset. Although opinions vary on taping – in measuring talar tilt in athletes with unstable ankles, Vaes *et al.* (1985) showed that taping was superior to adhesive bandages, while Larsen (1984) concluded that taping offered little or no support after 20 min exercise – we find taping produces subjective benefits to patients, especially during the early stages of healing. We also believe that conservative treatment for ATF and CF injuries result in good or excellent results in 85% of patients. Delayed ankle reconstructions are done in cases where conservative treatment has failed. Our experience is supported by Cass *et al.* (1985) who document no difference in final results on comparing primary repairs with delayed reconstruction. Their 10-year follow-up of Chrisman-Snook ankle reconstructions revealed that only three of 48 patients had fair or poor results; all three had severely re-injured their ankles after reconstruction.

For the rare instances of simultaneous rupture of the three ligaments, we usually do surgical repair.

Syndesmosis injury

The structures of the syndesmosis include the anterior and posterior tibiofibular, the inferior transverse and interosseous ligaments. Injury to the syndesmosis usually results from a pronation external injury. Symptoms are pain and swelling centred in the distal tibia and fibula. Diagnostic indicators are pain and characteristic widening between the tibia and fibula, best seen on the mortise radiograph. As Ramsey and Hilton (1976) have shown a 42% reduction in the area of contact between the tibia and talus with a 1 mm lateral shift of the talus, the importance of this injury cannot be overstated.

Patients with a reduced syndesmosis are placed in a non-weight-bearing cast for 6 weeks. If the distance between the tibia and talus is not reduced, we perform closed reduction under arthroscopic guidance followed by internal fixation with a 4.5 mm cortical screw placed through the fibula, the lateral cortex of the tibia, and approaching, but not capturing, the medial cortex. The cortical screw is never placed in a lag fashion. We advocate removal of the screw after 6–12 weeks, but we do not restrict weight-bearing while the screw is in place.

Ankle dislocation

Ankle dislocation is rarely without a related fracture. The mechanism of injury is inversion and axial loading in the maximally plantiflexed foot. Usually, it occurs posterior medially in the young, ligamentously lax patient. Closed dislocations can usually be treated non-surgically, but for open injuries incision, drainage, and primary repair of torn ligaments are required (Colville *et al.*, 1987).

Peroneal tendon dislocation

Peroneal tendon dislocation should not be mistaken for an ankle sprain. The dislocation may be caused by violent dorsiflexion with reflex contracture of the peronei, as described by Eckert and Davis (1976) and Escalas *et al.*, (1980), or by eversion as one edges a downhill ski turn (Escalas *et al.*, 1980). Afflicted patients usually complain of pain, swelling, popping, or the sensation of instability along the posterior lateral aspect of the ankle (Arrowsmith *et al.*, 1983). Palpation of the subluxed tendon is usually intolerable for the patient who exhibits retromalleolar pain and swelling. Frequently, the retinaculum avulses a piece of bone periosteum from the lateral malleolus; in 15–50% of cases, this shell of bone is visible on radiographs, especially from the mortise view (Murr, 1961). This finding is virtually pathognomonic for dislocation of the peroneal tendon.

Murr (1961) advocates operative treatment for all cases. Eckert and Davis (1976) also operated on all lesions. The conservative therapy of Escalas *et al.* (1980) failed in 28 of 30 patients. We manage all cases surgically, repairing torn structures or replacing avulsed periosteum to bone (Das and Balasubramaniam, 1985).

The shoulder

Procedures for evaluating shoulder injuries closely resemble those for other joints. Particular attention to the mechanism of injury and position of the arm on presentation often ensures accurate diagnosis. A full series of radiographs is mandatory. We prefer anteroposterior, trans-scapular and axillary views for each injured patient. After history, examination and X-rays have been done, the physician must determine whether other tests are required for an accurate diagnosis. Because of the complex anatomy of the shoulder, an arthrogram, computed tomography (CT) arthrogram or magnetic resonance imaging (MRI) scan may be needed for precise diagnosis.

Acromioclavicular separation

Injury to the acromioclavicular (AC) joint is often caused by a direct blow downwards over the shoulder. In the case of acute injury, the patient has pain, inability to lift the arm, and, frequently, obvious deformity. Radiographs may be normal or reveal varying degrees of clavicular displacement. Restraining structures include the AC ligament and two coracoclavicular ligaments – the conoid and trapezoid (Fukuda *et al.*, 1986). Injuries are classified as follows: grade I involves sprain to the AC ligament without ligament failure or laxity. Grade II designates AC ligament rupture with sprain to the coracoclavicular ligaments, diagnosed where there is disruption of the AC joint with maintained coracoclavicular distance. Grade III describes rupture of both groups of ligaments and is diagnosed in the presence of coracoclavicular distance 25–100% greater than the non-injured shoulder. Rockwood's (1984) schema expands classifications to grades IV–VI, wherein grade IV resembles grade III, excepting the posterior displacement of the distal clavicle; grade V describes the upward displacement of the distal clavicle into the base of the neck with the coracoclavicular interspace 100–300% greater than the interspace of the uninjured side; in grade VI injuries, the distal clavicle is displaced downwards.

Treatment for grade I and II injuries is conservative and includes use of a sling for several days. Grade III injuries elicit much controversy. Options include conservative treatment with a simple sling, use of a Kenny–Howard sling, or various operative reconstructions. In our experience, special slings to reduce dislocation have neither decreased pain nor deformity, so we do not use them. Operative repair has increased complications and delays return to work and sports more than non-operative treatment (Galpin *et al.*, 1985; Larsen *et al.*, 1986; Taft *et al.*, 1987). Moreover, the long-term results of operative repair are generally no better than results from conservative treatment. Larsen *et al.* (1986) support operative treatment in thin patients unwilling to tolerate deformity and in patients who perform heavy overhead work.

We perform acute reconstructions for patients with distal clavicular fractures or posterior dislocations. In addition, we do acute reconstructions in patients with severe cosmetic deformity or in those at risk of the skin sloughing. We choose a modified Weaver Dunn reconstructive technique using a Bosworth screw or dacron sling to aid reconstruction during the healing phase. Taft *et al.* (1987) have shown that resection of the distal clavicle improves results for patients with persistent pain, stiffness or post-traumatic osteoarthritis. We perform late reconstructions or distal clavicle resections in patients who have failed to respond to conservative care.

The necessity of reconstruction for grade IV–VI injuries is undisputed, and we employ the same procedure as that for grade III injuries.

Shoulder dislocation

Acute anterior shoulder subluxation or dislocation is best treated by early diagnosis and reduction. The shoulder is often externally rotated and adbucted and the humeral head palpated anteriorly. Radiographs confirm the diagnosis, rule out fracture, and facilitate evaluation of the size of the Hill–Sachs lesion. Pavlov *et al.* (1985) suggest three views, including an anteroposterior view of the shoulder in internal rotation, a Stryker notch, and a West Point or Didiee axillary X-ray. Reduction may be done using the Stimson method, i.e. with the patient prone, the arm flexed forward, and a 5lb (2.25 kg) weight attached to the hand. With relaxation, the shoulder then gently relocates. Otherwise, reduction may be achieved by gentle traction to the slightly abducted arm and by countertraction to the body, with a sheet around the thorax. Success with either method is achieved when the patient is relaxed, to which end intravenous medication or general anaesthesia may be required. Following reduction, the shoulder is immobilized. Practice regarding the length of time for immobilization varies. As Hovelius *et al.* (1983) have proven, lengthy immobilization does not appear to decrease the risk of subsequent dislocation. Hence, we immobilize the shoulder until comfort is achieved and advocate a strengthening programme with special focus on the internal rotators.

Although Aronsen and Regan (1984) report that the risk of subsequent dislocation can be reduced through adherence to a specified rigorous rehabilitation programme, it remains difficult to predict which patients chronically dislocate the shoulder. We know that age is the strongest predictive factor, but studies show much variation. Hovelius *et al.* (1983) reported that patients aged 17–19 years old had a 53% redislocation rate. Simonet and Cofield (1984) found a 66% rate in patients under 20, 40% in those 20–40, and no redislocations amongst those over 40 years old. Also, 82% of Simonet and Cofield's young athletes had redislocations versus 30% in young non-athletes. Therefore, we consider early repair in young athletic patients with dislocations.

To determine the type of anterior lesion and the status of the rotator cuff, we usually prescribe a CT arthrogram of MRI. Alternatively, diagnostic arthroscopy may be done prior to open ligament repair. This has the benefit of allowing direct cuff visualization from the superior and inferior surfaces and allows complete visualization of the labrum. The drawback of diagnostic arthroscopy prior to open reconstruction is the extravasation of large amounts of fluid which hinder easy dissection.

Arthroscopic shoulder stabilization is controversial. Its disputable reputation is the result of poor surgical technique and poor choice of candidates (Gross, 1989; Yahiro and Mathews 1989). In acute dislocations, we use staple capsulorhaphy with arthroscropically visualized anterior lesions. This technique eliminates the morbidity of open surgery, but the staple must be removed after 6 months to minimize the risk of the shoulder redislocating on to the staple.

Our approach to open reconstruction is based on the concept of anatomical repair using either the Bankart or modified Bankart repair (Rowe *et al.*, 1978; Loomer and Fraser, 1989; Thomas and Matsen, 1989). Instead of suturing through bony tunnels to affix the capsule to the glenoid, we use Mitek suture anchors. We find the suture anchors dependable, they are easier to use and positioning is more accurate.

Posterior dislocations are often misdiagnosed because of poor X-ray evaluation. This diagnosis must be considered in epileptic patients with shoulder pain. On physical examination the patient has a characteristic internal rotation deformity. Although the anteroposterior X-ray film may appear normal, the axillary view reveals the posterior position of the humeral head. Posterior dislocations are almost always treated successfully with closed reduction and immobolization until symptoms subside. Posterior subluxation is, however, much more common. Frequently associated with minimal symptoms, it is best treated initially by a programme of rotational and scapular strengthening.

Rotator cuff injury

Acute rotator cuff tear is characterized by pain in the shoulder and weakness of external rotation. Often the result of minor trauma, it is part of the continuum of impingement. Neer (1983) has stated that 95% of rotator cuff tears are caused by impingement and that trauma may enlarge the tear but is rarely its initiating factor. This is not entirely true, as young patients with no prior impingement do suffer traumatic tears. In addition to decreased strength in external rotation, the differential diagnosis may reveal acute bursitis, acromial clavicular arthritis and rotator cuff tear. Whenever acute arthritis is suspected a small amount of lignocaine is administered into this joint, and the amount of improvement is evaluated. To differentiate impingement from cuff tear, the impingement test described by Neer is performed. A small amount of lignocaine is injected into the subacromial bursa. If weakness persists after its injection, a cuff tear may be present, and will then be confirmed by either arthrogram or MRI. Those experienced in ultrasound will also be able to detect rotator cuff tears.

For suspected acute arthritis, we perform a technetium diphosphonate bone scan. If impingement is diagnosed, the subacromial bursa is then injected with a steroid–lignocaine mixture. The patient is started on anti-inflammatory medication, and physiotherapy is initiated with attention on stretching and strengthening the rotator cuff while avoiding activities which cause impingement. Should conservative treatment fail and other possible diagnoses be excluded (Hawkins *et al.*, 1989), anterior acromioplastry is performed (Neer, 1983; Bigliani *et al.*, 1989). In the presence of acute arthritis, the distal 1 cm of the clavicle is resected (Daluga and Dobozi; 1989; Watson, 1989).

We have found the arthroscopic approach to impingement very beneficial (Paulos and Franklin, 1990), allowing us to evaluate the glenohumeral joint and perform debridement as necessary. Arthroscopic subacromial decompression can be accurately done with minimal trauma to the deltoid. We proceed with shoulder arthroscopy for rotator cuff tears as with impingements, as long as patients fit the criterion of Post *et al.* (1983) – that is, have neither chronic lesions nor glenohumeral arthritis (Fig. 5.4).

Refinements in shoulder arthroscopy have changed our approach to rotator cuff repair. We no longer proceed with open anterior acromioplasty and cuff repair as suggested by Neer. Instead, we perform an arthroscopic subacromial decompression followed by open repair. This enables us to evaluate the glenohumeral joint at the time of cuff repair. Also, by performing the subacromial decompression arthroscopically, we repair most cuff tears through a 2-cm mid lateral deltoid-splitting approach. This minimizes surgical trauma to the deltoid and obviates the problems associated with removal and reattachment of the deltoid (Figs. 5.5 and 5.6).

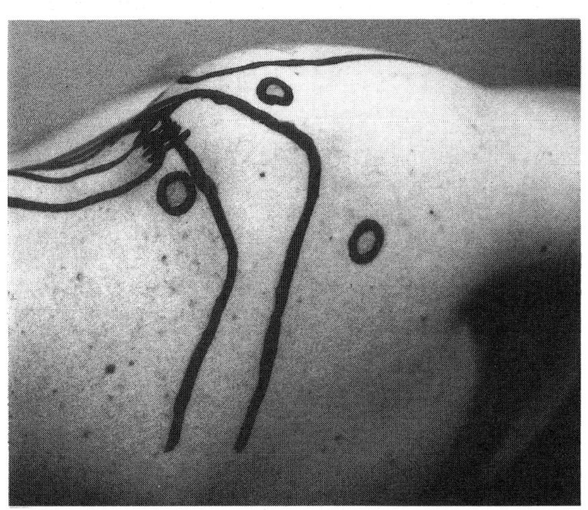

Fig. 5.4 Commonly used arthroscopic portals in shoulder surgery include the posterior, the mid lateral, and the superior portal, as shown here. The superior portal is rarely used and for anterior work we use an anterior portal located 1 cm inferior to the acromioclavicular joint.

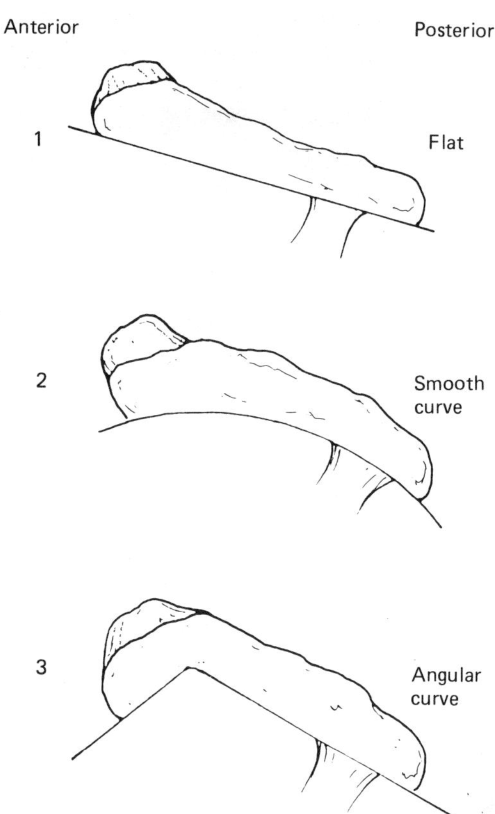

Fig. 5.5 The three common patterns of acromion shape. The incidence of impingement increases as one goes from a type 1 to type 3 acromion.

We also find suture and anchors effective in cuff repair. To affix the rotator cuff to a bony trough, we frequently use a combination of suture anchors and sutures placed through bony tunnels (Fig. 5.7). When massive or chronic cuff tears cannot be repaired through this simple means, we have recourse to an acromial-splitting approach. By lengthening the incision proximally and splitting the acromion with an oscillating saw, we can repair most massive tears. The acromion is then repaired with sutures through drill holes (Figs. 5.8 and 5.9).

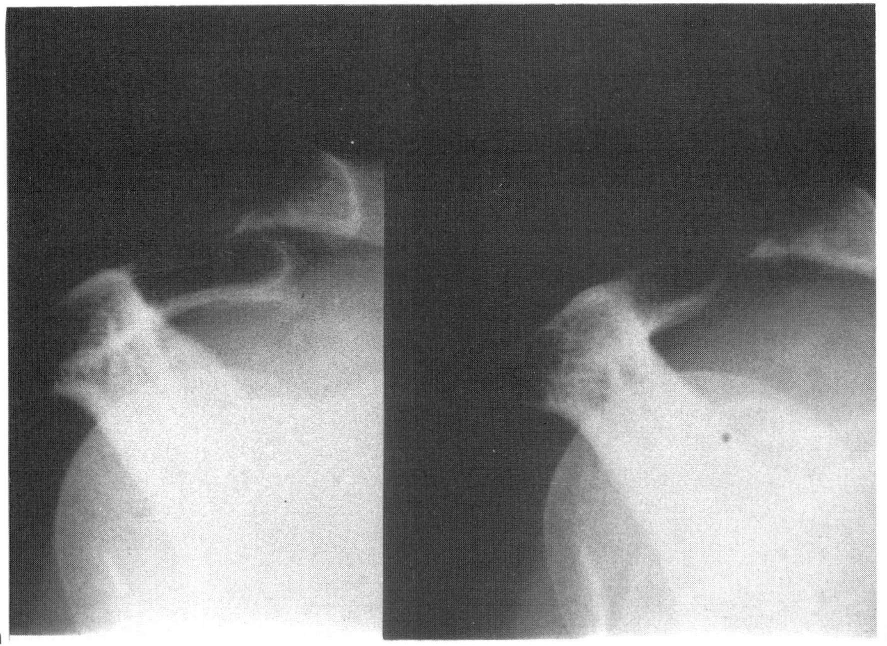

Fig. 5.6 (a) Pre- and (b) postoperative outlet views on a patient who underwent arthroscopic subacromial decompression for impingement. Note that the amount of bone resected is clearly visualized.

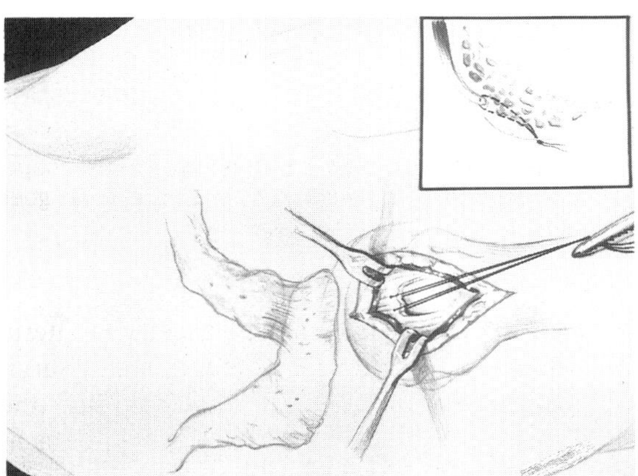

Fig. 5.7 The mini-approach for rotator cuff repair, utilizing a mid lateral deltoid-splitting approach.

Slap lesions

Advances in shoulder arthroscopy have shed light on a previously undescribed pathologic condition, the superior labral tear or SLAP lesion. Clinical complaints typically include catching or popping in the shoulder as well as pain with overhead activities. The mechanism of injury is often compression to the shoulder with the arm in slight abduction and forward flexion. Superior labral tears can be diagnosed with arthroscopy or sometimes with MRI. The tear extends from posterior to anterior with varying degrees of detachment of the biceps tendon from its insertion on the glenoid.

Treatment includes arthroscopic labral debridement with or without biceps tenodesis depending on the integrity of the biceps tendon's attachment. In selecting cases, labral repair is performed.

The knee

Patellar dislocation

A twisting injury may cause patellar dislocation. Patients report episodes of instability and often sense the patella on the lateral side of the knee. Usually, the patella will spontaneously reduce. If it is still dislocated at presentation, the knee is characteristically locked in flexion. Reduction is then easily accomplished with analgesia and knee

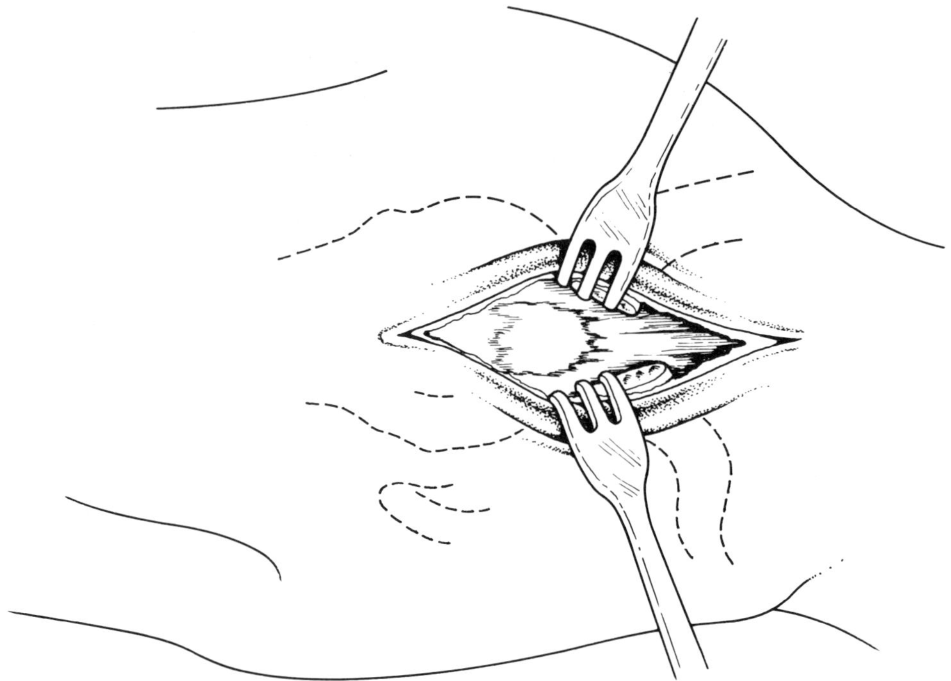

Fig. 5.8 If unable to visualize the torn rotator cuff adequately, extensile exposure is attained by splitting the acromion.

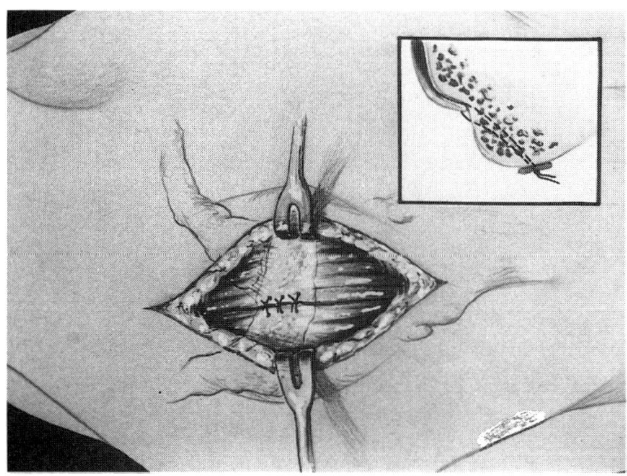

Fig. 5.9 After rotator cuff repair is complete, the acromion is repaired with sutures tied through drill holes.

extension. More often, the patient presents with medial parapatellar pain and swelling that may be mistaken for medial collateral ligament (MCL) strain.

Radiographic evaluation includes anteroposterior, lateral, and Merchant views. The Merchant view is obtained by directing the X-ray beam 30° inclined inferiorly from the horizontal with the patient supine, the knees flexed 45° and the cassette distal to the patella. Physical examination of the swollen knee is often too painful, so attention is turned to the opposite knee which is evaluated for patellar tracking, tilt, medial and lateral patellar glides at 30° flexion, and for Q or tuberosulcus angle. Patellar tracking is evaluated with the knee and hip flexed to 90°; attention is directed to the course of the patella with the knee extended and flexed. Tilt is evaluated by flexing the knee 20–30° and looking for elevation of the lateral pole of the patella. A zero or negative patellar tilt suggests excessive lateral retinacular tightness. Glides are tested by flexing the knee 30° and passively sliding the patella medially and laterally. A glide in either direction of more than half the width of the patella suggests laxity in the opposite reinaculum. For instance, a lateral glide exceeding two quadrants indicates deficiency in the medial retinaculum.

The Q angle is determined by estimating the vector of the quadriceps muscle and drawing a line to the centre of the patella and comparing it to a line from the centre of the patella to the tibial tubercle. As this angle is difficult to estimate, the tuberosulcus angle is often used and is measured with the knee at 90° to compare the tubercle patellar line with one drawn tangentially to the femoral condyles. Many examiners find the functional Q angle more helpful than static measurement. To assess this Q angle, we ask the patient to contract the quadriceps muscle as we observe the superior and lateral movement of the patella. If the patella moves more laterally than superiorly, the functional Q angle is increased.

Other predisposing factors to dislocation must be evaluated. These include genu valgum, shallow sulcus depth and external tibial torsion. Should this be the first instance of dislocation, if the patella is reduced on the Merchant view, and where the uninjured leg reveals no risk factors for dislocation, we treat the patient conservatively and prescribe a hinged knee brace and quadriceps rehabilitation programme. Operative measures are taken only to remove an osteochondral fragment interposed in the patellofemoral joint. For recurrent patellar dislocation, we proceed with operative reconstruction. If the patella is asymmetrically reduced in the trochlea or if the contralateral knee reveals serious biomechanical abnormalities, we consider performing acute proximal realignment as opposed to a proximal *and* distal procedure. Proximal realignment should lengthen the lateral retinaculum and reef or repair the medial retinaculum, whereas a distal realignment should only be done in skeletally mature patients with an abnormally increased tuberosulcus angle.

Cash and Hughston (1988) have reported on conservatively treated patellar dislocations grouped according to presence or absence of identified predisposing factors. Of the patients with identifiable signs, 52% responded successfully to conservative treatment compared to a 75% success rate in patients without predisposition to dislocation.

Extensor mechanism rupture

Rupture of the extensor mechanism is misdiagnosed frequently, yet it requires early surgical intervention for the best results.

Siwek and Rao (1981) found that 38% of the ruptures in their patient group were initially incorrectly diagnosed. Ruptures of the patellar tendon in the group occurred in patients 40 years old and younger, whereas quadriceps rupture occurred in an older age group. Kelly *et al.* (1984) reported on a group of athletes with patellar and quadriceps tendon ruptures found to be a complication of jumper's knee. Those with chondromalacia or patella alta had poor surgical results. Patients did well if the patellar tendon was repaired at the proper length; results with quadriceps tendon rupture were less satisfactory.

Violent quadriceps contraction upon knee flexion can rupture the extensor mechanism. If the rupture is in the quadriceps tendon, examination will reveal loss of extensor function, tenderness and swelling above the patella and, frequently, a palpable defect in the tendon. When diagnosis is uncertain, an arthrogram will show contrast in the quadriceps or an MRI will reveal the size and completeness of the rupture. Injury is most commonly at the tendon-to-bone junction and can often be repaired with suture anchors or through bony tunnels. For tendon-to-tendon repairs, augmentation can be achieved by turning down a flap of quadriceps tendon, a method described by Scuderi (1958).

A patellar tendon rupture is often the result of athletic activity. In addition to loss of active extension and a palpable defect, radiographs reveal patella alta. As mentioned above, operative reconstruction produces the best result. Should the tear be mid-substance, tendon-to-tendon repair is done using a Krackow-type suture. If the tear is an avulsion from the inferior pole of the patella, then Krackow sutures are tied to bony tunnels or suture anchors. Other techniques reinforce the repair with a wire that runs in circular fashion from the tibial tubercle through the patella. We believe this practice causes stress shielding of the tendon, so we now augment our repair with a Kennedy ligament augmentation device (LAD) fixed to bone at both ends in order to maintain length. The LAD is removed after 3 months. (The LAD is a device intended for implantation along with homologous grafts in ligament reconstructions. The concept is that by strengthening the graft with a synthetic stent the graft can be better tensioned and the stent can absorb stress during the early stages of ligament healing and collagen growth. The Kennedy LAD is a strip of braided polypropylene.)

Meniscal injury

The role of the meniscus as a load-bearing and stabilizing structure is only now being fully appreciated. Schoemaker and Markolf (1986) have documented its role in resisting anterior translation of the tibia on the femur in anterior cruciate deficient knees. Normally, the menisci may transmit 50–70% of the load on the knee (Ghosh and Taylor, 1987). Saving the meniscus by subtotal meniscectomy or other repair to avoid degenerative changes must be emphasized.

In the epidemiological study on 1515 meniscectomies of Baker *et al.* (1985), tears were three times more likely to occur in males, and there was a 4 to 1 predominance of medial versus lateral tears. Medial tears are more likely to be longitudinal, whereas lateral tears are most often radial and more frequently associated with meniscal cysts. Injury frequently occurs from twisting when the knee goes from flexion into extension. Often, the patient cannot recall a discrete injury. Certain types and tear sizes produce mechanical symptoms such as locking and popping.

Physical examination reveals joint line pain and effusion. Often the McMurray sign is positive. The McMurray test is performed by flexing the knee maximally and then extending the knee in forced internal and external rotation while feeling for the clunk of a catching meniscus. Patients will occasionally present with a locked meniscus which may be reduced by sedating the patient and gently manipulating the knee into extension. Radiographs are done to rule out fracture and degenerative changes. The MRI has replaced the arthrogram as the most sensitive test whenever more specific information is required. Mandelbaum *et al.* (1986) reported 90 and 91% accuracy in detecting medial, then lateral tears through MRI. We consider MRI if there is uncertainty after examination.

The only meniscal tears likely to heal without suturing are incomplete tears usually found on the meniscal undersurface. As the outer third of the meniscus is vascularized (Arnoczky *et al.*, 1988), there is much potential for healing. The study of Scott *et al.* (1986) shows that healing was statistically correlated with the width of the intact meniscal rim and the repair or reconstruction of the anterior cruciate ligament (ACL). Repair of avascular meniscal injuries with fibrin clot is currently being investigated. According to Arnotczky *et al.* (1988), the addition of fibrin clot to torn menisci in dogs has stimulated meniscal healing.

If the tear is in the peripheral portion of the meniscus, we use meniscal repair cannula with the suture knots tied over the capsule. Although we proceed with arthroscopic meniscectomy or repair in our young patients, we frequently start with conservative treatment in older, less athletic patients, using anti-inflammatories and therapy to allow symptoms to resolve. If there is worsening or no improvement after 6–12 weeks of conservative care, we perform arthroscopy.

Ligament injury

Evaluation of acute ligament injury is most complex. An adequate examination requires anatomical understanding and skilful physical examination. Because the structures of the knee work together to produce motion and share applied loads, natural knee motion and motions elicited during clinical laxity tests cannot occur independently. A number of active and passive constraints or stabilizers control these coupled motions and allow normal knee motion. Passive stabilizers include bone, menisci, the capsule and ligaments; active stabilizers are neuromuscular units providing stability by the nature of their insertion in or about the passive structures. Using the results of constrained cadaver studies, researchers have divided passive stabilizers into primary and secondary restraints to describe each knee motion, despite the fact that these motions do not occur independently.

With the popularization of MRI scanning, one may mistakenly depend on the scan as opposed to the physical examination. With practice, however, most ligament injuries can be diagnosed accurately through several laxity tests. The knee must be evaluated for effusion and areas of maximal tenderness. Radiographic evaluation will confirm or exclude fracture. The radiograph will occasionally reveal a small avulsion from the lateral tibial plateau, an occurrence Woods *et al.* (1979) have called the lateral capsular sign. This avulsion should alert the examiner of the high probability of ACL injury.

On every acutely injured knee we perform a minimum of four evaluative manoeuvres. These include valgus stress at 0 and 30°, varus stress at 0 to 30°, the Lachman test and the posterior drawer test, our goal being to classify the knee ligament injury according to terminology proposed by the International Knee Committee. Each test will be discussed as individual ligament injuries are detailed below.

Acute knee haemarthrosis is commonly associated with cruciate ligament disruption. Occasionally, however, examination reveals no instability, radiographs reveal no fracture, and no clear diagnosis can be made. Previously, diagnostic arthroscopy was indicated and advocated by DeHaven (1989). Today, other alternatives exist. Kannus and Jarvinen (1987) have suggested repeated clinical examination for ligament injury, a diagnosis often overlooked in the DeHaven study. We believe that virtually all ACL injuries can be documented by a well-performed examination and KT-1000 evaluation. With MRI, other possible causes of haemarthrosis such as meniscal tear, patellar dislocation or osteochondral fractures can be determined.

Medial collateral ligament injury

Injury to the MCL is one of the most common knee injuries. Its mechanism is valgus strain produced by a stepping inside manoeuvre or resulting from a blow directed over the lateral side of the knee. The examiner will discover medial pain and should attempt to locate the injury site at the femoral epicondyle, the tibial insertion, or at mid-substance, then examine the knee to valgus strain at 0 and 30°. Instability at 0° suggests grade III injury or complete MCL disruption with probable cruciate injury. Grade II injury is characterized by instability at 30° with a deserved end-point. A grade I injury is indicated where examination shows no increased laxity but the other characteristic findings are present. For all grades, the four knee tests mentioned above must be done to rule out concomitant injury. For example, approximately 20% of knees with MCL injury are associated with disruption of the medial retinaculum and vastus medialis. Also, patellar dislocations are frequently misdiagnosed as MCL strains.

Treatment for most isolated MCL injuries is conservative. Indelicato (1983) has proven that there is no benefit of surgery. For grade I injuries, the only treatment usually required is limitation of activities until tenderness disappears, followed by range of motion exercises. For grade II and III injuries, a hinged knee brace and crutches are prescribed for the first several weeks. After 3–6 weeks, crutches are discontinued; an additional 2–6 weeks later, brace use is discontinued. Therapy is directed towards strengthening and range of motion.

We repair grade III MCL injuries while performing an ACL reconstruction whenever the tears appear to be torn off the femur. We agree with the observation of Hunter *et al.* (1983) that the vastus medialis obliquus is often disrupted in the presence of this injury and repair the disruption while repairing the MCL. If the injury is grade II or judged principally interstitial, we proceed with ACL reconstruction only. The results of the rotation drawer and external rotation pivot–shift tests determine which patients require medial side repair. More complete discussion of these tests will appear in the section on the anterior cruciate ligament, below.

Lateral collateral ligament injury

Injury to this complex without disruption of the cruciate ligament is rare. The mechanism of injury is adduction of the knee with dissipation of forces prior to cruciate ligament disruption. Most adduction injuries are severe, causing disruption of both cruciates as well as the lateral side of the knee and are treated as knee dislocations. Disruption of all lateral ligaments and the posterior cruciate ligament results in acute straight lateral instability. In 1983 DeLee *et al.* studied 10 patients with acute straight lateral instability. The physical examination revealed lateral instability without rotation to varus stress with the leg in full extension. Surgical findings included complete lateral and posterior cruciate disruption as well as frequent ACL disruption. Primary surgical repair led to stable, functional knees in five of seven patients reviewed at 7 years post-injury.

Acute posterolateral instability results from injury to the arcuate ligament complex without disruption of the posterior cruciate ligament (PCI). Physical examination reveals a positive posterolateral drawer sign, a positive external rotation recurvatum test, or a positive reverse pivot–shift sign. The drawer test is done with the knee flexed 80° and the foot externally rotated 15°. A posteriorly directed force over the proximal tibia causes the lateral side of the tibia to move posteriorly, while the medial side stays in place. The external rotation recurvatum test is performed with the patient supine. The lower extremity is suspended with the knee extended by grasping the great toe. The test is positive if the knee falls into varus angulation, hyperextension and if there is external rotation of the tibia. The reverse pivot–shift test is done with the knee in 45% flexion and the leg in external rotation. In this position, the lateral tibial plateau displaces posterolaterally such that the lateral femoral condyle is in front of the summit of the convex lateral tibial plateau. During extension, the femoral condyle glides with the lateral tibial plateau until the lateral gastrocnemius muscle and posterolateral capsule tighten, causing the femur to snap as it returns to its normal position in extension. With early accurate diagnosis, repair of the injured ligament can be performed successfully. Surgical series done by Baker *et al.* (1983) and DeLee (1984) both indicate good results with early repair.

Anterior cruciate ligament injury

Injury to the ACL is often caused by valgus external rotation. Commonly, the patient can recall a distinct pop in the knee. This is followed by haemarthrosis within the several hours. The patient experiences varying degrees of pain related to other associated injuries. The Lachman and anterior drawer tests will be positive. The Lachman is done by grasping the distal femur in one hand and the proximal tibia in the other. The knee is flexed 20° as the tibia is drawn forwards on the fixed femur. An assessment of both the amount of anterior excursion and the quality of the end-point is made.

The anterior drawer test is done by flexing the knee to 90° and drawing the tibia forward. Butler *et al.* (1980) have shown that the ACL provides 86% of the resisting force to anterior tibial translation during this test. Successful testing requires the patient's relaxation, especially of the hamstring muscles. Whenever the knee is too painful to allow adequate examination, aspiration of the haematoma and injection of a small amount of lignocaine generally provide sufficient anaesthesia.

The studies of Zarins *et al.* (1983) and Larson (1983) have increased our understanding of rotatory instability in patients with ACL ruptures and are waiting for referral. In addition, we supplement physical exmination with a KT-1000 test performed by physiotherapists or trainers. Using the KT device, as Daniel *et al.* (1985) described, permits accurate diagnosis and quantitation of laxity. A complete ACL tear is verified by a 3 mm or greater increase in maximal anterior excursion as compared with the opposite limb. With the KT-1000, we can assess the patient's dependence on the ACL and the degree of ligament laxity. We believe that a patient with a maximal excursion of 7 mm on the uninvolved knee and 10–11 mm excursion on the involved knee is far less likely to require reconstruction than a patient with 10 mm on the normal and 16–17 mm excursion on the involved knee. It is our conviction that every ACL injury can be accurately diagnosed by these tests in one clinic visit.

Damage to secondary restraints such as an

ACL-MCL disruption is best treated with at least ACL reconstruction. For isolated ACL tears, we choose between operative reconstruction or a conservative leg press programme. The decision to proceed operatively or conservatively is based on factors including age, activity level and the patient's expectations. We usually prescribe ACL reconstruction for patients younger than 30 years old with high activity levels. Rehabilitation is suggested for older patients with a lower activity level. Older, very active patients and young patients who are less active present a dilemma which must be resolved to suit individual needs. Those we feel may be best treated conservatively are examined with MRI to rule out meniscal injury. A negative MRI is then a signal to proceed with therapy. If the MRI is positive for mensical injury, we suggest arthroscopy. For irreparable lesions, we perform meniscectomy; for reparable tears, we do meniscal repair if the patient has agreed to ACL reconstruction.

Before arthroscopy for ligament injury, we do a careful examination under anaesthesia. In all ACL patients, we perform the pivot–shift test in internal rotation to grade the laxity of the knee, as described by Bach *et al.* (1983) and Jakob *et al.* (1987). The leg is internally rotated by placing one hand on the ankle and the other hand posterolaterally behind the head of the fibula (Fig. 5.10). Valgus stress is applied to the knee in extension. In this position, the anterolateral aspect of the tibial plateau is subluxated anterolaterally with respect to the femoral condyle. As the knee is flexed, the tibia reduces at approximately 30–40°, the point at which the iliotibial band becomes a flexor of the knee. This is a positive sign for rupture of the ACL, and can be graded I–IV in accordance with the amount of ACL damaged and integrity of the secondary restraints. We also do the flexion rotation drawer test as described by Noyes *et al.* (1989). In this test, the leg is held in extension, allowing the femur to rotate externally and the tibia to sublux. As the knee is flexed with applied valgus force, the tibia will reduce in a positive test.

The rotary drawer test is performed with the knee at 90° in neutral, internal and external rotation. If there is a one-grade increase from neutral to external rotation, the brakestop mechanisms is injured, a signal that either the medial meniscus or the posterior medial corner is involved. A brakestop injury is verified by the external rotation pivot–shift test. This test is positive where there is an increase of two or more grades over the internal rotation pivot–shift test and a positive 90° drawer test with external tibial rotation. The external rotation pivot–shift test is done with the patient supine and the knee in extension (Fig. 5.11). The ankle is held in one hand, and the leg is externally rotated. The other hand is placed on the posterolateral aspect of the knee behind the fibular head, where valgus and anterior stress are applied to the tibia. With the leg in external rotation and the knee in near extension, the whole tibia is subluxated anteriorly; the anteromedial portion is subluxated to a greater extent than the anterolateral portion, in effect producing an anteromedial drawer sign in extension. As the knee is flexed, a reduction of this anteromedially subluxated tibia occurs at 30–40°, secondary to the cam effect of the iliotibial band and to the associated concavity of the medial tibial plateau.

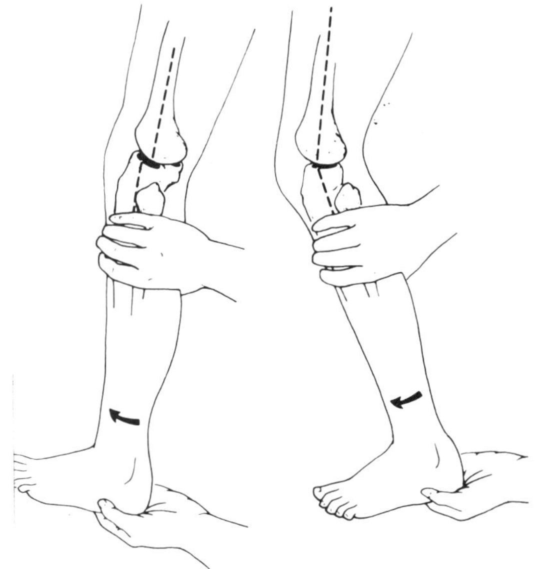

Fig. 5.10 The pivot–shift test. With the leg extended and the tibia internally rotated the leg is flexed with a valgus load; at 20–30° the tibia reduces with a 'clunk'.

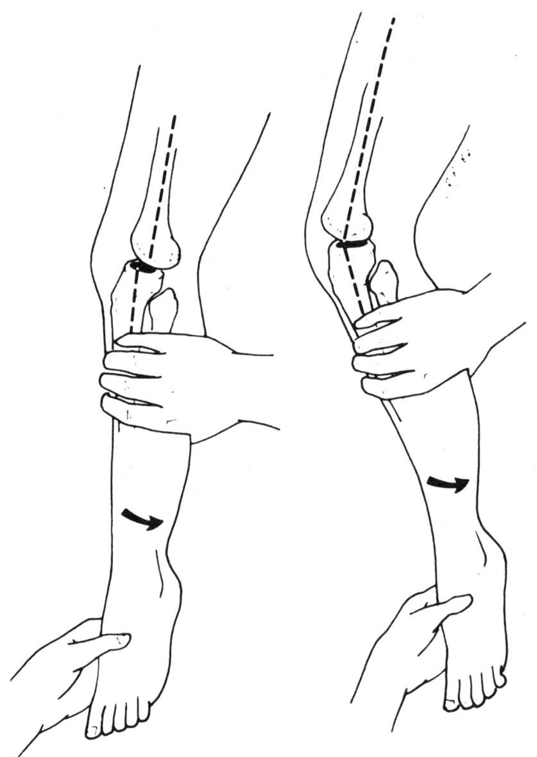

Fig. 5.11 The external rotation pivot–shift test. With the leg extended and the tibia externally rotated, the leg is flexed with a valgus load; at 20–30° the tibia reduces.

If an associated MCL injury exists, there will be 2–3+ valgus laxity at 5 and 30° of knee flexion. In this situation, the medial brakestop must be repaired in addition to the ACL reconstruction. The medial meniscal injury would be repaired, then the MCL and a reefing of the posterior oblique ligament done if necessary. If the anterior drawer sign fails to decrease upon neutral to internal rotation, the posterolateral corner is injured and may require lateral extra-articular repair or reconstruction.

The 4-year follow-up of Hawkin's *et al.* (1986) of 40 patients with isolated ACL reconstructions showed that only 14% achieved full return to athletics and 87.5% of the patients had only fair or poor results. With our candidates for ACL reconstruction, we first evaluate the integrity of the remaining ACL. For the rare avulsion injury without obvious interstitial haemorrhage, we perform ACL repair and augmentation. Clancy *et al.* (1988) also approve of augmentation. In our augmentation, we use sutures placed with a suture punch and augment the ACL with a double strand of semitendinosus. For patients undergoing ACL reconstruction, we offer several graft options. One option is fresh frozen allograft patellar tendon or achilles tendon. Ethylene oxide and freeze-dried grafts have been abandoned since Indelicato *et al.* (1990) showed that they were inferior to fresh grafts. Benefits of allograft include a large strong graft, no donor site morbidity and bone ligament fixation at both ends using the patellar tendon, and at one end using Achilles tendon. Concerns regarding the use of allografts include the risk of hepatitis or AIDS and the possibility of immunological graft rejection.

The central third of the patellar tendon is another graft option that excludes the risk of immunological rejection and disease transmission. Drawbacks include the small size of the graft, the risk of anterior knee pain or patellar tendinitis and a slightly more difficult rehabilitation. One case of patellar fracture following middle third patellar tendon harvest has been reported by McCarroll (1983). Another option is a graft using the semitendinosus and gracilis, both doubled over in a quadruple graft technique. This, too, is a small graft, and it does not allow bone-to-bone fixation at either end. However, it is probably superior to patellar tendon autograft for the patient with pre-existing patellofemoral pathology.

Since no clear evidence attests to the superiority of allografts over autografts, we leave the decision to the patient. If autograft is chosen, we use patellar tendon if there is no pre-existing patellofemoral pathology. Regardless of the graft chosen, ACL reconstruction is done endoscopically. The tibial tunnel is chosen with an arthroscopic guide and reamed over a guide wire. The femoral attachment site is chosen by fixing a suture to the estimated location in the notch and then checking for isometry. If 2 mm or less excursion with flexion and extension is found, the site is acceptable. A slotted pin is run through the isometric point, out of the anterolateral femur, and through the skin. The femur is then reamed with an endoscopic reamer the depth of the bone plug. The graft is held with a suture through the bone plug and is pulled into the femoral tunnel by attaching the sutures to the slotted pin. The graft is secured with a cannulated endoscopic screw and the suture slipped out through the skin. At the tibial side, fixation using patellar tendon grafts is done with another interference screw. Achilles tendon grafts are affixed to the tibia with two staples and hamstring grafts are attached with a screw and ligament washer.

With hamstring tendon use, one must make an incision over the femur, pull the hamstrings into the femoral tunnel by looping them over a dacron tape, then tie the tape over the screw and washer. We no longer perform extra-articular procedures like the Andrews mini-reconstruction or the iliotibial transfer. Such procedures are reserved for reinforcing primary intra-articular reconstructions in excessively lax patients who have damage to these specific structures.

If an ACL tear is associated with either a grade II or III MCL tear, we suggest ACL reconstruction. An intact ACL is required for adequate healing of the MCL.

We treat partial ACL tears with the same algorithm as an isolated tear. As Noyes *et al.* (1989) have shown, most partial ACL injuries progress to complete tears over time. Although many of these patients prefer conservative treatment initially, we often proceed with reconstruction when the patient is young and highly active.

Therapy has changed significantly in the last several years. Arms *et al.* (1984) demonstrated that strains in the ACL graft were highest in the terminal 40° of extension. This led investigators to immobilize the limb in flexion for various time lengths. This effort to protect the graft during early healing stages caused many patients to lose the terminal 5° of extension. Now that isometric intraoperative checking assures more precise placement of grafts, graft strain is largely avoided. Immediate full extension can be allowed with weight-bearing and a brace locked at 20°.

Evaluating the results of ACL reconstruction is very difficult. First, the literature is replete with varied operations to stabilize the knee. Also therapy protocols have changed so rapidly that few large patient groups have received the same therapy. Moreover, the expectations of patients differ widely. In light of these variables, Lyscholm and Gillquist (1982) have created a scale for evaluating patients which emphasizes instability. Nevertheless, comparing series of ACL reconstructions remains difficult, if not impossible.

Posterior cruciate injury

Surgeons have learned much in recent years about the function and injury of the posterior and posterolateral structures. Isolated injury to the PCL can occur as a result of sports injury or high-

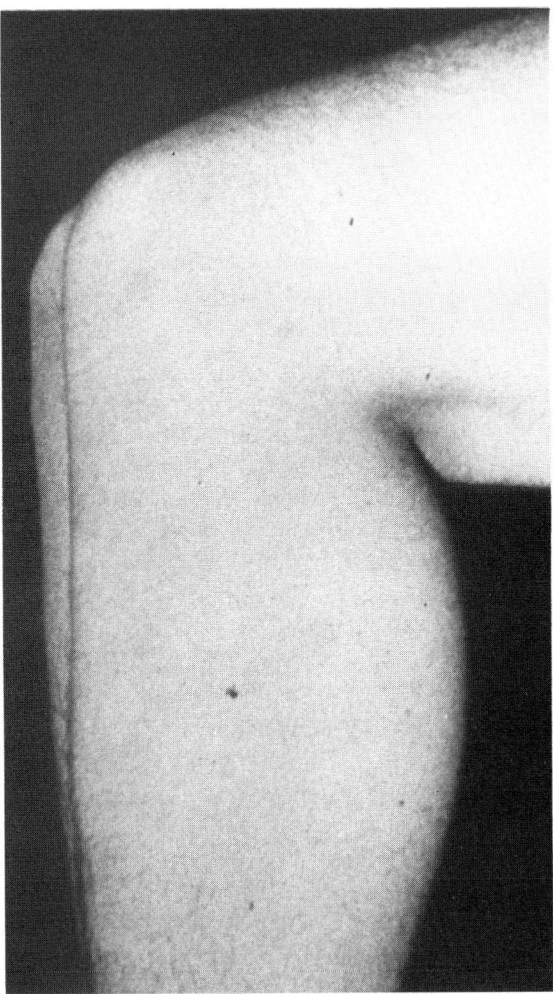

Fig. 5.12 The posterior sag test. By viewing across the flexed knees, the tibia of the posterior cruciate cdeficient knee rests more posterior than that of the normal knee.

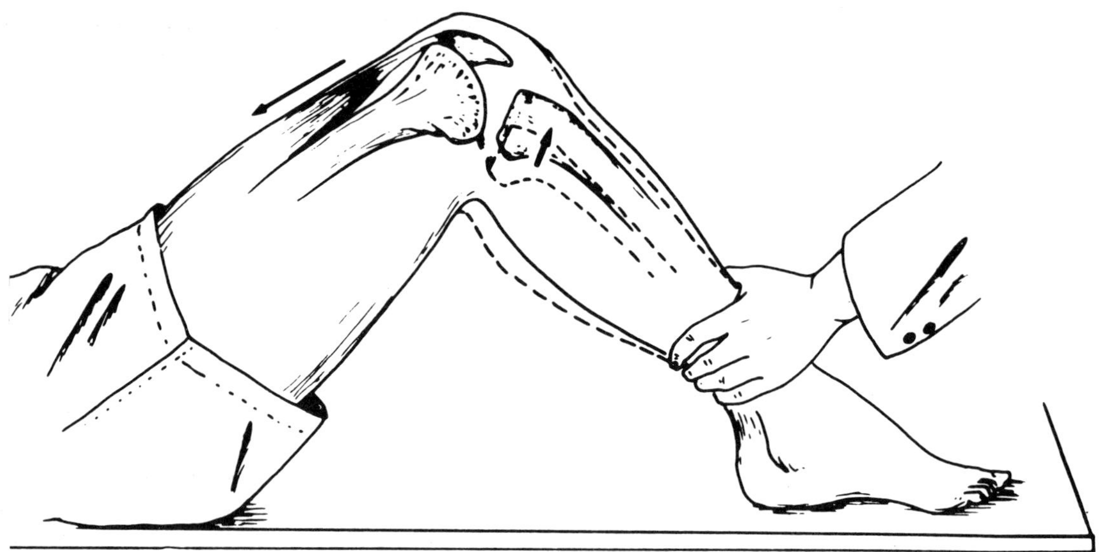

Fig. 5.13 The quadriceps active test. The examiner places a hand on the shin of the flexed knee and instructs the patient to slide the foot distally against resistance. In the posterior cruciate deficient knee the tibia will move forward on the femur.

energy vehicular trauma. A blow to the tibia of a flexed knee from a car's dashboard is a classic description of the isolated PCL injury mechanism. The patient presents with an effusion and posterior pain. The diagnostic examination begins with testing the tibia for a posterior sag by bending both knees to 90° and looking across the profile of the proximal tibia (Fig. 5.12). If a posterior sag is present, the involved knee will show posterior subluxation of the proximal tibia. The quadriceps active test is also done as described by Daniel *et al.* (1988). The knee is again flexed 90° and the patient is asked to contract the quadriceps (Fig. 5.13). The test is positive if the tibia is pulled forward by the quadriceps. The posterior drawer test is performed by flexing the knee to 90°, placing the tibia in its neutral point, and directing a posterior force over the proximal tibia. Any increase in posterior subluxation over the other limb is diagnostic for PCL disruption.

In 1986 Parolie and Bengfeld studied a series of isolated tears in atheletes and concluded that the majority of athletes who maintained strength were able to return to sports without functional disability. Dandy and Pusey (1982) and Cross and Powell (1984) have reported good functional results from non-operative treatment of PCL injuries. Clancy *et al.*'s (1983) study showed a high incidence of medial femoral condyle deterioration associated with PCL instability. They performed PCL reconstruction using patellar tendon. We individualize treatment and frequently treat the PCL non-operatively. Should the patient fail to regain an acceptable performance level, we perform PCL reconstruction using Achilles tendon allograft.

Patients with both posterior and posterolateral instability often respond much differently than those with isolated PCL tears. A common mechanism of injury is adduction internal rotation force to the flexed knee. Torn structures may include the PCL, fibular collateral ligament and the arcuate ligament complex. Varying degrees of injury also occur to the biceps femoris, the iliotibial band and the peroneal nerve. Frequently, however, this instability pattern is not recognized until it becomes a chronic problem. Tests for PCL disruption and the reverse pivot–shift test will be positive. These tests are performed by flexing the knee, externally rotating the foot to cause the lateral tibial plateau to sublux posteriorly and extending the leg under a mild valgus load (Fig.

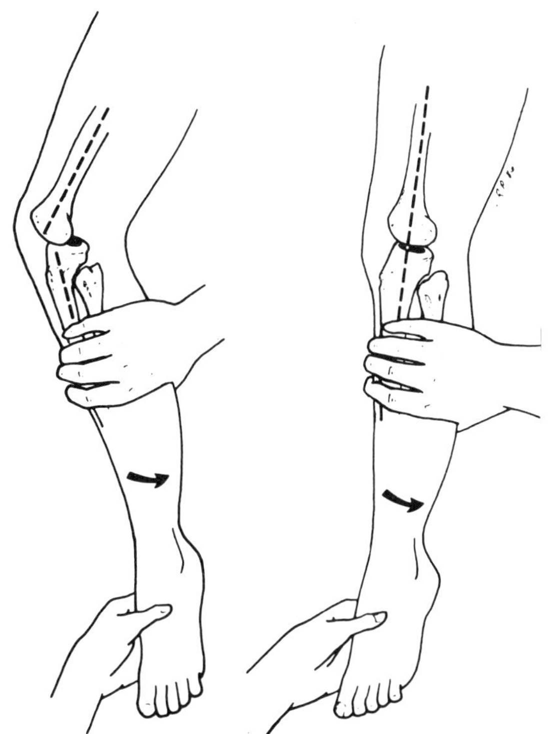

Fig. 5.14 The reverse pivot–shift test. With external rotation of the tibia the plateau subluxes posteriorly. As the leg is extended with a valgus load, the tibia reduces near full extension.

5.14). As the knee approaches 20° of flexion, the tibia will shift forwards into the reduced position, thereby proving posterolateral instability.

Another test is to flex the knee to 90° and measure the internal and external rotation of the normal and involved leg. Patients with posterolateral instability will have increased external rotation on the involved side and posterior subluxation of the tibia. [Gollehon *et al.*'s (1977) sequential sectioning of the lateral structures and the PCL has contributed to our understanding of our findings on examination.]

Treatment of patients with posterior and posterolateral instability is almost always surgical. The PCL is reconstructed with Achilles tendon allograft, and the fibular collateral ligament and arcuate complex are reconstructed with a double-limbed allograft fixed to the femur and routed through the tibia and the fibula. Further lateral reconstruction can be done with a biceps tenodesis if necessary. Baker *et al.*'s (1984) report on 13 patients treated with primary repair of all torn structures showed that 90% had good results.

Dislocation

Dislocation of the knee joint usually results from violent trauma. Diagnosis prior to reduction is easily made on the basis of clinical examination and obvious deformity. Most dislocations are anterior, i.e. the tibia displaces anterior to the femur. Nevertheless, dislocations in any plane are possible. Initial evaluation includes neurological and circulatory examination followed by radiography. Reduction with longitudinal traction is performed as soon after injury as possible. Following reduction, an angiogram is performed regardless of apparent circulatory status as anterior dislocations often result in intimal tears to the popliteal artery; posterior dislocations frequently result in arterial transection.

The lower leg is then examined for compartment syndrome and the reduction is maintained in a plaster splint. Reconstruction can be performed acutely with repair of the medial and lateral structures and cruciate reconstruction, or repair can be delayed until capsular scarring has provided some stability to the limb. If the patient requires vascular repair as well, we usually do repair or reconstruction during the initial surgery. If vascular repair is unnecessary, reconstruction is delayed to allow healing time. Arthroscopic cruciate reconstruction can be done once the capsule heals – a difficult procedure best performed by a rested surgical team during daylight hours. Failure to recognize a knee dislocation because the injury spontaneously reduced or was reduced at the scene of injury and prior to transport can result in devastating errors in treatment. This error can be avoided by careful examination of the varus, valgus and anterior posterior planes for ligamentous restraints in any direction. We emphasize again that circulatory monitoring and angiography are essential in the event of knee dislocation.

References

The ankle

Anderson KJ, Le Coq JF (1954) Operative treatment of injury to the fibular collateral ligament of the ankle. *Journal of Bone and Joint Surgery* **36A**, 825.

Arrowsmith SR, Fleming LL, Allman FL (1983) Traumatic dislocations of the peroneal tendons. *American Journal of Sports Medicine* **11**, 142.

Brostrom L (1966) Sprained ankles. V. Treatment and prognosis in recent ligament ruptures. *Acta Chirurgica Scandinavica* **132**, 537.

Cass JR, Morrey BF, Katoh Y, Chao EY (1985) Ankle instability: comparison of primary repair and delayed reconstruction after long-term follow-up study. *Clinical Orthopaedics* **198**, 110.

Colville MR, Colville JM, Manoli A (1987) Posteromedial dislocation of the ankle without fracture. *Journal of Bone and Joint Surgery* **60(A)**, 706.

Cox JS (1985) Surgical and nonsurgical treatment of acute ankle sprains. *Clinical Orthopaedics* **198**, 118.

Das SD, Balasubramaniam P (1985) A repair operation for recurrent dislocation of peroneal tendons. *Journal of Bone and Joint Surgery* **67B**, 585.

Eckert WR, Davis EA (1976) Acute rupture of the peroneal retinaculum. *Journal of Bone and Joint Surgery* **58-A**, 670.

Escales F, Figueras JM, Merino JA (1980) Dislocation of the peroneal tendons. *Journal of Bone and Joint Surgery* **62-A**, 451.

Evans GA, Hardcastle P, Frenyo AD (1984) Acute rupture of the lateral ligament of the ankle. *Journal of Bone and Joint Surgery* **66B**, 209.

Grace DL (1984) Lateral ankle ligament injuries. *Clinical Orthopaedics* **183**, 153.

Larsen E (1986) Experimental instability of the ankle. *Clinical Orthopaedics* **204**, 193.

Larsen E (1984) Taping the ankle for chronic instability. *Acta Orthopaedica Scandinavica* **55**, 551.

Murr (1961) Dislocation of the peroneal tendons with marginal fracture of the lateral malleolus. *Journal of Bone and Joint Surgery* **43–B**, 563.

Niedermann B, Anderson A, Anderson SB et al. (1981) Rupture of the lateral ligaments of the ankle: operation or plaster cast? *Acta Orthopaedica Scandinavica* **52**, 579.

Ramsey PL, Hamilton W (1976) Changes in tibiotalar area of contact caused by lateral talar shift. *Journal of Bone and Joint Surgery* **58A** 356.

Rasmussen O (1985) Stability of the ankle joint. *Acta Orthopaedica Scandinavica* **56** (suppl. 211).

Snook GA, Chrisman OD, Wilson TC (1985) Long term results of the Chrisman-Snook operation for reconstruction of the lateral ligaments of the ankle. *Journal of Bone and Joint Surgery* **67A**, 1.

Staples OS (1975) Ruptures of the fibular collateral ligaments of the ankle. *Journal of Bone and Joint Surgery* **57A**, 101.

Vaes P, DeBoeck H, Handelberg F, Opdecan P (1985) Comparative radiologic study of the influence of ankle joint bandages on ankle stability. *American Journal of Sports Medicine* **13**, 46.

The shoulder

Aronsen JG, Regan K (1984) Decreasing the incidence of recurrence of first time anterior shoulder dislocations with rehabilitation. *American Journal of Sports Medicine* **12**, 283.

Bigliani LU, D'Alessandro DF, Duralde XA, McIlveen SJ (1989) Anterior acromioplasty for subacromial impingement in patients younger than 40 years of age. *Clinical Orthopaedics* **246**, 111.

Daluga DV, Dobozi W (1989) The influence of distal clavicle resection and rotator cuff repair on the effectiveness of anterior acromioplasty. *Clinical Orthopaedics* **247**, 117.

Fukuda K, Craig EV, Kai-Nan A, Cofield RH, Chao EY (1986) Biomechanical study of the ligamentous system of the acromioclavicular joint. *Journal of Bone and Joint Surgery* **68A**, 434.

Galpin RD, Hawkins RJ, Grainger RW (1985) A comparative analysis of operative versus non-operative treatment of grade III acromioclavicular separations. *Clinical Orthopaedics* **193**, 150.

Gross RM (1989) Arthroscopic shoulder capsulorrhaphy: does it work? *American Journal of Sports Medicine* **17**, 495.

Hawkins RJ, Chris T, Bokor D, Kiefer G (1989) Failed anterior acromioplasty. *Clinical Orthopaedics* **243**, 106.

Hovelius L, Eriksson K, Fredin H et al. (1983) Recurrences after initial dislocation of the shoulder. *Journal of Bone and Joint Surgery* **65A**, 343.

Larsen E, Bjerg-Nielsen A, Christensen P (1986) Conservative or surgical treatment of acromioclavicular dislocation. *Journal of Bone and Joint Surgery* **68A**, 552.

Loomer R, Fraser J (1989) A modified Bankart procedure for recurrent anterior/inferior shoulder instability. *American Journal of Sports Medicine* **17**, 374.

Neer CS (1983) Impingement lesions. *Clinical Orthopaedics* **173**, 70.

Pavlov H, Warren RF, Weiss CB, Dines DM (1985) The roentgenographic evaluation of anterior shoulder instability. *Clinical Orthopaedics* **194**, 153.

Paulos LE, Franklin JL (1990) Arthroscopic shoulder decompression development and application. *American Journal of Sports Medicine* **18**, 235.

Post M, Silver R, Singh M (1983) Rotator cuff tear. *Clinical Orthopaedics* **173**, 78.

Rockwood CA Jr (1984) Subluxations and dislocations about the shoulder. Injuries to the acromioclavicular joint. In: Rockwood CA Jr, Green DP (eds) *Fractures*, 2nd edn, Vol 1. J. B. Lippincott, pp 860–910.

Rowe CR, Patel D, Southmayd WW (1978) The Bankart procedure. *Journal of Bone and Joint Surgery* **60A**, 1.

Simonet WT, Cofield RH (1984) Prognosis in anterior shoulder dislocation. *American Journal of Sports Medicine* **12**, 19.

Snyder SJ, Karzel RP, DelPizzo W, Ferkel RD, Friedman MJ (1990) SLAP lesions of the shoulder. *Journal of Arthroscopic and Related Surgery* **6**, 274.

Taft TN, Wilson FC, Oglesby JW (1987) Dislocation of the acromioclavicular joint. *Journal of Bone and Joint Surgery* **69A**, 1045.

Thomas SC, Matsen FA (1989) An approach to the repair of avulsion of the glenohumeral ligaments in the management of traumatic anterior glenohumeral instability. *Journal of Bone and Joint Surgery* **71A**, 506.

Watson M (1989) Rotator cuff function in the impingement syndrome. *Journal of Bone and Joint Surgery* **71B**, 561.

Yahiro MA, Matthews LS (1989) Arthroscopic stabilization procedures for recurrent anterior shoulder instability. *Orthopaedic Review* **18**, 1161.

The knee

Andrews JR, Sanders R (1983) A mini-reconstruction technique in treating anterolateral rotary instability. *Clinical Orthopaedics* **172**, 93.

Arms SW, Pope MH, Johnson RJ, Fisher RA, Arvidsson I, Eriksson E (1984) The biomechanics of anterior cruciate ligament rehabilitation and reconstruction. *American Journal of Sports Medicine* **12**, 8.

Arnoczky SP, Warren RF, Spivak JM (1988) Meniscal repair using an exogenous fibrin clot. *Journal of Bone and Joint Surgery* **70–A**, 1209.

Arnoczky SP, Warren RF (1982) Microvasculature of the human meniscus. *American Journal of Sports Medicine* **10**, 90.

Bach BR, Warren RF, Wicklewicz TL (1983) The pivot shift phenomenon: results and description of a modified clinical test for anterior cruciate ligament insufficiency. *American Journal of Sports Medicine* **16**, 571.

Baker CL, Norwood LA, Hughston JC (1984) Acute combined posterior cruciate and posterolateral instability of the knee. *American Journal of Sports Medicine* **12**, 204.

Baker CL, Norwood LA, Hughston JC (1983) Acute posterolateral rotary instability of the knee. *Journal of Bone and Joint Surgery* **65–A**, 614.

Baker BE, Peckham AC, Pupparo F, Sanborn JC (1985) Review of meniscal injury and associated sports. *American Journal of Sports Medicine* **13**, 1.

Butler DC, Noyes FR, Grood ES (1980) Ligamentous restraints to anterior-posterior drawer in the human knee. *Journal of Bone and Joint Surgery* **62–A**, 259.

Cash JD, Hughston JC (1988) Treatment of acute patellar dislocation. *American Journal of Sports Medicine* **16**, 244.

Clancy WG, Shelbourne KD, Zoellneer GB, Keene JS, Reider B, Rosenberg TD (1983) Treatment of knee joint instability secondary to rupture of the posterior cruciate ligament. *Journal of Bone and Joint Surgery* **65–A**, 310.

Clancy WG, Ray JM, Zoltan DJ (1988) Acute tears of the anterior cruciate ligament. *Journal of Bone and Joint Surgery* **70–A**, 1483.

Clancy WG, Nelson DA, Reider B, Narechania RG (1982) Anterior cruciate reconstruction using one-third of the patellar ligament, augmented by extra-articular tendon transfers. *Journal of Bone and Joint Surgery* **64A**, 352.

Cross MJ, Powell JF (1984) Long-term follow-up of posterior cruciate ligament rupture: a study of 116 cases. *American Journal of Sports Medicine* **12**, 292.

Dandy DN, Pusey RJ (1982) The long-term results of unrepaired tears of the posterior cruciate ligament. *Journal of Bone and Joint Surgery* **64–B**, 92.

Daniel DM, Stone ML, Barnett P, Sachs R (1988) Use of the quadriceps active test to diagnose posterior cruciate ligament disruption and measure posterior laxity of the knee. **70–A**, 386.

Daniel DM, Malcolm LL, Losse G, Stone ML, Sachs R, Burks R (1985) Instrumented measurement of anterior laxity of the knee. *Journal of Bone and Joint Surgery* **67–A**, 720.

Daniel DM, Stone ML, Sachs R, Malcolm L (1985) Instrumental measurement of anterior knee laxity in patients with acute anterior cruciate ligament disruption. *American Journal of Sports Medicine* **13**, 401.

DeHaven KE (1980) Diagnosis of acute knee injuries with hemarthrosis. *American Journal of Sports Medicine* **8**, 9.

DeLee JC, Riley MB, Rockweood CA (1983a) Acute straight lateral instability of the knee. *American Journal of Sports Medicine* **11**, 404.

DeLee JC, Riley MB, Rockwood CA (1983b) Acute posterolateral rotatory instability of the knee. *American Journal of Sports Medicine* **11**, 199.

Donaldson WF, Warren RF, Wickiewicz T (1985) A comparison of acute anterior cruciate ligament examinations. *American Journal of Sports Medicine* **13**, 5.

Engebretsen L, Benum P, Fasting O, Molster A, Strand T (1990) A prospective, randomized study of three surgical techniques for treatment of acute ruptures of the anterior cruciate ligament. *American Journal of Sports Medicine* **18**, 585.

Fried JA, Bengfeld JA, Weiker G, Andrish JT (1985) Anterior cruciate reconstruction using the Jones-Ellison procedure. *Journal of Bone and Joint Surgery* **67A**, 1029.

Ghosh P, Taylor TK (1987) The knee joint meniscus. *Clinical Orthopaedics* **224**, 52.

Gollehon DL, Torzilli PA, Warren RF (1987) The role of the posterolateral and cruciate ligaments in the stability of the human knee. *Journal of Bone and Joint Surgery* **69–A**, 233.

Gomes JL, Marczyk LR (1984) Anterior cruciate ligament reconstruction with a loop or double thickness of semitendinosus tendon. *American Journal of Sports Medicine* **12**, 199.

Hawkins RJ, Misamore GW, Merritt TR (1986) Follow-up of the acute non-operated isolated anterior cruciate ligament tear. *American Journal of Sports Medicine* **14**, 205.

Hughston JC, Andrews JR, Cross MJ, Moschi A (1976) Classification of knee ligament instabilities part I. The medial compartment and cruciate ligaments. *Journal of Bone and Joint Surgery* **58–A**, 159.

Hughston JC, Andrews JR, Cross MJ, Moschi A (1976) Classification of knee ligament instabilities part II. The lateral compartment. *Journal of Bone and Joint Surgery* **58–A**, 173.

Hunter SC, Marascalco R, Hughston JC (1983) Disruption of the vastus medialis obliquus with medial knee ligament injuries. *American Journal of Sports Medicine* **11**, 427.

Indelicato PA (1983) Non-operative treatment of complete tears of the medial collateral ligament of the knee. *Journal of Bone and Joint Surgery* **65–A**, 323.

Indelicato PA, Bittar ES, Prevot TJ, Woods GA, Branett TP, Huegel M (1990) Clinical comparison of freeze-dried and fresh frozen patellar tendon allografts for anterior cruciate ligament reconstruction of the knee. *American Journal of Sports Medicine* **18**, 335.

Jakob RP, Straubli HU, DeLand JT (1987) Grading the pivot shift. *Journal of Bone and Joint Surgery* **69–B**, 294.

Johnson RJ, Eriksson E, Haggmark T, Pope MH (1984) Five to ten year follow-up evaluation after reconstruction of the anterior cruciate ligament. *Clinical Orthopaedics* **183**, 122.

Jones KG (1980) Results of use of the central one-third of the patellar ligament to compensate for anterior cruciate ligament deficiency. *Clinical Orthopaedics* **147**, 39.

Kannus P, Jarvinen M (1987) Long-term prognosis of non-operatively treated acute knee distortions having primary hemarthrosis without clinical instability. *American Journal of Sports Medicine* **15**, 138.

Kelly DN, Carter VS, Jobe FW, Kenlan RK (1984) Patellar and quadriceps tendon ruptures – jumper's knee. *American Journal of Sports Medicine* **12**, 375.

Larson RL (1983) Physical examination in the diagnosis of rotatory instability. *Clinical Orthopaedics* **172**, 38.

Lyscholm J, Gillquist J (1982) Evaluation of knee ligament surgery results with special emphasis on use of a scoring scale. *American Journal of Sports Medicine* **10**, 150.

Mandelbaum BR, Finerman GA, Reicher MA et al. (1986) Magnetic resonance imaging as a tool for evaluation of traumatic knee injuries. *American Journal of Sports Medicine* **14**, 361.

McCarroll JR (1983) Fracture of the patella during a golf swing following reconstruction of the anterior cruciate ligament. *American Journal of Sports Medicine* **11**, 26.

Noyes FR, Modar LA, Moorman CT, McGinniss GH (1989) Partial tears of the anterior cruciate ligament. *Journal of Bone and Joint Surgery* **71–B**, 825.

Parolie JM, Bengfeld JA (1986) Long-term results of non-operative treatment of isolated posterior cruciate ligament injuries in the athlete. *American Journal of Sports Medicine* **14**, 35.

Scott GA, Jolly BL, Henning CE (1986) Combined posterior incision and arthroscopic intra-articular repair of the meniscus. *Journal of Bone and Joint Surgery* **68–A**, 847.

Schoemaker SC, Markolf KC (1986) The role of the meniscus in the anterior-posterior stability of the loaded anterior cruciate-deficient knee. *Journal of Bone and Joint Surgery* **68–A**, 71.

Scuderi C (1958) Ruptures of the quadriceps tendon: study of twenty tendons ruptures. *American Journal Surgery* **95**, 626.

Siwek CW, Rao JP (1981) Ruptures of the extensor mechanism of the knee joint. *Journal of Bone and Joint Surgery* **63–A**, 932.

Teitge RA, Indelicato PA, Kerlan RK et al. (1980) Iliotibial band transfer for anterolateral rotatory instability of the knee. *American Journal of Sports Medicine* **8**, 223.

Woods GW, Stanley RF, Tullos HS (1979) Lateral capsular sign: X-ray due to a significant knee instability. *American Journal of Sports Medicine* **7**, 27.

Zarins B, Rowe CR, Harris BA, Watkins MP (1983) Rotational motion of the knee. *American Journal of Sports Medicine* **11**, 152.

6

Tendon injuries with special reference to the hand

S. L. Knight

Introduction

Tendons and their surrounding structures may be injured in a single acute episode or the injury may occur more subtly by repetitive episodes of minor trauma that occur when the tendon is subjected to excessive use. In this chapter acute injuries to tendons, tenosynovitis and insertional tendinitis will all be considered. The basic principles may be applied to tendon injuries throughout the body, but most of the discussion specifically concerns the tendons in the hand.

Injury to the hand is a very common problem. It has been estimated that over 50% of all patients attending casualty departments have an injured hand. In many cases the injury will be trivial but in some an underlying tendon will be damaged. The best results follow prompt recognition and treatment of the injured tendon, so anyone who is likely to meet this problem in practice should have a thorough knowledge of the tendons of the hand and be able to examine the integrity of individual tendons with confidence.

Once the diagnosis of a tendon injury is made, most patients will require referral to a hand specialist. Emphasis is therefore placed on the diagnosis and immediate management of these injuries.

Aetiology

Acute tendon injuries may follow open or closed trauma. Open injuries to tendons may either be of a tidy or of an untidy nature. Most tidy wounds are simple lacerations, with glass the most frequent injuring agent. Untidy wounds are usually complex injuries involving many structures apart from the tendons themselves. Most of the mutilating industrial injuries fall into this last category.

Acute closed injuries to tendons usually result in an injury at the insertion of the tendon; a healthy tendon rarely ruptures along its length. The injury usually occurs when a tendon which is already loaded is suddenly subjected to an extra load. An example of this is a mallet finger, which usually occurs when the distal interphalangeal joint is forcibly flexed while the extensor is attempting to extend it. Other examples of this type of injury include the boutonnière deformity and the rupture of the flexor digitorum profundus insertion.

In addition to the acute injuries described above, tendons may also be injured by minor repetitive trauma. The site of this trauma is usually where the tendon is attached to the skeleton or where the tendon changes direction around a pulley or retinaculum, giving rise to insertional tendinitis and tenosynovitis respectively.

Insertional tendinitis is ill-understood and is probably due to numerous small tears in the collagen fibres, attaching either the insertion or origin of the tendon to the skeleton. In the upper limb, the most common site for this injury to occur is around the elbow, presenting as either medial or lateral epicondylitis. Acute calcific tendonitis is usually sited at the insertion of a tendon, particularly that of the flexor carpi ulnaris. Once again, the exact mechanism of the disorder is incompletely understood, but it is perhaps a form of insertional tendinitis where the minor trauma to the tendon insertion provokes precipitation of a calcium deposit.

Wherever tendons pass through pulleys or pass under retinacula they are protected from abrasion by synovial fluid, produced by the enveloping lining of synovium. Unaccustomed repetitive use of a particular tendon may result in transient inflammation or tenosynovitis. In addition to this, specific chronic disorders such as rheumatoid arthritis may affect the synovium primarily, leading to secondary damage of the tendon.

Acute injuries to the tendon sheath may also occur as a direct result of penetration, as occurs in flexor tendon sheath infection or, more dramatically, in hydraulic or grease gun injuries, where irritant hydrocarbons are injected into the sheath under high pressure.

Diagnosis

The diagnosis of tendon injury is usually straight forward provided that an accurate history has been obtained and the patient has been examined fully and logically.

Acute division and acute rupture of a tendon result in lack of function, which is usually obvious to both the patient and to the examining physician. However, pitfalls do exist; the integrity of an adjacent synergistic tendon may mask the signs. For example, division of the radial wrist extensors may be masked by the integrity of the extensors of the fingers, which also secondarily extend the wrist. Immediate diagnosis will only be made if the wrist extensors are specifically examined. Likewise, injuries to the flexor digitorum superficialis may be masked by an intact flexor digitorum profundus tendon. It is also important to note that tendon injuries rarely occur in isolation and adjacent nerves and vessels are often simultaneously injured. A systematic and complete examination of the injured part is therefore essential.

Examination of the injured hand is a very exciting and intellectually satisfying procedure. Many excellent texts are available on this subject. With practice, the diagnosis can usually be made from the history, the site of the wound and the posture of the hand.

Provided that the examiner has the necessary knowledge of anatomy, he or she will be well aware of the structures that may be divided deep to a wound on the forearm or hand. Where the injury has been caused by glass, it is safer to assume that any underlying tendon that may have been divided probably has been.

The relaxed hand assumes a characteristic position that is governed by the balancing tonic forces of the flexors and the extensors. With the palm uppermost, the wrist usually lies in a position of 30° of dorsiflexion and the thumb and the fingers are gently flexed. The fingertips lie on the same curve as they gently 'cascade' into increasing flexion from the index to the little finger. Interruption of this cascade signifies a tendon injury. For example, division of both flexor tendons to a digit causes that finger to lie in complete extension.

These general observations should be followed by specific examination of tendons. The flexor carpi radialis and the flexor carpi ulnaris tendons may be assessed by flexing the wrist against resistance and palpating the tendons. The flexor pollicis longus is tested by actively trying to flex the interphalangeal joint of the thumb. The flexor digitorum profundus tendons are assessed by flexing the distal interphalangeal joint of the fingers. The profundus tendon flexes not only the distal interphalangeal joint but will also flex the proximal interphalangeal joint, so in order to assess the integrity of the flexor digitorum superficialis, it is essential to place the flexor digitorum profundus out of action. This can be performed by recognizing the different properties of the two muscles: the

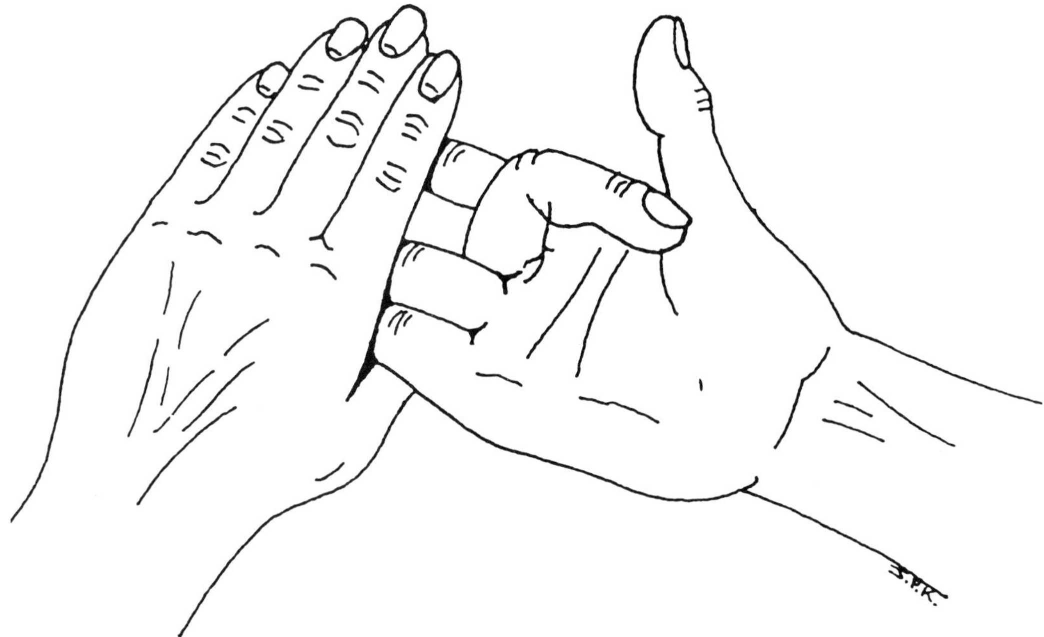

Fig. 6.1 Testing flexor digitorum superficialis.

superficialis muscle may flex the fingers individually, whereas the profundus cannot. By stretching the profundus tendons out to length in those fingers which are not being examined, the profundus tendon becomes slack in the remaining finger. Flexion at the proximal interphalangeal joint is produced solely by the superficialis tendon (Fig. 6.1).

The abductor pollicis longus and the extensor pollicis brevis can both be palpated on the radial side of the anatomical 'snuff-box' when the thumb is held in extension. On the ulnar side of the snuff-box the extensor pollicis longus can be felt. This may also be tested by actively extending the interphalangeal joint of the thumb. The extension of the metacarpophalangeal joints of the fingers confirms the integrity of the extensor digitorum communis. The index and little fingers each have an extra extensor tendon which allows them to extend independently. It is important to note that the prime function of the long extensors of the fingers is to extend the metacarpophalangeal joint. Extension of the interphalangeal joints requires the synergistic activity of the intrinsic muscles via the extensor expansion. The extensor carpi radialis longus and extensor carpi radialis brevis and the extensor carpi ulnaris may be palpated on the radial and on the ulnar sides of the wrist while dorsiflexing against resistance.

Where the main complaint is one of the pain associated with movement of a tendon, it is important to localize accurately the site of the pain and to try to elicit any other physical signs such as crepitus or synovial swelling, In both insertional tendinitis and in tenosynovitis, it may be possible to provoke the pain by the use of specific tests, which will be discussed under the separate headings.

A final complaint is that of clunking of a tendon. This may be due to triggering of a tendon nodule through a pulley, or it may be due to subluxation of a tendon over a bony prominence.

In some cases an X-ray will help clinch the diagnosis. Examples of this are the avulsion injuries of the tendon insertions, where the displaced bony insertion is diagnostic. X-rays may also be used to diagnose associated injuries or to eliminate other potential causes of pain.

Tendon healing

In order to function effectively, a tendon needs to glide smoothly in relation to the underlying skeleton. Full functional repair of a tendon therefore requires not only the apposition of its cut ends but also the restoration of its normal excursion.

Because of the relative acellularity of tendon, for many years it was assumed that tendon repair occurred by invasion of fibroblasts and blood vessels from the adjacent connective tissue (Potenza, 1969). Adhesion formation was considered to be an inevitable consequence of tendon healing. However, it is now evident that tendons do not rely on this mechanism and possess an intrinsic ability to heal by proliferation of the cells on the surface of the divided tendon (Lundborg, 1985). Arguments as to which is the predominant method of healing have continued for the last two decades. From the practical point of view it does not matter; almost certainly both methods of healing are important and occur simultaneously. Following an injury collagen is laid haphazardly throughout the wound and in the absence of any modifying factors the tendon and surrounding connective tissues will all heal as a solid block. The immature scar, however, possesses plasticity and the application of mechanical force to the repair in the postoperative period will modify this response. This is the basis of postoperative rehabilitation.

Traditionally tendons are repaired by approximating the ends of the tendon with a suture and immobilizing the injured part in such a manner that the tension on the tendon repair is minimal. However, such immobilization, while it allows the ends of the tendons to remain in contact with each other throughout the healing phase, also causes the tendon to remain in constant contact with the surrounding injured tissues. The end-result is a healed tendon which cannot glide. This is functionally useless. Intensive physiotherapy is then required to obtain differential movement between the tendons and the surrounding structures.

The results of such treatment vary from site to site. Where the tendon is surrounded by soft elastic tissues such as fat and muscle it may be possible to obtain a considerable excursion of the tendon despite its tethering, whereas injury of the tendon within a tight unyielding fibro-osseus tunnel, such as under the extensor retinaculum or within the digital flexor sheath, may result in a tendon repair which becomes completely stuck. At these sites, the results of tendon repair can be improved by either modifying the anatomy of the injury or by mobilizing the tendons throughout the healing phase.

In the case of injuries under the extensor retinaculum, the anatomy of the injury may be modified by excising the retinaculum so that the tendon repair adheres to more pliable overlying structures.

Excision of the digital flexor sheath is impractical, as intolerable bowstringing would result. These injuries therefore require a far more exacting postoperative regimen – that of immediate controlled mobilization of the repaired tendon. This relies on the intrinsic ability of the tendon to heal, and the aim is to produce the perfect tendon repair, where the tendon ends are spot-welded to each other without adhesions to the surrounding structures.

Principles of surgical treatment

Most tendon injuries will require referral to a specialist; there is now little place for the inexperienced surgeon to attempt even simple repairs. Where specialist advice is not immediately available, the injury should be fully documented and the wound cleaned, closed and dressed under local anaesthesia. The injured part should be splinted and arrangements made for specialist treatment as soon as possible. Ideally this delay should not exceed 24 hours. Obviously, problems such as ischaemia of the injured part, extensive skin loss or associated life-threatening injuries all have a greater priority than the individual tendon injury and need urgent treatment.

Bandaging and splintage of the acutely injured hand serve a number of important functions. The hand is immobilized, which makes the patient

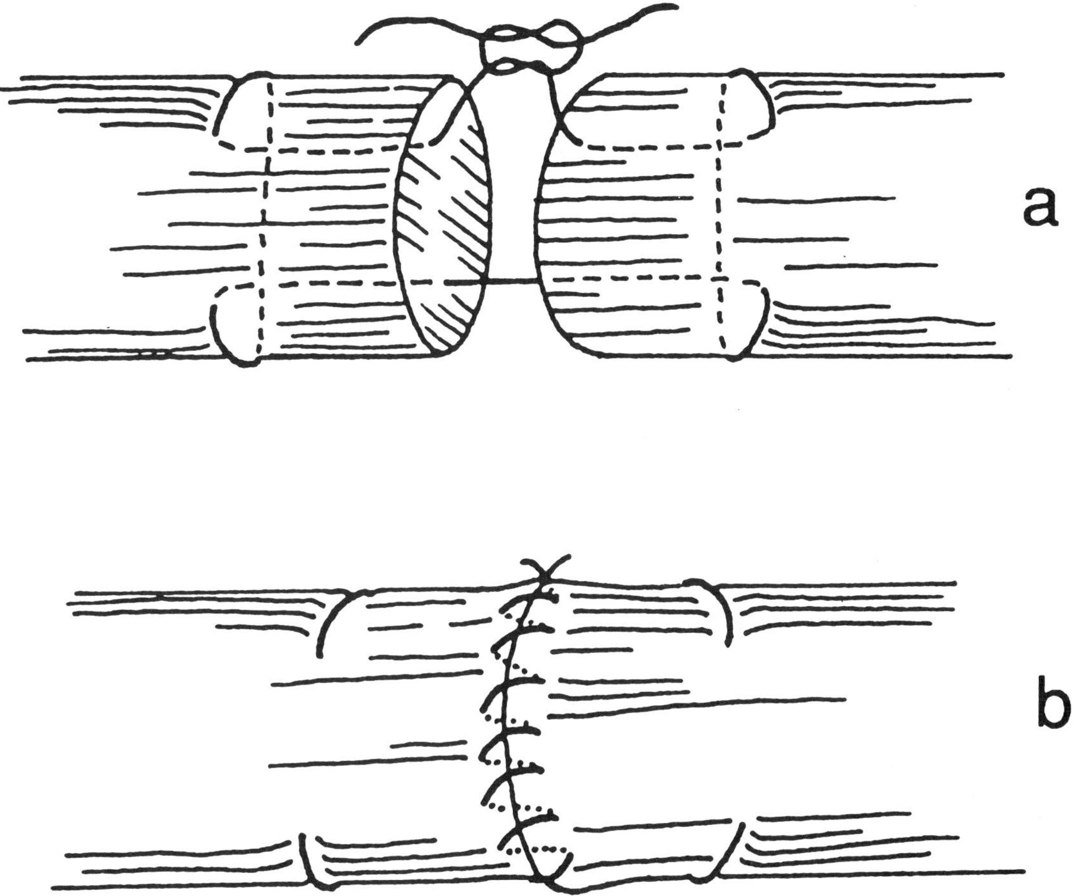

Fig. 6.2 Tendon sutures: (a) Kessler grasping suture augmented by (b) running epitendinous suture.

more comfortable and prevents further displacement of the cut tendon ends, and the gentle pressure exerted by the dressing reduces the bleeding and swelling. The simplest way to construct such a splint is to use a padded plaster of Paris slab which extends from the fingertips to the proximal forearm. Ideally the interphalangeal joints will be held in full extension, the metacarpophalangeal joints at 90° and the wrist should be dorsiflexed to 30°. The slab may be bandaged to the volar or dorsal aspects of the limb, depending on individual preference. A high sling should be worn.

Surgical treatment for most tendon injuries of the upper limb may be performed using a local or regional nerve block, although occasionally general anaesthesia may be preferred. The use of a tourniquet is essential.

The surgical technique is important. Every effort should be made to ensure that the blood supply to the tendon ends is not damaged; where present, the vinculae should be preserved and care should be taken not to strip the paratenon from the surface of the tendon. In order to minimize the adhesions to the surrounding structures, attention should be given to the siting of overlying skin incisions and dissection of the adjacent connective tissues should be kept to a minimum.

Before placing any sutures in the tendon, it is essential to relax the tendon in question by flexing or extending adjacent joints. Ideally the severed tendon ends should gently abut each other prior to the suture being placed. No attempt should ever be made to haul the ends of a tendon together; the sutures will cut out, cause the tendon to fray and make the repair progressively more difficult.

Tendon is made up of many longitudinally oriented fibres. In order to perform a strong repair, the configuration of the suture must be such as to grasp some of these fibres without strangulating the whole of the tendon. Flat tendons are usually repaired using a series of interrupted horizontal mattress sutures. For round tendons, the Kessler suture (Fig. 6.2a) is probably the most popular method of repair. Wherever a particularly smooth tendon repair is required, as in the digital flexor sheath, the Kessler suture may be augmented by a fine peripheral running suture (Fig. 6.2b).

The choice of suture materials will be subject to individual preference. The best results follow repair with non-absorbable, synthetic fibres. Braided polyester and monofilament nylon are the most popular choices. The strength of the required suture depends on the size of tendon being repaired: 4–0 is the size usually required to repair digitor flexor and extensor tendons. The larger tendons of the lower limb will require a stronger suture.

Following the tendon repair, the limbs should be splinted in a position that ensures relaxation of the repaired tendon, to minimize the chance of dehiscence of the repair in the postoperative period.

Splintage will normally be required for a period of 3–4 weeks. Following this, the splintage may be either discarded or modified so that a graduated programme of active mobilization may be commenced.

Some closed tendon injuries require operative repair, whilst others may be treated successfully with splintage alone. These will be discussed under their specific headings.

Open flexor tendon injuries of the hand

Flexor tendon injuries to the hand are conventionally classified according to the anatomical level at which they are divided (Table 6.1). As already discussed, the most difficult areas to deal with are those where the tendon is injured within a tight fibro-osseus tunnel. In these situations access to the tendon is difficult, accurate surgical repair is essential and the likelihood of resistant postoperative adhesions is very high.

Table 6.1 Classification of tendon injuries

Zone I	Distal to flexor digitorum superficialis insertion
Zone II	Digital flexor sheath containing superficialis and profundus tendons – 'no man's land'
Zone III	Mid-palm
Zone IV	Within carpal tunnel
Zone V	Proximal to carpal tunnel

The digital fibrous flexor sheath consists of five unyielding fibro-osseus tunnels placed in series along the course of the digit. These are named the annular pulleys and are labelled numerically (Fig. 6.3).

The fibrous tissue in the intervening portions of the sheath is arranged in a criss-cross fashion to enable the sheath to concertina when the finger is bent. These areas are misnamed the cruciate pulleys. A particularly busy and dangerous area for surgical repair of tendons is in the proximal part of the fibrous flexor sheath. In this area, the profundus tendon is encircled by the decussating fibres of the superficialis tendon and both are in turn encircled by the flexor sheath. The difficulties in operating in this particular area have long been recognized and for many years the territory defined by the proximal end of the A1 pulley to the insertion of the superficialis tendon was termed 'no man's land'.

The diagnosis of flexor tendon injury has been covered earlier. When both flexor tendons to the finger have been divided, the finger usually lies in an attitude of complete extension. It may be possible actively to flex the metacarpophalangeal joint using the intrinsic muscles but the patient cannot flex either of the interphalangeal joints. When a profundus tendon is injured, the patient is unable actively to flex the distal interphalangeal joint, which lies in an attitude of complete

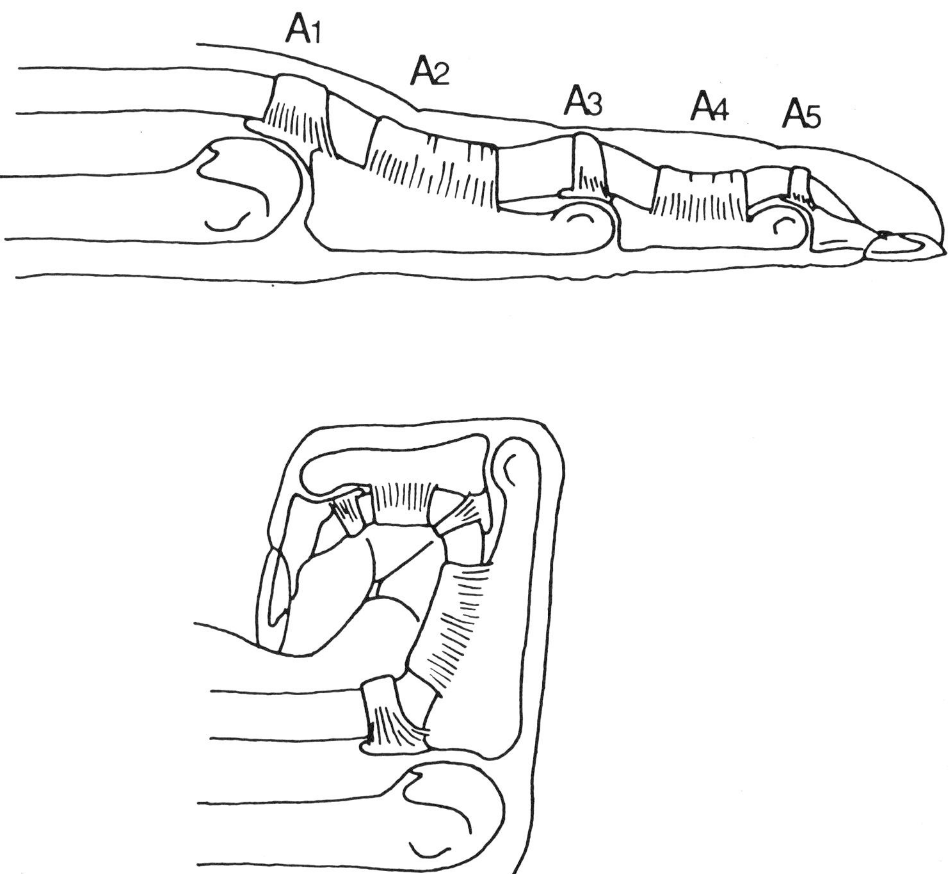

Fig. 6.3 Flexor tendon pulley system, demonstrating the five annular pulleys.

extension. When the flexor digitorum superficialis tendon alone is divided the diagnosis may be a little more difficult. The first clue to such an injury is the interruption of the normal digital cascade. Although the proximal and the distal interphalangeal joints are slightly flexed, the alteration in tone as a result of the division of the superficialis tendon results in the proximal interphalangeal joint lying in slightly greater extension than those of the uninjured fingers. The diagnosis can be confirmed by specifically examining the superficialis tendon. Close examination should then be performed to exclude injury to nearby nerves and vessels. It is important to make a point of specifically examining the flexor pollicis longus by asking the patient actively to flex the interphalangeal joint of the thumb. These injuries are often missed and are referred late. This is presumably because the examining physician accepts movement at the metacarpophalangeal joint as suggesting an intact flexor pollicis longus, when in fact this movement may be produced by the intrinsic muscles of the thumb alone. Finally it is important not to be lulled into a false sense of security by the size of the overlying skin laceration. Very extensive damage to tendons may occur through tiny external wounds.

Even in the very best hands, the results of flexor tendon repair are not predictable. There is no one recipe for success based on the anatomy of the injury alone. The treatment plan adopted by the specialist will also have to take into consideration such factors as the age, occupation, hobbies and intelligence of the patient. Other factors such as

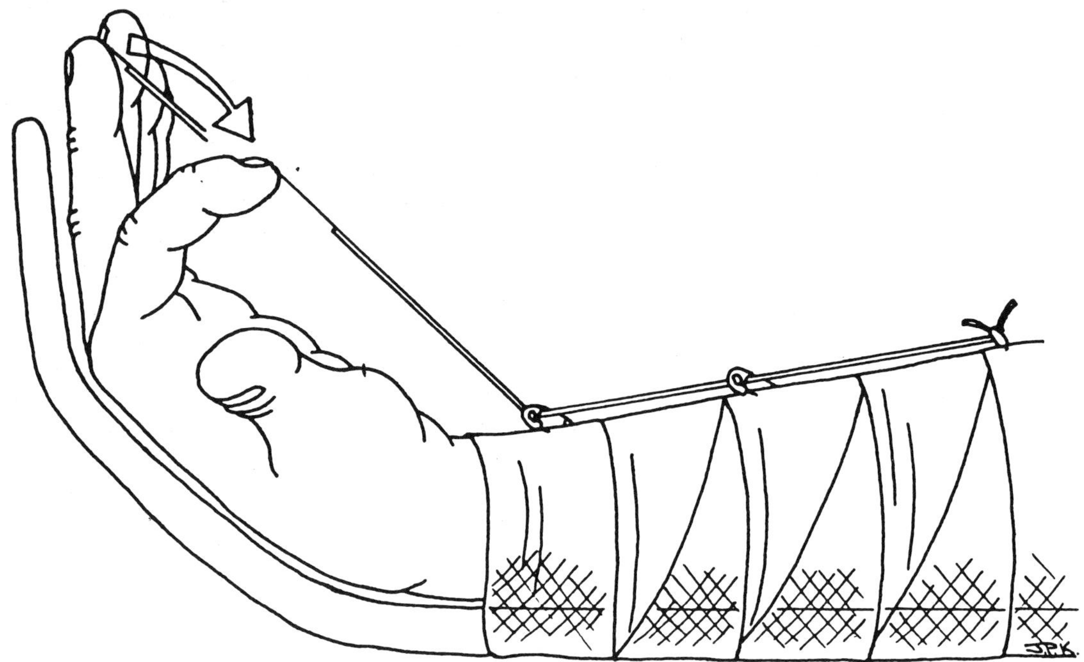

Fig. 6.4 The dynamic splint for controlled postoperative mobilization of flexor tendon injuries.

the ability of the patient to attend for postoperative rehabilitation need also to be considered. Under certain circumstances, the patient's interests may be best served by ignoring isolated profundus or isolated superficialis injuries. This decision, however, should be made by an experienced specialist with the full informed consent of the patient. In other circumstances, both tendons will be repaired in the manner already described.

Particular mention should be made of flexor tendon repair within the digital flexor sheath. This is technically very exacting. It is important to preserve the pulley system to the digit and this makes access difficult. The tendon repair can only be performed in the gaps between the pulleys and the position of the finger needs to be adjusted for this to be possible. The profundus tendon is repaired using a Kessler core suture and is augmented by a continuous peripheral running suture to tidy up the circumference of the repair. The superficialis tendon slips are flat and are repaired with mattress sutures. It is important that the repair does not increase the bulk of the tendon which should be able to glide within the sheath at the end of the repair. Further details of the operative repair at this site are beyond the scope of this chapter and operative texts should be consulted.

Following repair of a flexor tendon, the patient may undergo a number of postoperative rehabilitation regimes. For injuries outside fibro-osseus tunnels, static splintage for a month is followed by intensive physiotherapy. Elsewhere a more complicated postoperative regimen may be followed, whereby the tendon is gently moved throughout the healing period in an attempt to avoid adhesions. This is particularly suitable for tendon injuries within the digital flexor sheath. The most commonly used method of mobilizing the tendon in a controlled fashion is by using rubber band traction (Fig. 6.4) (Lister *et al.*, 1977). The injured finger intermittently extends the rubber band and is then drawn back into the flexed position. Another way of achieving this passive mobilization is by manipulating the injured fingers through their full range of movement (Strickland and Glogovac, 1980).

The foregoing account is mainly applicable to

tidy injuries where the tendon is cleanly divided. In untidy injuries a large segment of the tendon may be lost, the pulleys destroyed and there may be no overlying skin. These patients require staged treatment, involving the provision of adequate skin cover with local or distant flaps, pulley reconstruction and, later, tendon grafting.

Closed flexor tendon injuries

As already explained, healthy tendons rarely rupture along their length, and most ruptures occur at the insertion of the tendon. The flexor tendons are no exception. The most common site for the flexor tendon to rupture is that of the profundus insertion to the ring finger. This injury is most often seen during the game of rugby where the patient has tried to grasp a passing opponent's jersey (Burton and Eaton, 1973). The avulsion is associated with sudden pain and swelling of the finger. Bruising may be apparent throughout the length of the finger due to blood tracking down the tendon sheath. Sometimes part of the distal phalanx is avulsed with the tendon and becomes jammed at the decussation of the superficialis tendon. This may be felt as a lump. Alternatively the profundus tendon may be pulled completely out of the fibrous flexor sheath and a swelling may be felt in the palm at the base of the finger. In the acute phase, because of the pain and swelling it is often difficult to test for active motion at the distal and at the proximal interphalangeal joints. Frequently the patient assumes that he has simply sprained his finger and only presents after many days or many weeks when he notices that he cannot actively flex the distal interphalangeal joint. An X-ray should always be performed as this may demonstrate proximal displacement of a bony fragment attached to the profundus insertion.

If the injury is recognized acutely, immediate repair should be performed. This involves threading the tendon back through the pulley system and re-inserting it into the distal phalanx where it is maintained by a transosseus suture and a button over the nail on the dorsum of the finger (Fig. 6.5).

When the injury is noticed at a late stage serious consideration needs to be given as to whether anything needs to be done at all. In many cases there is little disability caused by the inability to bend the distal interphalangeal joint. Where the patient is keen on further treatment, is well-motivated and is prepared to undergo intensive postoperative rehabilitation, tendon grafting is a suitable procedure (Lunn and Lamb, 1984); it is usually impossible, at this stage, to re-introduce the original tendon back through the pulley system. Where patients are not prepared to invest a lot of their own time in their treatment, their interests may be best served by permanently fixing

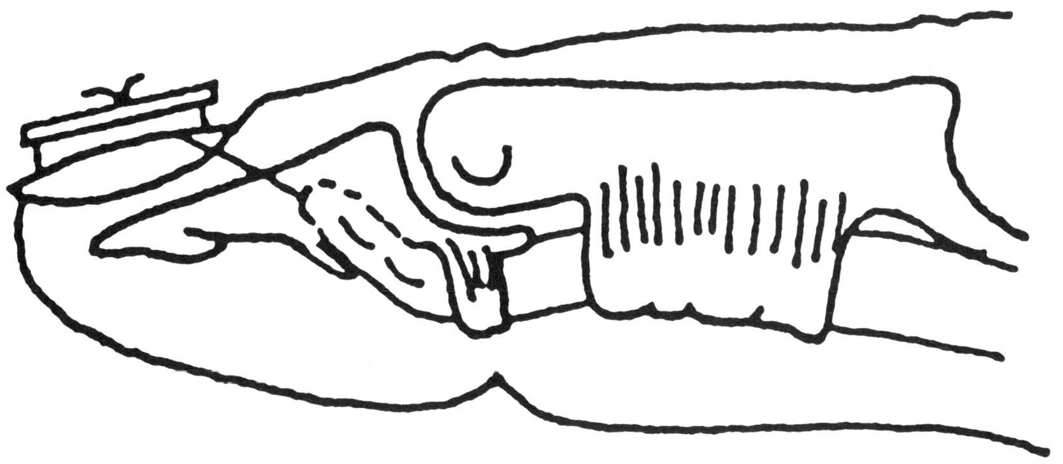

Fig. 6.5 Profundus tendon re-insertion.

the distal interphalangeal joint in an attitude of approximately 40° of flexion. This may be achieved by an arthrodesis of the interphalangeal joint.

Ruptures of flexor tendons elsewhere have been described and are usually associated with underlying chronic disorders, such as rheumatoid arthritis, which cause weakening of the tendon. The most usual site for the tendon rupture to occur is within the carpal tunnel.

Open extensor tendon injuries

Extensor tendons injuries over the dorsum of the fingers and hand are a very common injury and the diagnosis is usually easy to make. However a number of injuries deserve special mention.

The extensor digitorum communis tendons have tendinous attachments to each other on the dorsum of the hand. These are called the juncturae tendinae. Injury of one of the extensor tendons immediately proximal to this may result in only a few degrees' loss of active extension and the diagnosis may be overlooked.

Another site of diagnostic difficulty occurs when the central slip of the extensor tendon is divided over the dorsum of the proximal interphalangeal joint. This may be caused by tiny wounds over the dorsum of the finger. The diagnosis is not always easy and will be missed by cursory examination; a boutonnière deformity will then develop (Fig. 6.6). It is usually possible for these patients to extend the finger fully. The diagnosis will only be made if extension is performed against resistance or if a modification of Carducci's test is performed (Carducci, 1981). This test involves fully flexing the wrist and then passively flexing the metacarpophalangeal joint. This tightens the extensor apparatus and if the central slip is intact the interphalangeal joint will automatically extend. Failure of this to happen is diagnostic of central slip division.

The third injury that deserves special mention is that caused by punching an assailant in the mouth. In this injury, there is a laceration over the dorsum of the metacarpophalangeal joint caused by the assailant's tooth. This nearly always partially divides the extensor tendon and enters the metacarpophalangeal joint. The injury may occasionally cause damage to the articular surface of the head of the metacarpal which may be visible on X-ray. It is rare for these patients to be honest about the cause of the injury and any ragged laceration over the metacarpophalangeal joint should be treated with suspicion.

A final word of warning involves those injuries where the extensors on the dorsum of the forearm are divided. If this occurs proximally, the posterior interosseus nerve may be divided. If the

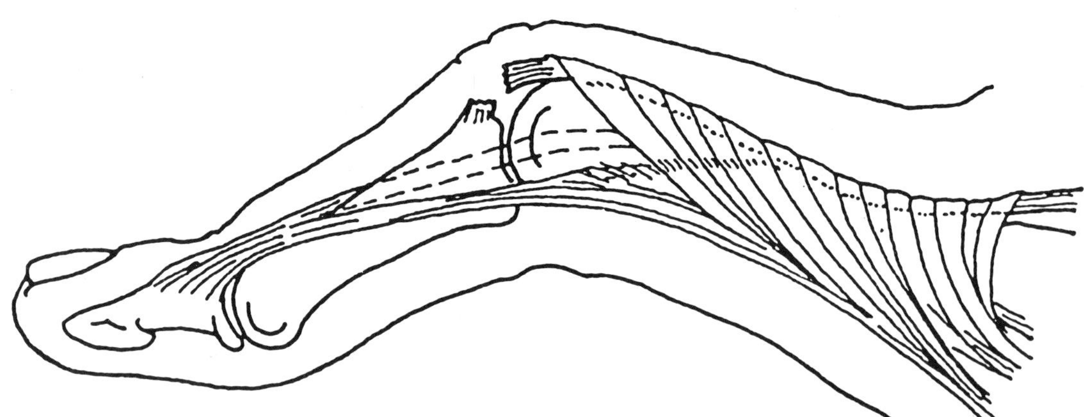

Fig. 6.6 Boutonnière deformity. The central slip rupture allows the proximal interphalangeal joint to 'button-hole' between the two lateral slips.

surgeon performing the repair is unaware of this, he or she will be surprised to note that the patient will be unable to extend the thumb or fingers when the splint is removed after a month.

The repair of extensor tendons is usually straightforward and is followed by a period of splintage of approximately 4 weeks, with the wrist firmly dorsiflexed and the metacarpophalangeal joints flexed to approximately 60°. At the end of this period of time, intensive physiotherapy is begun.

Where an injury occurs in the vicinity of the extensor retinaculum, it is permissible to resect either part or all of the retinaculum overlying the injured tendon. Bowstringing is rarely a problem. By opening up the fibro-osseus sheath, the likelihood of prolonged stiffness due to immobile and unstretchable postoperative adhesions is minimized.

Injuries caused by human teeth over the metacarpophalangeal joint should be treated with great care. These wounds need exploration and prolonged irrigation. The tendon injury is usually incomplete and no formal tendon repair is usually required. The wound should be left open and the hand splinted. A combination of antibiotics, such as flucloxycylin and metronidazole should be prescribed. Septic arthritis of the joint is not an infrequent complication of this injury. The wound should be reviewed every 2–3 days and splintage continued for approximately 3 weeks, before instituting rigorous physiotherapy.

Division of the extensor tendon over the distal and over the proximal interphalangeal joints requires exploration of the wound, repair of the tendon, and splintage of the joint in extension using a Kirschner wire. This should remain in place for approximately a month, followed by a period of 2–3 weeks' external splintage once the overlying wound has completely healed.

Closed extensor tendon injuries

One of the most common tendon injuries is that of the mallet finger. This is caused by the rupture of the extensor tendon at its insertion (Fig. 6.7a). Occasionally a small portion of the distal phalanx may be avulsed with the insertion of the tendon (Fig. 6.7b), which is visible on X-ray. As explained previously, this is usually caused by a sudden flexing force on a tense extensor tendon. Occasionally a much larger fragment of the distal phalanx appears to be avulsed with the extensor tendon. If this fragment is large enough, the distal phalanx will sublux in a volar direction (Fig. 6.7c). Although classified under mallet injuries, this particular injury has a completely different pathology and is usually caused by a very hard object such as a cricket ball hitting the end of an extended finger. The articular surface of the distal phalanx rather than the extensor tendon insertion bears the brunt of the force.

The first two injuries are best treated conservatively by splintage of the distal interphalangeal joint in extension (Burke, 1988). The splint may be either custom-made or alternatively a polypropylene Stack splint may be used. These are widely available in most casualty departments. The patient should be instructed that the splint needs to be worn for a period of 6–8 weeks. The splint

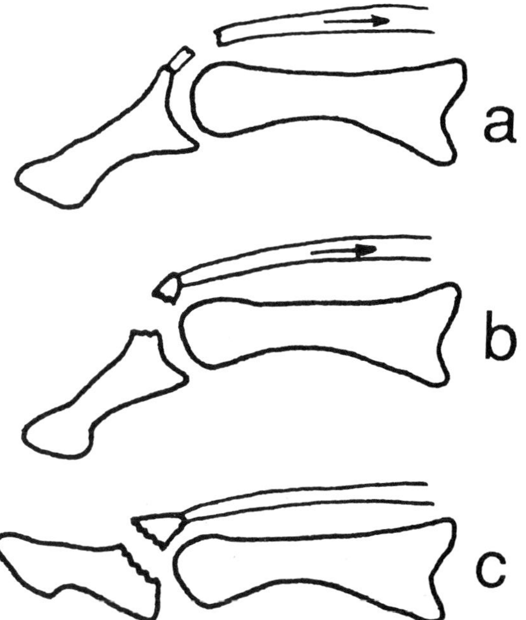

Fig. 6.7 Mallet finger due to (a) rupture of the extensor tendon, (b) avulsion of the extensor insertion and (c) associated with volar subluxation of the distal phalanx.

may be removed to wash the affected digit but the distal interphalangeal joint should be supported at all times. Following the period of splintage, it is advisable to replace the splint at night for a further 2–3 weeks to try to prevent the slight extensor lag that often develops once splintage is discarded.

This is not an uncommon injury amongst sports players who are always impatient to return to their activities very quickly. There is some evidence that the period of splintage may be slightly reduced if the tension in the extensor insertion is reduced. This may be performed by attaching a dynamic extension to the mallet splint, which keeps the proximal interphalangeal joint flexed (Evans and Weightman, 1988).

When the mallet fracture is associated with subluxation of the distal phalanx, operative treatment is required. This usually involves reduction of the subluxed distal phalanx and fixation with a longitudinal Kirschner wire.

Rupture of the central slip of the extensor may be difficult to diagnose in the acute phase and once again the modification of Carducci's test is useful. Treatment consists of static splintage of the proximal interphalangeal joint, in such a way that the distal interphalangeal joint is free to move. Once again this can be accomplished by the use of a short custom-made splint or alternatively mass-produced polypropylene splints are available. The month's static splintage should then be followed by a further period of splintage using a Capener dynamic splint. This splint allows flexion to occur at the proximal interphalangeal joint but its spring aids full extension of the joint.

If a central slip injury passes unnoticed the so-called boutonnière deformity will develop (see Fig. 6.6). This is caused by the proximal interphalangeal joint button-holing between the two lateral slips of the extensor tendon. The lateral slips now lie volar to the axis of the proximal interphalangeal joint and become flexors of this joint rather than extensors. As a result, a zig-zag deformity develops with flexion at the proximal interphalangeal joint at hyperextension at the distal interphalangeal joint. Treatment of the established deformity is unsatisfactory. Treatment is first aimed at trying to correct the deformity passively with dynamic and static splintage. Once this has occurred, central slip reconstruction is undertaken. Very many operations for this procedure are described – a multiplicity that suggests that none is ideal. These operations are beyond the scope of this chapter and operative texts should be consulted.

Rupture of extensor pollicis longus usually occurs as this tendon passes on its oblique course under the extensor retinaculum and around Lister's tubercle (Fig. 6.8). Rupture rarely occurs in the healthy tendon but usually follows a Colles fracture or disease such as rheumatoid arthritis. In the first case, the mechanism of injury is ill-understood. It is thought that the rupture occurs due to a combination of direct abrasion of the tendon at the time of fracture and to interference of the blood supply to that particular part of the tendon. In the second case, the tendon is damaged by the rheumatoid synovitis. In both cases, direct repair of the tendon is not feasible because of the diseased nature of the tendon. The most common method of repair of this tendon is to perform an indicis transfer whereby the extensor indicis propius is transferred to the distal healthy extensor pollicis longus tendon. This is a delightfully simple and elegant transfer and requires little re-education because simultaneous extension of the thumb and index finger is the normal pattern of movement when reaching out to grasp anything.

The extensor tendon is maintained in its position directly over the head of the metacarpal by an intact aponeurosis attached to either side of the tendon. This may be injured by sudden flexion and ulnar deviation of the finger, which results in a tear on the radial side of the expansion. This results in subluxation of the extensor tendon into the valley between the metacarpal heads. The diagnosis is usually missed acutely. The patient presents with sudden pain, swelling and bruising over the dorsum of the hand. Occasionally subluxation may be demonstrated immediately. More often, the injury is treated initially as a bruise and the patient returns complaining of a clicking sensation as the tendon flips over the metacarpal head on flexion and extension of the fingers. Treatment is exploration and repair of the ruptured extensor expansion followed by splintage for approximately 1 month.

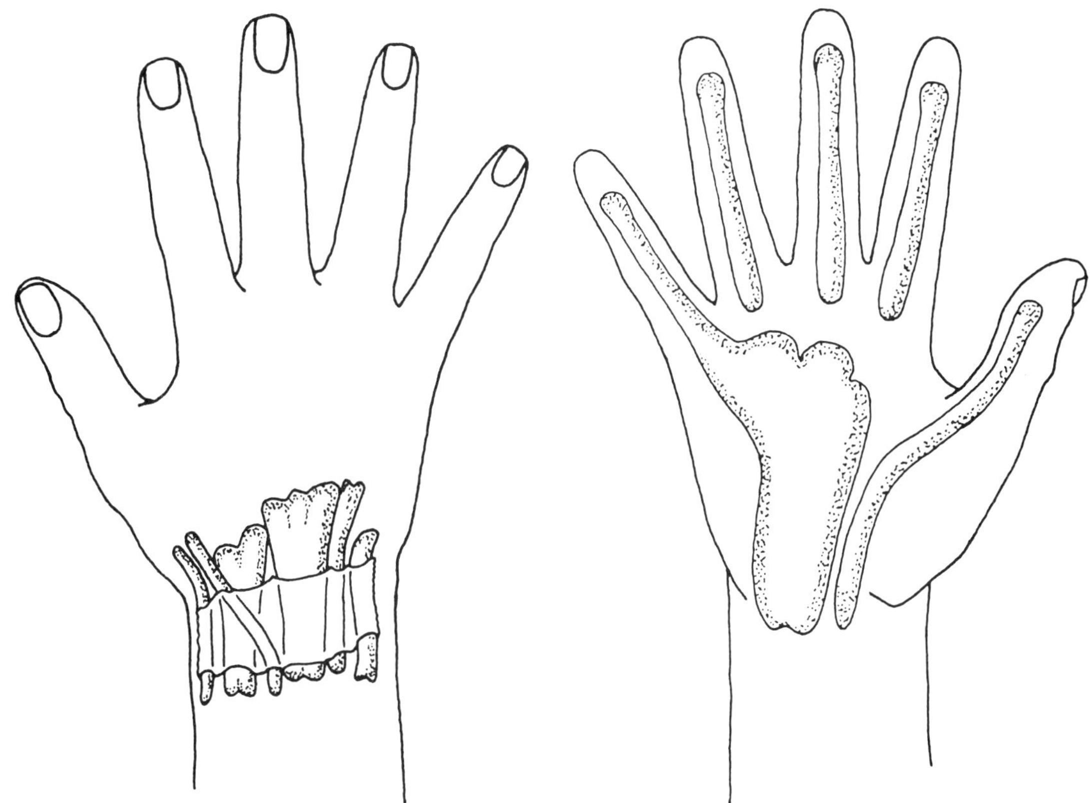

Fig. 6.8 Synovial sheaths.

Subluxation of the extensor carpi ulnaris tendon may occur following a closed rupture of its compartment under the extensor retinaculum. This usually occurs when the forearm is forcibly supinated and the wrist flexed at the same time (Osterman *et al.*, 1988). This may rip the fibrous extensor sheath, allowing the extensor carpi ulnaris tendon to sublux over the head of the ulnar when the forearm is supinated. Once again, these injuries are rarely diagnosed acutely and the patient usually returns complaining of a painful clicking sensation in the wrist when the forearm is supinated. On examination, it may be difficult to get the patient to perform this manoeuvre as he or she will be apprehensive. It can however usually be provoked by actively supinating the forearm and flexing or extending the wrist at the same time.

If the injury is seen and recognized acutely, it may be treated conservatively by placing the patient in a long arm plaster with the elbow at 90°, the forearm in neutral and the wrist in 30° of dorsiflexion. This position should be maintained for 4–6 weeks. If the injury is not recognized until much later, it may be necessary to explore the wrist and reconstruct the fibrous tunnel, using a flap of extensor retinaculum. Following the procedure, the patient will require immobilization as previously described for approximately 6 weeks.

Injuries to the peritendinous structures

Acute injuries to the pulley systems have been mentioned. It has been demonstrated that although the normal hand has five annular pulleys, it will function perfectly well on only two – the A2 and the A4 (Barton, 1969) pulleys. When the pulley systems are destroyed, only these two pulleys are specifically reconstructed. Numerous methods of reconstruction are available, but perhaps the most popular is to use a strip of extensor retinaculum which is passed around the relevant phalanx. These pulleys are subjected to extraordinary loads during the process of flexion and must be allowed to heal before they are stressed. These pulleys are usually repaired over a silastic rod which is left in place until it is replaced by a tendon graft at a second operation.

Chronic injuries to the annular pulleys have only recently become recognized (Bollen, 1990). They occur in top-class climbers who habitually submit their digital pulleys to extreme forces. Most of their hand grips involve acute flexion of the proximal interphalangeal joint. This eventually causes bowstringing between the distal end of the A2 pulley and the proximal end of the A4 pulley. This does not seem to hamper the climber's ability and treatment is unnecessary.

Triggering of a flexor tendon may occur due to a nodule in the profundus tendon which flips in and out of the A1 pulley, giving a triggering sensation. This usually affects the profundus tendons to the ring and middle fingers, although all the other fingers and thumb may be involved. In most cases, the cause is unknown but in a few there may be a prior history of trauma to that particular tendon or the patient may have rheumatoid arthritis. Injection of corticosteroid into the mouth of the affected sheath often allows the symptoms to subside. Resistant or recurrent cases may require division of the A1 pulley. As already explained, provided that the A2 pulley is not tampered with, bowstringing will not occur.

Tenosynovitis may follow excessive and unaccustomed use of the wrist and hand. This results in transient inflammation of the synovial sheaths and usually occurs in the region of the wrist. The patient usually complains of pain, localized to the synovial sheath. There may be associated swelling and crepitus. The symptoms usually subside with oral anti-inflammatory agents and simple analgesics and a period of splintage. It must be stressed that tenosynovitis is a frequently misused term (Semple, 1986) and should only be used to describe inflammation in the region of the synovial reflections (see Fig. 6.8).

A particular form of tenosynovitis which is prone to occur in middle-aged women and which affects the first extensor tunnel is called de Quervain's syndrome. This is a tenosynovitis affecting the abductor pollicis longus and extensor pollicis brevis tendons. As already described, it tends to occur following unaccustomed use and is associated with all the classic signs, namely swelling over the tendon as it passes under the extensor retinaculum, crepitus and pain on moving the tendons. Once again, the symptoms usually subside with a period of splintage and oral analgesics. Should they fail to do so, an injection of corticosteroid into the sheath may relieve the symptoms. Occasionally the diagnosis is difficult to make. When it occurs in middle-aged women it may be difficult to differentiate from osteoarthrosis of the basal joint of the thumb, which indeed may coexist with the syndrome.

One particular provocative test that may be of value in these circumstances is Finkelstein's test. This is performed by asking the patient to clasp the thumb in the palm and then force the wrist into ulnar deviation. A positive test elicits pain over the first dorsal compartment. Caution should be made in interpreting this test. It is uncomfortable in symptom-free patients. Perhaps the best aid to interpretation is to ask the patient to perform the test with the non-symptomatic hand and compare the two responses.

Complete examination should always include an X-ray to exclude osteoarthrosis of the basal joint of the thumb.

If the symptoms fail to subside with conservative measures, operative release of the extensor retinaculum over these tendons may be required. A small incision is made directly over the extensor sheath which is then completely divided. It is important to meticulously scrutinize the abductor pollicis longus and extensor pollicis brevis tendons, because they are often multiple and require incision of all the sheaths if the operation is to be successful. It is important not to damage the terminal branches of the radial nerve which pass directly over the tendon sheath and may be injured either by the incision or may be stretched during the retraction. Damage to these nerves may give rise to symptoms that are worse than the original problem.

Another cause of pain in this area, which may

be difficult to differentiate from de Quervain's syndrome, is the intersectional syndrome. This is so called because it occurs at the intersection where the tendons of the abductor pollicis longus and extensor pollicis brevis pass over the extensor carpi radialis brevis and longus. The two sets of tendons are normally separated from each other by a bursa and the area can be palpated on the reader's own arm immediately proximal to the extensor retinaculum. Symptoms occurring here have been particularly well-described as occurring in rowers and canoeists (Williams, 1977). It is differentiated from de Quervain's syndrome by the more proximal site of the pain and the swelling. The swelling in particular may be a conspicuous physical sign. Once again, these symptoms usually subside with a period of rest, splintage and analgesia. Should they fail to do so, decompression of abductor pollicis longus and extensor pollicis brevis has been demonstrated to cure the symptoms.

Infection of the synovial sheath may occur due to penetration of the sheath by any object such as a thorn. This results in swelling and intense pain in the finger, which adopts an attitude of slight flexion at all the digital joints. In the case of the little finger and the thumb, the synovial sheath continues into the carpal tunnel (see Fig. 6.8), and the signs of medium nerve compression may be added to the symptoms. Urgent incision of the sheath is required. The sheath is usually incised proximally and distally and irrigated until the fluid obtained is no longer turbid. Some authorities suggest leaving a drain within the sheath, to continue irrigation postoperatively. In the author's experience this is unnecessary provided that the irrigation at the time of surgery has been copious and prolonged. The patient is subsequently splinted, placed on intravenous antibiotics and the arm elevated until the infection has subsided. Following this a period of intensive physiotherapy is begun.

High-pressure injection injuries to the finger are dangerous conditions, particularly because their significance is often unrecognized. They occur in occupations dealing with hydraulics and high-pressure paint guns. The injection occurs through a tiny hole, which may be difficult to locate. The paint or hydraulic fluid is then passed proximally, either along the neurovascular bundles or along the fibrous flexor sheath. Once again, in the case of the thumb or the little finger, the extent to which the irritant material may travel is much greater. These cases all need urgent exploration and meticulous debridement. Following the surgery the wound should be very lightly tacked together, the hand splinted and elevated and intensive physiotherapy begun as soon as the inflammation has subsided.

Insertional tendinitis

In the upper limb the most common site for the pain of tendinitis to occur is at the lateral epicondyle, giving rise to the condition of tennis elbow. Its cause is obscure but is probably due to small tears in the muscles arising from the common extensor origin of the lateral epicondyle. The muscle primarily affected is the extensor carpi radialis brevis. The medial counterpart of this condition affects the muscles attached to the common flexor origin, particularly the flexor carpi radialis and the pronator teres muscles.

The condition usually affects patients in the fourth decade, of whom very few have ever played tennis. The diagnosis is made by eliciting tenderness over the lateral epicondyle and provoking the pain by passively flexing the patient's wrist and supinating the forearm while the elbow is held in extension.

In most patients, the symptoms will subside with conservative measures. The arm should simply be rested and anti-inflammatory analgesics prescribed. If this fails to alleviate the symptoms, a mixture of steroid and long-acting local anaesthetic should be injected into the tender spot. This may need to be repeated on several occasions. If the symptoms prove to be repetitive, a physiotherapy programme to strengthen the extensors of the wrist should also be commenced and if it is related to a racket playing sport, it may be necessary to modify the patient's technique (Leach and Miller, 1987). If all these efforts fail, it may be necessary to operate.

Many operations for the relief of this particular condition have been described. The most widely practised procedure is that of exploration of the lateral epicondyle, excision of the damaged part of the extensor carpi radialis brevis, removal of the superficial part of the lateral epicondyle and re-attachment of the extensor muscles to the raw bone. The arm is then immobilized in a long arm plaster for approximately 6 weeks, followed by a graduated programme of mobilization and strengthening.

Acute calcific tendinitis is a very unusual condition which usually presents as an unexplained acute inflammatory episode in the hand. Because of the intense pain it provokes and the overlying skin redness that occurs, it is often misdiagnosed as an infection and treated as such. The aetiology is ill-understood and thought to be due to acute deposition of calcium in areas of closed minor trauma. (Carroll *et al.*, 1955). In the hand, the most common areas involved are around the insertion of the flexor carpi ulnaris tendon and around the tendons of the intrinsic muscles. The accumulation of the calcium causes the lesion to behave like a sterile abscess which compresses the adjacent tissues and causes the pain. An X-ray is diagnostic and in most cases will demonstrate a fairly large deposit of calcium. If the diagnosis is made early, the condition should be treated by injection of local anaesthetic into the area to relieve the pain. The addition of steroids to the injection appears to confirm no extra benefit. The condition is self-limiting and after a 3-week period the calcium usually disappears.

Rehabilitation

After the period of splintage that follows tendon repair, it is very unusual for the patient to be able to move the affected part through its full range of motion. This is due to a combination of factors: the most important is adhesion of the tendon repair at the site of injury, but is also due to joint stiffness following prolonged immobility.

The timing of vigorous postoperative rehabilitation requires fine judgement. If it is begun too early, there is a risk of tendon rupture; if it is begun too late, the tendon adhesions lose their plasticity and are less easily attenuated. As a general rule, the tendon repair is usually strong enough after approximately 4 weeks to withstand active and passive mobilization under the supervision of a trained physiotherapist.

Transient joint stiffness is almost inevitable after prolonged splintage but the effects can be minimized by correct splintage of the injured hand. The ideal position from which full joint motion can recover is one where the capsular and ligamentous arrangements of the small joints of the hand is kept under tension so that contracture does not occur. The anatomy of the individual joints of the hands is such that the ideal position to keep these ligaments on the stretch is one where the interphalangeal joints are fully extended and the metacarpophalangeal joints are flexed to approximately 90°. The wrist should be maintained in approximately 30° of dorsiflexion and the thumb should be held in a position of palmar abduction. This position is very difficult to achieve and maintain, but nevertheless every effort should be made to try to achieve it when constructing splints. This 'ideal' position of splintage may have to be modified to cope with individual injuries, thus flexor tendon injuries require the wrist to be slightly flexed and extensor tendon injuries require the wrist to be slightly more extended, in order to take the tension of the individual tendon repairs. If splintage if necessary in a less than ideal position, the patient will need constant supervision throughout the postoperative period to ensure that joint contractures do not develop. This is particularly likely to occur when dynamic splintage is used following flexor tendon repair (see Fig. 6.4); if the patient is ill-motivated or the splint badly made, full extension of the finger at the interphalangeal joints may not occur for the whole month, inevitably leading to contractures of the interphalangeal joints.

On occasions it may not be possible for the physiotherapists to attenuate the adhesions around the tendon repair enough to regain a good range of motion. Under these conditions, tenolysis may be performed. This is an operation whereby the adhesions are mechanically divided from the surrounding tissues. Because the tendon repair has fully healed by this stage, it is permissible to immediately actively mobilize the patient following the operation. This is a very tedious operation, particularly when the tenolysis is performed within the digital flexor sheath. Division of all the adhesions surrounding the repair may also devascularize the segment of tendon, and rupture following tenolysis is not an uncommon event: the patient should be warned of this possibility.

Finally a look-out should always be kept for the possibility of reflex sympathetic dystrophy. This is a condition whereby the patient's hand becomes stiffer rather than more supple following surgery. The hand often exhibits colour changes, shows increased hair growth on the dorsum of the hand and may become painful. The aetiology is uncertain but is related to dysfunction of the sympathetic nervous system. It is particularly associated with injuries where adjacent nerves have been injured. Provided that it is recognized early, it may be treated successfully by aggressive sympathetic blockade and physiotherapy. The greatest danger lies in failure to diagnose the condition, when it becomes progressively more difficult to treat.

References

Barton NJ (1969) Experimental study of optimal location of flexor tendon pulleys. *Plastic and Reconstructive Surgery* **43**, 125.

Bollen SR (1990) Injury to the A2 pulley in rock climbers. *Journal of Hand Surgery* **15–B**, 268.

Burke F (1988) Editorial. Mallet finger. *Journal of Hand Surgery* **13–B**, 115.

Burton RI, Eaton RG (1973) Common hand injuries in the athlete. *Orthopaedic Clinics of North America* **4**, 809.

Carducci AT (1981) Potential boutonniere deformity – its recognition and treatment. *Orthopaedic Review* **10**, 121.

Carroll RE, Sinton W, Garcia A (1955) Calcium deposits in the hand. *Journal of the American Medical Association* **157**, 422.

Evans D, Weightman B (1988) The Pipflex splint for treatment of mallet finger. *Journal of Hand Surgery* **13–B**, 156.

Leach RE, Miller JK (1987) Lateral and medial epicondylitis of the elbow. *Clinics in Sports Medicine* **6**, 259.

Lister GD, Kleinert HE, Kutz JE, Atasoy E (1977) Primary flexor tendon repair followed by immediate controlled mobilization. *Journal of Hand Surgery* **2**, 441.

Lundborg G (1985) Flexor tendon nutrition and repair. In: *Recent Advances in Plastic Surgery* vol 3. Churchill Livingstone, pp 51–64.

Lunn PG, Lamb DW (1984) "Rugby finger" – avulsion of profundus of ring finger. *Journal of Hand Surgery* **9**, 69.

Osterman AL, Moskow L, Low DW (1988) Soft tissue injuries of the hand and wrist in raquet sports. *Clinics in Sports Medicine* **7**, 329.

Potenza AD (1969) Mechanisms of healing of digital flexor tendons. *The Hand* **1**, 40.

Semple C (1986) Editorial – Tenosynovitis *Journal of Hand Surgery* **11–B**, 155.

Strickland JW, Glogovac SV (1980) Digital function following flexor tendon repair in zone II: a comparison of immobilization and controlled passive motion techniques. *Journal of Hand Surgery* **5**, 537.

Williams JGP (1977) Surgical management of traumatic non infective tenosynovitis of the wrist extensors. *Journal of Bone and Joint Surgery* **59B**, 408.

7

Cold injuries

E. L. Lloyd

Introduction

Human beings are constantly losing heat through convection, radiation, conduction and evaporation, and the standard laws of physics apply. The sensation of cold is related to the lowered average skin temperature but humans are very sensitive to change in temperature, and cold applied to the skin is pleasant if the core temperature is raised but unpleasant if the core temperature is lowered. The severity of cold stress is not related to the absolute temperature alone but is also affected by air movement (wind or draughts) (Fig. 7.1) and moisture (humidity, rain or damp) (Lloyd, 1986). Since cold is a feature of the environment which every human being experiences, its contribution to injury, illness and death is often overlooked.

In the timber industry, and on building sites and farms, workers are exposed to all weathers. Because of cold, fishing is a particularly hazardous occupation, the accident rate being five times greater than the most dangerous land-based transport industry (Vanggaard, 1977). Cold is also a hazard for divers; the water temperature below 100 m depth is a constant 4°C dropping to −2°C in the Arctic (Lloyd, 1986). Deep-freeze stores are installed in large depots, individual shops (e.g. butchers), refrigerated lorries and in medical facilities (e.g. blood transfusion), and workers are exposed to temperatures of −20 to 40°C, sometimes with an additional fan-produced wind chill. Humans can also be exposed to potentially dangerous levels of cold at home, in poor-quality houses (Lloyd, 1986), during travel and following an accident.

Humans are also exposed to cold during sport and recreation. Any person in the hills whether as a climber, skier, or recreation walker is at risk, especially if there is an injury or a sudden change in weather. The temperature drops 1°C per 150 m rise in altitude (Lloyd, 1986) and at high altitude hypoxia compounds the problem. Sports people in winter are vulnerable whether in team sports, cross-country running or so-called winter sports. Water sports participants experience cold – Scuba divers and swimmers are immersed in cold water, and sailors suffer wind chill and wetting from spray and unexpected immersion. Cold can cause problems and injuries at any time of year: muscle tears can occur in 'cold' muscles, even in a heatwave.

While individual sections of this chapter may describe laboratory results or evidence from work environments, wartime experiences or recreational activities, all the details are applicable to any situation involving exposure to cold.

Guidelines

There is an ideal environment of temperature and humidity for the performance of mental tasks, and an increase in cold stress causes a decrease in performance, with an inverse relationship between cold discomfort and work rate. However some environmental stress is needed to provide

WIND SPEED		COOLING POWER OF WIND EXPRESSED AS "EQUIVALENT CHILL TEMPERATURE"																				
KNOTS	MPH	TEMPERATURE (°F)																				
CALM	CALM	40	35	30	25	20	15	10	5	0	-5	-10	-15	-20	-25	-30	-35	-40	-45	-50	-55	-60
		EQUIVALENT CHILL TEMPERATURE																				
3-6	5	35	30	25	20	15	10	5	0	-5	-10	-15	-20	-25	-30	-35	-40	-45	-50	-55	-60	-70
7-10	10	30	20	15	10	5	0	-10	-15	-20	-25	-35	-40	-45	-50	-60	-65	-70	-75	-80	-90	-95
11-15	15	25	15	10	0	-5	-10	-20	-25	-30	-40	-45	-50	-60	-65	-70	-80	-85	-90	-100	-105	-110
16-19	20	20	10	5	0	-10	-15	-25	-30	-35	-45	-50	-60	-65	-75	-80	-85	-95	-100	-110	-115	-120
20-23	25	15	10	0	-5	-15	-20	-30	-35	-45	-50	-60	-65	-75	-80	-90	-95	-105	-110	-120	-125	-135
24-28	30	10	5	0	-10	-20	-25	-30	-40	-50	-55	-65	-70	-80	-85	-95	-100	-110	-115	-125	-130	-140
29-32	35	10	5	-5	-10	-20	-30	-35	-40	-50	-60	-65	-75	-80	-90	-100	-105	-115	-120	-130	-135	-145
33-36	40	10	0	-5	-15	-20	-30	-35	-45	-55	-60	-70	-75	-85	-95	-100	-110	-115	-125	-130	-140	-150
WINDS ABOVE 40 HAVE LITTLE ADDITIONAL EFFECT		LITTLE DANGER					INCREASING DANGER (Flesh may freeze within 1 minute)						GREAT DANGER (Flesh may freeze within 30 secs)									
		DANGER OF FREEZING EXPOSED FLESH FOR PROPERLY CLOTHED PERSONS																				

ALCOM FORM 13b AUG 67 AAC - APO SEATTLE 98742

Chart courtesy of Director of Plans and Training, USARAL

Fig. 7.1 Wind chill chart showing the effect of wind on increasing the degree of cooling at any particular temperature and wind speed. From Mills (1973), with permission.

optimal peformance, and large slow swings of temperature have been shown to improve performance (Enander, 1984). The Factories Act 1961 and the Shops, Offices and Railway Premises Act 1963 both recommend environmental temperatures around 16°C, but these cannot be applied to many of the hazardous working situations described earlier. Nor are they applicable to outdoor sport or recreation.

Most of the studies of the adverse effects of work in extreme thermal environments have been concerned with heat (Holmer, 1988) and the so-called comfort criteria (Fanger, 1970) have not been validated for cold environments (Holmer, 1988). Cold as a hazard of work is often ignored in textbooks, and when 100 fatal accidents in the construction industry were examined and analysed (Health and Safety Executive, 1978) no attempt was made to include a consideration of cold as a factor and not even the time of year was given. There is in fact no generally acceptable definition of what constitutes cold working (Hassi, 1982).

Direct local cold injury

Frostbite

Local severe cold may cause the skin to freeze (Keatinge and Cannon, 1960) and this may progress to frostbite which, though it is most commonly associated with northern latitudes, may also occur in unexpected parts of the world, e.g. in the Sahara desert at night. (Barber, 1978).

Precipitating factors

Skin freezes at −0.5°C but true frostbite occurs when there is sufficient heat loss in the local area to allow ice crystals to form in the extracellular spaces, and extract cellular water (Mills, 1983), disturbing the enzyme mechanisms and causing cell death. Cold-induced vasoconstriction and stagnation increase cellular aggregation and sludging. Normally there is a decrease in local haematocrit and on rewarming vasodilatation occurs with immediate recovery of microvascular perfusion. However if there is pathological local vasodilatation without rewarming, e.g. because of histamine release, the part will be perfused with blood containing a high concentration of red cells. This will increase the risk of red cell aggregation and microvascular occlusion with complete stasis, and may result in gangrene and problems during rewarming (Schmid-Schonbein and Neumann, 1985).

Negroid people are more susceptible than caucasians, and the risk is increased in smokers, in some medical disorders, including peripheral vascular disease and Raynaud's syndrome, and by a previous episode of frostbite. The risk is also increased by dehydration (Mills, 1983; Foray and Salon, 1985), which can often occur during exposure to cold (Lloyd, 1986), by alcohol, excess tiredness (Hassi, 1982) and at altitude, where local haemoconcentration and dehydration are increased, and hypoxia blunts mental function, so that proper preventive measures may be forgotten. If the body temperature is lowered, a small cold skin stimulus which normally has no effect will cause an intense vasoconstriction in the fingers and feet (Grayson and Kuehn, 1979).

Though the ears, nose and the distal extremities of the limbs are most commonly affected, with frostbite of the ears increasing if short hairstyles are fashionable (Mills, 1983), the site of frostbite is influenced by physical immobility, position, pressure, lack of insulating fat, liability to wetting (including overflow incontinence), or by contact with cold metal, e.g. penile frostbite from metal zips (Wilkerson *et al.*, 1986). Inadequate or tight clothing worn during skiing or running in extreme cold can also produce penile freezing (Travis and Roberts, 1989). Anything which restricts the circulation increases the risk of frostbite and worsens the outcome. For example, training shoes and similar shoes used for cross-country skiiing are dangerous especially if too tightly laced, and snow boots have felt liners which shrink and freeze if they become wet. A similar compression can occur if neoprene boots are worn during ascent to altitude (Mills, 1983).

Classification

Frostbite can be classified into a number of different grades of severity but three divisions are enough for practical purposes (Ward *et al.*, 1989). In *frostnip* the exposed skin, which has been painful, blanches and loses sensation, but remains pliable. In *superficial frostbite* the skin becomes white and frozen, with the deep underlying tissues remaining fairly pliable. In *deep frostbite*, muscle, bone and tendons are involved as well as the skin and subcutaneous tissues. The part is insensitive, wooden and grey-purple or marble white. Because tendons are less sensitive to cold and the associated muscle groups are distant from the injury, the part can still be moved voluntarily.

Even if the damage is only superficial (Fig. 7.2), the initial assessment of severity is often inaccurate (Mills, 1973; Flora, 1985) because the part is hard, cold, white and anaesthetic and appears

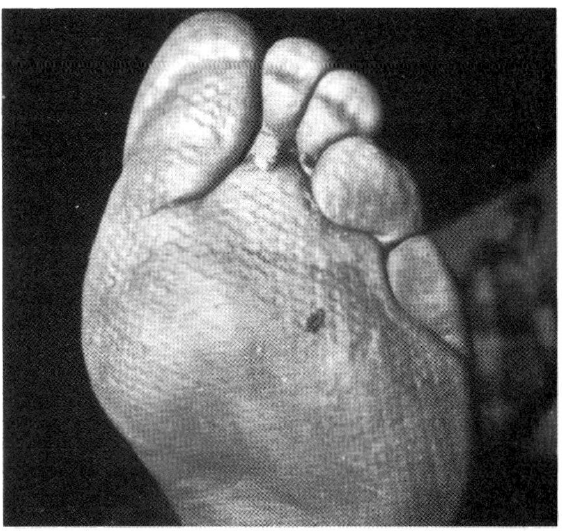

Fig. 7.2 A cold rigid forefoot without sensation or digital motion. Tissue compression and sock marks are obvious. From Mills (1973), with permission.

solidly frozen through. Tissue viability may be assessed by using Doppler ultrasound (Foray and Salon, 1985), by the injection of technetium-99 isotopes with perfusion examined radiologically (Mills, 1983), or by comparing the temperature differential between the frostbitten area and a reference unaffected area before and after thawing. In practice the extent of the final damage is determined by the changes occurring during rewarming as well as during freezing, and there is no evidence that decisions about treatment are best determined by the severity of the damage (Mills, 1973).

Thawing

Frostnip can be rewarmed in the field by placing the affected part in the armpit or under clothing. The part tingles and becomes hyperaemic, and within a few minutes sensation is restored and normal working can be resumed. There may be some skin desquamation several days later. No attempt should be made to thaw frostbite if there is the likelihood of the part being refrozen, because refreezing causes much more damage than continuous freezing (Keatings and Cannon, 1960; Mills, 1983). It is possible, and better, to walk to safety on frozen feet, as has been done for up to 74 hours (Mills and Rau, 1983).

The current recommended method (Mills, 1983; Foray and Salon, 1985) is rapid rewarming by immersion of the part or the whole person in a whirlpool or bubble bath (38–41°C) until the distal tip of the thawed part flushes. If clear blebs develop over the next 48 hours (Fig. 7.3), there is the greatest degree of tissue preservation and the most adequate early function, especially in deep injury (Fig. 7.4). If the part remains cyanotic and cold and blebs do not develop (Fig. 7.5), there is no chance of tissue recovery (Fig. 7.6). (Rapid rewarming should not be used if the part has been thawed previously.)

After thawing the extremities should be elevated, and kept exposed on sterile sheets with cradles to avoid damage. To remove necrotic and infected tissue without causing any damage to healthy tissue, treatment is continued with whirl-

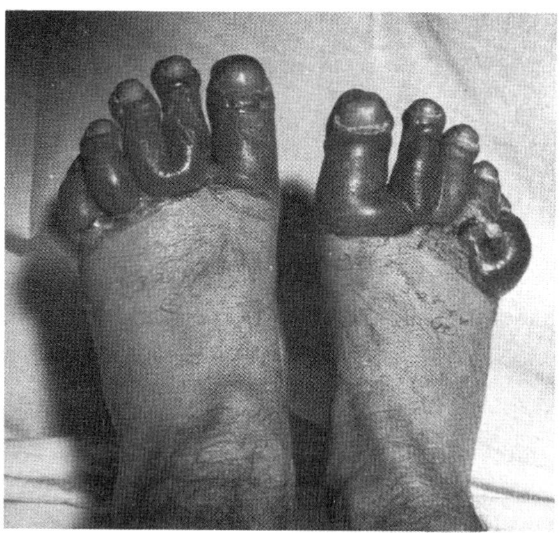

Fig. 7.3 36 hours post-thawing by rapid rewarming in warm water showing clear blebs reaching to the ends of the toes. Patient complained of severe pain. From Mills (1973), with permission.

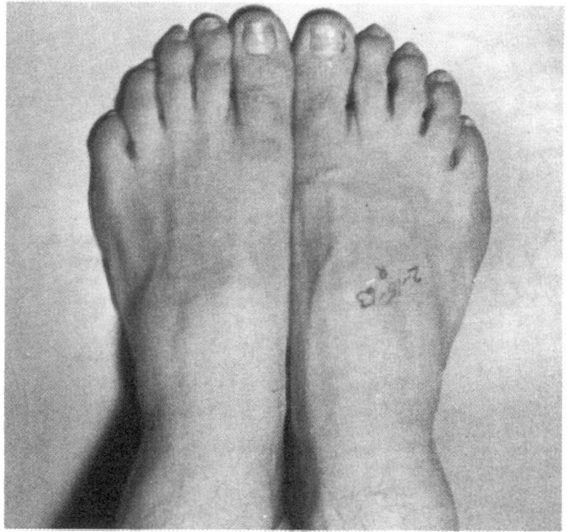

Fig. 7.4 Four months post injury and rewarming in warm water. Epithelialisation is complete and the anatomy has been preserved, but the changes of deep injury included volar fat pad loss, early interphalangeal joint contracture nail changes, hypaesthesia and hyperhydrosis, and some are obvious. At the end of one year the extremity had adequate sensation, there was mild subcutaneous loss and interphalangeal contracture, with a few interphalangeal subarticular lesions present on X-Ray. Increased sweating was still present. From Mills (1973), with permission.

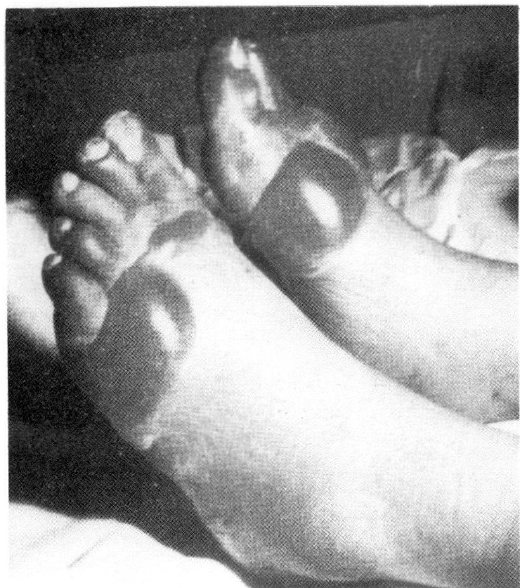

Fig. 7.5 The feet are approximately five days post-freezing and 48 hours post thawing, which was by rubbing with ice and snow. A very poor prognostic sign is evident. The blebs are all proximal and are dark, while the toes and distal tissues are without blebs or blistering, and are dusky, œdematous, painless and insensitive. Phalangeal amputation is generally unavoidable with this pattern and may be predicted as early as 24 hours post thaw, see Fig. 7.6. From Mills (1973), with permission.

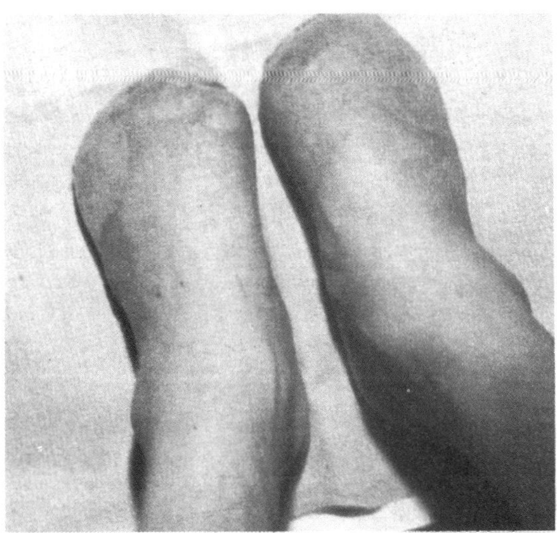

Fig. 7.6 Amputation at the distal metatarsal level. Despite this the patient was back in the Arctic the following winter and continued trapping and hunting for many years. From Mills (1973), with permission.

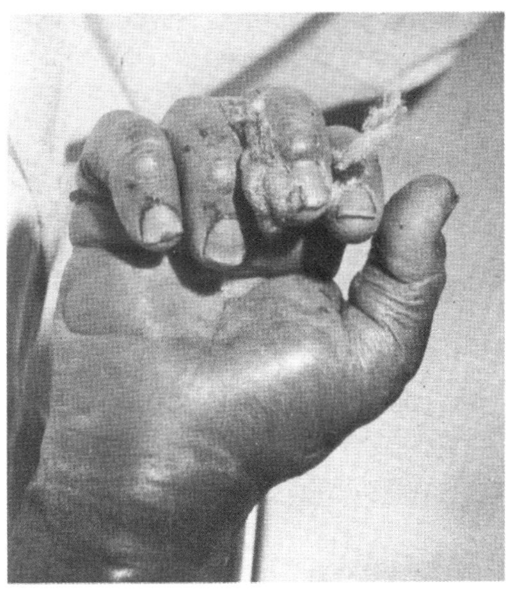

Fig. 7.7 The extremity less than 24 hours after thawing frostbite by using excess heat (boiling water in this case). The hand is cyanotic, painful and foul smelling and there are no blebs. From Mills (1973), with permission.

pool or bubble baths (35°C) twice daily for 20 min with an antiseptic, e.g. hexachlorophane or Betadine, added to the water.

Gradual spontaneous thawing is probably satisfactory for superficial frostbite but not for deep injury. Delayed thawing or using ice or snow-rubbing often results in marked tissue loss. The worst results follow thawing with excessive heat (Figs. 7.7–7.9) at or above 50°C – temperatures produced by diesel exhausts, stoves or wood fires, or scalding water (Mills, 1983; Flora, 1985; Foray and Salon, 1985). Rapid internal rewarming might produce good results but intra-arterial lines could cause more damage than they prevent (Mills, 1983).

Surgery

Blebs should be protected but drained if infected. When the escher is dry, escharotomy releases splinting of the digits (Mills, 1983). After thawing, the formation of oedema may result in a compartment pressure syndrome and fasciotomy is then

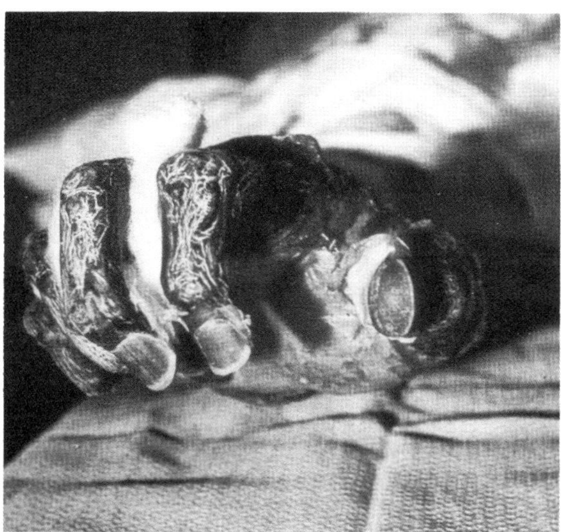

Fig. 7.8 At three weeks the digits show tissue death, being hard and rigid with the soft tissue completely mummified. There is evidence of infection, superficial only, at the area of tissue demarcation. From Mills (1973), with permission.

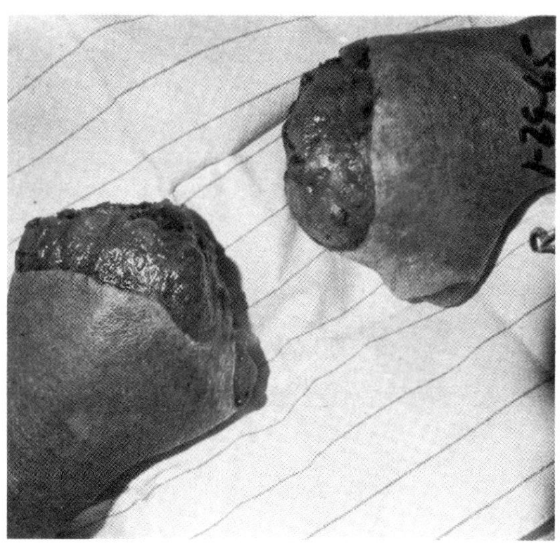

Fig. 7.9 Spontaneous amputation at the metacarpophalangeal junction at six weeks. This is typical of the extent of tissue loss and the hopelessness for recovery when gangrene is caused by "cooking" frozen tissues with excessive dry or wet heat. From Mills (1973), with permission.

essential to avoid extensive tissue necrosis (Franz *et al.*, 1978), and clinical judgement should not be over-ruled by sophisticated technology in deciding whether or not a fasciotomy is necessary (Mills, 1983). Dislocations should be reduced immediately the part has been rewarmed but fractures are treated conservatively. Since the gangrene of frostbite is much more superficial than it appears, debridement or amputation should be delayed up to 90 days till mummification and tissue demarcation are complete (Mills, 1983; Ward *et al.*, 1989). After the blackened areas have separated, the underlying tissue is raw, shiny, tender and unduly sensitive, and there may be abnormal sweating. This should return to normal in 2–3 months (Ward *et al.*, 1989).

Other measures

The treatment of hypothermia, if present, takes precedence (Mills, 1983; Foray and Salon, 1985). Most patients with frostbite and/or hypothermia are dehydrated, and rehydration with warmed fluids is very important. Low molecular weight dextran may reduce the cellular aggregation and sludging through haemodilution, and may be worth continuing for 10–12 days in the post-rewarming phase (Foray and Salon, 1985). Sedatives and analgesics should be given as required. Sympathectomy reduces pain, decreases oedema and there is less infection but, despite more rapid tissue demarcation, it does not result in increased tissue preservation (Mills, 1973). Current management includes alpha-adrenergic blockade using phenoxybenzamine hydrochloride 10 mg daily, increasing to 20–60 mg depending on effect and need, though the patient must be well-hydrated after sympathetic blockade (Mills, 1983). There is disagreement as to the effectiveness of vasodilators used in the post-thawing period, but smoking is prohibited because of its vasoconstrictor effect.

To counteract severe drying, splitting and separation of the eschar, silver nitrate may be used as 0.5–1% solution lavaged over the area of frostbite after the whirlpool treatment (Mills, 1983). Frostbite and thermal burns may both be present in the same lesion, and there may be other injuries. Therefore thrombolytic enzymes and anticoagulants are risky, especially if there is the possibility of a head injury. Hyperbaric oxygen and biofeedback training have not been adequately evaluated (Mills, 1983), and there is disagreement about antibiotic policy.

The patient should be nursed in a pleasant environment and fed with a high-protein and high-calorie diet. Digital exercises are encouraged throughout the day and, for the lower limbs, Buerger's exercises 4 times daily (Mills, 1983).

Trench foot

Cold can also cause tissue damage without freezing – Trench foot, immersion injury, non-freezing cold injury (NFCI). There is sometimes confusion between frostbite and NFCI, though NFCI is likely to be present proximal to areas of frostbite. NFCI was frequent during the wars, among soldiers living in wet trenches, and among sailors after long periods spent in lifeboats. Even in the Falklands campaign in 1982, NFCI accounted for 20% of the men received on the hospital ship Uganda (Francis, 1984). Prolonged trekking through boggy terrain in northern countries could result in NFCI.

Running barefoot on frozen ground, though painless during the run due to cold-induced neuropathy, has resulted in considerable loss of tissue on the soles of the feet (Reichl, 1987).

Risk factors

NFCI requires longer exposure than does frostbite (Mills, 1973), and develops when the legs are exposed to the wet and cold above 0°C, though wet conditions are not absolutely necessary. If the part is wet, tissue damage may occur even with skin temperatures above 16°C (Maclean and Emslie-Smith, 1977), and even up to 29°C (Francis, 1984). As in frostbite (and hypothermia), predisposing factors include dehydration, inadequate nutrition, fatigue, stress, intercurrent illness and injury. Damage is more likely to occur and be more extensive if the limb is dependent, immobile or is constricted by footwear. If footwear has been soaked in sea water the incidence of NFCI is higher because the salt crystals attract water, and in the mountains, NFCI can develop if the boots are impervious to water because the build-up of sweat inside the boot is the equivalent of immersion (Francis and Golden, 1985).

Signs and symptoms

The troops in the Falklands described their symptoms:

> Numbness began to develop after about 7 to 10 days. At night in their sleeping bags, the numbness would be replaced by paraesthesia or pain, or both – described by some as being like electric shocks running up the legs from their toes. In some cases the pain was enough to keep them awake. On weight-bearing in the morning the pain was sometimes almost unbearable for the initial 5 or 10 minutes, but would gradually wane and once again be replaced by numbness on re-exposure to cold. Some – particularly those with very severe nocturnal pain – found their feet had swollen to such a degree in the morning that they had difficulty in putting on their boots; or if it had been necessary for them to sleep with their boots on, they had difficulty in tying their laces (Payne, 1984).

There is a sensation of 'walking on cotton wool' and when first examined the typical case has cold, swollen and blotchy pink-purple or blanched feet which feel heavy and numb. This is succeeded by hyperaemia, with hot, red, swollen feet, and pain which may be severe. This phase may last for days or weeks (Mills, 1973). There may be bleeding into the skin and severe injury is indicated by large blisters. The damage may progress to gangrene which tends to be deeper than in frostbite.

Treatment

This involves removing the person from the hostile environment, bed rest, and analgesics for the pain. Whole-body warming and sympathectomy are controversial. Unfortunately at present there is no satisfactory treatment for the many late manifestations of NFCI (Francis and Golden, 1985).

After-effects of local cold injury

There is a large overlap in the pathology and late sequelae of frostbite and NFCI. All nerves degenerate if kept below freezing for more than a few seconds, with complete necrosis of all structures within the perineurium except the endothelium lining of the blood vessels, though regeneration does occur (Peyronnard *et al.*, 1977; Nukuda *et al.*, 1981). However even at temperatures above freezing, demyelination of nerves may occur. In freezing cold injury, the degree of muscle damage depends on the amount of exposure. There is coagulation necrosis in the superficial coldest layer, slow necrosis in the intermediate zone and muscle atrophy in the deepest layer. Repair is by fibrous tissue (Lewis and Moen, 1952).

After recovery there may be persistent after-effects with vasomotor paralysis, analgesia and paraesthesia, which may be permanent, and early anhydrosis or late hyperhydrosis. Epiphyseal cartilage is more sensitive to cold than bone cells which are more sensitive than skin. Even following complete return of function, X-rays may show typical changes (Fig. 7.10). Other late problems may include toe rigidity and fallen arches, and osteoporosis, though new bone formation usually restores the normal X-ray appearance. Epiphyseal damage and eroded joints predispose to osteoarthritis. There may be hardening and atrophy of soft tissues. Some victims suffer permanently from intermittent local ulceration of the skin with fissuring and chronic infection. Obliterative endangiitis may occur and Raynaud's syndrome, with the feet in particular tending to develop a marked and persistent vasospasm when presented with cold stimuli, and the vasospasm persists long after the cold stimulus has been removed. This cold hypersensitivity of the feet may persist for years or even be permanent, and re-exposure to cold is very liable to cause relapse. Finally there may be weakness and deformity because of muscle damage and/or amputation (Mills, 1973; Francis and Golden, 1985).

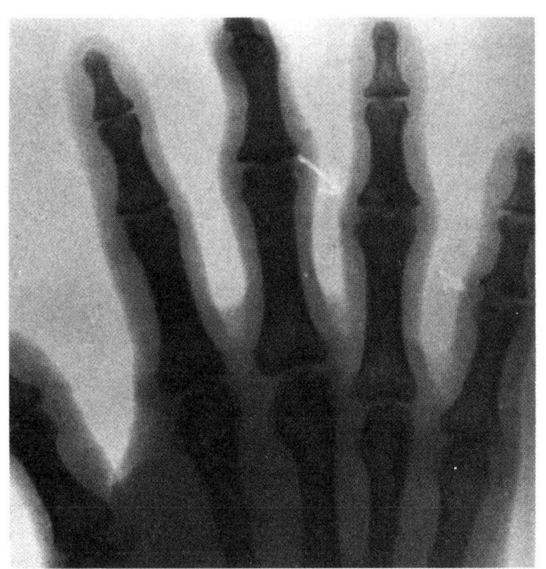

Fig. 7.10 X-Ray showing fusiform enlargement of the proximal interphalangeal joints, and the sub and intra articular lytic areas. Severe freezing 3 years previously, thawed rapidly in warm water. From Mills (1973), with permission.

Prevention of local cold injury

There should be adequate fluid intake to prevent dehydration. The disappearance of pain is an early warning of incipient cold injury (Vanggaard, 1985) and, where practicable, the feet and hands should be warmed at intervals, especially if there is total anaesthesia on attempting to move the fingers and toes. No current boot or shoe will prevent NFCI or frostbite, because the many functions shoes and boots have to perform cause conflict in design. The way forward may be to design footwear on the modular pattern with a variety of inner, middle and outer components to be combined as required to fulfil the needs of any particular situation (Oakley, 1984). The most useful preventive measures are:

1. to limit the time the person is exposed to the hazardous environment;
2. taking a hot drink whenever possible – of thermal and hydration benefits;
3. adequate foot care to keep the feet as dry and abrasion-free as possible;
4. 'buddies' can keep a close watch on each other for early signs.

These measures were used in World War II by the British troops but not by the American troops and the result was that, even under identical conditions, the US troops suffered 10 times the incidence of cold injuries incurred by the British (Francis, 1984).

Unfortunately accidents and the exigencies of modern warfare mean that the preventive measures are not always possible in practice, and it is important for the future to look at ways of breaking the vicious pathogenetic circle of cooling and vasoconstriction accompanied by a high level of sympathetic tone (Francis and Golden, 1985).

Other conditions

Conjunctivitis due to cold and cold injury to the cornea have been seen in downhill skiers and ice skaters unprotected by goggles (Ward *et al.*, 1989).

Chilblains (British Medical Journal, 1975; Lahti, 1982) are local cold-induced inflammatory lesions which are more frequent in humid conditions than in a cold dry climate. Inadequate clothing is an important predisposing factor in the cooling, and women are more often affected than men. Central heating reduces the incidence of chilblains but increases the problem of *winter itch* (asteatotic eczema), because the low relative humidity causes water loss, decreased sweating and sebum secretion, and the skin becomes dry, brittle and itchy, and cracks develop. Treatment involves humidification of the room, emulsifying skin ointments and the avoidance of too much washing (Lahti, 1982).

In *Raynaud's syndrome* a cold stress, whose severity does not affeet normal people, produces severe arterial vasoconstriction and the normal reactive hyperaemia following arterial occlusion is virtually absent (Holti, 1985). Even in the warm, there is an altered pulse contour (Sumner and Strandness, 1972). Raynaud's phenomenon is most marked in the fingers and toes, but the tips of the tongue, nose and ears may also be involved, and the vasospasm may affect the internal organs (Belch, 1990). Raynaud's syndrome is more readily induced if the core temperature is below 36°C (Holti, 1985). Raynaud's phenomenon is associated with a large number of connective tissue, and other, disorders (Belch, 1990). However a large percentage of patients have detectable antinuclear antibodies without any other evidence of autoimmune disease but those without antinuclear antibodies have lower noradrenaline levels than controls but higher cortisol levels, which increase vasomotor reactivity (Surwit *et al.*, 1983). In idiopathic Raynaud's disease the vasospastic attacks are precipitated by either cold or emotional stress or both together, whereas in scleroderma attacks are precipitated by cold provocation alone (Freedman and Ianni, 1983). Trauma, hormones and chemicals, including those in tobacco smoke, may provoke an attack, and also a number of drugs including beta-blockers, ergot and other antimigraine drugs, cytotoxic agents, bromocriptine and sulphasalazine (Belch, 1990).

Raynaud's syndrome from exposure to arsenic in mining (Linderholm and Lagerkvist, 1984), and the hand vibration syndrome, e.g. from pneumatic drill usage (Kinnersley, 1974), or by driving snowmobiles (Hassi *et al.*, 1984), both cause increased sensitivity to cold, as does previous local cold injury. Smoking should be stopped. Protection from cold exposure can be applied through suitable clothing, shoes and gloves, but if the attacks of digital ischaemia are incapacitating, portable electrically heated gloves should be considered (Kempson *et al.*, 1983).

Drug treatment is possible and calcium channel blockers and prostaglandins are the most promising. Unfortunately side-effects and practical problems of administration are severe with all drugs. Sympathectomy may be effective, but only in the lower limbs (Belch, 1990). Biofeedback training may be of value (Kappes and Mills, 1984), especially in the group without antinuclear antibodies.

Acrocyanosis is a symmetrical permanent cyanosis with normal peripheral pulses. The aetiology is unknown, there are no complications and no treatment is needed (Lahti, 1982).

Some people have a genuine *allergy* to cold. Exposure of the skin to cold causes degranulation of sensitized mast cells in the skin (Wasserman *et al.*, 1977). The clinical features are malaise with shivering, aching joints and generalized urticaria (Eady *et al.*, 1978). The local effects include wheals, and even cold drinks may produce lesions in the mouth and on the lips (British Medical Journal, 1975). In mild cases wading or swimming in cold water may produce a transient localized rash (personal observation). Treatment using doxentrazole (Bentley-Phillips *et al.*, 1978) or an H_1-receptor histamine antagonist, e.g. cyproheptadine (Ting, 1984), may be of value. The susceptibility is transmitted as a genetic dominant (Ting, 1984). The diagnosis of familial cold urticaria should not be missed since it may occur on any immersion, even in an indoor swimming pool. Proper counselling and prevention of exposure to cold may save the life of a susceptible person, since some deaths which occur within a few minutes of entering cold water may be due to anaphylaxis in a person with previously unsuspected cold urticaria (British Medical Journal, 1975).

Other soft tissue effects of cold

Oedema

Exposure to cold normally results in dehydration through diuresis and respiratory moisture loss, and exercise increases the loss through both routes (Lloyd, 1986). However if the body cools very slowly, fluid shifts from the intravascular to the intracellular space and this may produce oedema (Lloyd, 1986). Oedema may also occur within 12–24 hours of rewarming due to plasma passing through cold-damaged capillaries into the interstitial tissue (Ward *et al.*, 1989). As has been seen in mountains, associated exercise may cause swelling of the feet (Williams *et al.*, 1979).

Backache

The muscles of the back are very powerful, and heat production rises by increased muscle metabolism and tone. Therefore in a cold environment the back muscles may have to be constantly generating heat. Backache was certainly found to be a symptom associated with cold housing (Platt *et al.*, 1989) and its mechanism may be similar to that of an overuse injury.

Cold and muscle injury

Movement is the final action of a complex series of processes starting with the brain receiving information from peripheral senses, and culminating in a muscle contraction which alters the position of two bones in relation to each other. Impairment of function at any point in the system will affect the efficiency of a movement.

Peripheral injury

Injury can occur in muscle or tendon, or at the junctions of muscle, tendon and bone. The more power the muscle can develop, the greater the risk of injury to the muscle–tendon system. Joints can be dislocated causing damage to the ligaments and joint capsule, and even bones can fracture if the muscle contractions are too powerful.

Injury is more likely if muscle activity is unco-ordinated; for example, the powerful hamstring muscles are a common site of injury. Because they act across two major joints, the hip and knee, simple contraction of the hamstrings would result in the knee bending and the hip being extended backwards. In sprinting, movement starts with the knee and hip both flexed. The hamstrings extend the hip but, to straighten the knee, there must be quadriceps contraction and partial or relative hamstring relaxation. The potential for some degree of inco-ordination is therefore very high.

The contribution of cold to muscle injury

On exposure to cold, constriction of the peripheral and limb vessels reduces heat loss by limiting blood flow to the periphery. Though the skin is at a temperature only a few degrees above that of the environment, there is a very steep temperature gradient and, even in fingers immersed in water at 0–4°C, the internal finger temperature remains about 20–25°C (Greenfield *et al.*, 1950), though this is still very low when compared with the normal core temperature of 37°C. The muscles themselves are therefore cold with a reduced blood supply.

Effect on muscles

Cold decreases the power and duration of muscle contraction (Clarke *et al.*, 1958; Fox, 1961; Foldes *et al.*, 1978; Horvath 1981), e.g. handgrip strength is reduced by immersion of the forearm in 10°C water (Coppin *et al.*, 1978) through a direct effect-on the muscle fibres (Guttman and Gross, 1956).

As muscles cool, there is a delay in the onset of the contraction, the contraction time is prolonged (Tuttle, 1941), the twitch size is reduced and relaxation time is prolonged (Lakie *et al.*, 1986). When the muscle temperature drops below 25°C continuing physical activity becomes impossible (Freeman and Pugh, 1969). Normally impairment is temporary and full recovery can occur within 40 min of removal from the cold (Coppin *et al.*, 1978).

Cold muscles become stiffer and this increased tone is not due to nerve impulses. It is as if the muscle state changes from a 'sol' when warm to a 'gel' when cold and, with cold muscles, the greater the force producing passive movement, the greater the stiffness (Lakie *et al.*, 1986). One swimmer developed such severe muscle rigidity that he was unable to move after 33 min in 16°C water (Pugh and Edholm, 1955). If the muscle is cold, slow movement is possible but rapid alternating movements cannot be made (Lakie *et al.*, 1986).

Effect on joints

On exposure to cold the temperature in the joints falls faster than the temperature in the muscles and the viscosity of synovial fluid increases (Hunter *et al.*, 1952). This increases joint stiffness and resistance to movement.

Effect on nerves

As nerves are cooled conduction slows progressively (Vanggaard, 1975) until at 4°C reversible paralysis occurs (Holdcroft, 1981). However prolonged exposure of nerves below 10°C causes sensory and motor damage (Paton, 1983). Myelinated nerve fibres are more susceptible than non-myelinated (Ward *et al.*, 1989). Exposure of the hands to a very cold environment may impair the function of the nerves after as short a time as 15 min, even though there may have been no freezing of the skin. This impairment is not reversed by immediate rewarming of the hands in hot water but may occasionally persist for periods in excess of 4 days (Marshall and Goldman, 1976).

Failure of muscle function may also be due to failure of neuromuscular transmission (Katz and Miledi, 1965; Foldes *et al.*, 1978) and/or impairment of muscle receptor activity (Hassi, 1982).

Cold muscles are, understandably, notoriously liable to tears, and the more sudden or explosive the movement, the greater the danger, and the risk is increased by cold stiff joints and by any inco-ordination within an individual muscle or muscle groups from impaired nerve conduction. Other effects of cold on the body (see Cold and the increased risk of accidents) can result in a person getting into an unexpected or dangerous situation which requires sudden violent exertion to correct, and therefore increasing the risk of muscle tears.

Prevention

The most effective way of trying to reduce the risk of injury is for the person to do warm-up exercises before exercising hard. This principle is accepted in sport but it should also be applied to workers in a similar situation, though unfortunately it never is.

The warm-up

This must be sufficiently energetic and prolonged to ensure that the whole body is warm, including the joints, and the junctions between muscles, tendons, and bone, and also the muscles used in breathing. A hot shower is useless because it only warms the skin. The real value of the active warm-up may be because it involves the cells which are going to be used in moving and in breathing, and therefore the biochemical assembly line which produces energy, including heat, has been brought into full function. During the warm-up the blood vessels to the active muscles have also opened up, which helps to spread the heat and means that, when the exercise starts, there is no problem with the transport of food and oxygen to the muscle or of the waste products away.

Protective clothing should be worn initially and the warm-up should be taken to the point where sweating is about to start. Once this stage has been reached, the person can shed the protective clothing, and will remain warm in minimal clothing provided he or she continues exercising vigorously.

The warm-down

When the activity is over, the person should put on warm clothes and warm down. This eases the stiffness out of the muscles, reduces the risk of injury and allows the body to adjust the rate of heat production. This avoids sweating and will help to prevent chilling or even hypothermia developing.

Treatment

If a person is unlucky enough to develop an acute muscle injury, the emergency treatment is RICE – rest, apply ice or very cold water to the site of injury, compress and elevate the part. The ice causes vasoconstriction and reduces the amount of bleeding into the injury, thus reducing the immediate disability and helping the chance of early repair and recovery. If the weather is cold, it is important to provide warmth and protection from the elements to prevent hypothermia.

Cold and the increased risk of accidents

In factories the incidence of injury due to accidents is less at an environmental temperature of 18°C than at lower (or higher) temperatures (Vernon, 1939, Goldsmith and Minard, 1976), and in the construction industry, cold weather causes an increased incidence of accidents and a drop in work output (Taylor, 1975). This could be due to a number of factors (Lloyd, 1986). No comparable figures are available for accidents during leisure activities.

Peripheral effects

As the skin temperature drops, the skin receptors lose sensitivity. Pain is caused when the skin temperature drops to somewhere in the range of 10–16°C (Hassi, 1982; Enander, 1984) and subjective discomfort caused by cold is greater if certain areas, e.g. the forehead or feet, are cold, and the discomfort is increased by shivering (Enander, 1984).

Manual performance

Cold reduces manual performance and dexterity (Provins and Clarke, 1960; Clark and Jones, 1962), even when the rest of the body is kept warm (Lockhart, 1960). The effect on manual performance of cooling the body plus hand is greater than the effect of cooling the hand alone, which in turn is greater than the effect of cooling the body alone (Enander, 1984). Initially although the hands may feel cold, performance is little affected. This is followed by a numbing of cutaneous sensation and a reduction in sensitivity followed by an attenuated manual dexterity. Finally there is a precipitous decline in performance affecting the muscle spindle mechanism, proprioceptors or the joints of the hand and wrist. Slow cooling may impair function at a higher temperature than does rapid cooling, and following slow cooling the impairment persists after the hands are rewarmed to normal (Enander, 1984; Lockhart, 1960). The duration of the cold stress as well as its magnitude are of prime importance in determining reaction to cold.

The effects of cold on nerves, joints and muscles discussed earlier are factors which are all liable to cause clumsiness, loss of manual dexterity and an impairment of co-ordination.

Effects of cold on the higher cerebral function

Visual perception efficiency is impaired in proportion to the degree of cold stress experienced (Poulton *et al.*, 1965). Even sleeping in the cold causes a decrease in vigilance and reaction times, and test performances were worse after a very cold night (Angus *et al.*, 1979). Cold causes a decrease in word recognition ability (Davis *et al.*, 1975); reasoning is slower but remains accurate (Coleshaw *et al.*, 1983); powers of judgement are impaired, and the ability to judge the passage of time is significantly affected, resulting in underestimates of elapsed time (Baddeley, 1966). There is an impairment of memory, especially recent memory (Coleshaw *et al.*, 1983), e.g. when someone reaches safety from a hypothermia situation, he or she is often unable to give the exact location of the party (Pugh, 1964, 1966).

Among workers in a coldstore, Andrew (1963) has also detected low-grade euphoria, personal irritability and a reduction in the ability to concentrate. Cold causes anxiety and apathy, and also discomfort, which has both a distracting and an arousal effect. Reports suggest that cold exposure may cause depression, apathy, fear, panic or suicide (Lloyd, 1986), and apparent madness has been reported during Antarctic expeditions (Brent, 1974; Bickel, 1977).

During cold exposure there is an increase in errors (Teichner, 1958; Enander, 1984) which can be clerical, verbal or mechanical, and may seem silly. Unfortunately a person developing hypothermia is unaware of the development of mental impairment, and often feels that a test has been done particularly well when in fact the results showed the greatest impairment.

Hallucinations in cold stress

It is said that hallucinations occur when the core temperature drops below 32°C (Hiroven, 1982) but in incidents (Gray, 1970; Lee and Lee, 1971; McOwan, 1979; Lloyd, 1986) where the weather conditions suggested that cold stress was present, if the core temperature had been below 32°C when the hallucination occurred, it is unlikely that the person would have survived. Hallucinations probably occur when there is a specific change in the neurochemistry of the brain, and cold may act synergistically with other hallucinogenic factors. These include hypoxia from altitude or medical disorders, drugs, sensory deprivation, monotony, sleep deprivation or fatigue, aggravated by mental or physical stress (Lloyd, 1986). Some hallucinations are obviously triggered by misinterpretation of distance, natural objects or unusual natural sounds, but this does not explain all the case reports of people seeing figures, talking to non-existent people, feeling fear or a presence, or seeing things or hearing sounds or irregular footsteps (Gray, 1970; Lee and Lee, 1971; McOwan, 1979; Lloyd, 1986). As in some of the case reports, if a person responds to a hallucination, any actions will be inappropriate to the person's situation and may lead to the death of the individual or of others. In these circumstances the death has traditionally been attributed to 'pilot error' and the true cause, cold stress or hypothermia, has been overlooked (Lloyd, 1986). Confusingly, the symptoms and signs of alcohol intoxication are similar to those of hypothermia (Pugh, 1968) and hypothermia, or the other effects of cold stress, may be the main factor in an accident even though alcohol has been consumed and the person has appeared drunk.

A related phenomenon is that of paradoxical undressing in the cold, first reported in 1952 (Wedin, 1976) and many cases have since been reported (Lloyd, 1986). The death of Petty Officer Evans recorded in Scott's Antarctic diary (Brent,

1974) is probably the first recorded and best-observed (if unrecognized) case of paradoxical undressing.

Interestingly, a century ago Hans Anderson in the *Little Match Girl* and Charles Dickens in *A Christmas Carol* gave vivid fictional accounts of cold-induced cerebral disorientation. Similarly, polar Eskimos have long recognized a hysterical mental condition which occurs in winter and which they call *pibloctoq*. In this the person suddenly goes berserk, rushing out of the house, throwing the arms in the air and doing a number of other irrational actions such as taking their clothes off, jumping in the sea or climbing icebergs (Simpson, 1972). These effects are obviously of critical importance to climbers, divers and long-distance swimmers since they may cause death through accidents or errors of judgement.

Prevention of cold injury

The specific problems in the prevention of frostbite and trench foot have already been discussed.

Adaptation to cold

Performance under normal conditions is no guide to likely performance in the cold which is affected by motivation, the state of arousal and the emotional state of the person (Teichner, 1958; Enander, 1984). Unfortunately the effect of cold cannot be assessed by monitoring ambient temperature and other climatic variations, or even by measuring skin temperature. Performance in the cold is also task-dependent: complex tasks are more affected than simple (Thomas *et al.*, 1989). Conditioning, training and familiarity will enable tasks to be performed at a low level of hand and finger sensitivity (Clark and Jones, 1962), but the progressive effects of cold results in a significant deterioration in motor performance. With continued exposure there is a degree of physical adaptation, e.g. the person learns to use movements of the arms and shoulders to compensate for the impairment caused by cold hands, and there is also a psychological adaptation to cold (Enander, 1984).

Maintaining the work environment

People who are employed to work in a coldstore environment should be carefully selected on certain physical and psychological criteria (Andrew, 1963).

Where applicable, special measures, such as heated cabs for crane operators and tractor drivers, can allow work to continue safely in the cold (Andrews, 1963). All knobs, levers, handles and seats should be made of materials with low thermal conductivity (Andrew, 1963), and equipment intended for use in the cold should be designed so that all controls can be handled with thick gloves (Provins and Clarke, 1960) since the hands will remain warmer and therefore more efficient, but the use of gloves will also avoid the risk of frostbite or freeze/burn which may occur if the equipment has to be handled with bare hands in extreme cold. This is also important for skiers, climbers and other outdoor sports or sports involving freezing conditions.

Moving from a room at −30°C into a room at 0°C gives a feeling of warmth and comfort, i.e. perceived warmth, but the risk of hypothermia is still present. Welfare recommendations are that work in coldblast stores should be limited to 45 min followed by a 15-min break with a hot drink in a warm room before returning to the cold room. These recommendations do not apply if workers are constantly moving in and out of a cold store, e.g. with food. Unfortunately a person may fail to recover total body heat while outside the cold room, and may slowly become hypothermic without shivering or feeling cold. Perceived warmth has clinical implications in other situations, e.g. divers (Lloyd, 1986).

All coldroom doors should be capable of being opened from the inside and there should also be an alarm lever in the room. However, the door may jam, the alarm system may fail or there may be no one present to notice the alarm. To cover this contingency, emergency protective gear should be kept inside the cold room. This equipment should include an arctic-quality sleeping bag with an integral insulated hood, inside a large polythene bag of the type used by climbers to keep out the wind, and a face mask with a condenser humidifier device (Lloyd, 1986) since this will not only provide insulation to reduce or eliminate the heat lost through breathing but will also trap the exhaled moisture and prevent it wetting the inside of the sleeping bag.

Education and training

Panic during an emergency may cause people to take wrong or delayed actions, and therefore compromise their survival. Education can prevent many problems (Andrew, 1963), but training must be specific to the conditions during work or leisure activities in which the activity is to be done (Enander, 1984). The disproportionately high proportion of English climbers involved in accidents in the Scottish hills (MacGregor, 1988) may be due to a failure to appreciate the much greater cold and general severity of the weather conditions present in Scotland as compared with hill areas in England and Wales. The selection of appropriate equipment, e.g. crampons and ice axes for winter climbing, is important but inadequate training in their use may result in accidents and death (MacGregor, 1988). Unfortunately even education is not sufficient without common sense.

Education outdoors includes training in the assessment of the weather (Adam, 1981), i.e. listening to forecasts, observing the sky and, on land, observing the vegetation which will indicate the general climate of the region. Education should also persuade climbers that turning back or taking shelter early in the face of deteriorating weather conditions is a mark of maturity whereas pressing on is often a sign of weakness. Every participant in boating should have and wear a flotation device (Hayward, 1982).

Food

Maintaining a high blood sugar level prevents any deterioration of performance during severe exercise, thus reducing the risk of accidents, and also prevents prolonged post-exercise exhaustion.

Clothing

This is an obvious precautionary measure and inadequate clothing is an important factor in accidents in the hills in summer as well as in winter (MacGregor, 1988). In every situation clothing should provide varying combinations of thermal insulation, wind protection and waterproofing (Cena and Clark, 1979) but the principles are often badly understood.

The insulating potential of clothing is usually expressed as clo units, which is a purely arbitary term. One clo unit is roughly the clothing which keeps an average person comfortable while sitting at rest in a room of 21°C with 50% relative humidity (Burton and Endholm, 1955; Maclean and Emslie-Smith, 1977). The clo insulation values for typical clothing ensembles are readily available in the literature (Holmer, 1988), but unfortunately these basic insulation values are measured dry and on a thermal manikin which is standing, static and when there is no wind. The actual insulation of clothing is dynamic, being modified by posture, intensity and type of activity, moisture content of the clothing and the extent to which wind penetrates the clothing. Movement produces a bellows effect, causing heat and moisture to be lost from within the protective barrier of the clothing (Lloyd, 1986; Holmer, 1988). The insulation value of clothing is reduced by 30% while walking, by 50% through wind or wetting, and by 90% if there is wind and wetting (Pugh, 1968; Holmer, 1988). From calculations of heat loss through various routes, a protection factor has been developed, the insulation required index (IREQ) (Holmer, 1988). This is not the same as clo insulation but is the resultant insulation when all other factors are considered. To provide comfort the clo value of clothing should be 30–80% higher than normally predicted.

Because IREQ is only applicable to the whole body, hands and feet must be considered separately. Adequate gloves impair manual performance (Enander, 1984) and where only thin protective covering of the hands is possible, the use of limited auxiliary heating to raise the temperature around the cold exposed part can minimize or even eliminate the incapacitating effects of cold on hand and finger dexterity, and improve the strength and speed of movement (Lockhart and Keiss, 1971). Unfortunately if the hands and feet are too well-insulated, vasoconstriction may not occur because of lack of cold stimulus, and warm hands and feet may be accompanied by shivering and a falling core temperature. If the hands and feet are kept cool or cold, the core temperature remains high and the person is comfortable (Kaufman, 1983). Physical exercise, at 40–60% of maximum aerobic capacity, can increase the temperature of covered hands and feet even in the cold, though rewarming is delayed in unprotected limbs, and toes are more difficult to warm than fingers (Hellstrom *et al.*, 1966). From personal experience, it often seems that the extremities warm most in the first few minutes after the exercise has stopped.

In a cold environment there is a steep vapour pressure gradient within clothing with the surface layers becoming wet from condensation. Wet clothing is inefficient and difficult to dry under field conditions. Clothing which is suitable at rest is excessive if the person is going to exercise since he or she will overheat and sweat, causing increased condensation. A waterproof outer layer will increase condensation, though some fabrics e.g. Goretex, allow most of the sweat vapour to escape while preventing rain penetration.

In practical terms several thin layers of clothes provide better insulation and are more flexible than one thick layer. In an emergency, paper, especially newspaper, between the layers of clothing will provide a remarkable degree of thermal insulation and windproofing. Natural wool, because of its crimped fibre, retains 40% of its insulation value when wet as compared with 10% for wet cotton (Danzl, 1983). However some synthetic fibres may be better because they are hydrophobic and do not retain moisture (Stephens, 1982). Clothing has to be adjusted to the situation and the needs and preferences of the person involved, but where conditions are likely to change, as in climbing or hill walking, clothing ensembles should be flexible in the degree of insulation, and in protection from wind and rain.

The head has minimal vasoconstrictor activity and, while this has a protective effect against frostbite, the rate of heat loss through the head increases in a linear manner between 32°C and −20°C; indeed at rest at −4°C the heat loss from the head may equal half the total heat production (Froese and Burton, 1957). Therefore protective clothing should include the head.

Protection in the water requires special garments, which should be brightly, luminously coloured to aid rescue. Wetsuits of closed-cell neoprene insulate by trapping a thin layer of water between the garment and the person and must therefore be body-hugging. A neoprene kidney belt improves insulation by eliminating the looseness which is usual around the waist, but it is nonsense to claim, as advertised, that it protects the kidneys from damage due to cold.

Wetsuits are of greatest benefit when the person is totally immersed but they are often used by sailors e.g. windsurfers, when they are less effective because of wind chill and evaporation. In this situation a windproof cagoule and trousers over a wetsuit have a marked thermal benefit.

Wetsuits compress under pressure and therefore will not give adequate protection during deep diving. Drysuits prevent the entry of water and insulation is provided by the clothing under the suit.

All protective suits at present available have disadvantages – they reduce mobility, are expensive and uncomfortable, may cause heat stress if worn before the immersion occurs (White and Roth, 1979; Hayward, 1982) and when worn they are not flattering for the person. Price is no guide for recommendations, and survival suits should be assessed in practical use (White and Roth, 1979) because the best in theory may be easily damaged, which will make it ineffective. For survival, buoyancy is also necessary but if buoyancy and survival suits are separate, this will cause delay in an emergency and increase the chance that one or other will be missing.

Action to be taken if isolated in a hostile environment

In the hills shelter is important, e.g. in bothys, tents, survival bags or snow holes, but it requires maps and navigating ability to locate bothys, and knowledge of how to build a snow hole is valueless if there is insufficient snow. In all hill areas, irrespective of wind strength or direction, it is possible to find 'dead areas' – localized areas of calm – and even the lea of a large boulder may be of value in an emergency (Lloyd, 1986). At sea, the modern covered life-rafts, with the doors closed properly, are extremely effective at raising the temperature of the internal environment (Pugh, 1968; Gavshon and Rice, 1984) but if a raft has many fewer people than the intended number, the thermal benefit can be reduced. Unfortunately in an emergency it is rarely possible to launch all the available liferafts or lifeboats.

In cold water there are no conditions in which activity would prolong survival, and under most conditions exercise will accelerate hypothermia (Keatinge, 1969) because physical activity increases the surface area of warm skin exposed to the cold, through the increased blood supply to the muscles and the bellows effect in the clothing. Deliberate inactivity markedly decreases cooling rates and may increase the survival time by up to an hour (Hayward, 1982), which gives the rescuers more time.

If immersion occurs, people should stay near the wreck as long as possible, especially if the boat is still afloat, because this will save energy, and it is also easier for the rescue services to find a wreck rather than bodies in the water.

Posture is also important in the survival situation. A person sitting fully flexed reduces the exposed surface area of the body by 30–40% (Pugh, 1968). This is the basis for the heat escape lessening posture (HELP) recommended for water immersion, and a number of people, by huddling together, will decrease the heat loss by trapping water between them (Wilkerson *et al.*, 1986). This will be aided if the survivors are roped together and would prevent an unconscious person drifting away, though the rope should be long enough to allow the survivors some movement.

Conclusions

Cold exposure can contribute to soft tissue injury in a variety of ways, directly or indirectly. However, many injuries in cold conditions are not due to cold, and summer may be more hazardous than winter, partly because the cold stress present in summer is often unexpected and unsuspected. In the Scottish mountains the commonest cause of injury is a simple slip or a stumble – more accidents take place in the summer than winter (MacGregor, 1988). This cannot be entirely attributed to cold since the long grass during summer may be more treacherous underfoot than snow.

Many specific winter injuries, e.g. from ice skates or lower limb fractures in skiing, are related to the equipment in use, and would also occur if the activity could be done in a warm environment. Similarly, head injuries from falling rocks during climbing are not specifically cold-related. This caveat even applies to avalanches, which are an important cause of injury (Lloyd, 1986; MacGregor, 1988).

Though the subject of this chapter is cold as related to soft tissue injury, it is important to remember that cold has other dangers. Hypothermia is a hazard which can cause death, though many deaths are in fact caused by inappropriate methods of rewarming. Submersion in very cold water, e.g. an outdoor skater or curler falling through the ice, may produce death through the so-called diving reflex. Full recovery is possible, especially in children, after up to 40 min total submersion, but resuscitation must start immediately on rescue (Lloyd, 1986). Cold exposure is also related to some diseases of the respiratory system, e.g. asthma and bronchitis, heart disease and strokes (Lloyd, 1986).

The systemic or whole-body effects of cold can occur in many situations and may coexist with soft tissue injuries. Some of the local effects of cold may cause death, as when cold-induced muscle spasm in a swimmer may cause death through drowning. Diving into cold water, such as on a warm day in spring, may cause drowning from muscular incapacity even in very competent swimmers. Cold water in the nose may cause vagal-induced cardiac arrest and in the ears it may cause caloric labyrinthitis and disorientation. The sympathetic mediated surge in heart rate and blood pressure may cause myocardial infarction or stroke with immediate death or death through drowning. The cold-induced uncontrollable hyperventilation may cause drowning directly or as a result of unconsciousness secondary to hypocapnia (Lloyd, 1986).

References

Adam JM (1981) Cold weather: its characteristics, dangers and assessment. In: J M Adam (ed) *Hypothermia Ashore and Afloat*. Aberdeen: University Press, pp. 6–14.

Andrew HG (1963) Work in extreme cold. *Transactions of the Association of Industrial Medical Officers* **13**, 16–19.

Angus RG, Pearce DG, Buguet AGC, Olsen L (1979) Vigilence performance of men sleeping under arctic conditions. *Aviation and Space Environmental Medicine* **50**, 692–6.

Baddeley AD (1966) Time estimation and reduced body temperature. *American Journal of Physiology* **70**, 475–579.

Barber SG (1978) Drugs and doctorings for trans-Saharan travellers. *British Medical Journal* **ii**, 404–6.

Belch JJF (1990) Management of Raynaud's phenomenon. *Hospital Update* **16**, 391–400.

Bentley-Phillips CB, Eady RAJ, Greaves MW (1978) Cold urticaria; inhibition of cold induced histamine release by doxantrazole. *Journal of Investigative Dermatology* **71**, 266–8.

Bickel L (1977) *This Accursed Land*. London: Macmillan.

Brent P (1974) *Captain Scott and the Antarctic Tragedy*. London: Weidenfeld and Nicolson.

British Medical Journal (1975) Cold hypersensitivity. *British Medical Journal* **i**, 643–4.

Burton AC, Edholm OG (1955) *Man in a Cold Environment*, London: Edward Arnold.

Cena K, Clark JA (1979) Transfer of heat through animal coats and clothing. In Robertshaw D (ed) *Environmental Physiology III*. Baltimore: University Park Press, pp 1–42.

Clark RE, Jones CE (1962) Manual performance during cold exposure as a function of practice level and thermal conditions of training. *Journal of Applied Physiology* **46**, 276–80.

Clarke RSJ, Hellon RF, Lind AR (1958) The duration of sustained contractions of the human forearm at different muscle temperature. *Journal of Physiology (London)* **143**, 454–73.

Coleshaw SR, van Someren RNM, Wolff AH, Davis HM, Keatinge WR (1983) Impaired memory registration and speed of reasoning caused by low body temperature. *Journal of Applied Physiology* **55**, 27–31.

Coppin EG, Livingstone SP, Kuehn LA (1978) Cold-decreased grip strength: effects on handgrip strength due to arm immersion in a 10 deg C water bath. *Aviation and Space Environmental Medicine* **49**, 1322–6.

Danzl DF (1983) Accidental hypothermia. In: Rosen P, Baker FJ, Braen GR, Dailey RH, Levy RC (eds) *Emergency Medicine, Concepts and Clinical Practice* vol 2: *Trauma*. Boston: Mosby, pp 477–96.

Davis FM, Baddeley AD, Hancock T (1975) Diver performance: the effect of cold. *Undersea Biomedical Research* **2**, 195–213.

Eady, EA, Bentley-Phillips CB, Keahey TMk, Greaves MWN (1978) Cold urticaria vasculitis. *British Journal of Dermatology* **99** (suppl 16), 9–10.

Enander A (1984) Performance and sensory aspects of work in cold environments – a review. *Ergonomics* **27**, 365–78.

Fanger PO (1970) *Thermal Comfort. Analysis and Applications in Environmental Engineering*. New York: McGraw-Hill.

Flora G (1985) Secondary treatment of frostbite. In: Rivolier J, Cerretelli P, Foray J, Segantini P (eds) *High Altitude Deterioration*. Basel: Karger, pp 159–69.

Foldes FF, Kuze S, Vizi ES, Deery A (1978) The influence of temperature on neuromuscular performance. *Journal Neural Transmission* **43**, 27–45.

Foray J, Salon F (1985) Casualties with cold injuries: primary treatment. In: Rivolier J, Cerretelli P, Foray J, Segantini P (eds) *High Altitude Deterioration*. Basel: Karger, pp 149–58.

Fox RH (1961) Local cooling in man. *British Medical Bulletin* **17**, 14–18.

Francis TJR (1984) Non-freezing cold injury: a historical review. *Journal of Royal Navy Medical Service* **70**, 134–9.

Francis TJR, Golden F St C (1985) Non-freezing cold injury: the pathogenesis. *Journal of Royal Navy Medical Service* **71**, 3–8.

Franz DR, Berberich JJ, Blake S, Mills WJ (1978) Evaluation of fasciotomy and vasodilators for treatment of frostbite in the dog. *Cryobiology* **15**, 659–69.

Freedman RR, Ianni P (1983) Role of cold and

emotional stress in Raynaud's disease and scleroderma. *British Medical Journal* **ii**, 1499–502.

Freeman J, Pugh LGCE (1969) Hypothermia in mountain accidents. *International Anesthesiology Clinics* **7**, 997–1007.

Froese G, Burton AC (1957) Heat losses from the human head. *Journal of Applied Physiology* **10**, 235–41.

Gavshon A, Rice D (1984) *The Sinking of the Belgrano*. London: New English Library, p 106.

Goldsmith R, Minard D (1976) Cold, cold work. *Occupational Health and Safety*, vol 1. Geneva: International Labour Office, pp 319–20.

Gray A (1970) *The Big Grey Man of Ben Macdhui*. Aberdeen: Impulse Books.

Grayson J, Kuehn LA (1979) Heat transfer and heat loss. In: Lomax P, Schonbaum E (eds) *Body Temperature: Regulation, Drug Effects, and Therapeutic Implications*. New York: Marcel Dekker, pp 71–87.

Greenfield ADM, Shepherd JT, Whelan RF (1950) The average internal temperatures of fingers immersed in cold water. *Clinical Science* **9**, 349–54.

Guttman R, Gross MM (1956) Relationship between electrical and mechanical changes in muscle caused by cooling. *Journal of the College of Comparative Physiology* **48**, 421–30.

Hassi J (1982) Working in cold conditions. *Nordic Council for Arctic Medical Research* **30**, 20–22.

Hassi J, Virokannas H, Auttonen H, Jarvenpas I (1984) Health hazards in snow mobile usage. Presentation at Sixth International Symposium on Circumpolar Health May 13-18 1984. Anchorage Alaska. Abstracts p. 142. University of Alaska, Anchorage.

Haywards JS (1982) Protection against immersion hypothermia. In: Koch P, Kohfahl M. (eds) *Unterkuhlung im Seenotofall. 2nd Symposium* Cuxhaven: Deutsche Gesellschaft zur Rettung Schiffbruchiger, pp 72–9.

Health and Safety Executive (1978) *One Hundred Fatal Accidents in Construction*. London: Health and Safety Executive, HMSO.

Hellstrom B, Berg K, Lorentzen FV (1966) Human peripheral rewarming during exercise in the cold. *Journal of Applied Physiology* **29**, 191–9.

Hirvonen J (1982) Accidental hypothermia. *Nordic Council for Arctic Medical Research* **30**, 15–19.

Holdcroft A (1981) *Body Temperature Control in Anaesthesia, Surgery and Intensive Care*. London: Baillière Tindall.

Holmer I (1988) Assessment of cold stress in terms of required clothing insulation – IREQ. *International Journal of Industrial Ergonomics* **3**, 159–66.

Holti G (1985) Vascular reactivity in patients with Raynaud's phenomenon. *Scottish Medical Journal* **30**, 120–1.

Horvath SM (1981) Exercise in a cold environment. *Exercise, Sport Science Review* **9**, 221–63.

Hunter J, Kerr EH, Whillans MG (1952) The relation between joint stiffness upon exposure to cold and the characteristics of synovial fluid. *Journal of Canadian Medical Science* **39**, 367–77.

Kappes BM, Mills WJ (1984) Thermal biofeedback training with frostbite patients. *Presentation at Sixth International Symposium on Circumpolar Health*, May 13–18, 1984. University of Alaska, Anchorage. Abstracts p 100.

Katz B, Miledi R (1965) The effect of temperature on the synaptic delay at the neuromuscular junction. *Journal of Physiology (London)* **181**, 656–70.

Kaufman WC (1983) The development and rectification of hiker's hypothermia. In: Pozos RS, Wittmers LE (eds) *The Nature and Treatment of Hypothermia*. London: Croom Helm, pp 46–57.

Keatinge WR (1969) *Survival in Cold Water*. Edinburgh: Blackwell.

Keatinge WR (1977) Accidental immersion hypothermia and drowning. *Practitioner* **219**, 183–7.

Keatinge WR, Cannon P (1960) Freezing point of human skin. *Lancet* **i**, 11–14.

Kempson GE, Coggan D, Acheson ED (1983) Electrically heated gloves for intermittent digital ischaemia. *British Medical Journal* **i**, 268.

Kinnersly P (1974) *The Hazards of Work: How to Fight Them*. Pluto Press: Surrey.

Lahti A (1982) Cutaneous reactions to cold. *Nordic Council for Arctic Medical Research* **30**, 32–35.

Lakie M, Walsh EG, Wright GW (1986) Control and postural thixotropy of the forearm muscles: changes caused by cold. *Journal of Neurology Neurosurgery and Psychiatry* **49**, 69–76.

Lee ECB, Lee K (1971) *Survival and Safety at Sea*. London: Cassell.

Lewis RB, Moen PW (1952) Further studies on the pathogenesis of cold induced muscle necrosis. *Surgery, Gynecology and Obstetrics* **95**, 543–51.

Linderholm H, Lagerkvist B (1984) Increased tendency to cold induced vasospasm in the fingers (Raynaud's phenomenon) in copper smelter workers exposed to arsenic (As). *Presentation at Sixth International Symposium on Circumpolar Health*, May 13–18, 1984. University of Alaska, Anchorage. Abstracts p 72.

Lloyd EL (1986) *Hypothermia and Cold Stress*. London: Croom Helm.

Lockhart JM (1960) Extreme body cooling and psychomotor performance. *Ergonomics* **11**, 249–60.

Lockhart JM, Keiss OK (1971) Auxilliary heating of hands during cold exposure and manual performance. *Human Factors* **13**, 457–65.

MacGregor AR (1988) *The Nature and Causes of Injuries Sustained in 190 Scottish Mountain Accidents*. Research Report RR1. The Scottish Sports Council, Edinburgh.

Maclean D, Emslie-Smith D (1977) *Accidental Hypothermia*. Edinburgh: Blackwell.

McOwan R (1979) The hills are alive. *The Scots Magazine*, 258–67.

Marshall HC, Goldman RF (1976) Electrical response of nerve to freezing injury. In Shephard RJ, Itoh S (eds) *Circumpolar Health*, Toronto: University Press, p 77.

Mills MJ (1973) Frostbite. *Alaska Medicine* **15**, 27–47.

Mills WJ (1983) Frostbite. *Alaska Medicine* **25**, 33–8.

Mills WJ, Rau D (1983) University of Alaska, Anchorage – section of high latitude study, and the Mt McKinley project. *Alaska Medicine* **25**, 21–8.

Nukuda H, Pollock M, Allpress S (1981) Experimental cold injury to nerve. *Brain* **104**, 779–813.

Oakley EHN (1984) The design and function of military footwear: a review following experiences in the South Atlantic, *Ergonomics* **6**, 631–7.

Paton BC (1983) Accidental hypothermia. *Pharmacology Therapy* **22**, 331–77.

Payne R (1984) Lessons of the Falklands. *World Medicine* **19**, 26–7.

Peyronnard JM, Pednault M, Aquayo AJ (1977) Neuropathies due to cold. Quantitative studies of structural changes in human and animal nerves. In: *Proceedings of 11th World Congress of Neurology*. University of Amsterdam, Amsterdam, pp 308–29.

Platt SD, Martin CJ, Hunt SM, Lewis CW (1989) Damp housing, mould growth, and symptomatic health state. *British Medical Journal* **1**, 1673–8.

Poulton EC, Hutchings NB, Brooke RB (1965) Effect of cold and rain upon the vigilance of lookouts. *Ergonomics* **8**, 163–8.

Provins KA, Clarke RSJ (1960) The effect of cold on manual performance. *Journal of Occupational Medicine* **2**, 169–76.

Pugh LGCE (1964) Deaths from exposure on Four Inns walking competition. *Lancet* **i**, 1210–12.

Pugh LGCE (1966) Accidental hypothermia in walkers, climbers and campers: report to the medical commission on accident prevention. *British Medical Journal* **i**, 123–9.

Pugh LGCE (1968) Isafjordur trawler disaster. Medical aspects. *British Medical Journal* **i**, 826–9.

Pugh LGCE, Edholm OG (1955) The physiology of channel swimmers. *Lancet* **ii**, 761–8.

Reichl M (1987) Neuropathy of the feet due to running on cold surfaces. *British Medical Journal* **ii**, 348–9.

Schmid-Schonbein H, Neumann FJ (1985) Pathophysiology of cutaneous frost injury: disturbed microcirculation as a consequence of abnormal flow behaviour of the blood. Application of new concepts of blood rheology. In: Rivolier J, Cerretelli P, Foray J, Segantini P (eds) *High Altitude Deterioration*, Basel: Karger, pp 20–38.

Simpson HW (1972) The exploring scientist. *British Journal of Sports Medicine* **6**, 100–7.

Stephens DH (1982) Sleeping snugly in cold damp bedrooms. *Journal of the Royal Society of Health* **6**, 272–5.

Sumner DS, Strandness DE (1972) An abnormal finger pulse associated with cold sensitivity. *Annals of Surgery* **175**, 294–8.

Surwit RS, Allen LM, Gilgor RS, Schanberg S, Kuhn C, Duvic M (1983) Neuroendocrine response to cold in Raynaud's syndrome. *Life Science* **32**, 995–1000.

Taylor G (1975) Men at risk from cold. *Viewpoint* 2, November.

Teichner WH (1958) Reaction time in the cold. *Journal of Applied Physiology* **42**, 54–9.

Thomas JR, Ahlers ST, House JF, Schrot J (1989) Repeated exposure to moderate cold impairs matching-to-sample performance. *Aviation and Space Environmental Medicine* **60**, 1063–7.

Ting S (1984) Cold-induced urticaria in infancy. *Pediatrics* **73**, 105–6.

Travis S, Roberts D (1989) Arctic willy. *British Medical Journal* **ii**, 1573–4.

Tuttle WW (1941) The effects of decreased temperature on the activity of intact muscle. *Journal of Laboratory and Clinical Medicine* **26**, 1913–19.

Vanggaard l (1975) Physiological reactions to wet-cold. *Aviation and Space Environmental Medicine* **46**, 33–6.

Vanggaard L (1977) Occupational hazards in the Danish North-Sea fishing. *Nordic Council for Arctic Medical Research* **18**, 31–7.

Vanggaard L (1985) Cold-induced changes. In: Rey L (ed) *Arctic Underwater Operations*. London: Graham & Trotman, pp 41–8.

Vernon HM (1939) *Health in Relation to Occupation*. London: Oxford University Press.

Ward MP, Milledge JS, West JB (1989) *High Altitude Medicine and Physiology*. London: Chapman and Hall.

Wasserman SI, Soter NA, Center DM, Austen KF (1977) Cold urticaria. Recognition and characterization of a neutrophil chemotactic factor which appears in serum during experimental cold challenge. *Journal of Clinical Investigation* **60**, 189–96.

Wedin B (1976) Cases of paradoxical undressing by people exposed to severe hypothermia. In Shephard RJ, Itoh S (eds) *Circumpolar Health*. Toronto: Toronto University Press, pp 61–71.

White ER, Roth NJ (1979) Cold water survival suits for aircrew. *Aviation and Space Environmental Medicine* **50**, 1040–5.

Wilkerson JA, Bangs CC, Hayward JS (1986) *Hypothermia, Frostbite and other Cold Injuries*. Seattle: The Mountaineers.

Williams ES, Ward MP, Milledge JS, Withey WR, Older MJW, Forsling ML (1979) Effect of the exercise of seven consecutive days hill-walking on fluid homeostasis. *Clinical Science* **56**, 305–16.

Part II

Diagnostic Methods and Problems in Practice

8

Imaging of the soft tissues

R. C. Evans

In recent years there have been many significant advances in imaging techniques. As a result we are now capable of visualizing, often in startling detail, most of the tissues of the human body.

No longer does a structure have to be ossified before it can be captured on film and neither does it have to be static. Techniques are now available to study dynamic processes such as blood flow and the movement of heart valves as well as to picture soft tissues such as tendons and menisci.

Whilst ionizing radiation still plays a major part in the production of images in any radiology unit, other modalities are becoming increasingly commonly used. Foremost amongst these are electromagnetism and ultrasound, both of which are particularly helpful in the diagnosis of soft tissue problems.

Imaging techniques are expensive, high-performance tools, to be used with economy and precision. Their use should be dictated by the information obtained from a careful history and a painstaking examination. The blunderbuss approach to the injured sports player in which every possible radiological investigation is fired at him or her is the way of the dilettante and to be deprecated.

Head injuries

Usually the bones which make up the vault of the skull are solidly constructed and require a significant blow to fracture them. Concussive injuries to the brain are common in the contact sports but skull fractures and associated significant intracranial injuries are rare. Their incidence however is increasing with the introduction of more and more high-risk sports such as hang-gliding and racing in all-terrain vehicles. The majority of fractures to the vault are usually easily demonstrated by plain radiography, though suture lines and vascular markings can cause confusion.

Whilst depressed skull fractures to the vault are demonstrable by plain X-ray, depending upon the site of the injury, tangential views may be needed. Small depressions may be difficult to spot and under these circumstances computed tomography (CT) scanning is a useful complementary technique.

Base-of-skull fractures are notoriously difficult to demonstrate on normal plain films and depending upon their extent can even be difficult to pick out after narrow-section CT scanning of the area.

Associated with damage to the skull may be injury to the intracranial soft tissues. Most commonly this is due to intracranial bleeding, sometimes from a torn intracerebral vessel but also – more importantly, as it is potentially treatable – bleeding from an extracerebral source. This may be a subdural or an extradural (epidural) haematoma.

Though occasionally plain X-rays will raise a suspicion of intracranial bleeding if calcified structures such as the pineal are seen to be shifted laterally, CT is the investigation of choice (Gentry *et al.*, 1988). At present scanning times with CT are quicker than with magnetic resonance imaging (MRI), this is important when patients are unco-operative, CT also picks out bony damage more accurately. Occasionally MRI is useful, e.g. in posterior fossa problems where good pictures are difficult to obtain using CT.

Due to the potentially disastrous consequences of delay in diagnosis, CT scanning should be undertaken promptly whenever there is clinical suspicion of an intracranial bleed. It should be remembered that worldwide around 6000 people a year die from the effects of a head injury sustained in some type of sporting activity (Wallace, 1988).

Whilst acute compression of the brain by an intracranial haematoma can cause death or result in severe permanent neurological problems, recurrent less severe injuries also cause cumulative damage.

Where athletes, most particularly boxers, sustain frequent concussive injuries, a chronic progressive post-traumatic encephalopathy can result (punch-drunk syndrome/dementia pugilistica). This is characterized by slurred speech, ataxia, various Parkinsonian features and progressive dementia (Corsellis *et al.*, 1983).

CT scanning reveals tears or splits in the septum pellucidum (a cavum septum pellucidum) together with cortical atrophy. Post-mortem studies confirm these abnormalities and demonstrate other characteristic features such as depigmentation in the substantia nigra.

Facial bones

Fractures to the light bones of the facial skeleton are seen in many of the contact sports. Whilst they can be the result of genuine accidents on occasions, they are also sometimes caused by deliberate foul play. Due to the complexity of the facial skeleton small fractures can be difficult to pick out on the set of films normally produced (occipitomental 15° and 30° and a submentrovertical). Various other specialized views are available which can be coned down on to an area of particular interest and other plain film techniques such as panoramic zonography, a process which 'opens out' the facial skeleton, have been found to be very useful.

Fractures to the facial skeleton can be associated with damage to various soft tissue structures, e.g. the infraorbital nerve. In this instance there will be numbness over the area innervated by that nerve.

Where the floor of the orbit is fractured extra-ocular muscles can be entrapped and this results in an ophthalmoplegia with diplopia in certain directions of gaze. Orbital floor fractures can best be detected by CT scanning (Gentry *et al.*, 1983).

Conventional tomography is used only occasionally as CT has been developed to the extent that it is now used frequently where not enough detail has been demonstrated on plain films.

Mandible

Fractures to the mandible are commonly bilateral, e.g. ramus on the left together with condylar neck on the right, and it is easy to miss the second fracture in the self-congratulatory phase after having spotted the more obvious lesion. The most common fracture site is the body or angle of the mandible (approximately 60%) and about 20% involve the condyle.

Where blows to the mouth have caused damage to the teeth with associated labial lacerations, it is important to obtain soft tissue films of the lips. This is done in order to ascertain if any of the broken pieces of tooth have been retained in the substance of the wound. If this is the case they will need to be removed prior to wound repair – if this is not done sepsis is almost inevitable.

Spinal injuries

The most important point to be made with regard to the investigation of spinal injuries is that it is vital to ensure that damage of the spinal cord is not made worse by insensitive handling of the sports player, during procedures which are, of necessity, often undertaken hurriedly. Do not forget that in up to 15% of spinal injuries damage to the cord is made worse by poor technique during initial management, transportation and investigation. When dealing with a patient in whom the index of suspicion with regard to injury is high, movement should be kept to a minimum and any necessary manoeuvres should be carried out carefully under experienced medical supervision.

Cervical spine

The basis of the diagnosis of cervical spine injuries from a radiological point of view is provided by the three views – anteroposterior, lateral and open-mouth view of the odontoid peg – normally obtained. Occasionally these are supplemented by oblique films and, rarely, conventional tomography.

Straightforward contrast studies (myelography) are only undertaken occasionally these days as CT and MRI have superseded them. However, contrast is still used combined with CT and is probably the investigation of choice at the moment. MRI, whilst it is better than myelography alone, has not yet achieved the accuracy of CT myelography (Cantu, 1988).

It is vital when imaging the neck that the whole of the cervical spine from C1 to the C7–T1 junction is visualized. Cases of medical negligence which hang on a failure to obtain views of the whole cervical spine still occur with depressing regularity.

Whilst plain X-rays cannot directly demonstrate damage to the supporting ligaments of the cervical spine, where rupture has occurred with resultant instability, screening the neck and obtaining flexion and extension views will demonstrate the fact that these structures have been ruptured. This investigation should never be undertaken without *experienced* medical supervision.

In association with plain films, MRI images allow you to evaluate damage to the intervertebral discs (Fig. 8.1) and ligaments as well as demonstrating paraspinal haematomata and injuries to the spinal cord itself. With plain films one indicator of a cervical spine injury is the soft tissue shadowing produced by a prevertebral haematoma, though how well this shows up depends on the exposures used. Modern developments in MRI scanning have allowed the radiologist to differentiate between simple oedema of the cord and intramedullary or perimedullary haemorrhage. MRI also graphically illustrates a prevertebral haematoma (Fig. 8.2).

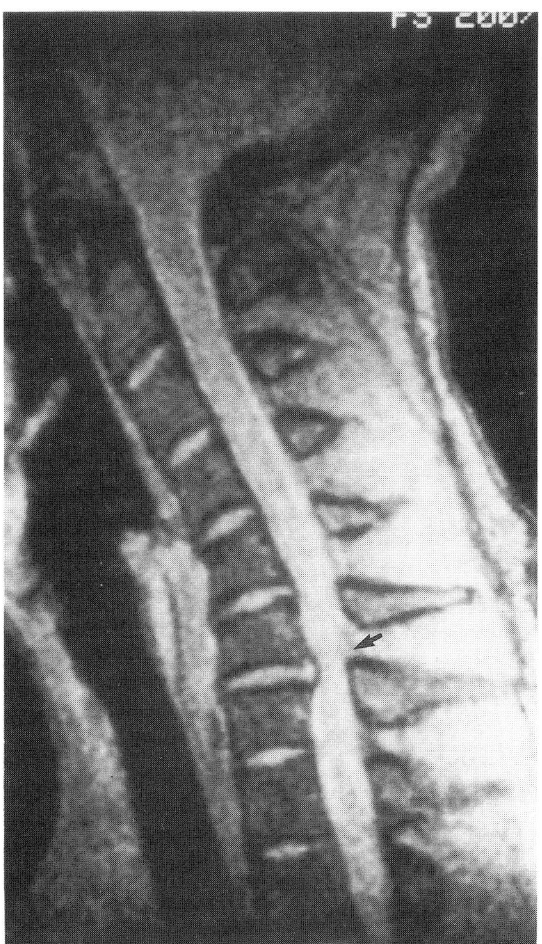

Fig. 8.1 MRI of the neck of a 27-year-old back-row forward who injured his neck in a tackle. He was complaining of pain in the neck radiating down his right arm. The film shows a prolapsed disc at the C6–7 level (arrowed).

Occasionally traction injuries or blunt trauma may damage some of the trunks of the brachial plexus during athletic activities. Imaging of the plexus is difficult but some information can be gained from CT myelography and MRI. Using

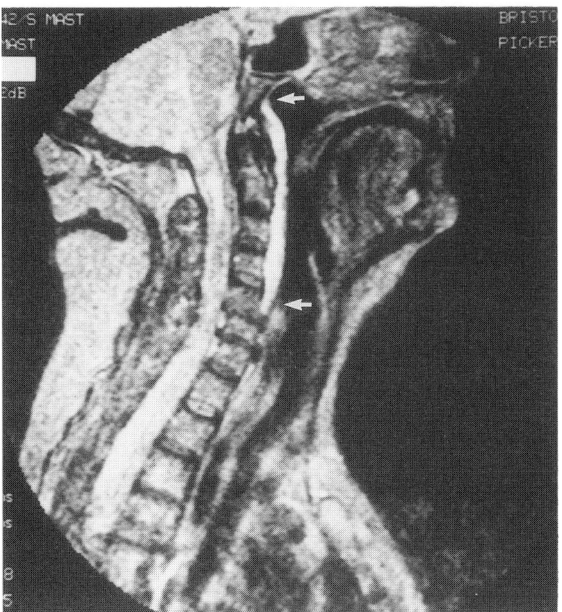

Fig. 8.2 MRI of the cervical spine showing a prevertebral haematoma (between arrows) secondary to a fracture of C1.

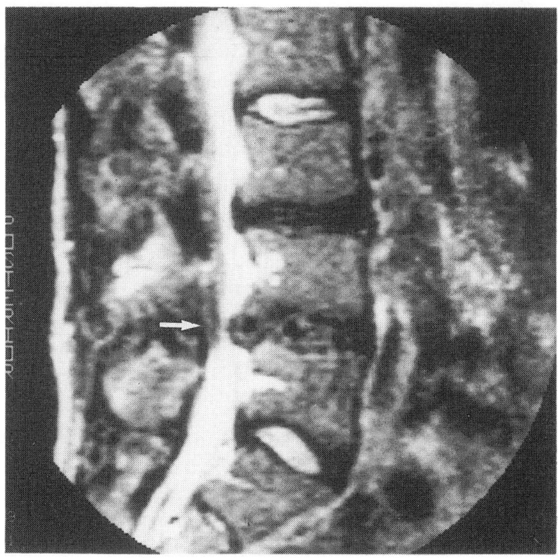

Fig. 8.3 MRI of the lumbar spine of an oarsman. There is a loss of signal from the L3–4 and L4–5 discs indicating disc degeneration. There is a central protrusion of the L4–5 disc (arrowed).

these techniques we can for instance identify such things as root avulsion.

Whilst 60% of spinal injuries occur in the cervical region, the remaining third are found in the dorsal and lumbar spine. Injuries to this area occur in the high-risk and vehicular sports and occasionally in the brute sports (American football, rugby, wrestling etc.). Whilst these areas are more stable than the cervical spine, the dorsolumbar junction is the site most commonly affected and here the investigation of choice following plain X-rays is MRI (Modic *et al.*, 1984).

More commonly, problems in the lumbar region are due to chronic damage to the intervertebral discs and here again MRI is the investigation of choice as discs which are degenerate but not yet prolapsing can be differentiated from normal ones (Fig. 8.3). Both MRI and CT are better than myelography in detecting prolasped intervertebral discs; the diagnosis provided by MRI correlates well with the surgical findings (83%). The results with CT are very comparable with 82% correlation with the findings at surgery.

The thorax

The shoulder and upper limb

Injuries to the shoulder region may result in calcification to structures around the joint, e.g. supraspinatus tendon. Such lesions can usually be easily picked up on plain films of the joint or on screening the area. Evidence of previous damage to the acromiocalvicular joint may similarly be pinpointed by demonstrating ossification of its securing ligaments, e.g. conoid and trapezoid (Fig. 8.4).

Previous dislocations (usually anterior) to the shoulder joint may be indicated on plain films by the presence of a Hill–Sachs and/or a Bankart's lesion. The extent of the damage to the capsule can be shown by CT arthrography. MRI has been shown to demonstrate tears of the rotator cuff well and this modality will probably be the investigation of choice as it becomes more widely available.

Tears of the rotator cuff can be demonstrated using high-definition ultrasound (Middleton *et al.*, 1985) and where the tear is due to an impingement

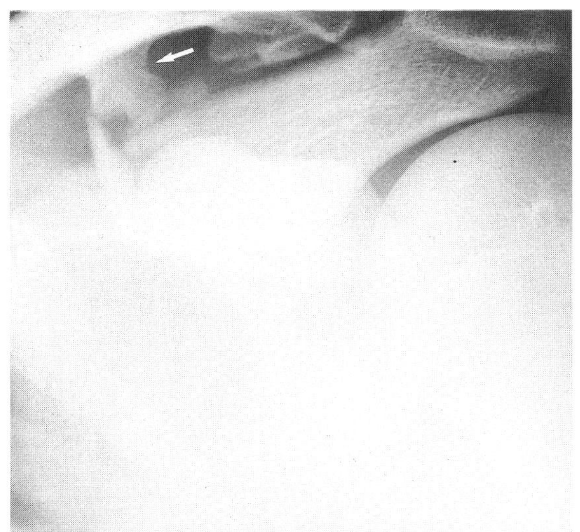

Fig. 8.4 Plain X-ray of the shoulder of a 29-year-old American footballer who has sustained several shoulder injuries in the past. The damage sustained by the ligaments has resulted in them becoming ossified (arrowed).

syndrome there may be radiological changes on the plain films such as the presence of a subacromial spur. The diagnosis of impingement may be confirmed by screening the patient whilst abducting the arm in external rotation.

Ultrasound has the advantage over MRI in that it is more widely available, though the quality of the picture is to a large extent dependent upon the presence of a radiologist who is experienced in the procedure.

Other shoulder problems such as tendinitis, subacromial bursitis, etc. have also been demonstrated by MRI. The images produced will no doubt improve as more experience is gained with the wider availability of the equipment.

As with the shoulder joint, evidence of past injury to the elbow (e.g. posterior dislocation) can often be found on plain films where calcification has taken place in part of the damaged joint capsule.

The chest

The most commonly traumatized of the soft tissues within the bony cage of the thorax are the lungs. The damage usually takes the form of a pneumothorax secondary to a rib fracture or a pulmonary contusion. A small pneumothorax can be difficult to detect and should be carefully sought at the apices. Films need be obtained in full inspiration and full expiration.

The abdomen

The structures most commonly involved in intra-abdominal trauma are the kidneys and the spleen.

The spleen

As far as radiology is concerned the evaluation of splenic injuries is based on contrast-enhanced CT and ultrasound. These would be the first line of attack before embarking on angiography. Occasionally scintigraphy has proven useful.

Some authorities have suggested that the accuracy of images produced by CT, particularly those which are contrast-enhanced, is now good enough to enable, where it is appropriate, patients with splenic trauma to be managed non-operatively (Buntain *et al.*, 1988).

Renal trauma

Damage to the kidney can be picked up using non-invasive methods such as ultrasound and CT but intravenous pyelography remains the investigation of choice and is only minimally invasive. Rarely is it necessary to proceed to arteriography.

The lower limb

The pelvis

Damage to muscles originating from the pelvis can sometimes be demonstrated by avulsed fragments of bone. Where these have occurred in childhood, quite impressively large fragments can be seen on plain films, though these usually do not significantly interfere with lower limb function.

The thigh

The muscles of the thigh are often subject to contusions with intra- and extramuscular haematomata. Intramuscular bleeding as well as muscle tears can be detected on MRI images and also by ultrasound. It is useful for both therapeutic and prognostic reasons to have an accurate idea of the extent of, for instance, a hamstring tear.

Occasionally, if inappropriately treated, such haematomata calcify and the consequent myositis ossificans can usually be easily detected on plain films and also on ultrasound (Fig. 8.5).

It is possible to decide whether or not such lesions are still actively calcifying by using scintigraphy. Where bone is still being laid down, a

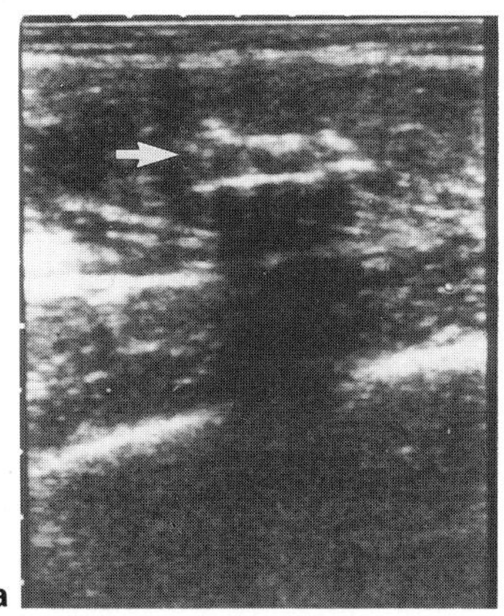

Fig. 8.5 (a) Ultrasound and (b) plain X-ray of the thigh of a 26-year-old soccer player who presented with recurrent muscle tears. There is an area of myositis ossificans (arrowed) which is well-demonstrated by both techniques.

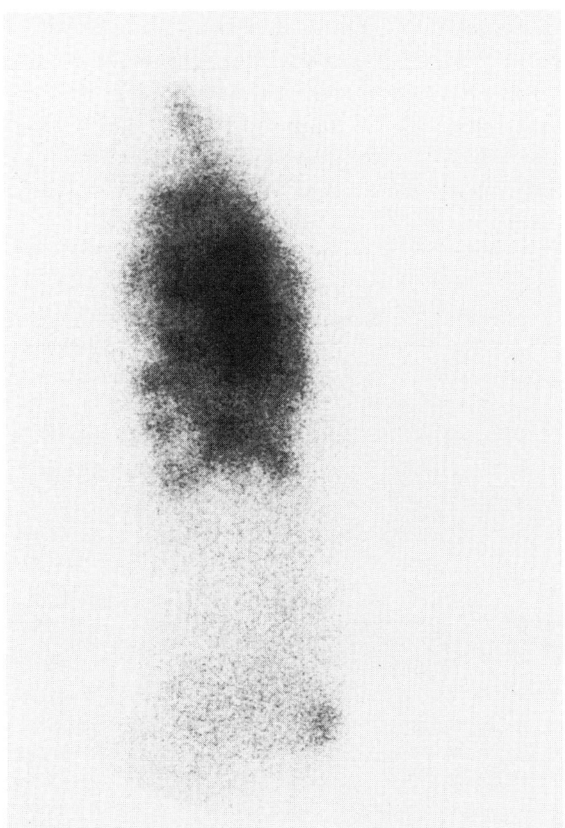

Fig. 8.6 Triple-phase technetium-99m bone scan in a case of myositis ossificans, showing avid uptake of the isotope by the lesion which is still obviously very active.

large 'hot' area will be noticed on the triple-phase bone scan (Fig. 8.6).

The knee

Injury to the intra- and extra-articular soft tissue structures about the knee is a major problem facing any physician with an interest in sports medicine.

The advent of arthroscopy as a diagnostic and therapeutic manoeuvre has transformed the management of knee injuries, though it is an invasive procedure and inevitably as such has its complications, e.g. infection. Fortunately we now have a wide range of radiological techniques which, if used, judiciously can often provide a diagnosis.

Plain films of the knee can reveal ligamentous damage where small pieces of bone have been avulsed as, for instance, the proximal tip of the fibula (lateral collateral ligament) or tibial spines (cruciate ligaments).

Past injuries may be shown by calcification in the damaged ligament, e.g. the so-called Pellegrini–Stieda lesion (Fig. 8.7).

Where a ligament has been ruptured but has remained uncalcified, this deficit can be demonstrated by stress views of the knee. For instance, where the lateral ligament has been ruptured, applying varus stress to the knee causes the joint to 'open up' laterally. Complete rupture of the anterior cruciate ligament can be demonstrated similarly by X-raying a knee subjected to an anterior draw test. The tibia will be drawn forward to the extent that the femoral condyles are often seen to be just resting on the back of the tibial plateau (Fig. 8.8).

It should be remembered that attempting to stress damaged ligaments in the acute phase of the injury is intensely painful. If an attempt is to be made to obtain radiographic confirmation of liga-

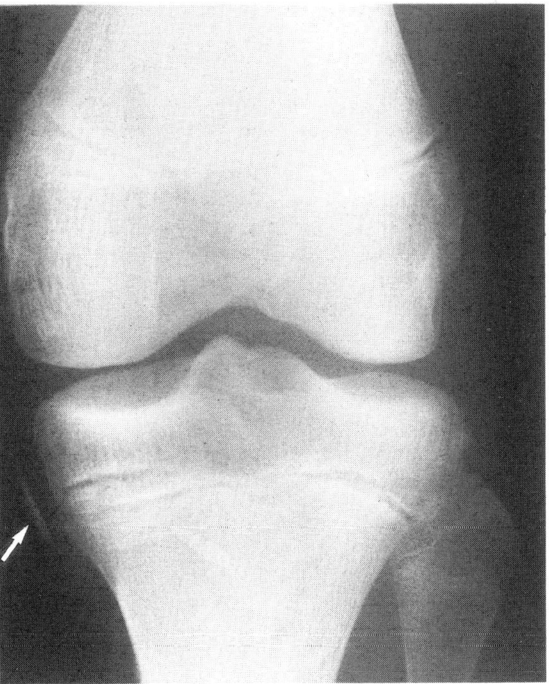

Fig. 8.7 Pellegrini–Stieda lesion (arrowed) indicative of previous injury to the medial collateral ligament.

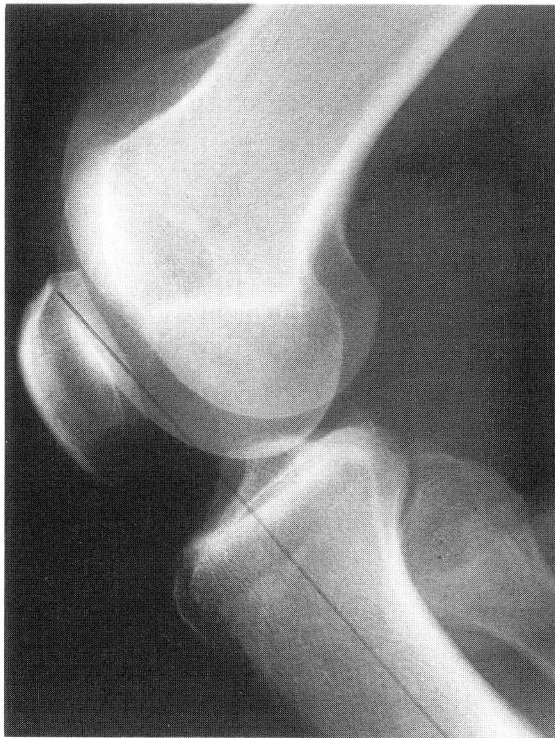

Fig. 8.8 An anterior drawer test being performed on the knee of a 24-year-old rugby player who had a complete rupture of the anterior collateral ligament. As can be seen on this stress view, the tibia has been drawn forward and the condyles of the femur are barely resting on the back of the tibial plateau. The line drawn through the middle of the shaft of the tibia should in fact bisect the condyles.

ment rupture shortly after the injury has occurred then it should only be done as part of an examination under anaesthetic.

Early stress films can be produced by infiltrating the damaged area with a local anaesthetic but this is a technique which is rarely used these days.

Attempts have been made to visualize the cruciate ligaments using CT; however, this has proven impracticable for routine use. However, MRI using a knee coil can demonstrate anterior cruciate tears, though the appearances produced will vary with the age of the lesion and the extent of the damage. Recent work has shown that use of this technique is >95% accurate in its assessment of the damage to an anterior cruciate ligament (Mink *et al.*, 1988).

Similarly, lesions of the posterior cruciate can be demonstrated, though not yet with the sensitivity of those in the anterior cruciate.

Both acute and chronic damage to the collateral ligaments has been demonstrated using MRI; most work so far has been done on the medial collateral ligament.

Lesions to the tendons (quadriceps and patellar) around the knee, e.g. haematomata, inflammation and rupture, can be diagnosed by ultrasonography which demonstrates such problems elegantly, e.g. the thickening of the tendom with areas of hypogenicity which are found in patellar tendonitis. An alternative method of diagnosis is with MRI, which can delineate the damage with great accuracy.

Pain close to and around the knee, e.g. the insertion of semimembranosus on the medial aspect of the tibia, can be due to stresses at the site of insertion produced by athletic activity. They can be well-demonstrated by triple-phase bone scanning using technetium-99m. These lesions are only exceedingly rarely demonstrable by plain X-ray or CT.

Previously damage to menisci could only be well-shown by the use of double-contrast arthrography where a radio-paque dye is injected into the joint cavity. The medial meniscus can usually be demonstrated fairly easily. However, it requires an experienced arthographer to demonstrate all of the lateral meniscus with clarity, particularly the posterior horn. The congenital abnormality of a discoid menuscus can also be picked up on an arthrogram (Williams *et al.*, 1989).

In all probability arthrography will be overtaken in the next few years by MRI for the diagnosis of meniscal tears. In a recent paper MRI was noted to be 93% accurate in diagnosing mensical tears and this figure is expected to be exceeded soon (Fig. 8.9).

The tibia and fibula

Shin splints, a rather vague term for a clinical entity which some authorities feel will proceed to a

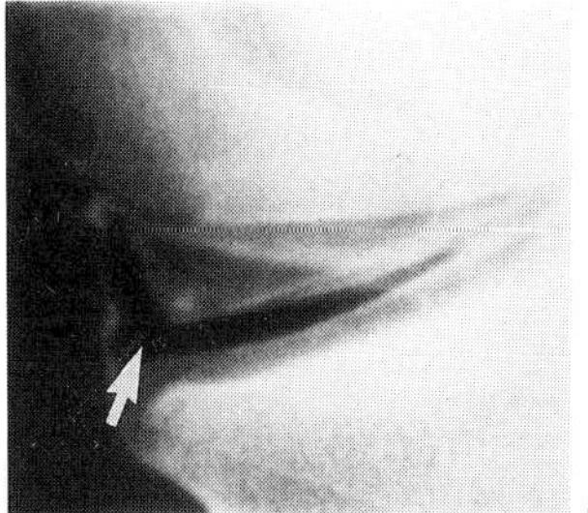

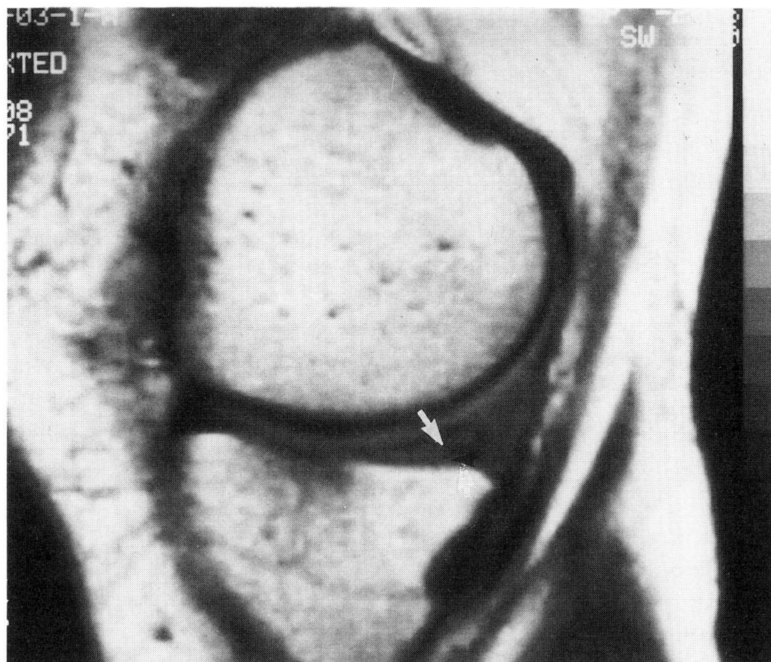

Fig. 8.9 (a) Arthrogram and (b) MRI of the knee of a 22-year-old ice hockey player. They illustrate the tear to the posterior horn of the medial meniscus.

stress fracture if untreated, can be well-shown by scintigraphy. The area of abnormal uptake tends to be much more diffuse, superficial and sometimes linear compared to the more localized 'hot spot' which picks out a stress fracture.

Compartment syndrome in the calf has been diagnosed using MRI, particularly if the other calf is normal so that comparative views can be produced.

Ruptures of the tendo-Achilles should be diagnosable on clinical grounds, though the use of both ultrasound (Fig. 8.10) and MRI (Rosenberg *et al.*, 1988) to demonstrate the lesion precisely prior to surgery, if that is to be undertaken, is becoming more common. It is also useful to be able to demonstrate partial tears and tears of the gastrocnemius, which often occur at the musculotendinous junction.

The ankle

The most common structure around the ankle joint which is damaged in sporting activity is the lateral ligament complex (usually the anterior talofibular ligament or the calcaneofibular ligament).

Occasionally such damage may be indicated by tiny avulsion injuries to the tip of the fibula,

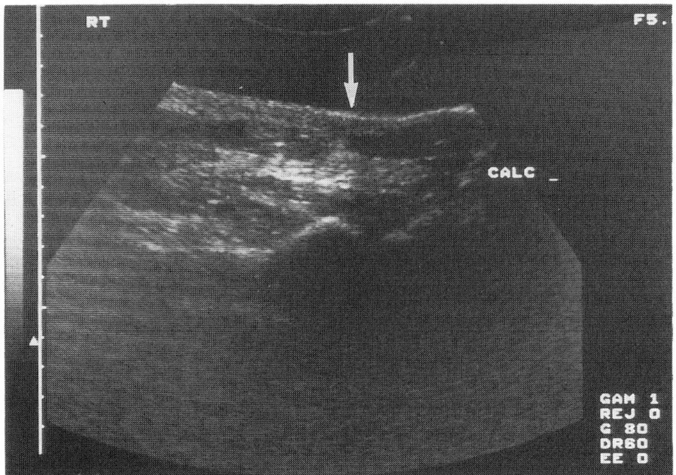

Fig. 8.10 Ultrasound of a torn tendo-Achilles in a 28-year-old netball player.

though usually there is nothing to see on the plain films.

After the acute phase has settled stress X-rays may be obtained. The X-rays are regarded as being positive if the talus has tilted more than 7° from the horizontal (Fig 8.11).

An investigation that is occasionally performed and which if positive indicates that significant lateral ligament damage has occurred is the peroneal tenogram. This involves injecting contrast medium into the peroneal tendon sheath under local anaesthetic. A positive result is indicated by medium entering the ankle joint.

The occasional case of posterior tibial tendon rupture which is seen most commonly in middle-aged women runners or joggers can now be picked out on both CT and MRI scanning. These woman usually present with pain and an inability to stand on the ball of the foot. The arch of the foot on the affected side is lost and the athlete looks flat-footed

Arthrography of the ankle joint is helpful in the evaluation of ligamentous damage, particularly if undertaken in the first day or two following the injury. Less traumatic for the patient however is MRI of the ligaments and the anterior talofibular ligament, which is the one most often damaged, can be well-deomonstrated, as can the calcaneofibular ligament.

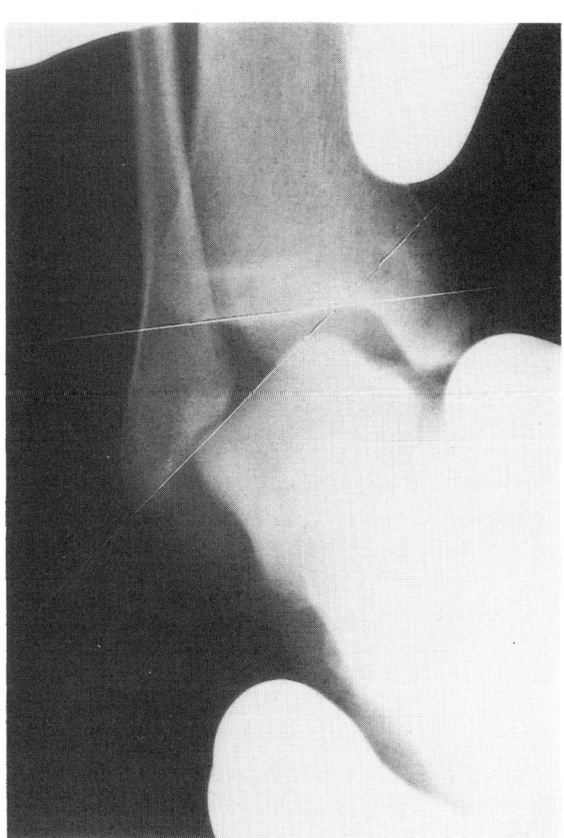

Fig. 8.11 Stress view of the ankle of a 27-year-old soccer player who has sustained a complete rupture of the lateral ligaments with consequent instability.

Bony injuries

Most acute bony injuries are still best demonstrated by normal plain X-rays as long as appropriate views are requested. The injured area needs to be pictured in at least two different planes, e.g. anteroposterior and lateral. Occasionally additional oblique or specialized views are required, for instance to demonstrate injuries to the scaphoid or small fractures to the head of the radius.

References

Buntain WL, Gould HR, Maull KI (1988) Predictability of splenic salvage by computed tomography. *Journal of Trauma* **28**, 24–34.

Cantu RC (1988) Head and spine injuries in the young athlete. *Clinical Sports Medicine* **7**, 459–72.

Corsellis J, Bruton C, Freeman-Browne D (1983) The aftermath of boxing. *Psychological Medicine* **3**, 270.

Gentry LR, Godersky JC, Thompson B (1988) Prospective comparative study of intermediate field MR and CT in the evaluation of closed head trauma. *American Journal of Roentgenology* **150**, 673–82.

Gentry LR, Manor WF, Turski PA et al. (1983) High resolution CT analysis of facial struts in trauma: 2. Osseous and soft tissue complications. *American Journal of Roentgenology* **140**, 533–41.

Middleton WD, Edelstein G, Reinus WR et al. (1985) Sonographic detection of rotator cuff tear. *American Journal of Roentgenology* **144**, 349.

Mink JH, Levy T, Crues JV (1988) Tears of the ACL and menisci of the knee: MR imaging evaluation. *Radiology* **196**, 769.

Modic MT, Pavlicek MS, Weinstein MA et al. (1984) Magnetic resonance imaging of intervertebral disc disease. *Radiology* **152**, 103.

Rosenberg ZS, Cheung Y, Jahss MH (1988) Computed tomography scan and magnetic resonance imaging of ankle tendons: an overview. *Foot Ankle* **8**, 297.

Wallace RB (1988) Application of epidemiologic principles to sports injury research. *American Journal of Sports Medicine* **16** (suppl), S22–4.

Williams LA, Evans R, Shirley PD (1989) *Imaging of Sports Injuries*. London: Baillière Tindall.

9

Physiological testing in sport performance

P. A. Butlin

The assessment of performance is a skill which is continually being carried out during a sporting event. The most common and valuable tool to a coach is the ability to observe and make subjective assessments of performance. However, whether the result of the performance was the outcome of skill, fitness or mental attitudes can be difficult to discern. The problem with subjective assessment is that its accuracy is subject to the knowledge and the experience of the assessor. Even with the most experienced observer there are many times when inaccurate judgements have been made because one of the dominant factors, governing performance, has been compensated for an inadequacy in another. Objective assessments are more valuable for they give some dimension to the result, e.g. time, distance, score. The means by which a coach can assess the present state of a performers capacity would be to administer certain tests which would provide objective measurements relating to total performance. In order to do this, the specific component of performance would have to be objectively measured independently of the others, thus providing a more accurate insight to its value.

The intention of this chapter is to concentrate on physiological fitness and how it can be objectively assessed within the laboratory. Whilst making the reader aware that this is an important factor of performance, it does not wish to detract from the importance of the other factors such as skill and mental attitude and will show, at a later stage, how both of these important factors can affect the validity of results in a test. Likewise, field testing is a useful means of acquiring the results of fitness parameters for it is often simple to administer and requires inexpensive equipment. Unfortunately, it has many drawbacks in producing reliable results. The laboratory setting eliminates some of these deficiencies and although it may have its own related problems, it does provide a suitable environment in which testing procedures can be standardized to provide greater accuracy in the results.

Before any method of assessing fitness can be carried out certain important considerations must be accounted for, these include:

1. Pre-test procedures
2. The purpose and intention of the test
3. The suitability of the test and the equipment used
4. The statistical criteria for the test
5. The use of the test results

Pre-test procedures

The test must be preceded by an ethical screening questionnaire. (B.A.S.S. 1988) (Lange-Anderson *et al.*, 1971). This document should contain general information such as name, date of birth, age, occupation and sport (event or position), it should ascertain certain features relating to the subject's lifestyle and hereditary factors concerning cardiovascular disease and the related risks of smoking, drugs and alcohol. It is important that it be known to the tester any reason why the subject is presently being treated for injury or taking any form of medication. Before continuing with the next stage the questionnaire must be approved by the tester and signed by the subject to its accuracy.

The next procedure is to take certain measurements of the subject relating to spot health checks. These include height, weight, body fat, blood pressure, lung function and haemoglobin tests. The upper limits for systolic and diastolic blood pressures which have been approved by the ethical committee for testing of athletes must be adhered to and tests which would be of a potential danger to a subject with hypertension must not be carried out. If possible, prior visits to the laboratory before the actual tests are to be administered provide an opportunity for habituation to the facility and the equipment, a chance to establish a friendly relationship between the performer and the test administrators and a time for reinforcing the procedures of the tests.

Safety of the subject must be of paramount importance, equipment must be checked and calibrated, blood sampling must follow a strict code of practice and where tests are to be carried out to maximal limits of exhaustion a medical practioner must be present or resuscitation equipment made available, with someone having the knowledge of how to use it. An efficient laboratory will have facilities for first aid, medical support and knowledgeable laboratory technicians.

Purpose and intention of the test

Total fitness is comprised of certain components:

1. Strength
2. Speed
3. Flexibility
4. Endurance

Strength and *speed* are products of *power*.
i.e. Power = strength × speed (watts)
= force × velocity

It would seem simple enough to state that the intention of a test was to measure '*Fitness*'. However, when it is known that fitness is made up of several components, one test alone cannot fulfil the requirements. It is usual that if one wishes to establish an assessment of total fitness, that a physiological profile is built up which consists of a battery of tests, (AAHPER, 1965) each one reflecting the measurement of a fitness component. In many cases this is unnecessary as one or two tests may reflect the demands of the performance and the effects of exercise and training. The intention of any test becomes more apparent when the physiological demands of the performance is known and the magnitude to which each component of fitness is required. Therefore, the purpose and intention of any fitness test is to choose one which relates to the physiological profile of the performer and reflects the physiological demands of the performance.

The tests and equipment

Prior to a fitness component test the true definition and an understanding of the component must be established. This will enable the tester to choose the most appropriate test and equipment.

Strength

Strength is the maximum force which a muscle can exert in a single contraction. However, muscles can contract either isometrically, isotonically or isokinetically and tests for these types of muscle contraction can be performed using strength dynamometers, free weights and isokinetic strength testing machinery respectively. The method by which this gross strength can be ascertained is to perform one single, maximal contraction. Strength testing is essential in sports and events which demand great amounts of strength e.g. shot-putting. It is necessary also in certain muscle groups which are constantly in use.

Isokinetic strength testing

For many years the ultimate tests for maximum gross strength was the one maximum repetition

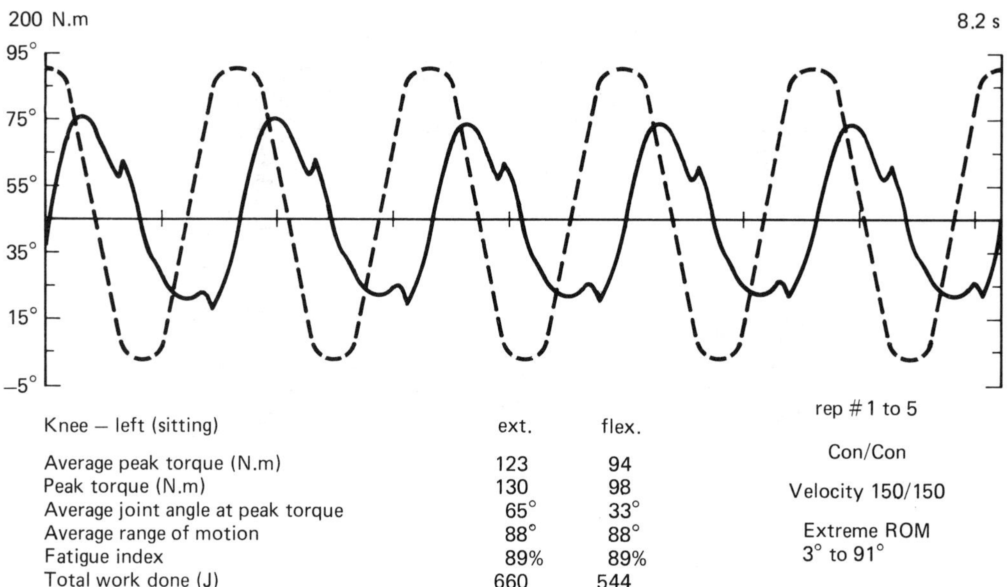

Fig. 9.1 Using the Lidoactive isokinetic rehabilitation system. Trace from isokinetic machine of left knee in extension and flexion. Peak torque of quadriceps group above the horizontal line and peak torque of hamstring group below the line. Dashed line indicates joint angle.

method (1RM). However, the dynamics of muscular strength involve far more than the final outcome of moving (1RM). Since the emergence of microprocessor technology sensitive instrumentation has provided sports physiologists with an opportunity to measure muscular force, acceleration and velocity of different body segments in different positions. (McArdle *et al.*, 1991). An isokinetic dynamometer is an electro-machanical instrument that contains a speed-controlling mechanism that accelerates to a pre-set speed when any force is applied. When the constant speed is attained, the isokinetic loading is operated to provide a counterforce in opposition to the force generated by the muscle. This means that for all phases of the movement at a constant velocity both the maximum force and any percentage of maximum effort can be measured. The subject performing such a test on an isokinetic machine must push against a lever which will be moving at constant velocity. The dynamometer measures the torque applied by the subject to the lever. Based on the ratio between force and contraction speed, the greater the speed of the moving lever, the smaller the force applied and vice versa. An isokinetic test can be performed on a variety of joint articulations and their movements and on certain machines can examine the peak torque and the angle of incidence between paired muscle action e.g. flexion and extension of the knee (quadriceps and hamstrings), Figs. 9.1 and 9.2.

The information obtained from such tests can provide the medic, the exercise physiologist or the sports physiotherapist with a range of valuable data for the purpose of testing, evaluation and prescription in the training or rehabilitation of muscular function. (Dirix *et al.*, 1988).

Speed

This can be defined as the minimal movement time of a single limb 'limb speed' or the total body 'body speed' between two fixed points. It can be recorded simply as a time (seconds) or if the distance is known can be given in units of velocity. The time for a short sprint (less than 60 m) or a karate chop are examples of speed tests and when technical equipment is used such as lasers or light sensors linked to either a multisecond timer or computer, greater precision and accuracy is guaranteed.

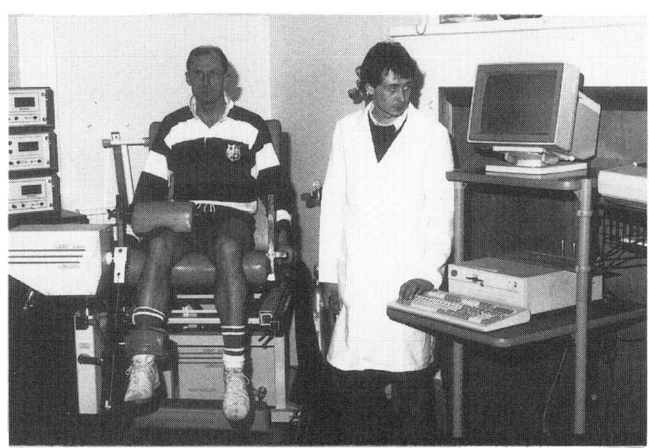

Fig. 9.2

Flexibility (Montoye, 1978)

This is the range of movement of a given joint or combination of joints. Various pieces of equipment which are used to measure this component range from simple protractors to highly sophisticated goniometers. The procedures involve recording the displacement of a bone, in a linear or angular dimension, to the adjacent bone with which it articulates. In sports where great amounts of flexibility are demanded the testing of this component is essential, e.g. gymnastics. However, tests on an injured joint compared to its counterpart can give an indication of limited movement.

Endurance

Endurance is defined as the ability to repeat muscular contractions without fatigue. Fatigue is a decline in the level of performance. The performance in this case relates to muscular contraction and as all our skeletal muscles depend upon different energy sources, which in turn depend upon the duration and intensity of the contractions, appropriate tests must reflect the predominant energy source used for these contractions.

Aerobic endurance

This is the ability of the body to supply oxygen to the working muscles and extract waste products which are transported in the bloodstream and the airways, to the atmosphere. The ultimate test for measuring the ability to perform areobically is the maximal oxygen uptake test (MAX.$\dot{V}O_2$). (Sinning, 1975). The test is designed to elicit the highest possible oxygen uptake a performer can achieve and can be administered using various work ergometers, the two most commonly used being the Cycle ergometer and the Treadmill. The protocol, which can be continuous or discontinuous, is similar irrespective of the work machine used. The continuous method is the most widely used especially when testing sport performers. It consists of the subject working at a constant rate whilst measurements of the volume of expired air are being taken during the steady state of work (Fig. 9.3). The expired air is then analysed for oxygen content and from the results the amount of oxygen used can be calculated. This procedure is repeated for further increments in work load and the test is terminated when the subject reaches a state of exhaustion and can no longer continue. If the values for oxygen uptake are plotted against their corresponding values of work or power the graph should be linear to a point where there is no

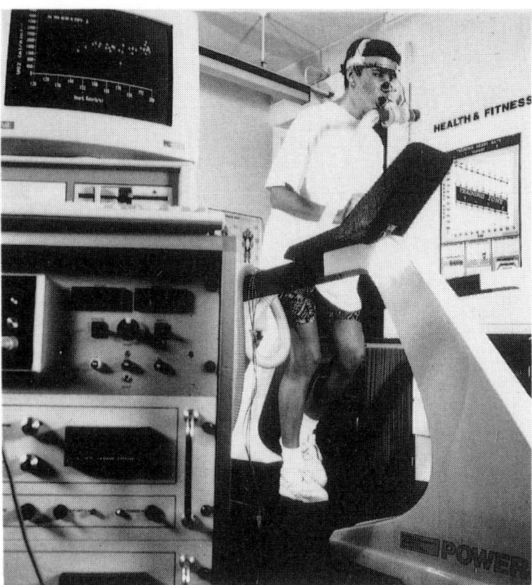

Fig. 9.3 A subject performing in a Max.$\dot{V}O_2$ test on a treadmill using an on-line computerized system for gas analysis.

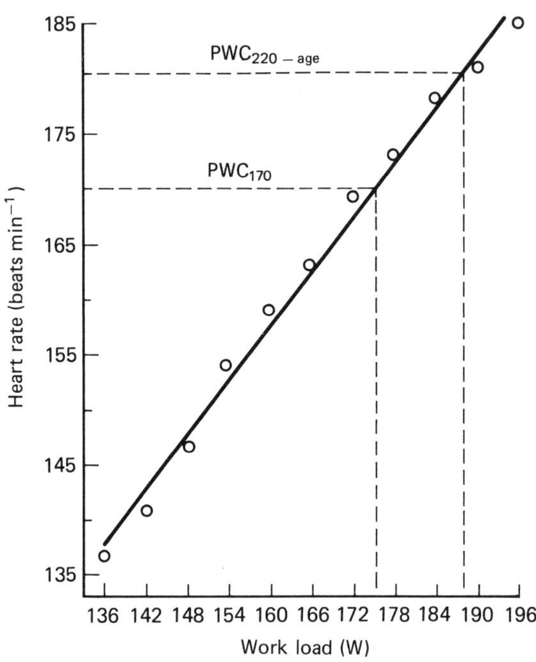

Fig. 9.4 The relationship between heart rate and work load for subject CL, ♂, age 40 years.
$PWC_{220-age} = PWC_{180} = 187$ W
$PWC_{170} = 175$ W

further increase in oxygen uptake with further increases in work load. This point of deflection is known as the MAX.$\dot{V}O_2$.

The equipment used for gas analysis and collection can range from a sophisticated on-line, fully computerised system or the more reliable and accurate on-line collection bag system. The latter involves collecting the expired air at each increment of work within a large plastic bag or rubber balloon. An extract from each bag is then analysed for oxygen content using either a modern electronic gas analyser or the more accurate, yet time consuming, chemical analyser.

The estimates for the value of MAX.$\dot{V}O_2$ are often made by measuring heart rate (HR) at the same point as oxygen uptake ($\dot{V}O_2$). If several measurements are made at submaximal levels the value of HR can be plotted on a graph against its corresponding value of $\dot{V}O_2$. From the linear relationship which these two measurements form, the estimated value for MAX.$\dot{V}O_2$ can be extrapolated using the criterion of MAX.HR = 220 − age. When gas analysis equipment is not available an estimated value of MAX.$\dot{V}O_2$ can be made by recording the HR at the appropriate level of work and plotting this figure on an Astrand Nomogram (Astrand, 1986).

Another test which does not give direct value for MAX.$\dot{V}O_2$ but which is widely used and related to the aerobic efficiency of the performer is the physical work capacity test (PWC). This can be taken at any level of HR but the most common is the PWC test which relates to the physical work capacity extrapolated at a heart rate of 170 beats/min (Wahlund, 1948). This is a value which is considered for the majority of people to be a high but well tolerated working level. However, for sport performers an extrapolation would be more applicable if taken at MAX.HR = 220 − age (Fig. 9.4).

Lactate endurance

This is the ability of the muscle to rely on anaerobic metabolism at any given point of submaximal

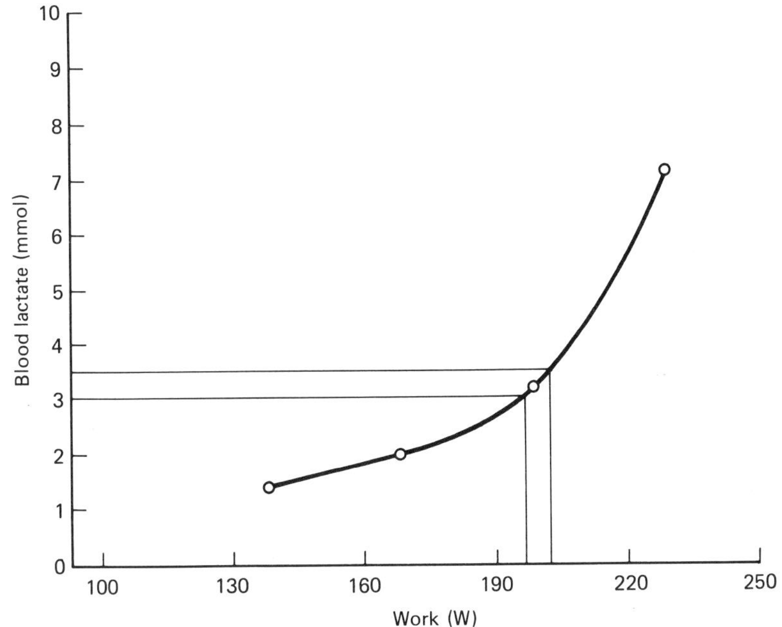

Fig. 9.5 Subject AB, ♂. The curve indicates an anaerobic threshold (OBLA) at 202 W.

intensity of exercise. The end product of this anaerobic metabolism is lactic acid and if not removed then muscle fatigue will inevitably occur. The test which ascertains the work level at which there is a dramatic increase in blood lactate is known as 'The onset of blood lactate accumulation test' (OBLA). This term is preferred to the old term of anaerobic threshold (Brooks and Fahey, 1984). The test can be administered in conjunction with the MAX.$\dot{V}O_2$ test. Blood sampling (finger prick of 50 microlitres) commences at a work load corresponding to 60% of the maximum and a further three collections made up to approximately 90% of maximum work load. When the figures for blood lactate are plotted against the corresponding values of % MAX.$\dot{V}O_2$ it can be seen that between blood lactate levels of 2 and 4 mmol these are the limits between which there is a sudden and steep rise in blood lactate concentration (Fig. 9.5).

This sudden rise in blood lactate level indicates a rapid rate of muscle glycogenolysis. This can result in glycogen depletion and consequent muscle fatigue. A rise in blood lactate levels indicates that the lactate entry into the blood is higher than can be removed and kept at reasonable levels. A failure to cope with lactate production during a performance will cause the pH of the blood to fall thus causing an additional fatigue factor during aerobic endurance activity.

Therefore, it is important to realise, that when testing an endurance athlete the MAX.$\dot{V}O_2$ test is not the sole criteria for assessing the aerobic capabilities of the performer (Skinner, 1980). Ultimately the MAX.$\dot{V}O_2$ test gives an indication of the performer's potential but does not indicate the level at which the performer can operate without high levels of fatigue setting in.

Estimation of anaerobic threshold from a non-invasive test of ventilatory threshold

Because blood acidity is one of the factors that increase expired ventilation ($\dot{V}_E$,) it has been hypothesized that an abrupt increase in VEQ could be used to suggest that the reason for this rise was due to an insufficient O_2 delivery to the muscle. (Wasserman *et al.*, 1973). This hypothesis is particularly attractive because it could suggest

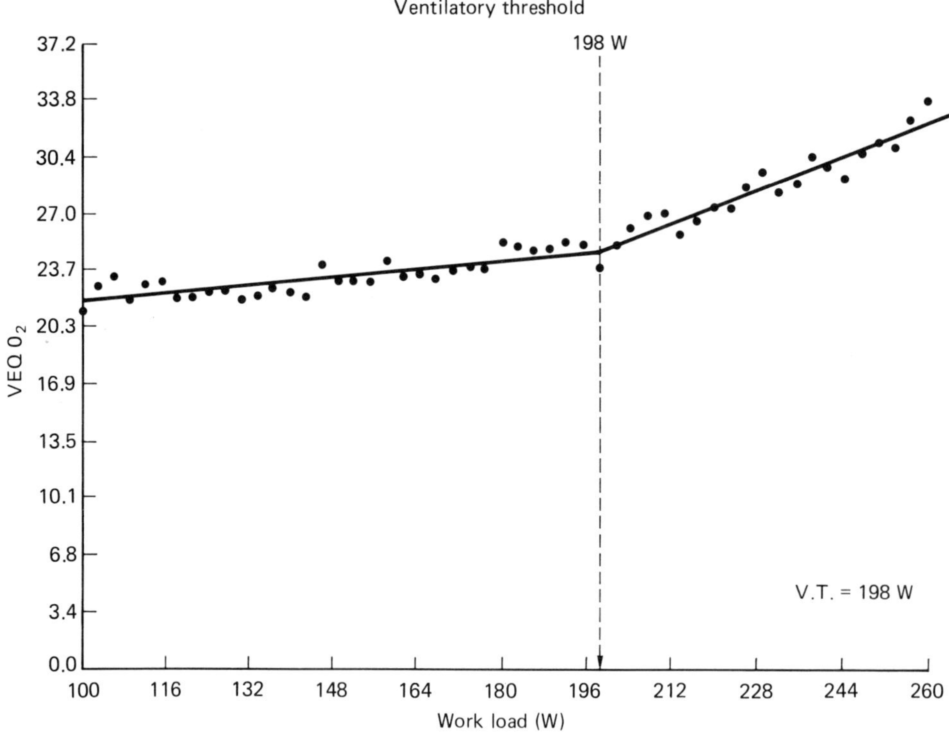

Fig. 9.6 VEQ vs. work for the same subject as in Fig. 9.5.

that the inflation point on the $\dot{V}_E/\dot{V}O_2$ graph where $\dot{V}$EQ increases sharply from its linear relationship with increases in work load is the same point as the sharp rise in blood lactate. Thus the ventilatory threshold (VT) and the anaerobic threshold (AT) or onset of blood lactate accumulation (OBLA) are one and the same point (Figure 9.6).

The test is carried out using a cycle ergometer together with appropriate expired gas collection and analysing equipment. Knowing that the steep rise in blood lactate with increasing work load occurs at a point approximately between 60–70% of MAX.VO the subject after a brief warm-up of light pedalling commences at a work rate equating to 30% of estimated MAX.VO. Thereafter the work rate is increased in increments of 22 W until volition fatigue or 80% of MAX.VO is reached. At each work load the V and $\dot{V}O_2$ are recorded and when plotted on a graph against each other they show a linear relationship until a point at which there is a deviation away from this relationship, this being taken as the ventilatory threshold (VT).

Other research has shown that work rate is influenced by other gas exchange kinetics (Cassaburi, 1989) and that a significant rise in $\dot{V}CO_2$ against $\dot{V}O_2$ could also be taken as the point of anaerobic threshold (AT). The association of changes in ventilatory gas exchange with that of steep increases in blood lactate (OBLA) is not yet fully resolved and an excellent review of this work is given in a paper by Gladden (1984). In some subjects, favourable results have been reported whilst in others there remains much scepticism (Brooks, 1984). A classic piece of research which supports the latter group is the work carried out on patients with McArdles disease (Hagborg, 1990). These patients lack muscle phosphorylase and therefore do not increase their blood lactate levels. However, when tested under the same conditions as control subjects they show a ventila-

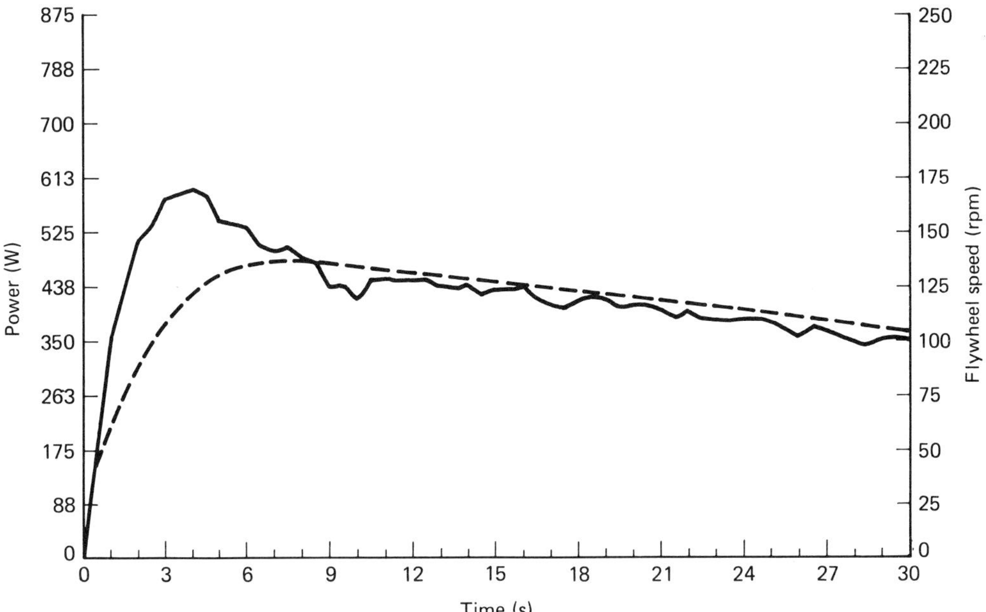

Fig. 9.7 Power output vs. time in a 30 s test. The dashed curve represents the speed of the flywheel.

tory threshold (VT). This would indicate a complete dissociation with the increase in blood lactate levels found in the control group.

In conclusion, if methods of ventilatory and gas exchange kinetics are to be used in measuring levels of fatigue during work performance, they must be used with caution, due to the interpretation of precisely what it is, that the final results refer.

Anaerobic endurance

This is the ability to maintain high levels of work intensity. In order to recover from such bouts of activity ultimately will depend on the performers tolerance to high levels of lactate produced locally within the muscle. The test most widely used to ascertain this ability is the Wingate anaerobic test (Bar-Or *et al.*, 1980). This test consists of pedalling a front loaded cycle ergometer which has a special timing device attached to the flywheel in order to measure fractions of a revolution of the flywheel and which is linked to a computer. On command, the subject pedals the cycle at maximum speed and with a fixed load previously worked out according to body weight (Dotan, 1983). The number of revolutions is fed into the computer which, on termination of the test, prints out the results in a graph form of power, calculated by the fixed load and distance travelled in intervals of time, against the time interval up to a maximum of 30 s (Figure 9.7) (Table 1).

Instantaneous power

This is the ability of the body to explode into immediate action and relies exclusively upon the high energy phosphates stored within the muscles. Short bouts of high speed performances are synonymous with instantaneous power generation and the tests which are used to indicate this ability are of 10 s or less in duration. A simple test is the standing vertical jump which requires very little expensive equipment other than a vertical board marked in centimetre height intervals. The purpose of the jump board is to measure the standing vertical jump from standing reach, to jump and reach. The height obtained combined

Table 9.1 Results of Wingate power test

Name: AB (male) Date: 12/5/1992
Load: 3.5 kg Weight: 84.6 kg

Time (s)	Power (W)	W/kg	Energy (J)
3.0	407.0	4.8	1221.1
6.0	565.8	6.7	1697.4
9.0	484.3	5.7	1452.9
12.0	444.2	5.3	1332.6
15.0	439.6	5.2	1318.9
18.0	421.0	5.0	1263.1
21.0	413.2	4.9	1239.6
24.0	389.7	4.6	1169.0
27.0	375.4	4.4	1126.1
30.0	354.8	4.2	1064.3

Maximum power recorded = 597.16 W
Maximum power at time = 4.00 s
Minimum power recorded = 345.40 W
Minimum power at time = 28.50 s
Fatigue index = 10.28 W/s

with the weight of the performer can indicate the explosive power output. A more sophisticated piece of equipment used to measure this component is the force platform. This registers the maximum downward force exerted by the subject at take-off. A sprint cycle of a 10 s duration administered in an indentical way to the 30 s Anaerobic endurance test will provide the maximum peak power output.

Statistical criteria

Having decided upon the test and the equipment to be used the next stage is to make certain that the test procedures follow certain statistical criteria:

Validity
Reliability
Objectivity

Validity

This is a fundamental requirement of all testing procedures and asks whether the test measures what it is intended to measure. It indicates the relevance of the test and should take into consideration the principle of specificity (Sharkey, 1988) of measurement, i.e. that the test corresponds as closely as possible with the purpose and mode of the exercise or training which it is intending to assess. Testing can be quite meaningless if the procedures employed are not specific to the sport in which the performer competes or that the pattern and speed of movement of the various used muscle groups are not reconstructed within the tests. A good example of non-specificity would be for a sprint cyclist to be tested on a treadmill for an aerobic assessment. Whether or not the principle of specificity can be adhered to will ultimately depend upon the type of equipment available within the laboratory and the different sports in which participants are wanting to be assessed. Swimmers for example are very difficult to assess specifically, because they should be measured within the water and swimming at their own particular stroke. This would involve the use of a swimming flume – a very expensive piece of equipment.

A great deal of innovative design has gone into the specificity of laboratory testing equipment. This has helped to simulate the various sports such as rowing, canoeing, skiing and skating (International Olympic Committee, 1988). The obvious location for testing would take place in the environment in which the performance takes place and without restricted equipment such as tubing and mouthpieces. A system of telemetry overcomes this problem but the environmental changes which cannot be controlled make it difficult for accurate results to be obtained.

As mentioned in the first part of this chapter a skill performance does not depend on fitness alone, for skill and mental attitudes play a significant role. As all physical tests measuring performance demand a certain level of skill the movement patterns of the performer must be reflected in the test. Running on a treadmill necessitates a different skill to running on the track and a test on a cycle ergometer is alien to a cyclist who is accustomed to a racing machine. Similarly, if a performer is not motivated enough to do well in a test this will reflect the results. It is important that the tester is aware of the precise reasons why test results have not achieved their expected limits.

Reliability

Providing that the control of variables is accounted for and the tests do measure what they are supposed to measure, the next criteria is, can the tests follow the same procedures under the same conditions and produce similar results? If this is so, they are said to be *reliable*. In order to accept the reliability of a test a certain level of correlation must exist between the two sets of test scores.

Laboratory assessments score high on this criteria because there is a greater control over the environmental variable.

Objectivity

One of the problems which exists with the testing of sport performance is that one laboratory may have different equipment, procedures and trained personnel from another. This may affect the results of a subject who decides to be tested at two different venues. However, if the two sets of results are shown, as in reliability, to be highly correlated then the *objectivity* criteria is satisfied. The Sports Council in conjunction with the National Coaching Foundation have made considerable effort to eliminate some of the objectivity problems. They asked members from the physiological section of the British Society of Sports Medicine (BASS) to develop test procedures and to recommend how testing centres may be staffed, equipped and managed. As a result of this exercise, BASS produced an excellent document which states the guidelines to assist laboratories in ensuring that adequate precision and reliability of measurement is achieved and ensures consistency of procedures between different testing centres is available. They recommend that centres who may wish to implement the testing of human performance apply for creditation, thus ensuring that this criteria is satisfied on a national network. Only when a reliable network of national testing centres is established will there be a national data bank of reliable information available. This information will provide sport scientists and coaches a set of norms on which to compare the results of their tests.

The use of test results

Providing the tests, the procedures and the criteria for testing have all been satisfied one of the most important questions remains to be asked; what will the results of the tests be used for? The results of a fitness test, as sound as the intentions may have been, are quite meaningless if they are presented to the coach as a set of statistical data. The following criteria can be used as guidelines for the use of test results.

1. If reliable national norms are available and the tests satisfy the criteria of objectivity, then the results can be compared to similar performers in the same sport, age and gender categories.
2. If the tests are reliable and repeated at regular intervals then the results can be compared to the performer's own, previous test results. This is particularly useful in assessing the benefits of training programmes and performance before and after injury.
3. If national norms are not considered to be reliable, or the laboratory uses different procedures, then the results can be compared to other performers under identical conditions in the same laboratory.

Whichever one of these criteria is chosen for the use of the results, the final outcome must provide the sport scientist, the coach, the performer, the medical practitioner and the physiotherapist with vital information from which they can evaluate the essential aspects of their important work in preparation of sport performance. A combination of the information acquired before and after the tests provides an educational base from which all concerned can work together in gaining a greater understanding of the improvement in sporting performance.

References

AAHPER (1965) *Youth Fitness Test Manual* (Revised Edition), Washington DC. N.E.A. Publication.

Astrand PO and Rodahl K (1986) *Textbook of Work Physiology*, (3rd Edn), McGraw Hill, New York.

Bar-or O (1987) The Wingate anaerobic test: an update of methodology, reliability and validity. *Sports Medicine* **IV**, 381–394.

BASS (1988) *Position Statement on the Physiological Assessment of the Elite Competitor* (2nd Edn), White Line Press.

Brooks GA and Fahey TD (1984) *Fundamentals of Human Performance*, Macmillan, New York.

Cassaburi *et al.* (1989). Influence of work rate on ventilatory and gas exchange kinetics, *Journal of Applied Physiology* **67**(2), 547–555.

Dirix A *et al.* (Ed) (1988) *The Olympic Book of Sports Medicine*, Vol. 1, Blackwell Scientific, Oxford, pp. 121–150.

Dotan R and Bar-Or O (1983) Load optimisation of the Wingate anaerobic test. *European Journal of Applied Physiology* **51**, 409–417.

Gladden LB (1984) Current 'anaerobic threshold' controversies. *The Physiologist* **27**, 312–317

Hagberg JM (1990) Exercise and recovery ventilation and VO responses of patients with McArdle's disease. *Journal of Applied Physiology* **68**(4), 1393–1398.

Lange-Anderson K *et al.* (1971) *Fundamentals of Exercise Testing*, World Health Organisation.

McArdle WD *et al.* (1991) *Exercise Physiology – Energy, Nutrition and Human Performance*, Lee and Febiger.

Montoye HJ (1978) *An Introduction to Measurement in Physical Education*, Allyn and Bacon Inc.

Sharkey BJ (1988) Specificity of Testing taken from Advances in Sports Medicine and Fitness, Vol. 1, Year Book Medical Publishers, pp. 25–43.

Sinning WE (1975) *Experiments and Demonstrations in Exercise Physiology*, W.B. Saunders.

Skinner JS and McLellan TH (1980) The transition from aerobic to anaerobic metabolism. *Research Quart Exercise Sport* **51**, 234–248.

Wahlund H (1948). Determination of physical working capacity. *Acta Medica Scandinavica* (Suppl.), 132, 1.

Wasserman *et al.* 1973. Anaerobic threshold and respiratory gas exchange during exercise. *Journal of Applied Physiology* **25**, 236–243.

10

Gait analysis

M. W. Whittle

Introduction

Gait analysis is the systematic examination of the way in which a person walks. It may be conducted either for clinical purposes or for research. In the clinical area, it may be used for diagnosis, assessment or for monitoring the results of treatment. Research uses cover a wide range of disciplines including clinical medicine, biomechanics, physiology and human performance.

Historical development

Although the observation of human gait is undoubtedly as old as the human race itself, the earliest known systematic descriptions of walking are those by Leonardo da Vinci, Galileo, Newton and especially Borelli. In *De Motu Animalum*, published in 1679, Borelli described how balance is maintained by moving the centre of gravity of the body over each foot in turn. During the Victorian era, the gait cycle came to be largely understood, thanks to the work of the Weber brothers in Germany, Muybridge in California and Marey in Paris. The mechanical processes involved in walking were studied in Germany, by Braune and Fisher, and described by them in 1895. The early development of gait analysis was reviewed by Steindler (1953).

Progress in gait analysis during the 20th century has occurred in three areas: the development of measurement technology, the use of mathematical modelling to understand the mechanics of the walking process, and the recognition of the value of detailed information on gait in the clinical setting. These topics will be discussed further, later in this chapter.

The walking process in normal individuals is now understood from a mechanical point of view. It is possible to measure the movements of the joints and the limb segments, and to calculate the force and timing of the muscular contractions required to achieve these movements. Areas which are not fully understood are the neurophysiological control mechanisms and the strategies used to decide which combinations of muscles to use at different times. Pathological gait is not understood to the same extent as normal gait, particularly when spasticity is present, which may result in the co-contraction of antagonistic muscles.

Terminology used in gait analysis

The gait cycle is defined as the interval between two successive occurrences of the same event, typically the initial contact between one foot and the ground. Figure 10.1 shows the sequence of events between successive heel contacts by the right foot in a normal individual: heel contact – foot flat – mid-stance – heel off – toe off – mid-swing. The cycle is completed by the next heel contact. The stance phase, from heel contact to toe off, is the time the foot is on the ground. The swing phase, from toe off to the next heel contact, is the time the foot is swinging forward through the

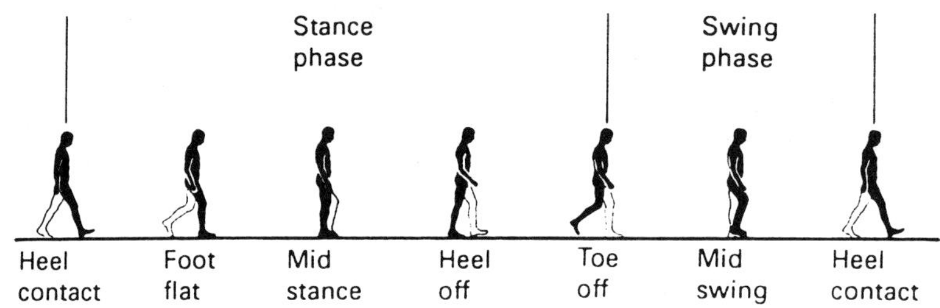

Fig. 10.1 Positions of the legs during a single gait cycle from right heel contact to right heel contact. From Whittle (1991), with permission.

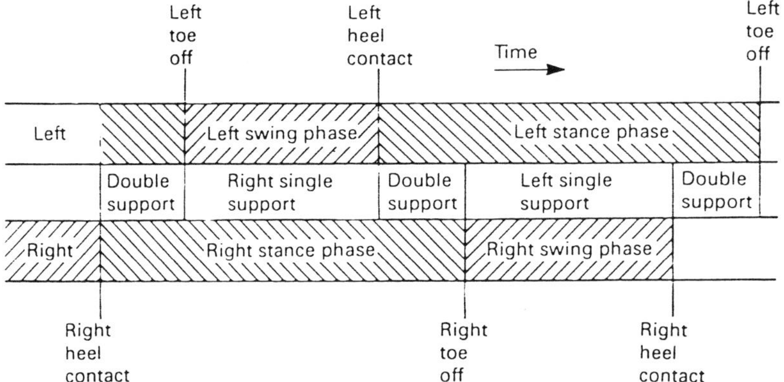

Fig. 10.2 Timing of single and double support during a single gait cycle from right heel contact to right heel contact. From Whittle (1991), with permission.

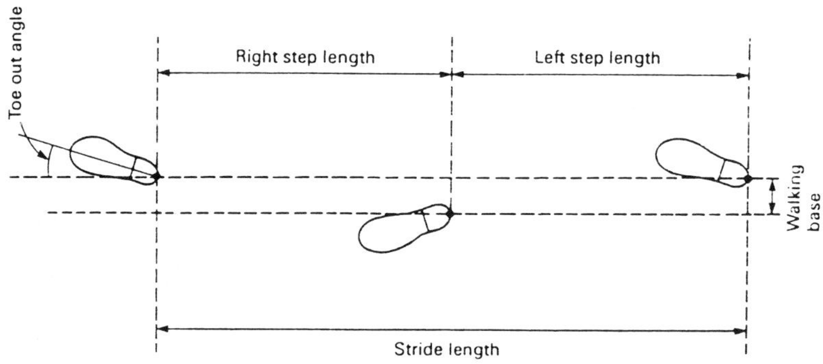

Fig. 10.3 Terms used to describe foot placement on the ground. From Whittle (1991), with permission.

air. Figure 10.2 shows the sequence of events for both feet. In each gait cycle there is a time when each foot is on the ground by itself (single support), and two occasions when both feet are on the ground (double support). The single support phase on one side corresponds to the swing phase on the other.

Figure 10.3 shows the terms used to describe the positioning of the feet on the floor during walking. Although the terms 'step' and 'stride' mean much the same thing in normal speech, in gait analysis they have more precise meanings, step referring to the movement of one foot, and stride to the movement of both. The step length is the distance that one foot moves forward in front of the other one. The stride length is the distance that either foot moves forwards in one gait cycle, so that the stride length is the sum of the two step lengths. The walking base is the lateral separation between the two feet during walking, measured as the distance between the lines joining the midpoints of the heels. Step and stride lengths are measured in metres, walking base in millimetres.

A number of parameters can be measured to provide objective information on some aspect of gait. The most easily measured are the general gait parameters, of which there are three: cadence, velocity and stride length. The cadence is the rate at which the individual feet contact the ground, measured in steps per minute. The velocity is the distance the whole body moves forwards in a given time, measured in metres per second. The three general gait parameters are related to each other by the formula:

velocity (m/s) = stride (m) × cadence (steps/min)/ 120

The division by 120 is needed because there are two steps in a stride, and 60 seconds in a minute. Tables 10.1–10.3 show the normal ranges for the general gait parameters at different ages in both sexes.

Table 10.1 Approximate range (95% limits) for general gait parameters in free-speed walking by normal female subjects of different ages

Age range (years)	Cadence (steps/min)	Stride length (m)	Velocity (m/s)
13–14	103–150	0.99–1.55	0.90–1.62
15–17	100–144	1.03–1.57	0.92–1.64
18–49	98–138	1.06–1.58	0.94–1.66
50–64	97–137	1.04–1.56	0.91–1.63
65–80	96–136	0.94–1.46	0.80–1.52

From Whittle (1991), with permission.

Table 10.2 Approximate range (95% limits) for general gait parameters in free-speed walking by normal male subjects of different ages

Age range (years)	Cadence (steps/min)	Stride length (m)	Velocity (m/s)
13–14	100–149	1.06–1.64	0.95–1.67
15–17	96–142	1.15–1.75	1.03–1.75
18–49	91–135	1.25–1.85	1.10–1.82
50–64	82–126	1.22–1.82	0.96–1.68
65–80	81–125	1.11–1.71	0.81–1.61

From Whittle (1991), with permission.

Table 10.3 Approximate range (95% limits) for general gait parameters in free-speed walking by normal children

Age (years)	Cadence (steps/min)	Stride length (m)	Velocity (m/s)
1	127–223	0.29–0.58	0.32–0.96
1.5	126–212	0.33–0.66	0.39–1.03
2	125–201	0.37–0.73	0.45–1.09
2.5	124–190	0.42–0.81	0.52–1.16
3	123–188	0.46–0.89	0.58–1.22
3.5	122–186	0.50–0.96	0.65–1.29
4	121–184	0.54–1.04	0.67–1.32
5	119–180	0.59–1.10	0.71–1.37
6	117–176	0.64–1.16	0.75–1.43
7	115–172	0.69–1.22	0.80–1.48
8	113–169	0.75–1.30	0.82–1.50
9	111–166	0.82–1.37	0.83–1.53
10	109–162	0.88–1.45	0.85–1.55
11	107–159	0.92–1.49	0.86–1.57
12	105–156	0.96–1.54	0.88–1.60

Partly based on Sutherland *et al.* (1988); from Whittle (1991), with permission.

The normal movements of walking

Walking is achieved primarily through the movement of the legs, although in normal individuals it also involves movements of the trunk and the arms. Murray (1967) and Perry (1974) both gave excellent descriptions of normal gait.

The most important movements are those taking place at the hips, knees and ankles. Figure 10.4 shows the angular excursions of these joints in the sagittal plane, in a normal individual. The movement of the hip is close to being a simple

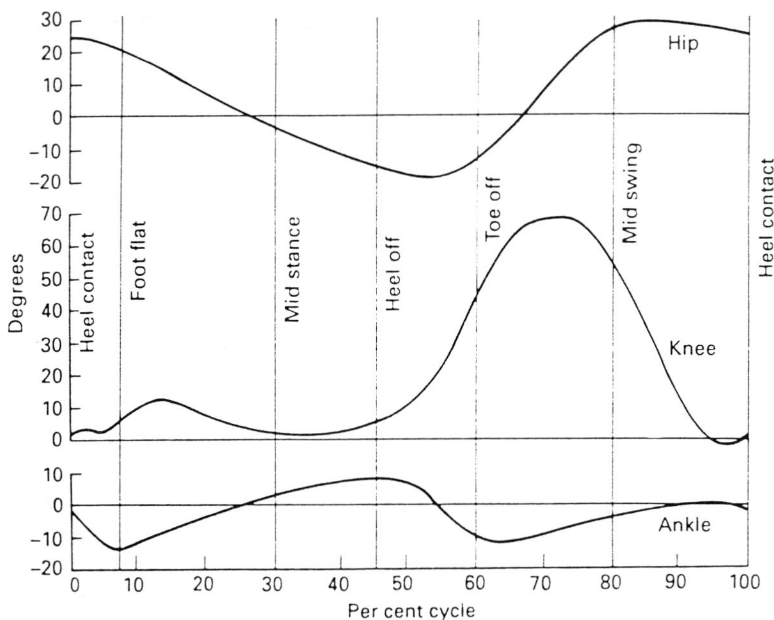

Fig. 10.4 Sagittal plane angles during a single gait cycle of hip (flexion positive), knee (flexion positive) and ankle (dorsiflexion positive). From Whittle (1991), with permission.

flexion/extension cycle. It is flexed at the time of heel contact, bringing the leg forwards. During the stance phase the hip extends, reaching the peak of extention a little before the end of the stance phase. It then flexes again, reaching its peak around the centre of the swing phase. There is a slight hesitation at this point, before the hip starts to extend again, around the time of the next heel contact.

The knee has a more complicated motion, with two waves of flexion and two of extension. At heel contact, the knee is close to being fully extended. In the movement known as stance-phase flexion, it flexes to about 20° then extends again, during the first half of the stance phase. Later in the stance phase, it begins to flex again, producing the swing-phase flexion peak of about 60°, just before mid-swing. The knee extends again just before the next heel contact.

The ankle motion also involves two flexion/ extension movements during the gait cycle. Around the time of heel contact, the ankle is close to its neutral position. Soon after heel contact, plantarflexion occurs, to achieve foot flat. As the body moves forwards, the tibia rotates over the foot, and the ankle angle changes from plantar-flexion to dorsiflexion. This motion is reversed about three-quarters through the stance phase, at heel off, when there is active plantarflexion of the ankle (known as the push-off phase of gait), lifting the heel off the ground. As soon as the rest of the foot leaves the ground, the ankle joint returns towards the neutral position, so that the toes are able to clear the ground during the swing phase.

The movements in the coronal and transverse planes are normally much smaller in magnitude than those in the sagittal plane, although they may be exaggerated in pathological gait. The most important coronal plane movement in normal gait is a tilting of the pelvis, keeping it lower on the side of the swing-phase leg. This helps to reduce the up-and-down motion of the centre of gravity. In the transverse plane, the pelvis rotates to bring the hip joint on each side forwards at heel contact, and backwards at toe off. This increases the stride length, without a corresponding increase in the angles of flexion and extension at the hip (Saunders *et al.*, 1953).

Pathological gait

There is clearly insufficient space in this chapter to give a complete description of all the many forms of pathological gait. However, some of the commonest abnormalities will be described very briefly. Fuller descriptions can be found in the publications by New York University (1986) and Whittle (1991).

Lateral trunk deviation

The trunk leans over the affected limb during its stance phase, producing a pattern known as Trendelenburg gait. It is used to stabilize the pelvis without the need to contract the gluteus medius muscle, either because it is weak, or because contracting it causes pain in the hip joint.

Anterior trunk deviation

The trunk leans forwards at the time of heel contact on the affected side, to bring the line of force in front of the knee, thus compensating for weak knee extensors.

Posterior trunk deviation

The trunk leans backwards at the time of heel contact on the affected side, to bring the line of force behind the hip joint, thus compensating for weak hip extensors.

Increased lumbar lordosis

If the hip joint is unable to move into extension, for example because of an arthrodesis or a flexion contracture, the femur can still be brought into the vertical or extended position by rotating the pelvis forwards. This rotation causes an increase in the lumbar lordosis.

Functional leg length discrepancy

The length of the leg will be inappropriate for a particular phase in the gait cycle if it is unable to shorten in the swing phase or to lengthen in the stance phase. Four gait abnormalities may be used to overcome this problem:

1. Circumduction, in which the swing-phase leg takes a curved path, swinging away from the stance-phase leg, thereby increasing its ground clearance.
2. Vaulting, where the stance-phase leg is lengthened by going up on tiptoe.
3. Hip-hiking, in which the pelvis, and thus the whole leg, is raised on the side of the swinging leg.
4. Steppage, where the swing phase leg is effectively shortened by increased flexion at both the hip and the knee.

Abnormal hip rotation

The thigh may be excessively rotated, either internally or externally, due to an imbalance of the rotator muscles about the hip, or due to severe hip joint disease.

Excessive knee extension

People with weak or paralysed quadriceps muscles who walk with anterior trunk deviation (see above) fully extend or hyperextend the knee during the stance phase. This gait pattern is also present when using an above-knee prosthetic limb. Unusual extension of the knee may also be seen during the push-off phase of gait, as a compensation for weak plantar flexors of the ankle.

Excessive knee flexion

Where a flexion contracture of the knee exists, the limb will be too short for the stance phase, and one of the compensations for functional leg length discrepancy will be required. A sudden and unexpected excessive flexion of the knee can also occur as a reflex response to pain, such as that caused by a torn meniscus.

Inadequate dorsiflexion control

The anterior tibial muscles are responsible for elevating the toes during the swing phase. Should they be paralysed or weak, toe drag will occur, unless one of the compensations for functional leg length discrepancy is used. The anterior tibial muscles are also responsible for lowering the foot gently to the ground following heel contact, and foot slap will occur if they are unable to control this motion.

Abnormal foot contact

The normal pattern of foot-to-ground contact consists of heel contact followed by forefoot contact. This may be altered in a number of pathological conditions. Equinus deformity will result in a flat-footed ground contact, or in more severe cases in a primary toe strike. The heel may not contact the ground at all during the whole of the gait cycle. Anterior tibial weakness, with a drop foot, may cause one of three initial contact patterns: foot slap, mentioned above, flat-footed initial contact, or a primary toe strike, rapidly followed by heel contact. A calcaneous deformity of the foot will result in a heel contact with little or no subsequent loading of the forefoot. Other severe foot deformities, such as talipes equinovarus, may cause the load to be taken on other areas of the foot, such as the lateral border, or occasionally even the dorsum.

Insufficient push-off

Weakness or paralysis of the soleus and gastrocnemius, or rupture of the Achilles tendom, may make it impossible to achieve push-off, which depends on active plantarflexion. The push-off may also be absent when there is pain under the forefoot, for example that caused by metatarsalgia.

Abnormal walking base

The width of the walking base may be increased where there is joint deformity, such as an abduction contracture of the hip or a valgus knee. It may also be increased to provide greater lateral stability, especially in neurological conditions such as cerebellar ataxia. A reduced walking base, including a negative one in which the feet are crossed over or scissored, may result from an adduction contracture of the hip or a varus knee.

Rhythmic disturbances

Normal gait has a symmetrical rhythm, the two halves of the gait cycle being of equal length. Each successive gait cycle is also of approximately the same duration. In pathological gait, the rhythm may be asymmetrical, with uneven step durations. This is particularly noticeable in the antalgic or pain-relieving gait pattern, in which weight is borne on the painful side for a shorter period of time than on the sound side. The rhythm may also be irregular, with step-to-step variations, as in the inco-ordination of cerebellar ataxia, or in the gait of parkinsonism, in which the cadence may increase over the course of the first few strides.

Other gait abnormalities

A number of other gait abnormalities may be observed, either alone or in combination with some of the gait patterns described above. They include rapid fatigue, and also abnormal movements of the head and neck, trunk, arms or legs. Common abnormal movements include intention tremors, athetoid movements, or a failure to swing the arms.

Methods of gait analysis

The techniques used to perform gait analysis form a spectrum, from the simple and inexpensive at one end to the complex and costly at the other. As a general rule, the more complicated systems give better-quality objective data, but the type of information provided is often of more value in a research setting than for routine clinical management. An important point, which must always be borne in mind, is that it is uneconomical to use a complicated and expensive measurement system unless the information it provides is both useful and unobtainable in any other way. Although many of the major advances in understanding have come from the use of expensive systems in research laboratories, the lessons learned can often then be applied, for the benefit of patients, by clinicians using much simpler equipment.

The techniques will be described in three groups: those which need little or no equipment, and which are suitable for routine use in a clincial setting; those which need a moderate amount of equipment, but might be expected in at least one hospital in a reasonable-size town, and those which need a lot of expensive equipment, which will probably be found only in a major laboratory, either in a university research setting, or in a specialized clinical facility.

Inexpensive methods for routine clinical care

Visual gait analysis

It is tempting to call visual gait analysis simple, because it can be performed without any equipment. However, since it relies on the formidable abilities of the human eyes to see and the brain to analyse, it is without doubt the most complex of all the methods currently in use. The patient is asked to walk up and down in front of the observer, who systematically looks for a series of gait abnormalities, such as those listed above. Since some abnormalities show up best when viewing from the side, and others are more visible from the front, the patient should be viewed while walking towards and away from the observer, as well as from each side.

When a patient has a locomotor disorder, most doctors and therapists will watch him or her walk as part of their clinical examinations. Where this differs from visual gait analysis is that such an assessment is usually unsystematic, and the most that can be obtained is a general impression of how well the patient walks, and perhaps some idea of one or two particular problems. To turn this into a true gait analysis requires two things. Firstly, it needs to be carried out carefully and systematically, with the aim of identifying all deviations from the normal pattern. Secondly, having identified the abnormalities, they need to be explained in terms of the underlying pathology. In this regard it is important to realize that what is observed is not the direct result of the pathology – it is the combined effect of the pathology and the patient's compensations. Putting it another way, what is observed is what is left over after the patient's ability to cope has been exhausted (Rose, 1983).

Videotape

The most valuable single piece of equipment for use in gait analysis is the video cassette recorder (VCR), which enhances visual gait analysis in a number of ways. Firstly, it greatly reduces the number of individual walks which the patient needs to make. This may be very important if he or she is in pain or easily fatigued. Secondly, it allows the clinician much more time to study the gait pattern, by watching and rewatching the tape, and it also makes it easier to obtain the opinion of colleagues. The ability to view the tape in slow motion makes it much easier to identify those events which occur too quickly to be seen by the unaided eye. Finally, the tape provides a permanent record, which may be reviewed after a period of time, or following therapeutic intervention. A reasonable-quality domestic camera-recorder (camcorder) is quite suitable for gait analysis, so long as the picture tube uses a charge-coupled device, which prevents blurring during rapid movements. The device used to replay the tapes, whether it be the camcorder itself or a separate VCR, needs to be able to provide a steady picture when used in slow motion or frame by frame.

General gait parameters

The simplest objective measurements which can be made are the general gait parameters: cadence, velocity and stride length. Cadence is measured by counting the number of individual footfalls in a given period of time, such as 10 or 15 seconds. The reduction in accuracy caused by timing for less than a full minute is unlikely to be of practical significance. Velocity is most easily determined by measuring the time taken to cover a known distance, such as that between two marks on the floor, or between two pillars in a corridor. Any length above about 5 m is acceptable. Stride length can be determined in three ways: by direct measurement, described in the section on foot positioning below, by counting the number of strides in a given distance, or by calculation from the cadence and the velocity, using the relationship:

stride (m) = 120 × velocity (m/s)/cadence (steps/min)

In making these measurements, it is important that the subject should be allowed a few steps at the beginning and end of the walk for speeding up and slowing down, so that the timing and counting are made under steady-state conditions. While ideally all the parameters should be measured on the same walk, little error will result from making the measurements on different walks, unless the patient's speed varies a great deal from walk to walk.

If a videotape of the patient's gait is being made for the purpose of visual gait analysis, it is convenient to determine the general gait parameters when replaying the tape. All that is required is that the patient should walk past two clearly visible markers, whose separation is known, and which cover a steady-state part of the walk, as described above. It is unnecessary to determine the exact instant at which the subject passes the two markers – both the counting and the timing can start and end with the first ground contact *after* passing each of the two markers. If the distance between the markers is d meters, the number of individual steps (not full strides) taken between them is s, and the time taken is t seconds, the general gait parameters are given by:

cadence (steps/min) = $60 \times s/t$
velocity (m/s) = d/t
stride (m) = $2 \times d/s$

Foot positioning

The positioning of the feet on the ground during walking can be obtained by having the patient walk along a polished floor, after stepping with both feet in a shallow tray filled with talcum powder. The two step lengths, the stride length and the walking base can be measured with a tape measure, as shown in Fig. 10.3. It is also possible to measure the angle of toe out (or toe in), and the approximate area of contact between the foot and the ground. This simple test gives a great deal of useful information, even if it does involve mopping up the floor afterwards!

Methods for use in a clinical laboratory

Time-and-distance measurements

A number of systems have been developed to measure the timing of the events of gait. Typically, such systems use either switches fixed beneath the shoes, or a conductive walkway which detects contact between the foot and the floor. The simpler systems, which only detect heel contact and toe off, give the cadence and the durations of the single-support phases on each side and the two double-support phases (see Fig. 10.2). Systems with separate switches or contacts beneath different parts of the foot also give the timing of foot flat and heel off. Photoelectric cells at the ends of the walkway are commonly used to measure the duration of the walk, from which the velocity may be calculated, and hence, knowing the cadence, also the stride length (but not the individual step lengths).

Other systems have been developed which measure either the position of the two feet on the ground, or the distance each foot moves forwards at each step. These systems are able to give the step and stride lengths, as well as the cadence, velocity, and the single and double-support times.

Electrogoniometers

The angular excursion of a joint during walking may be measured by the electrogoniometer, which is fixed to the limb and aligned to the joint axis. The commonest type is based on a rotary potentiometer, and gives an output voltage which depends on the joint angle. Other designs are based on the deformation of a thin strip of metal, or the change in resistance of a column of mercury, contained in a thin elastic tube, as the tube is stretched. Electrogoniometers may be used to measure the motion of any joint, in any axis, although they are most commonly used for the sagittal plane motion of the hip, knee and ankle joints.

Pressure beneath the foot

Several systems exist which are able to measure the pressure beneath different regions of the foot. This information may be of great value in a number of pathological conditions (Lord *et al.*, 1986). In diabetic neuropathy, both sensory and motor nerves are damaged, causing anaesthesia and foot deformity, which readily lead to ulcer formation. Measurement of the pressure beneath the foot makes possible early diagnosis and treatment, prior to ulcer formation.

Electromyography

The measurement of the electrical activity of the muscles during walking may give valuable information about the motor causes underlying certain gait abnormalities (Shiavi, 1985). Electromyography is also essential prior to some forms of specialized treatment, such as muscle transplantation in cerebral palsy. For clinical purposes, electromyography is normally performed using surface electrodes, although where necessary more detailed information can be obtained by inserting fine wires directly into the muscle.

Methods for use in a major gait analysis laboratory

Energy consumption

A consequence of many abnormal gaits is that the normal energy-conserving mechanisms are lost, leading to an increased energy cost of walking, with rapid fatigue and a limitation of activity. Some idea of the energy cost of walking can be obtained by measuring the increase in heart rate. This may be quantified using the physiological cost index (PCI) described by Steven *et al.* (1983):

PCI = (heart rate walking − heart rate resting)/ velocity

More accurate determination of energy cost of walking requires the measurement of the subject's oxygen consumption, by collecting the expired air as he or she walks, by means of a face mask or mouthpiece.

Force platforms

The force exerted by the foot on the ground can be measured by means of a force platform (also called a forceplate). Modern designs measure not only the vertical force, but also the horizontal forces, both in the direction of progression and from side to side (Fig. 10.5). They also give the position on the ground of the centre of the applied force, and the torque about the vertical axis. Such information is of limited value by itself, but is sometimes used empirically for monitoring progress, since the pattern of the force and the magnitude of the force components may indicate the severity of particular disabilities.

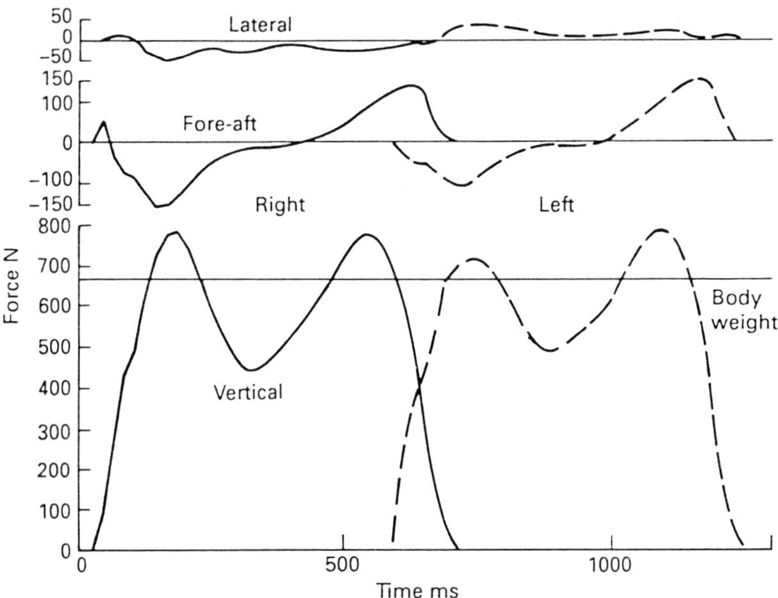

Fig. 10.5 Lateral, fore-aft and vertical components of the ground reaction force, in newtons, for right foot (solid line) and left (dashed). From Whittle (1991), with permission.

Kinematic systems

Kinematics is the study of movement, and systems which make measurements of the movements of the body during walking are essential for scientific gait analysis. Earlier kinematic systems used cine photography, but this has now largely been replaced by electronic optical techniques, based either on television, or on special-purpose cameras or scanners. Many systems are three-dimensional, and provide information on the limb positions and joint angles in all three planes.

Combined kinetic/kinematic systems

The most advanced gait analysis laboratories use a kinematic system combined with one or more force platforms, as in Figure 10.6. The system shown consists of a three-dimensional kinematic system, using four television cameras, and two force platforms.

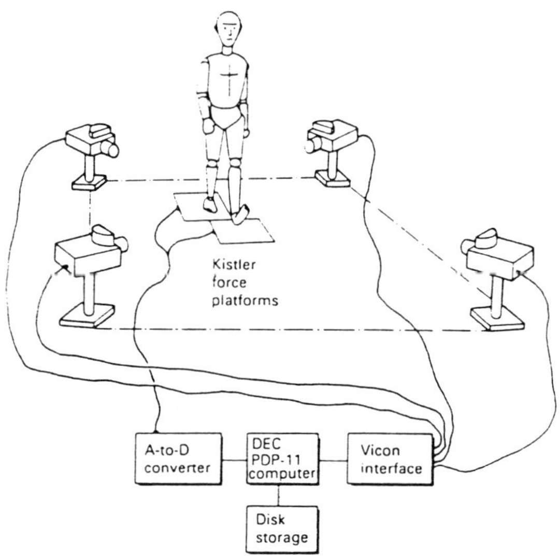

Fig. 10.6 The Oxford University gait analysis laboratory, with a four-camera Vicon kinematic system and two Kistler force platforms. From Whittle (1991), with permission.

Mathematical modelling

Using data from a combined kinetic/kinematic system, it is possible to make mechanical calculations on the joint moments of force, the energy exchanges taking place during walking, and the forces within the joints. These calculations are made using a mathematical model – a series of equations which take as their inputs the measured parameters, such as limb position and ground reaction force. In order to make these calculations, a number of assumptions have to be made, including which muscles are active at particular times.

Clinical applications of gait analysis

The applications of gait analysis may conveniently be divided into clinical applications, which are aimed at benefitting an individual patient, and scientific applications, which have as their main aim the furtherance of knowledge. This chapter will concentrate on the former.

Clinical gait analysis is best regarded as one type of special investigation, which contributes to the overall assessment of a patient. The information on gait is interpreted along with that from the history, physical examination and other special investigations, such as radiographs and biochemistry (Rose, 1983). Gait analysis may contribute to diagnosis, decision-making, and to documentation.

Diagnosis

In most patients referred for gait analysis, the general diagnostic category is already known (cerebral palsy, parkinsonism, hemiplegia, etc.). Where gait analysis may be of value, however, is to provide a detailed diagnosis of a motor deficit (Winters *et al.*, 1987). It is very important to be able to distinguish between a number of different possible causes for the same gait abnormality, and also between the original motor deficit and a patient's coping responses (Winter, 1985). For example, a child with cerebral palsy may be vaulting on one side because of an inability to flex the opposite knee in the swing phase. If the vaulting is erroneously ascribed to a tight heel cord, and treated by a heel cord lengthening, the gait would be made worse, not better.

Gait analysis may also be useful in distinguishing between a pathological gait and a habit pattern. An example of this is in the diagnosis of toe walking, where gait analysis may be used to differentiate between the relatively harmless and self-limiting condition of idiopathic toe walking, and more serious conditions, such as cerebral palsy (Hicks *et al.*, 1988).

Gait disorders in the elderly are frequently thought to be the inescapable consequence of age, whereas many are due to an underlying – and treatable – pathological cause. The use of gait analysis to identify such a cause could result in an improved life for the patient, with a reduced risk of falls and fractures (Cunha, 1988).

Decision-making

The use of gait analysis in clinical decision-making involves four separate stages (Rose, 1983). Firstly, a clinical assessment is performed, with gait analysis as one of the special investigations. Secondly, a hypothesis is formed as to the exact cause of the observed gait abnormalities, based on all of the information available. Thirdly, that hypothesis is tested, and revised if necessary. Testing the hypothesis may be done in various ways, including further measurements, such as fine-wire electromyogram, or some form of intervention, such as fitting an orthosis or paralysing a muscle with local anaesthetic. Finally, a decision is made as to what treatment (if any) is appropriate. Considerable progress has been made in recent years by adopting this approach in the management of cerebral palsy (Gage, 1983), but it is also appropriate for many other conditions which affect gait.

Gait analysis may also be useful in making decisions on the management of patients with joint disease. It may indicate which joint needs to be operated first in multiple joint disease, and it may also be used to differentiate between those patients who will do well and those who will do badly following a particular procedure. For example, gait analysis may be used to predict the success of high tibial osteotomy, for osteoarthritis of the knee with a varus deformity (Prodromos *et al.*, 1985).

In a number of neurological conditions, notably hemiplegia, a detailed gait analysis may be used as the basis for planning either physiotherapy or some form of surgical treatment (Perry, 1969). Hemiplegic patients tend to walk very inefficiently, and measuring their joint moments and powers may suggest ways in which training could be used to reduce their energy expenditure.

Mention has already been made of the value of measuring the pressure beneath the foot, particularly in diabetic neuropathy, to detect high pressures before ulcer formation occurs. This information may be used for the prescription of pressure-relieving insoles, and for measuring the success of this form of treatment (Lord *et al.*, 1986).

The alignment and adjustment of prosthetic limbs may be improved by using objective measurements of gait, particularly if repeat trials are performed with different adjustments (Murray *et al.*, 1983). Orthotic prescription may also be improved, if the gait can be monitored with the patient wearing different orthoses. For example, measurements may be made with different ankle alignments on an ankle–foot orthosis for drop foot. Trials of different orthoses may also form part of the process of hypothesis testing, described above.

Documentation

It is frequently of value to record the current state of a patient's condition, either to quantify the disability on a single occasion, or to monitor it over a period of time. Assessing the degree of disability may be particularly important in medicolegal work. Measuring the changes which take place over a period of time may be useful to follow the progress or deterioration of the patient's condition, or to quantify the effects of a particular form of treatment. The general gait parameters provide a simple means of obtaining useful objective data for these purposes. The results of the analysis may be used to identify areas where the treatment is ineffective, or it may define an end-point for stopping treatment, when progress appears to have ceased.

These examples, which have been limited to the uses of gait analysis in direct patient management, form only a small part of the total utilization of the techniques. Over the years, gait analysis has been far more important as a research tool than as a clinical technique. It remains an extremely powerful tool for monitoring the effects of different forms of treatment, and for performing fundamental research on the musculoskeletal system and its nervous control. However, it is important to realize that gait analysis is not the exclusive prerogative of research scientists, but that it may also make a significant contribution in day-by-day patient management.

References

Borelli GA (1679) De Motu Animalium. Rome.

Braune W and Fischer O (1889) Uber die lage des schwerpunkt des menschlichen Korpers. Abh Math Phys Klasse d. Kgl Saschen, Ges d. Wiss **15**.

Cunha UV (1988) Differential diagnosis of gait disorders in the elderly. *Geriatrics* **43**, 33–42.

Gage JR (1983) Gait analysis for decision-making in cerebral palsy. *Bulletin of the Hospital for Joint Diseases Orthopaedic Institute* **43**, 147–63.

Hicks R, Durinick N, Gage JR (1988) Differentiation of idiopathic toe-walking and cerebral palsy. *Journal of Pediatric Orthopaedics* **8**, 160–3.

Lord M, Reynolds DP, Hughes JR (1986) Foot pressure measurement: a review of clinical findings. *Journal of Biomedical Engineering* **8**, 283–94.

Marey EJ (1895) *Movement*. New York: Appleton.

Murray MP (1967) Gait as a total pattern of movement. *American Journal of Physical Medicine* **46**, 290–333.

Murray MP, Mollinger LA, Sepic SB, Gardner GM, Linder MT (1983) Gait patterns in above-knee amputee patients: hydraulic swing control vs constant-friction knee components. *Archives of Physical Medicine and Rehabilitation* **64**, 339–45.

Muybridge E (1901) *The Human Figure in Motion*. London: Chapman and Hall.

New York University (1986) *Lower Limb Orthotics*. New York: Prosthetics and Orthotics, New York University Postgraduate Medical School.

Perry J (1969) The mechanics of walking in hemiplegia. *Clinical Orthopaedics and Related Research* **63**, 23–31.

Perry J (1974) Kinesiology of lower extremity bracing. *Clinical Orthopaedics and Related Research* **102**, 18–31.

Prodromos CC, Andriacchi TP, Galante JO (1985) A relationship between gait and clinical changes following high tibial osteotomy. *Journal of Bone and Joint Surgery* **67A**, 1188–94.

Rose GK (1983) Clinical gait assessment: a personal view. *Journal of Medical Engineering and Technology* **7**, 273–9.

Saunders JBDM, Inman VT, Eberhart HS (1953) The major determinants in normal and pathological gait. *Journal of Bone and Joint Surgery* **35A**, 543–58.

Shiavi R (1985) Electromyographic patterns in adult locomotion: a comprehensive review. *Journal of Rehabilitation Research and Development* **22**, 85–98.

Steindler A (1953) A historical review of the studies and investigations made in relation to human gait. *Journal of Bone and Joint Surgery* **35A**, 540–2.

Steven MM, Capell HA, Sturrock RD, MacGregor J (1983) The physiological cost of gait (PCG): a new technique for evaluating nonsteroidal antiinflammatory drugs in rheumatoid arthritis. *British Journal of Rheumatology* **22**, 141–5.

Sutherland DH, Olshen RA, Biden EN, Wyatt MP (1988) *The Development of Mature Walking*. London: Mac Keith Press.

Weber W and Weber EF (1836) Mechanik der menschlichen gehiverkzeuge. Dietrich: Gottingen.

Whittle MW (1991) *Gait Analysis: An Introduction*. Oxford: Butterworth–Heinemann.

Winter DA (1985) Concerning the scientific basis for the diagnosis of pathological gait and for rehabilitation protocols. *Physiotherapy Canada* **37**, 245–52.

Winters TF, Gage JR, Hicks R (1987) Gait patterns in spastic hemiplegia in children and young adults. *Journal of Bone and Joint Surgery* **69A**, 437–41.

11

The effect of ultrasound on the biology of soft tissue repair

M. Dyson

Introduction

Ultrasound therapy (UT), exposure of injured tissues to high-frequency mechanical vibrations, is used at present mainly to stimulate the repair of soft tissue injuries and to relieve pain. It introduces absorbable energy into the tissues, providing stimuli to which cells involved in the reparative process can respond.

In this chapter the cellular events which follow soft tissue injury and which result in repair are summarized, the characteristics of UT is described and its effects on the cellular responses to soft tissue injury considered and compared.

Cellular events involved in soft tissue repair

When applied in an appropriate fashion, both ultrasound and light can produce cellular changes which modify the process of soft tissue repair, frequently accelerating it. However, if used incorrectly it can be ineffective, or even damaging. To ensure that treatments are effective and, ideally, optimized, their effects on the cells involved in the repair of soft tissue should be appreciated. As a necessary preliminary to considering these effects and the mechanisms by which they take place, the main cellular events which occur during the repair of the soft connective tissue of the dermis will be described. Similar events occur during the repair of other forms of soft tissue injury.

Phases of repair

The repair of the injured dermis is generally described as consisting of three overlapping and inter-related phases, namely acute inflammation (early and late), proliferation and scar tissue maturation or remodelling. The first two are involved in the production of highly cellular and vascular granulation tissue, whereas in the last phase this is gradually replaced by a relatively less cellular and less vascular scar.

Inflammatory phase

When soft connective tissue is injured the degranulation of platelets, mast cells and basophils results in the release of agents, some of which trigger the acute inflammatory response, whereas others are involved in its resolution. The degranulation of mast cells, for example, results in the release of mediators of inflammation such as histamine and arachidonic acid metabolites and heparin which has an angiogenic role in wound healing (Trabucchi *et al.*, 1988). During acute inflammation local blood clotting occurs and blood vessel permeability increases temporarily; neutrophils and monocytes leave the vessels and are attracted to the wound site by chemotactic agents released from platelets, mast cells and basophils (Fernandez *et al.*, 1978).

The neutrophils phagocytose bacteria at the wound site, leaving it when this is completed. The cessation of neutrophil invasion of the wound site marks the end of the early part of acute inflammation (Clark, 1985). Monocytes, however, develop into macrophages on entering the injured tissues, and remain there throughout the entire inflammatory phase and during the early part of the proliferative phase. Like neutrophils they are phagocytic, but as well as debriding the wound site by removing dead and damaged tissue from it, they also synthesize and release mitogenic and angiogenic growth factors, together with chemotactic agents, which collectively initiate and help to control the proliferative phase of the dermal repair process. In contrast to chronic inflammation, which delays healing and must be suppressed, acute inflammatory is a normal, and necessary, part of the healing process. Ideally, acute inflammation should be accelerated, so that the proliferative and remodelling phases are entered, and healing completed, more rapidly. When used in an appropriate fashion, UT can achieve this acceleration.

Proliferative phase

In response to factors released, mainly by macrophages, during the later part of the acute inflammatory phase, granulation tissue begins to develop within the bed of the wound. Granulation tissue is a highly cellular and vascular material, rich in macrophages, lymphocytes, fibroblasts, multipotent pericytes and endothelial cells. These cells are surrounded by a matrix containing fibronectin, hyaluronic acid, other glycosaminoglycans and collagen. At first the collagen produced within the granulation tissue is mainly type III but later type I predominates. The collagen appears to be deposited initially in a haphazard fashion.

Granulation tissue is formed when macrophages, fibroblasts and the blood capillaries formed by the endothelial cells migrate into the wound bed as an interdependent unit, termed a wound module (Hunt and Van Winkle, 1979). The macrophages, which lead the migration, are closely followed by fibroblasts and endothelial cells, attracted by chemotactic agents and growth factors which the macrophages liberate. The fibroblasts produce a matrix through which cells can readily move, in response to chemotactic factors. Endothelial cells become arranged to form capillary loops which, as they become patent and functional, supply the developing granulation tissue with the nutrients needed for maintenance and further development of granulation tissue within the wound bed. The macrophages appear to have a controlling role in the development of granulation tissue. If their migration into the wound bed is curtailed, for example by the application of anti-inflammatory steroids, or if those present are destroyed by interaction with antimacrophage serum, the development of granulation tissue is inhibited (Liebovich and Ross, 1975). In addition to producing direct effects on the cellular components of the granulation tissue, there is evidence that UT can affect fibroblast and endothelial cell activity indirectly, via growth factors released from macrophages.

Remodelling phase

During remodelling the degree of orderliness in the arrangement of the collagen increases, as fibres are removed from some locations and newly synthesized fibres are deposited in others. The more regular pattern of fibres which gradually emerges is considered to be related to the mechanical forces to which the tissue is subjected during physical activity. Some of the type III collagen is replaced by type I. During remodelling the cellularity and vascularity of the newly formed tissue at the wound site are gradually reduced, as the granulation tissue is replaced by scar tissue. Although the remodelling process continues for years, the scar tissue never achieves the structural and functional attributes of the connective tissue at the wound site before injury. Evidence will be presented that UT, if used early in the repair process, can modify the fibre pattern and improve the physical characteristics of scar tissue.

Characteristics and effects of ultrasound therapy

Ultrasound is a mechanical vibration or wave which is repeated at a frequency above the limit of human hearing. At low intensities, it can stimulate the repair of injured tissues (Dyson *et al.*, 1976).

Media that can transmit ultrasound, such as water and the soft tissues of the body, oscillate or vibrate at the frequency of the applied ultrasound. The compressional waves produced are, when travelling through soft tissues and liquids, longitudinal in type, that is the molecular displacement produced by the waves is parallel to the direction of wave propagation. In solids, however, such as bone, ultrasound is transmitted as transverse or shear waves, that is, molecular displacement is in a direction at right angles to the direction of wave propagation. This difference in wave type is of importance clinically because the mode conversion which occurs when ultrasound reaches the interface between soft tissues and bone results in a local increase in temperature (Williams, 1987) which may be sufficient to cause periosteal pain and localized tissue damage. The higher the intensity of the ultrasound, the greater the possibility of tissue damage occurring. Because of this, it is recommended that the intensity of ultrasound applied to the tissues should not exceed the low level found to be therapeutically effective.

The frequency, wavelength and amplitude of the ultrasound applied therapeutically can affect the outcome of treatment. *Frequency* (f) is the number of times per second that a molecule displaced by the ultrasound completes a cycle of movement, returning to its original position; it is expressed in hertz or cycles per second. The frequencies used to accelerate soft tissue repair are typically from 0.5 to 3.0 MHz, where 1 MHz is one million cycles per second. The higher the frequency, the more readily the ultrasound is absorbed; thus 3.0 MHz is suitable for treating superficial tissues, whereas lower frequencies are more penetrative. *Wavelength* (ℓ) is the shortest distance, measured parallel to the direction of propagation of the ultrasound, between molecules at equivalent points in the cycle of movement which constitutes a wave. It is dependent upon the frequency and velocity (c) of ultrasound in that $\ell = c/f$. Since the velocity of ultrasound in soft tissue is virtually the same as that in water, i.e. approximately 1500 m/s, at a frequency of 1 MHz the wavelength is $1500/10^6$ m, i.e. 1.5 mm. *Amplitude* is the maximum disturbance, in terms of molecular displacement or pressure, caused by passage of a wave of ultrasound through a transmitting medium such as soft tissue; it increases with intensity (usually measured in W/cm^2). Whether or not the application of ultrasound to injured soft tissues assists in their repair, is ineffective, or produces further injury, is dependent upon the levels of these parameters, since they determine the types of interactions which occur with the various components of the tissues.

Production of therapeutic ultrasound

The high-frequency ultrasound used therapeutically to accelerate the repair of injured tissue is generally produced by a piezoelectric transducer. The transducer is usually a disc of a ceramic such as lead zirconate titanate (PZT) which expands and contracts at the rate at which an alternating electric charge is applied across it. If the rate of oscillation or vibration of the disc is sufficiently rapid (at or over 20 kHz), the waves of pressure and rarefaction emanating from the transducer are, by definition, ultrasonic. The frequencies used therapeutically to stimulate soft tissue repair are typically between 0.5 and 3.0 MHz. Ultrasound at this frequency is reflected from the interface between the transducer and air, but can be transmitted into any suitable solid or liquid applied to it. The discoid transducer is mounted in an applicator or treatment head in such a way that the interiorly directed surface of the face is in contact with air, while the exteriorly directed surface is bonded to the metallic face of the applicator. When a high-frequency oscillating voltage is applied across the transducer via electrodes attached to these surfaces, electrical energy is transduced into mechanical energy; since reflection occurs at the air-backed interiorly directed surface of the transducer, virtually all of this mechanical energy is transmitted externally through the face of the applicator into any ultrasound-transmitting material which is in contact with it. Users of ultrasound should be aware, however, that some ultrasound can be transmitted laterally into the side walls of the applicator, and thence, unless suitable precautions are taken, into the operator. Although the amounts of energy involved are small (Hoogland, 1986), their effects may be cumulative. It is advisable either to avoid holding the active applicator near to the transducer or to do so only if wearing air-trapping gloves which will reflect the ultrasound away from the user's hands.

The transducer is powered and controlled by a therapeutic ultrasound generator linked by a coaxial cable to the applicator within which the transducer is housed. The generator usually contains the following:

1. A circuit which produces the oscillating voltages needed to drive the transducer.
2. A controlling circuit which can switch the oscillator on and off to give pulsed ultrasound.
3. A means of rectifying the power supply.
4. A means of measuring and varying the intensity.
5. A controlling microcomputer.

Continuous and pulsed ultrasound

When ultrasound is being used primarily to heat tissue, then it is most efficiently delivered in continuous mode. Pulsing is used when the intention is to exploit its non-thermal effects. Pulsing allows the ultrasound to be used at higher intensities during the pulse than would be thermally appropriate if the ultrasound was being applied continuously. It reduces the temporal average intensity, and hence the total amount of energy being delivered to the tissue during a treatment session in comparison to the total energy when delivered continuously at the same spatial average, temporal peak, intensity (Dyson, 1990). Since the total amount of energy available for absorption, and transduction to heat, is reduced, the amount of tissue heating is also reduced.

The pulses (or marks) are typically from 0.5 to 2.0 ms long, and are separated by pauses (or spaces), typically from 0.5 to 8.0 ms. Most therapeutic ultrasound generators produce pulses of 2 ms and vary the time separating them. Mark : space ratios of 1 : 1 (2 ms pulse, 2 ms pause) and 1 : 4 (2 ms pulse, 8 ms pause) are commonly available; the former gives a duty cycle of 50% and the latter one of 20%, duty cycle being the term used to describe the percentage of the total treatment time that the transducer produces ultrasound.

Transmission of ultrasound

When the metal plate of the applicator, to which the transducer is attached, is caused to vibrate at high frequencies, a stream of compression waves is produced. The reflective air-backing of the transducer ensures that these waves, which comprise the ultrasonic beam, are transmitted away from the applicator, provided that it is in contact with an ultrasound-conducting medium. Because the wavelength of the ultrasound is considerably smaller (0.5 mm at a frequency of 3.0 MHz and 3.0 mm at a frequency of 0.5 MHz) than the diameter of the discoid transducer (usually at 1 cm or more), the ultrasonic beam is approximately cylindrical and the same diameter as the transducer. Users of ultrasound should be aware that the ultrasonic beam lacks uniformity, particularly close to the applicator, in the so-called near field or Fresnel zone. This is because compression waves reaching the same point from various parts of the transducer travel by different paths and arrive out of phase, sometimes cancelling and sometimes reinforcing each other. Beyond it, in the far field or Fraunhofer zone, the beam begins to diverge and becomes more regular.

The length of the near field is directly proportional to the square of the radius of the transducer and inversely proportional to the wavelength of the ultrasound; for a 3 cm diameter transducer operating at 1 MHz in water and soft-tissue, the near field extends approximately 15 cm from the applicator (Low and Reed, 1990). At higher frequencies, where the wavelengths are shorter, the near field is even longer. Since most of the soft tissues exposed to ultrasound are in the irregular near field, it is recommended that the applicator be moved throughout treatment, thus increasing the chance of treating all the tissues exposed to the ultrasound in a similar fashion and reducing the risk of accidental overdose at spatial peaks within the near field. It is also safer to use applicators with a low beam non-uniformity ratio (BNR), that is, the ratio of spatial peak intensity in the near field to spatial average intensity; this avoids exposure to high, and potentially damaging, spatial peak intensities.

For ultrasound to produce effects in tissues it has to reach them and be absorbed by them. Its transmission involves wave progression at a velocity which is characteristic for each medium through which the wave passes. This velocity depends on the density and elasticity of the medium, the product of which gives the acoustic impedance of the medium. When the ultrasonic compression waves meet the interface between two media of differing acoustic impedance, e.g. soft tissue and bone, some of the waves will be reflected and others transmitted. There is also a change in direction of transmission at the boundary due to refraction. The more different the acoustic impedance of the adjacent media, the greater the amount of both reflection and refraction. The acoustic impedances of water and soft tissue are virtually similar, while that of air and soft tissue, bone and soft tissue, and metal and soft tissue, differ greatly. It will be appreciated, therefore, that knowledge of the location, type and shape of such interfaces is essential if the energy levels to which tissues are exposed are to be predicted. It is also important that appropriate coupling media are used to transmit ultrasound from the applicator into the soft tissue (Docker *et al.*, 1982). These media must be free of ultrasound-reflecting material such as air bubbles, and should have similar acoustic properties to soft tissues. Degassed water, ultrasound-transmitting gels and some aqueous gel-based wound dressings are suitable (Brueton and Campbell, 1987).

Reflection at an interface can also result in the formation of standing waves in the medium through which the ultrasound travels first. In these circumstances the original or incident wave and the reflected wave travel in opposite directions, and the peaks and troughs of the two travelling waves may interact to produce a stationary or standing wave in which the peaks and troughs remain at fixed positions, unless the applicator is moved, when they alter. The formation of standing waves should be avoided when ultrasound is used therapeutically because they can have damaging consequences; the flow of blood cells can be interrupted and vessel endothelia may be damaged (Dyson *et al.*, 1974); the possibility of locally damaging transient cavitation (see below) and free radical formation occurring can also be increased (Crum *et al.*, 1986).

As a beam of ultrasound travels through any medium it increases the motion and collisions of molecules in its path, resulting in the transduction of its kinetic energy into heat. The kinetic energy of the beam decreases exponentially with the distance travelled as absorption of the energy by the medium occurs. The distance at which the amount of energy remaining in the beam is half that when the beam entered the medium is termed the half-value depth of penetration. This varies with the absorption coefficient of the medium and with the frequency of the ultrasound. The greater the absorption coefficient and the higher the frequency, the shorter is the half-value depth of penetration. Thus, according to Hoogland (1987), the half value depth of penetration in fat is 50 mm for 1 MHz ultrasound and 16.5 mm for 3 MHz ultrasound, while that in tendon is 6.2 mm for 1 MHz ultrasound and only 2 mm for 3 MHz ultrasound. In skeletal muscle the equivalent distances, again according to Hoogland, are 9 mm and 3 mm. Tissues with a high protein and low water and fat content, such as tendon and muscle, absorb ultrasound, and are thus heated by it more readily than tissues in which the protein content is low and the water and fat content high, such as areolar tissue and adipose tissue (Frizzel and Dunn, 1982). The clinical relevance of this is that ultrasound can deliver energy at the site of deeply located lesions of soft connective tissues with a high protein content, such as joint capsules and tendons, without excessive heating of intervening areolar and adipose tissues. The deeper the tissue, the lower the frequency which should be used, while for superficial soft tissue lesions such as those of the dermis, the more readily absorbed higher frequencies are indicated.

It should be appreciated that the amount of tissue heating is affected not only by the characteristics of ultrasound and the chemical composition of the tissue, but also by blood flow and heat conduction, both of which carry the deposited heat away from the tissues. In highly vascularized tissue such as skeletal muscle, heat is dissipated rapidly, while in the less well-vascularized densely fibrous tissues of tendons and ligaments, and avascular tissues such as cartilage, greater temperature rises occur. In the absence of vascular dissipation of heat, it has been calculated that exposure of soft tissues to an ultrasonic intensity of 1 W/cm^2 produces a temperature rise of the order 0.8°C/min (ter Haar, 1987). Should the temperature exceed 45°C then tissue damage will occur.

It should be noted that ultrasonic energy is lost from the beam not only by absorption, but also by being scattered from the beam by reflection and refraction. Collectively these processes constitute *attenuation*.

Clinically relevant variables in ultrasonic therapy

Variables whose levels should be known and recorded when ultrasound is administered as a therapeutic agent include power, intensity, exposure duration, frequency and the position of the target tissues relative to the applicator. The time of onset and spacing of treatments are also important (Dyson, 1990).

1. *Power* is the total energy in the ultrasonic beam, measured in watts.
2. *Intensity* is the amount of energy divided by the effective radiating area (ERA) of the applicator, where ERA is the area in front of the applicator face over which the power of the output, measured with a pressure-sensitive detector, is more than 5% of the spatial maximum output. The intensity can be averaged in space over the face of the applicator; this is termed spatial average intensity or I(SA). With pulsed ultrasound the pulse average intensity or I(PA), that is, the average intensity during the duration of the pulse, should be measured. For continuous ultrasound the spatial and temporal average intensity I(SATA) should be recorded, while for pulsed ultrasound both I(SATA) and I(SAPA) should be stated. If heating is required, then ultrasound is generally used in the continuous mode; this is not recommended, however, if the circulation is impaired and excess heat cannot be dissipated by it, for in such circumstances thermal injury could ensue. Pulsing can be used to reduce the temporal average intensity [I(TA)], and thus the amount of heating, while ensuring that the pulse average intensity [I(PA)] is maintained sufficiently high to permit the beneficial non-thermal effects required (see below). An I(SAPA) of 0.5 W/cm^2, pulsed 2 ms on, 8 ms off, giving an I(SATA) of 0.1 W/cm^2, is usually adequate to accelerate the repair of soft tissue injuries (Dyson, 1990). Increasing the intensity above this level is not recommended as this can have proinflammatory effects (Hashish, 1986).
3. *Exposure duration* is the total time of irradiation in minutes. It is usually based, empirically, on the surface area to be treated. Oakley (1978) recommended dividing this area into zones each 1.5 times the active area (ERA) of the applicator, and allowing 1 or 2 min for treating each zone. Hoogland (1986) recommended a maximum total treatment time of 15 min with at least 1 min of treatment time for each area of 1 cm^2.
4. *Frequency* is, as stated previously, the number of times per second that a molecule displaced by the ultrasound completes a cycle of movement; it is measured in hertz. UT at 3 MHz is recommended for superficial injuries and at 1 MHz for deeper injuries, since the latter is the more penetrative.
5. *Position of the target tissues*, in terms of their anatomical location and distance from the transducer, should be noted and taken into consideration when selecting the output level, because the acoustic properties of any intervening substances and the distance the

ultrasound travels through them affects the amount of mechanical energy to reach the target. If the energy level is reduced to such an extent that it is subthreshold when it reaches the target, then treatment will be ineffective.

6. *Onset and spacing of treatments* can affect the efficacy of UT. It is recommended that acute injuries be treated as soon as possible (Oakley, 1978; Patrick, 1978), ideally within 24 hours of their occurrence, so that the inflammatory phase of repair can be accelerated, with the result that the proliferative phase begins more rapidly (Dyson, 1990). Treatment once or twice a day until pain and swelling are diminished, followed by treatment on alternate days until the condition is resolved, has been found to be effective (McDiarmid and Burns, 1987). Chronic conditions are usually treated less frequently, for example once a week (Callam, 1987) or three times a week (Dyson *et al.*, 1976); in the case of chronic ulceration of the skin, the treatments are not restricted to the inflammatory phase, but are continued throughout the proliferative phase, since it has been shown that low-intensity (primarily non-thermal) UT can stimulate angiogenesis (Young, 1988) and fibroblast activity (Mummery, 1978; Webster, 1980; Dyson, 1987), which are essential elements of this stage of repair.

Clinically significant physical effects of ultrasound therapy

When ultrasound interacts with cells and tissues it can affect their activity. Some of its effects are therapeutic, resulting in the acceleration of tissue repair, whereas others are potentially damaging and must be avoided. An understanding of the physical mechanisms underlying these changes is essential if UT is to be used with confidence in its efficiency and safety. These physical mechanisms are generally classified as being either primarily thermal or non-thermal.

Thermal

The local tissue temperature increases when ultrasound is absorbed. The extent of the increase in temperature depends on a variety of factors, including the frequency of the ultrasound, the effectiveness of the local microcirculation in removing the heat generated, and the types of tissues in the path of the ultrasound. Clinically significant effects of a local increase in temperature to between 40 and 45°C include hyperaemia and decreased pain. Temperature increases in excess of this can, however, induce thermal necrosis and must be avoided. It should be appreciated that some structures absorb ultrasound preferentially, for example the periosteum, and care should be taken to ensure that such tissues are not heated excessively by it.

Non-thermal

Non-thermal mechanisms are responsible for many of the clinically significant changes which UT can produce in tissues. These mechanisms include cavitation (stable and transient), acoustic streaming and standing wave formation. The thresholds required for these primarily non-thermal physical phenomena can be below those needed to induce clinically significant heating. They can interfere, either constructively or destructively, with the thermal effects of ultrasound, and may occur at levels below those which produce clinically significant heating. Therefore, UT can never be used solely to heat tissue. Although there is evidence that the effects of stable cavitation and acoustic streaming can be therapeutically useful, others, such as those resulting from transient cavitation and standing wave formation, are damaging.

1. *Cavitation*: Exposure to ultrasound can result in the formation of minute cavities, a few microns in diameter, in gas-containing fluids. At the low-pressure amplitudes associated with low-intensity UT, these 'bubbles' vibrate in response to the cyclical pressure changes of the ultrasound (stable cavitation), and may modify, in a reversible fashion, the permeability of the plasma membranes of adjacent cells (Mortimer and Dyson, 1988), acting as a signal for their increased activity. However, if the pressure amplitude is sufficiently great, then the cavities implode violently (transient

cavitation); this produces local mechanical and chemical damage, the latter as a result of free radical formation in excess of that which can be removed by naturally occurring free radical scavengers. Although there is no evidence that the levels of ultrasound currently used therapeutically can induce transient cavitation *in vivo*, it has been detected *in vitro* in blood plasma exposed to ultrasound at the upper extreme of the range of available intensities produced by UT equipment used under standing wave conditions (Crum, 1986). There is no evidence for transient cavitation occurring either *in vitro* or *in vivo* at the levels currently used in UT in the absence of standing waves. It has been suggested, however, that stable cavitation can be induced at lower intensities, and hence at lower pressure amplitudes, both *in vitro* and *in vivo* (ter Haar and Daniels, 1981), although the interpretation of the evidence for this occurring *in vivo* has recently been challenged (Watmough *et al.*, 1991). Mechanical stresses induced around the pulsating bubbles formed during the process may be responsible for the increased uptake of calcium ions observed in fibroblasts exposed to ultrasound *in vitro*. It is of interest that this modification in plasma membrane permeability did not take place when the cells were exposed to ultrasound under conditions which suppressed cavitation (Mortimer and Dyson, 1988).

2. *Acoustic streaming*: This is the unidirectional circulatory movement of fluid induced by radiation forces. High-velocity gradients are produced next to boundaries between the fluid and discontinuities produced by cells and bubbles. The high viscous forces associated with these gradients can modify membrane structure; by temporarily altering membrane permeability to second messengers such as calcium ions, cell activity can be affected in a manner which could be of therapeutic value (Dyson, 1985). The transport of some molecules across the plasma membrane may also be accelerated. It has been suggested that increased uptake of calcium ions by fibroblasts following exposure to 1 MHz ultrasound, at I(SAPA) of 0.5 W/cm^2, pulsed 2 ms on, 8 ms off, *in vitro* may be due to shear forces produced by acoustic streaming. This is probably associated with stable cavitation (Mortimer and Dyson, 1988), but can occur in its absence as a result of radiation torque (Nyborg, 1985). As indicated earlier, temporarily increased calcium ion concentration could be an intracellular signal for a cascade of events in a range of cells involved in, and resulting in the acceleration of, the repair process. In fibroblasts an increase in protein synthesis would be expected. It could also explain the observed increase in the liberation of serotonin (and possibly chemotactic agents) from platelets (Williams, 1974), of histamine (and possibly angiogenic heparin and other chemotactic agents) from mast cells (Fyfe and Chahl, 1982), and of growth factors from macrophages (Young, 1988). All these effects could collectively assist in producing the observed acceleration of tissue repair which can follow exposure to ultrasound therapy.
3. *Standing waves*: These can be formed when ultrasound is reflected at the interface between two acoustically different media, for example soft tissue and bone or soft tissue and air. In a standing wave the pressure peaks (or pressure antinodes) of the incident and reflected waves are superimposed, stationary in position, and separated by half a wavelength. Midway between the pressure antinodes are nodes at which the pressure is zero. Cells in suspension collect at the nodes while gas bubbles collect at the antinodes (NCRP Report No. 74, 1983). The enhanced acoustic streaming (or microstreaming) occurring around the bubbles could, if excessive, irreversibly damage the membranes of immobile cells such as the endothelial cells of blood vessels, producing the damage which has been observed in these cells after exposure to standing waves (Dyson *et al.*, 1974); reversible blood cell stasis has also been observed, the cells forming bands, half a wavelength apart, centred on the pressure nodes. Although reflection from appropriate interfaces is inevitable, tissue damage can be avoided if the applicator is moved continuously during exposure to UT, so that the positions of the nodes and antinodes are never stationary.

In summary, both thermal and non-thermal effects may produce clinically significant changes in injured soft tissues. If the heating achieved raises the tissue to between 40 and 45°C this may be beneficial, provided that transient caviation and standing wave formation are avoided. The stimulation of tissue repair can also be achieved at intensities too low to induce a clinically significant amount of heating, suggesting that predominantly non-thermal mechanisms, such as acoustic streaming and/or stable cavitation, may be involved in their production.

To ensure that observed effects can be repeated, it is essential that all relevant information on exposure is measured and recorded. Where thermal mechanisms are implicated, intensity is a particularly important parameter, whereas for non-thermal mechanisms other variables are of greater significance. For example, the incidence of cavitation is related to the extent of the pressure changes induced by ultrasound; it may therefore be more appropriate to measure output in terms of acoustic pressure amplitude (in atmospheres or megapascals) than intensity (NCRP Report No. 74, 1983).

Effects of therapeutic ultrasound on injured soft tissues

As indicated previously, soft tissue injury is generally followed by repair – a complex series of interrelated cellular events, subdivided for descriptive convenience into three overlapping phases: inflammation, proliferation and remodelling. The effect of ultrasound on each of these phases is considered below.

1. *Inflammatory phase*: If therapeutic levels of ultrasound are applied to injured tissues shortly after injury, the inflammatory phase can be reduced in duration and the repair process thereby accelerated, provided that the inflammatory stimulus is removed (Dyson, 1987). A single treatment of ultrasound at an output level of I(SAPA) = 0.5 W/cm^2 can stimulate mast cell degranulation in injured tissues (Fyfe and Chahl, 1982), liberating chemotactic agents which attract polymorphonuclear leukocytes and monocytes to the wound site and in doing so ensure that wound healing begins. This is far lower than the level required in intact tissue (Dyson and Luke, 1986), indicating that the prior exposure of the cells to injury causes an increase in the sensitivity of the cells to ultrasound. Ultrasonic stimulation of the release of chemotactic agents and other repair-stimulating materials from mast cells may, at least in part, explain why the early treatment of soft tissue injuries is so effective. Degranulation of mast cells is generally a response to changes in membrane permeability which permit increased transport of calcium ions into the cells (Yurt, 1981). Although it is not known if therapeutic ultrasound affects the transport of calcium ions into mast cells, there is evidence that it does so in fibroblasts (Mortimer and Dyson, 1988) and, presumably, also in other cell types.

In response to chemotactic factors released at the wound site, monocytes leave the circulating blood, enter the injured tissue and develop into macrophages. Polymorphonuclear leukocytes are also attracted to the injured tissue, and, together with the macrophages, these cells remove bacteria and debris phagocytically, and also release other chemotactic materials and growth factors which stimulate pericytes, fibroblasts and endothelial cells to form granulation tissue at the wound site. It has been shown by Young and Dyson (1990) that exposure to therapeutic levels of ultrasound can result in the release of factors which can stimulate fibroblast proliferation from U937 cells, a type of macrophage which can be maintained *in vitro*. The results obtained suggest that UT should be applied shortly after injury, provided that bleeding has ceased, and should be continued throughout inflammation and into the proliferative phase, i.e. whenever there are macrophages at or near the wound site.

Although treatment with therapeutic levels of ultrasound reduces the duration of the inflammatory phase of repair, so that the proliferative phase begins earlier, it is not an anti-inflammatory agent. Research on the resolution of postoperative oedema clinically (Hashish, 1986) has demonstrated that what appeared to be an anti-inflammatory effect of low-intensity ultrasound was primarily a placebo effect, spatial average pulse average intensities of 0.5 W/cm^2 and higher being proinflammatory, although this was masked to some extent by the 'anti-inflammatory' placebo effect of treatment with ultrasound.

2. *Proliferative phase*: In addition to reducing the length of the inflammatory phase of repair, possibly by encouraging the release of growth factors and other agents which stimulate fibroblast and endothelial cell activity, non-thermal levels of ultrasound can also affect these cells directly. When fibroblasts are exposed to therapeutic levels of ultrasound *in vitro* their secretion of collagen can be stimulated (Harvey *et al.*, 1976). It is possible that this is in response to a temporary increase produced by the ultrasound in the calcium ion content of the cells resulting from reversible changes in membrane permeability. It has been suggested that shear stresses associated with acoustic streaming (microstreaming) and/or stable cavitation may be responsible for these effects *in vitro* (Mortimer and Dyson, 1988). There is evidence that non-thermal levels of ultrasound can also stimulate fibroblast activity *in vivo* (Webster, 1980), and may produce what is presumably stable cavitation within the tissues (ter Haar and Daniels, 1981), but whether or not these are causally related is as yet uncertain.

   Wound contraction, which is initiated during the inflammatory phase of repair and continues during the proliferative phase, can be accelerated by non-thermal levels of ultrasound (Dyson and Smalley, 1983). The activity of the myofibroblasts, the specialized contractile and secretory cells which are responsible both for wound contraction and the secretion of matrix materials of granulation tissue (Gabbiani *et al.*, 1971), is presumably affected. Myofibroblasts resemble smooth muscle cells, the contraction of which can be induced by exposure to therapeutic levels of ultrasound (ter Haar *et al.*, 1978). It is possible that myofibroblasts are affected in a similar manner, although they could also be affected indirectly via the ultrasonic induction of growth factor secretion from macrophages. Interestingly, no reports have been found of abnormally excessive contraction, that is, of contracture, following treatment with ultrasound therapy. Contraction occurs more rapidly, but remains under the control of local factors.

   The hypothesis that the stimulation of dermal repair by non-thermal levels of ultrasound applied in the inflammatory and early proliferative phases of repair is due to an acceleration of these processes has been supported experimentally. Quantitative assessments made of the different types of cells present at the wound site have shown that macrophages move into the wound site more rapidly following exposure to therapeutic levels of ultrasound than in control, sham-irradiated wounds, and that they are followed more rapidly by fibroblasts and endothelial cells (Young, 1988). This indicates that wounds treated with low-level ultrasound [0.1 W/cm^2 I(SATA)] have a shorter inflammatory phase than do sham-irradiated controls, and that the proliferative phase begins more rapidly.

   As well as affecting mast cells, macrophages and fibroblasts, exposure to low levels of ultrasound can also encourage angiogenesis, stimulating endothelial cell activity directly and/or indirectly. It has been observed that in chronically ischaemic muscle, capillaries develop more rapidly when the tissue is treated with ultrasound (Hogan *et al.*, 1982). The development of blood capillaries and other vessels in granulation tissue at the site of excised lesions of the skin is also accelerated following exposure to ultrasound (Hosseinpour, 1988). This stimulation of angiogenesis may be due to the enhanced release of angiogenic growth factors from mast cells and macrophages, the degranulation of both of which is stimulated by low levels of ultrasound (Fyfe and Chahl, 1982; Young, 1988).

3. *Remodelling phase*: Attempts at improving the mechanical properties of scar tissue by treatment with therapeutic levels of ultrasound

during the remodelling phase of repair have been met with variable degrees of success (Bierman, 1954; Lehmann *et al.*, 1961). More impressive results have been obtained when treatment is commenced shortly after injury, during the early part of the inflammatory phase, and continued during the proliferative phase. When full-thickness excised skin wounds were exposed to low levels of ultrasound [0.1 W/cm^2 I(SATA)] three times a week for the first 2 weeks after injury, the scar tissue which developed at the wound site was significantly stronger and also more elastic than that of sham-irradiated wounds (Webster, 1980). The increased tensile strength and energy absorbance before rupture found in the ultrasonically treated wounds is associated with the observed increase in collagen synthesis in such wounds, while the increased elasticity may be associated with a change in collagen fibre pattern. The pattern in ultrasonically treated scar tissue resembled the three-dimensional lattice arrangement found in uninjured dermis, whereas that in sham-irradiated scar tissue was less regular (Dyson, 1981). It has been suggested that reversible changes in fibre angle in the lattice arrangement in response to the application of a tensile force to the tissue would permit a limited amount of extension and subsequent recoil when the force was reduced and the fibres returned to their original position, as well as increasing the amount of energy which the scar tissue could absorb before rupturing (Forrester, 1973). Similar improvements in the mechanical properties of injured tendons have been observed following exposure to therapeutic levels of ultrasound (Enwemaka, 1988).

In conclusion, treatment with therapeutic ultrasound, when applied correctly, can accelerate the repair of soft tissue injuries and improve the mechanical properties of the scar tissue; effects are greatest when treatment is during the inflammatory and early proliferative phases of repair. Low levels of ultrasound accelerate the inflammatory phase, and appear to do so by modifying the permeability to calcium ions of the plasma membranes of growth factor-secreting cells such as macrophages. It is suggested that this reversible increase in intracellular calcium ions acts as a second messenger, triggering growth factor synthesis and secretion by the cells affected. The ultrasonically induced release of growth factors from mast cells and macrophages can stimulate the activity of other cells involved in the reparative process, for example, fibroblasts and endothelial cells. Ultrasound may also affect these cells directly, again via reversible changes in the permeability of their membranes, and in doing so could lead to the enhanced synthesis and secretion of matrix materials such as collagen (Webster, 1981) and changes in cell motility (Mummery, 1978) which have been recorded following exposure to UT, and which can result in improved healing.

References

Bierman W (1954) Ultrasound in the treatment of scars. *Archives of Physical Medicine* **35**, 209–213.

Brueton RH and Campbell B (1987) The use of Geliperm as a sterile coupling agent for therapeutic ultrasound. *Physiotherapy* **73**, 653–654.

Callam MJ, Harper DR, Dale JJ, Ruckley CV and Prescott RJ (1987) A controlled trial of weekly ultrasound therapy in chronic leg ulceration. *Lancet* **ii**, 204.

Clark RAF (1985) Cutaneous repair: basic biologic considerations. I. *Journal of the American Academy of Dermatology* **13**, 701–725.

Crum LA, Daniels S, Dyson M, ter Haar GR and Walton AJ (1986) Acoustic cavitation and medical ultrasound. *Proceedings of the Institute of Acoustics* **8**, 137–146.

Docker M, Foulkes DJ and Patrick MK (1982) Ultrasound couplants for physiotherapy. *Physiotherapy* **68**, 124–125.

Dyson M (1981) The effect of ultrasound on the rate of wound healing and the quality of scar tissue. In *Proceedings of the International Symposium on Therapeutic Ultrasound* (Manitoba, 1981) (eds. A. M. Mortimer and N. Lee), Canadian Physiotherapy Association, Winnipeg, pp. 110–123.

Dyson M (1985) Therapeutic applications of ultrasound. *Clinics in Diagnostic Ultrasound* **16**, 121–134.

Dyson M (1987) Mechanisms involved in therapeutic ultrasound. *Physiotherapy* **73**, 116–120.

Dyson M (1988). The use of ultrasound in sports

physiotherapy. In International Perspectives in Physical Therapy. (series eds. I Bromley and N Watts), *Sports Injuries* (ed. V Grisogono), Churchill Livingstone, Edinburgh, pp. 213–232.

Dyson M (1990) Role of ultrasound in wound healing. In Contemporary Perspectives in Rehabilitation (series ed. S Wolff), *Wound Healing: Alternatives in Management* (eds. LC Kloth, J Feeder and J McCullough), FA Davis Company, Philadelphia, pp. 229–285.

Dyson M and Luke DA (1986) Induction of mast cell degranulation in skin by ultrasound. *Institute of Electrical and Electronic Engineers, Transactions on Ultrasonics, Ferroelectrics and Frequency Control*, URRC-33(2), 104–201.

Dyson M and Smalley D (1983) Effects of ultrasound on wound contraction. In *Ultrasound Interactions in Biology and Medicine* (eds. R Millner and U Corbet), Plenum, New York, pp. 121–158.

Dyson M, Pond J, Woodward B and Broadbent J (1974) The production of blood cell stasis and endothelial cell damage in the blood vessels of chick embryos treated with ultrasound in a stationary wave field. *Ultrasound in Medicine and Biology* **1**, 133–148.

Dyson M, Franks C and Suckling J (1976) Stimulation of healing of varicose ulcers by ultrasound. *Ultrasonics* **14**, 232–236.

Dyson M, Webster DF, Pell R and Crowder M (1979) Improvement in the mechanical properties of scar tissue following treatment with therapeutic ultrasound *in vivo*. In: *Proceedings of the Fourth European Symposium on Ultrasound in Biology and Medicine* (ed. P Greguss), Vol. 1, Technical University, Budapest, pp 129–134.

Enwemaka C (1989) The effects of therapeutic ultrasound on tendon healing. A Biomechanical Study. *American Journal of Physical Medicine and Rehabilitation* **68**, 283–287.

Forrester JC (1973) Mechanical, biochemical and architectural features of surgical repair. *Advances in Biological and Medical Physics* **14**, 1–34.

Fyfe MC and Chahl LA (1982). Mast cell degranulation: a possible mechanism of action of therapeutic ultrasound. *Ultrasound in Medicine and Biology* **8**(Suppl. 1), 62.

Gabbiani G, Ryan GB and Majno G (1971) Presence of modified fibroblasts in granulation tissue and their possible role in wound contraction. *Experientia* (Basel), **27**, 549.

Harvey W, Dyson M, Pond J and Grahame R. (1975). The *in vitro* stimulation of protein synthesis in human fibroblasts by therapeutic levels of ultrasound. In *Proceedings of the Second European Congress on Ultrasonics in Medicine*, Excerpta Medica Congress Series No. 363, Excerpta Medica, Amsterdam, pp. 10–21.

Hashish II (1986) The effect of ultrasound therapy on post-operative inflammation. PhD Thesis, University of London.

Hogan RD, Burke KM and Franklin TD (1982) The effect of ultrasound on microvascular hemodynamics in skeletal muscle: effects during ischemia. *Microvascular Research* **23**, 370.

Hoogland R (1986) *Ultrasound Therapy*, Delft. Enraf-Nonius, Holland.

Hosseinpour AR (1988) The effects of ultrasound on angiogenesis and wound healing. BSc Thesis. University of London.

Hunt TK and Van Winkle Jr W (1979) Normal repair. In *Fundamentals of Wound Management* (eds. TK Hunt and JE Dunphy), Appleton-Century-Crofts, New York, pp 2–67.

Lehmann JF *et al.* (1961) Clinical evaluation of a new approach in the treatment of contracture associated hip fracture after internal fixation. *Archives of Physical Medicine and Rehabilitation* **42**, 95.

Liebovich SJ and Ross R (1975) The role of the macrophage in wound repair. *American Journal of Pathology* **78**, 71–92.

Low J and Reed A (1990) *Electrotherapy: Principles and Practice*, Heinemann Medical, Oxford.

McDiarmid T and Burns PN (1987) Clinical applications of therapeutic ultrasound. *Physiotherapy* **73**, 155.

Mortimer AJ and Dyson M (1988) The effect of therapeutic ultrasound on calcium uptake in fibroblasts. *Ultrasound in Medicine and Biology* **14**, 499–506.

Mummery CL (1978) The effect of ultrasound on fibroblasts *in vitro*. PhD Thesis, University of London.

NCRP Scientific Committee 66 (1983) *Biological effects of ultrasound: mechanisms and clinical implications.* NCRP Report No. 74. National Council on Radiation Protection and Measurements, Bethesda, MD.

Nyborg WL (1985) Acoustic streaming. In *Physical Acoustics*, Vol. 2, part B. Academic Press, New York, p. 265.

Oakley EM (1978) Application of continuous beam ultrasound at therapeutic levels. *Physiotherapy* **64**, 103.

Patrick MK (1978) Applications of therapeutic pulsed ultrasound. *Physiotherapy* **64**, 169.

ter Haar GR (1987) Basic physics of therapeutic ultrasound. *Physiotherapy* **73**, 110.

ter Haar GR and Daniels S (1981) Evidence for ultrasonically induced cavitation *in vivo*. *Physics in Medicine and Biology* **26**, 1145–1149.

ter Haar GR, Dyson M and Talbert D (1978) Ultrasonically induced cavitation *in vivo*. *Ultrasonics* **16**, 275–276.

Trabucchi E, Radaelli E, Marazzi M *et al.* (1988) The role of mast cells in wound healing. *International Journal of Tissue Reactions*. **X**(6), 367–372.

Watmough DJ, Davies HM, Quan KM, Wytch R and Williams AR (1991) *Ultrasonics* **29**, 312–318.

Webster DF (1980) The effect of ultrasound on wound healing. PhD Thesis, University of London.

Williams AR (1974) Release of serotonin from human platelets by acoustic microsteaming. *Journal of the Acoustic Society of America* **56**, 1640–1643.

Williams AR (1987) Production and transmission of ultrasound. *Physiotherapy* **73**, 113.

Young SR (1988) The effect of therapeutic ultrasound on the biological mechanisms involved in dermal repair. PhD Thesis, University of London.

Young SR and Dyson M (1990) Macrophage responsiveness to therapeutic ultrasound. *Ultrasound in Medicine and Biology* **16**, 809–816.

Yurt RW (1981) Role of mast cells in trauma. In: *The Surgical Wound*. (ed. B Dineen and G Hildick-Smith). Philadelphia, Lea and Febiger, p. 125.

12

Injuries to the head and spine

J. A. Vafidis

Introduction

Minor injuries to the head and neck are commonplace in sport, as in life itself. The odd bang on the head, sprained neck or pulled back are generally considered to be part and parcel of an active sporting life. Serious injury thankfully is rare but may result in permanent paralysis or death. However while these can be seen as opposite ends of the spectrum of severity, the mechanisms of injury are much the same, the sports and circumstances of injury often identical. In this sort of injury we can recognize three different elements. First, the actual injuring episode, in this case almost always a collision involving a blow to the head or body resulting in among other things a forced flexion, extension or twisting of the spine. Second, the injury produced by this, and last, the resulting disability. The relationship between these elements involves several factors which must be understood. These include the force and direction of the blow as well as its site and the anatomical and functional defences of the victim.

At the end of the day all such injuring episodes are potentially dangerous and the outcome will vary from the commonest benign musculoskeletal injury to severe neurological disability. Somewhere in the middle and largely unrecognized are those injuries which predispose to further injury, which weaken defences without in themselves producing a bad outcome, or if repeated and taken cumulatively, result in chronic problems, both neurological and structural. This intermediate group is the subject of much study and controversy. The stakes are high – sport is a recreational activity and permanent disability is a very high price to pay for it.

Incidence

The incidence of such injuries is hard to calculate. Most undoubtedly remain unreported because they are transient, mild and not considered to be more than the normal result of sporting activity. Furthermore it can be difficult to estimate the total number of both organized and informal participants in any particular sport. The level at which one participates does not seem to influence the vulnerability, except that the less well-regulated the sporting event and the less well-disciplined the player, the more likely the injury. Certainly, when reviewing risk factors (Davies, 1980), it has been shown that foul play in rugby was relevant in about a third of cases. The rules are often framed with one eye on player safety. Lack of fitness and familiarity with the sport seem to increase the risk further; there tends to be a higher incidence early in the sporting season.

No particular sport is entirely immune to the risk of head and spinal injury. All that is needed is a potential for impact at speed. However, some sports are recognized as particularly prone to such injuries. Notable among these are the team contact sports, rugby and American football. It seems that in Rugby football over 50% of participants when asked by confidential questionnaire, admitted to a head injury involving a period of amnesia, in many cases on more than one occasion. It seems therefore that brain injury is both common and unreported in a majority of cases. What information there is about cervical injury is hampered by similar under-reporting of minor injuries; severe injuries are reported in rugby in about one per 333 000 player–match exposures. (Burry and Gowland, 1981). Typically, perhaps, more thorough studies can be found relating to American football (Maroon *et al.*, 1980), which suggests that perhaps one in 20 experience a head injury resulting in some degree of concussion, while for serious spinal injuries a rate of about 1/60 000 participants per year is reported. The value of statistics is to highlight the frequency of injury but it must be realized that serious injury can occur at any time, and no sport or sporting occasion is guaranteed not to produce one. What is more valuable than the statistics is the light thrown on the mechanisms of injury by these studies.

Other team games carry the risk of accidental collision but the incidence of serious damage is very low. In association football, for example, the actual risk of damage is relatively low but because so many people play the sport it accounts for a fairly high proportion of injuries. Studies have used football as an example of a sport providing the opportunity for repeated minor injuries, some not even severe enough to classify as injuries in the accepted sense. Evidence is growing that both accelerated cervical spine degeneration (Sortland *et al.*, 1982) and even cerebral atrophy (Sortland and Tysvaer, 1989) may be seen in professional participants. This does not seem to be clinically evident (Tysvaer and Storli, 1981; Sortland *et al.*, 1982), but it can be seen on X-rays and scans.

Sports which have accidental collision, not with other players but with the ground, often at high speeds, such as horse riding (Barber 1973; Ilgren *et al.*, 1984) and skiing (Sahlin, 1988), have a high incidence of head and spinal injuries and in particular of serious injuries. In these cases the injury generally is accidental or the result of foul play but in the case of boxing the aim in part is to inflict a brain injury. This sport is out on its own both in terms of moderate head injury and chronic side-effects of repeated minor injuries (Lancet, 1973).

Mechanisms of injury

Head injuries

Head injuries are usually the result of impact, the blow being to the head. There are two components of this capable of doing damage. The first is the blow itself. The skull is a very good defence against this and unless the force and implement are such that the skull is fractured and the underlying brain directly contused – very uncommon in both sport and civilian life – this is not usually a cause of much damage. What is more common and a potent cause of brain injury is the sudden jarring of the head as a result of the blow. The whole head is accelerated, causing the brain to impact against the inside of the skull and dural partitions, producing surface contusions. In addition the force tends to produce shearing between those parts of the brain which are mobile and those which are fixed, as well as between parts of the brain with different densities. This disrupts brain pathways and tears small blood vessels, with the result that the damage may be both widespread and severe. The torn blood vessels may be of such a calibre that the resulting bleeding can cause a sizeable clot within the brain or subdural space. Clots within the extradural space are the result of skull or dural damage and in adults especially are generally associated with a skull fracture.

Although the force required to fracture the skull often results in a degree of brain injury as well, where the blow is directed to an area of the skull where the bone is thin and relatively easily fractured, for example the temple, the amount of jarring of the head and resulting diffuse brain injury may be relatively slight and its effects transient. Several factors influence the extent of the damage: first the magnitude of the blow and to some extent the direction; that producing rotation is particularly dangerous. Secondly, there is the degree to which the head is fixed – the amount of bracing of the neck in anticipation of the blow, which reflects the awareness of the victim of the threat of injury. In boxing this can be seen quite graphically. The recipient of the knockdown blow is either distracted by a feint or incapacitated by a

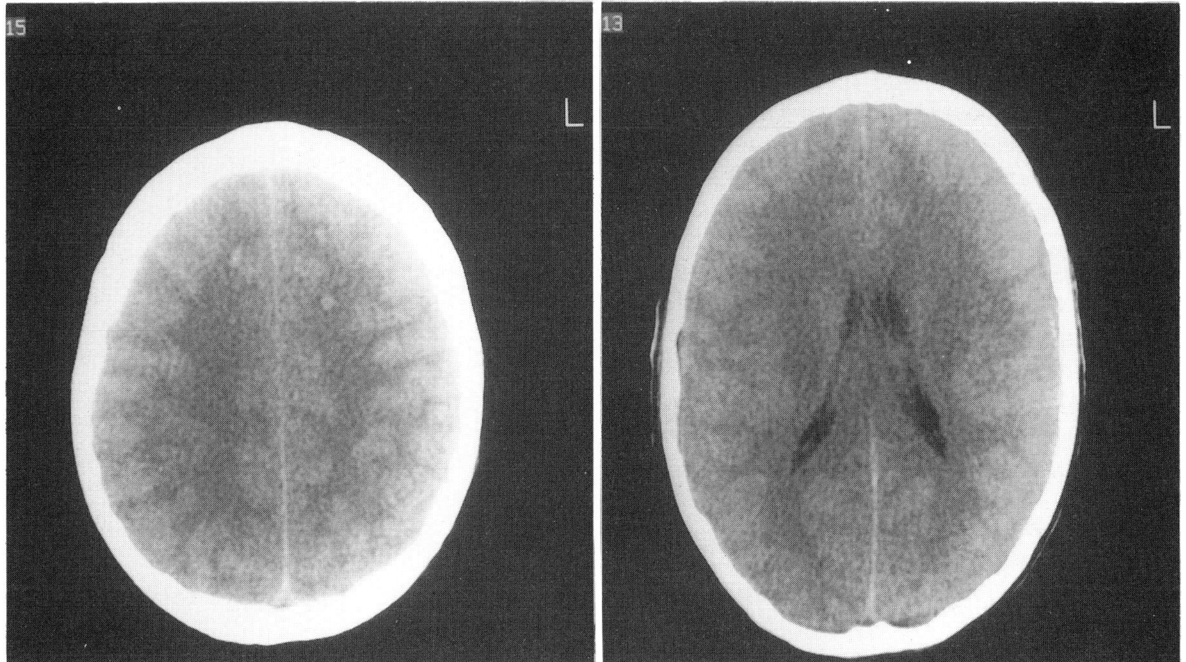

Figs. 12.1 and 12.2 Computed tomography scans of acute brain swelling following deceleration injury. Note the lack of cerebral sulci and the pinched ventricles implying raised pressure. Furthermore there are small haemorrhages in the white matter (arrowed).

previous battering and cannot anticipate the blow. The head, previously held steady to receive blows, is jolted violently by the punch. On falling to the ground, all protective reflexes gone, the head strikes the canvas hard, thus accelerating the contents in the opposite direction. Thus the brain receives two or three accelerations within a very short time, each tending to compound the effect of the others. This is the recipe for severe widespread injury (Figs. 12.1–12.3).

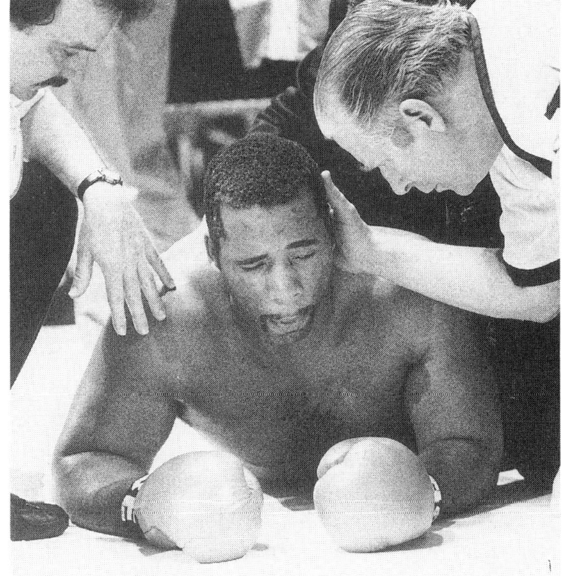

Fig. 12.3

Cervical spine injuries

Similar circumstances accompany cervical spine injuries. The anatomy of the area is so designed to produce a mobile structure and at the same time to protect the upper spinal cord which runs throughout the length of it. The cervical vertebrae are thus tightly connected to each other by the shape of their articulating surfaces, the strength of the intervertebral ligaments – in particular the nuchal ligament – and by the numerous strong muscles. Direct blows to the neck rarely cause damage to the vertebral complex and its contained spinal cord. It must be remembered, however, that some of the structures in the neck are vulnerable to direct blunt injury, for example the larynx, the carotid arteries and even the upper branchial plexus.

However most injuries are caused by blows to the head causing forced hyperflexion, extension, lateral flexion or rotation of the whole neck. Often this is accompanied by force applied along the axis of the neck itself. The most dangerous situation seems to be collision, with the force being applied to the top of the head when the neck is flexed. In flexion the neck is at its most unstable with regard to the bony articulation and the soft tissue elements; the strong extensor muscles and major ligaments are at full stretch. Thus both bony dislocation and disruption of stabilizing mechanisms can occur. In flexion with force applied along the axis of the cervical spine there is, in theory, a risk of rupture of the intervertebral disc when the posterior annulus is stretched and the nucleus pulposus is under tension, but in practice this seems to be relatively uncommon. Especially in young people the intervertebral disc is a very strong structure and unlikely to rupture in the absence of severe disruption of other elements. With less severe forces muscles and ligaments are vulnerable to sprain and partial rupture, which may not however materially affect the mechanical strength of the neck. Extension injuries are less dangerous from the purely mechanical point of view because the structure is more stable in this position and perhaps behavioural reflexes are more relevant: the victim receives a blow from in front and from this angle he or she is more aware of it. Severe lateral flexion may disrupt the lateral masses of the cervical vertibrae but tend to produce crush fractures rather than soft tissue injuries. Thus while the magnitude of the force is important it is the interplay of direction of impact and anatomical features which determines the nature and severity of injury and behavioural responses are relevant.

Neurological injury may occur in assocation with mechanical disturbance or may be seen in the absence of any apparent residual abnormality of either alignment or stability. Where gross dislocation or associated disc prolapse occurs the cord may be directly damaged, producing severe and often permanent deficit. Where there is no structural damage of the spinal column, neural injury can still occur; this usually tends to recover and is termed, somewhat loosely, spinal cord concussion (Schneider, 1973). The mechanism of this is unknown but it is suggested that it is akin to brain concussion with jarring of the cord producing transient loss of function. Anatomical studies show that between flexion and extension there is considerable movement up and down by the cord (Adams and Logue, 1971) and it may be that concussion is a stretch phenomenon.

The brachial plexus is vulnerable in contact sports and those involving heavy falls, such as skiing and horse riding. This is not so much a result of its vulnerable position in the supraclavicular fossa, although it may be theoretically contused by direct blows immediately above the clavicle and lacerated in the same area. However the commonest cause of injury is a blow to the shoulder, producing a traction injury. The plexus leads to the nerves of the arm and when the upper limb is forcibly depressed it is stretched between its origin at the cervical spine and the arm, where it is tethered. The peripheral nerves are mechanically tough structures which resist stretching and, in the case of the brachial plexus, the weakest point is the insertion of the nerve roots into the spinal cord, from which they are avulsed, causing as well as root deficit a varying degree of intrinsic spinal cord damage mostly from bleeding into the cord. In this respect the upper roots (C5 and C6) are the most often damaged but forced abduction of the arm can avulse the lower roots by a similar mechanism (C8 and T1).

Lumbar spine

The lumbar spine is similar to the cervical spine in its anatomy but differs in the context of acute injury in that it is much stronger, better protected by the muscles of the posterior abdominal wall and less mobile. The forces required to disrupt it are therefore much greater and generally beyond those of most sports injuries. However where forces are great, as in equestrianism, skiing, hang-gliding and motor sports, such magnitude may be achieved. The line of force is usually in the axis of the lumbar spine, causing crush fracture of the upper lumbar vertebrae. The fragments may encroach on the vertebral canal, causing direct injury to what is at this level the conus medullaris or upper cauda equina. Severe forces in flexion, unlike in the cervica spine, tend to cause fractures rather than rupture of ligaments or muscles, such is the relative strength of the structural elements at this level. Most acute injuries of the lumbar spine are muscular sprains caused by twisting and perhaps flexion movements. There are various ways of producing this injury but usually it is caused by the momentum of the body with the legs held, as in a rugby tackle. It must be noted that serious injuries in this area are rare and the majority are acute exacerbations of chronic injury. The uncommon prolapsed intervertebral disc is similarly not the immediate result of injury but more a case of a particular movement provoking a prolapse in an already degenerate disc. The role of a vigorous sporting life in contributing to the degenerative process is a matter of debate.

Assessment of injury

History

As with all medical assessment, an accurate history is important. This should be sought from witnesses as well as from the victim. What must be established is the exact circumstances of the injury and the condition of the victim in the immediate aftermath. In particular it is important to obtain any history of apparent unconsciousness and subsequent disorientation. Further, any abnormal posturing, however brief, is significant in suggesting neurological damage. Questioning the patient should seek to show any period of amnesia, indicating brain injury. The presence – even transiently – of tingling, electric shock-like sensations, numbness or pain away from the injured area will raise the possibility of spinal or nerve root damage.

Examination

It is not necessary to outline in detail what is involved in examining the patient. It should be noted, however, that until the possibility of spinal injury has been excluded the patient should not be moved. Essentially what is required is a quick assessment of the conscious state and the limbs to demonstrate any paralysis or areas of numbness.

Conscious level

This is the cornerstone of the assessment of brain function. Conscious level is difficult to define unambiguously but full consciousness in the clinical situation could be defined as the state of spontaneous eye opening, with coherent and appropriate speech and ability to obey commands. Degrees of unconsciousness are assessed by the Glasgow Coma Scale (Table 12.1). This is used in most hospitals and therefore should be applied from the outset so that there is a continuum of compatible observations from the time of injury. This must be assessed separately from the examination of focal deficit. Thus if one shows a paralysed arm it is the response in the normal arm which should be noted. This gives an overall guide to the functioning of the brain. In the context of acute concussive head injury, however, it is perhaps slightly crude and should be enlarged to take account of the degree of orientation. This can be gained from brief questioning of the patient, asking about immediate events and places. Merely to know one's name and address is not necessarily evidence of full awareness.

Movements

The examination of the motor system must establish as much as possible that the patient can move all muscle groups with normal strength. Clearly to be complete, this will be time-consuming and is not practicable in the immediate first-aid situation. Fortunately, in the immediate post-injury

Table 12.1 The Glasgow Coma Scale

Eye opening
4 Spontaneous eye opening
3 Eye opening to command
2 Eye opening to pain
1 No eye opening

Verbal response
5 Coherent appropriate response
4 Coherent inappropriate response
3 Incoherent speech
2 Non-speech noises, moans, groans etc.
1 No vocalization

Motor response
6 Obeying commands
5 Localizing purposeful response to pain
4 Purposeful withdrawal to pain, non-localizing
3 Reflex flexion to pain (arms; decorticate posturing)
2 Reflex extension to pain (arms; decerebrate posturing)
1 No motor response to pain

Notes
1. While it is possible to evaluate conscious or unconscious level in terms of numbers (from 3 to 15), this does not aid communication. Stick to brief descriptions.
2. Observe the best response only.
3. This scale is designed to be quick and easy, to require no specialized examination skills, have little interobserver variation and be widely known. Arguably it is the last factor which has let it down; it is poorly taught, even among medical students.

phase, weakness tends to be profound and usually asking the patient to perform arm and leg movements will indicate weakness.

Sensation

Perhaps testing sensation by eliciting awareness of light touch is easier. If an abnormality is found by comparison with the other side or with other areas of the body it can be refined using pinprick and joint position sense.

In practice, exhaustive motor and sensory testing can be prolonged; in fact, what neurologists do is look for evidence of recognizable patterns of deficit. One can tell a great deal about any focal abnormality by the company it keeps. Without pretending to be in any way exhaustive, the major patterns are as follows.

From brain abnormality
Weakness is usually confined to one side – hemiplegia, often with involvement of the face, arm, and maybe the leg. Sensory abnormality is often mild, affecting the same side. In the absence of drowsiness focal abnormality from damage to the brain is very unlikely in the acute phase.

Spinal deficit
Here we seek evidence of a level, that is a point above which there is no abnormality and below a varying degree of weakness and numbness. Usually in the case of spinal injury the findings will be bilateral. The other feature of spinal lesions, especially when partial, is that different sensory modalities are transmitted through different pathways, thus there can be evidence of dissociated sensory loss – areas numb to pinprick but with preserved joint position sense and vice versa. The most dramatic finding in unilateral spinal lesions is that the numbness to pinprick (spinothalamic sensation) is on the opposite side to the weakness, whereas the loss of joint position sense (posterior column sensation) is on the same side. This is the Brown–Séquard syndrome.

Nerve root deficit
In this case there is usually weakness of a specific movement, depending on the root involved and numbness within a specific dermatome, the area supplied by that particular root. However these sensory zones overlap considerably and with a single root lesion the numbness may be confined to a small area in the middle of the dermatome or may be absent altogether. The numbness will be to all sensory modalities. In brachial plexus injuries an additional finding may be a Horner's syndrome, ipsilateral ptosis, small pupil and absence of sweating on the ipsilateral half of the face. This is probably a result of local spinal damage caused by the avulsion. Apparent bilateral root lesions are more than likely to be spinal damage.

Peripheral nerve lesions
Here the pattern of sensory and motor loss will conform to the destination of the nerve distal to the damaged segment. It will rarely conform to dermatomal or myotomal distribution and in the

case of sensory loss there is much less overlap between nerves than with nerve roots, so one can usually identify a clear area of complete numbness.

In practice the deficits produced by trauma are not usually subtle and a recognition of the pattern of loss will usually make the site of damage clear. The significance of upper and lower motor neuron weakness may be mentioned only to state that it is not particularly relevant in acute injuries. The classical picture of an upper motor neuron weakness, that from a lesion above the anterior horn cell and characterized by hypertonicity, increased reflexes and absence of wasting, does not occur acutely. All weaknesses will tend to be flaccid and the reflexes lost, although in some cases of hemiplegia from a brain lesion there may be more typical findings.

Management of head and spinal injuries

In this context, management can be defined as any measure which improves outcome. Recognizing the crucial feature of neurological trauma – that once damaged, the system may not mend itself nor can even the most sophisticated treatment repair it – it is clear that prevention is extremely important. Indeed it is not overstating the situation to say that prevention is the main aim – prevention if possible of the potentially injuring incidents, prevention of injury to those involved in those incidents and prevention of avoidable neurological damage to those injured. A clear-minded assessment is therefore important to recognize the damaging potential of any situation, to identify the possibility of injury to any involved individual and pinpoint the evidence of injury when it does occur. Management thus begins at the very starting point of any sport, deciding how and under what rules it should be played.

Avoidance of potentially injuring incidents

It is probably the case that if safety were taken to the ultimate degree there would be very few sporting activities. However in deciding rules and regulations the nature of both injury-prone situations and injury-prone participants should and has been taken into account. Thus the lessons learnt from analysing cervical injuries in rugby and American football have resulted in training stressing the dangerous nature of tackling head-on with the neck flexed (Williams and McKibbin, 1977; Maroon *et al.*, 1980). Similarly, rules on the collapsed scrum have resulted from the same observations. Most are agreed that it is those episodes where contact is made – the scrum ruck, but most often the tackle – that account for most injuries (Addley and Farren, 1988).

Avoidance of injury to participants

This is a large area of study, given that in sport there will always be potentially injuring situations. There are two aspects of this: the formulation of rules outlawing dangerous practices and, equally important, the visible enforcement of these. It is of little use to punish a violator when the victim is rendered disabled. The rules should act as a deterrent to injury. With this must come a concerted effort to educate participants in both the mechanisms of injury as well as their effect. The sometimes heroic achievements of paraplegics, tetraplegics and brain-injured people can often detract from the realization of the devastating effect of these disabilities. It cannot be overstressed that in terms of individual and collective suffering, neurological injury is utterly horrible and is not a prospect to be taken lightly. It is important to make it totally unacceptable to take risks which might visit this horror on either one's opponent or oneself, and in consequence spouses, children and society in general. Thus there is no doubt that education is of the first order of importance.

These situations will probably always exist in sport and participants cannot be expected to be able to take avoiding action. What do our studies tell us of how serious injury can be avoided? It is often noticed that injuries tend to occur early in the season (Sparks, 1985), suggesting that physical fitness and lack of immediate match experience may predispose to such injuries. General fitness is important before anyone participates in these dangerous pastimes. Further attention to the strength of the neck muscles and indeed exclusion of those whose physical characteristics might render them more vulnerable is valuable. In particular, consideration of the basic musculature of the neck before allowing anyone to take to rugby or American football, while perhaps extreme, is entirely justified (Maroon *et al.*, 1980).

Further consideration must be given to protective devices, in particular helmets. Considering the mechanisms of injury it would seem that their use is perhaps of marginal value. Given that the cause of much neurological injury is the acceleration/deceleration of the head as a whole, it would seem to make little difference if the head is encased in a helmet, since the internal forces are much the same. However there is evidence that the wearing of helmets and protective head gear does coincide with greater protection from injury. In horse riding, for example, there seems little doubt that in head-injured patients those wearing properly fitting and up-to-standard head gear that remained on their heads tended to have less severe injuries (Barber, 1973; Ilgren *et al.*, 1984). However, are these the more conscientious and sensible riders in the first place? Given that severe head injuries result from acceleration/deceleration forces from a blunt injury it is hard to see how a hard helmet can have more than a marginal effect on the injury. Furthermore if wearing a helmet gives the participant a feeling of being protected this might tend to make him or her more reckless. There is a suggestion that in American football (Maroon *et al.*, 1980) helmets are a mixed blessing, in that they do tend to impart an impression of protection from all injury; also, as the face guard can be grabbed or may catch on the ground when falling, helmets may predispose to the frequency with which contact is made with a flexed neck. Thus while protective aids are to be encouraged, the benefits of protection from the greatest dangers must be weighed against the disadvantages of giving a false sense of security and how they might with their hardness cause injury themselves. Nothing can replace the participant's awareness of the dangers lurking round every corner in sport.

Avoidance of neurological damage after injury

Given that neither the dangerous situations nor the vulnerability of the sports player can be eradicated, it is necessary to consider how neurological damage can be either avoided or at least reduced. This is the role of the medical attendant. From what has been described above it is clear that it would be optimistic to suggest that pre-existing neurological damage can be reversed. However one need not be nihilistic about the value of appropriate treatment after the injury. First, there will always be a possibility of spontaneous recovery and this must be facilitated by good resuscitation. Secondly, deterioration must be avoided.

Head injury

The initial stage here is recognition that a brain injury has taken place and an assessment of the extent of recovery. Injury to the brain is not a one-off event. The injury itself causes damage which is commensurate with the nature of the injuring force in the context, anatomically and neurologically, of its victim. If severe enough it will set up a chain of events within the head. These include swelling of the brain, progressive compression by clot and because of general anoxia or high pressure inside the head failure of the brain cells to receive enough oxygen. This last will in itself cause brain swelling. Thus an injury can set up a vicious circle, culminating in a swollen, anoxic and irreversibly functionless brain. To some extent these secondary effects can be forestalled by adequate resuscitation. However more aggressive measures such as surgery to remove clots or damaged swollen brain may be indicated. The sooner the need for these is recognized and action taken, the better. In this situation it becomes a matter of close observation and speedy response on the part of medical attendants to either failure to recover or deterioration, particularly of the conscious level. The immediate management will depend on the state of the patient.

The unconscious patient

The first-aid rules of resuscitation cannot be bettered: ABC – airway, breathing and circulation. Taking into account the possibility of a concomitant neck injury, the airway must be rendered patent. This is most easily achieved by putting the patient in the recovery position. Since this also puts the neck in extension this is safe even with a neck injury, as discussed below. Otherwise a plastic airway should be inserted. The commonest cause of inadequate breathing is obstruction of the airway. Either as a result of brainstem dysfunction or chest injury, adequate ventilation may still not be maintained and the patient may become cyanosed. In this situation assisted ventilation is necessary, whether mouth-to-mouth, bag and mask or, if there are facilities, by endotracheal intubation and mechanical ventilation. The recognition and correction of hypotension can be difficult in the field. One should check for the presence of the palpable peripheral pulses and an adequate heart rate.

Unconsciousness is clear evidence of brain failure and as such is a medical emergency. The overriding imperative is to avoid delay in diagnosis and treatment, since this in itself can lead to prolonged damage and disastrous results. Thus, while immediate resuscitation is crucial, transfer of the injured person to an appropriate hospital must also be achieved without delay. Delay and failure of resuscitation are the two commonest potentially avoidable factors contributing to poor results from head injury. The sports field is no place to treat this sort of injury and the sooner the patient is transferred to hospital, the better. It is important therefore that the means for calling the emergency services are immediately to hand and utilized when unconsciousness is recognized. The ambulance should then be directed to a hospital which has appropriate facilities for handling head injuries. The unconscious patient is at imminent risk of dying and this fact over-rides all other considerations. Being knocked out is not a benign event – it is very serious. A half-hearted response to this is always wrong, usually dangerous and often disastrous.

Conscious but disoriented patient

The first necessity is to recognize that there has been a head injury with transient brain dysfunction and that recovery is not complete. The patient must be removed from the sporting arena and observed until full recovery has occurred. This may not be easy. The victim by virtue of the disorientation may not be able to cooperate by leaving the field and indeed colleagues and team management may similarly feel that he or she should continue. The medical imperative however is paramount. Partially recovered patients are at greater risk from further and probably more serious injury. Even if recovery has occurred it is always correct not to allow the player to continue; indeed many sports have a mandatory period of rest after any head injury involving unconsciousness. This is entirely justified from the head injury point of view; the after-effects render the victim more vulnerable to repeated and potentially severe further injury. Two injuries in a short period of time are likely to have a combined and more serious outcome. Close observation, directed specially at conscious level, must be instituted and failure to recover or, worse, deterioration requires immediate transport to a hospital. Disorientation is, like unconsciousness, evidence of brain dysfunction and if prolonged requires correct and urgent investigation and treatment. It is difficult to state how long one should wait for recovery, but my preference is to play safe and transfer immediately.

Fully recovered but evidence of transient dysfunction

Given that a hiatus in memory is evidence of a period when the brain was not functioning properly, this should be actively sought in all cases. If present the patient should be taken off. There is no such thing as a minor brain injury – only some which are more severe than others. Perhaps in some circumstances this is an over-reaction but while the personal judgement of the person on the spot must be considered, it is the long-term well-being of the sportsman or woman which is the prime concern and which is potentially at risk after even minor head injuries.

Recent tragic sequelae to brain injury, mostly from the boxing arena, have focused attention on the management of brain injury in sports. These serve to demonstrate many of the principles mentioned above. The first is the mechanism of injury – the violent jerking of the head both from the blow and immediately afterwards from striking the floor or rope around the boxing ring. The second is the sequence of events which in different circumstances is familiar to neurosurgeons. The injured person can recover from the immediate effects of the injury, improve from being unconscious – albeit for a very short time – is able to walk and perhaps talk before the secondary chain of events, pressure from clot or brain swelling, produces a further neurological deterioration. It is tempting to point out that in theory this secondary deterioration is avoidable. Of course in practice this is not so but from the moment of the second collapse speed is absolutely crucial. The patient is not unconscious from the blow but from a continuing process set in action as a consequence. The urgency with which this must be identified and treated cannot be overstated. Every minute that treatment is delayed erodes the chance of recovery.

The last and most important fact is that once brain dysfunction occurs, no matter why or where, its victim becomes a patient who may be invalided or die if not treated with extreme urgency. It is the role of the medical attendent to insist that the sports player receives care commensurate to the danger.

Spinal injuries

These may be divided into those with evidence of neurological deficit and those without. In the latter it can be very difficult to decide purely clinically whether there is any disruption of the stability of the bony spinal column, which would of course increase the risk of serious neurological injury after even innocuous trauma. The nature of the injuring incident and a history of neurological symptoms suggest this possibility, as would marked painful limitation of movement of the spine or the presence of distant pain or tingling at the extremes of the range of active movement – that which the patient will perform him or herself. If in doubt it will always be prudent to play safe; Bert Troutman may have got away with it but many will not.

Spinal injury with deficit

In this case one should assume that the spine is unstable and therefore strive to establish and maintain normal alignment. Unless one knows exactly the alignment at the time, this will be difficult. The main rules are to avoid movement, especially into spinal flexion, which is the least stable position. Holding the head in neutral or slight extension is the safest way to move the patient (Fig. 12.4).

In addition, like the brain, the spinal cord will recover better if provided with adequate blood with normal blood gases, thus the ABC of resuscitation must not be neglected. High cervical cord lesions above the roots of the phrenic nerve (C3–5) will cause paralysis of the respiratory muscles, so the patient will need external ventilation from the outset. Similar lesions will also interrupt the pathways involved in the maintenance of blood pressure control and such patients must be nursed flat or slightly head-down. The recovery position remains desirable for the protection it gives to the airway, but in the spinal injury situation the extension of the neck should be maintained and reinforced by a collar, or rolled-up towel or newspaper.

Patients with paralysed limbs cannot feel or move and the role of protection from injury must be taken by the attendant who must be careful to avoid the distortion of applying pressure to or causing burns of the limbs. These patients must therefore be moved in one piece and very carefully, three or four people usually move the patient while another supervises (Fig. 12.5).

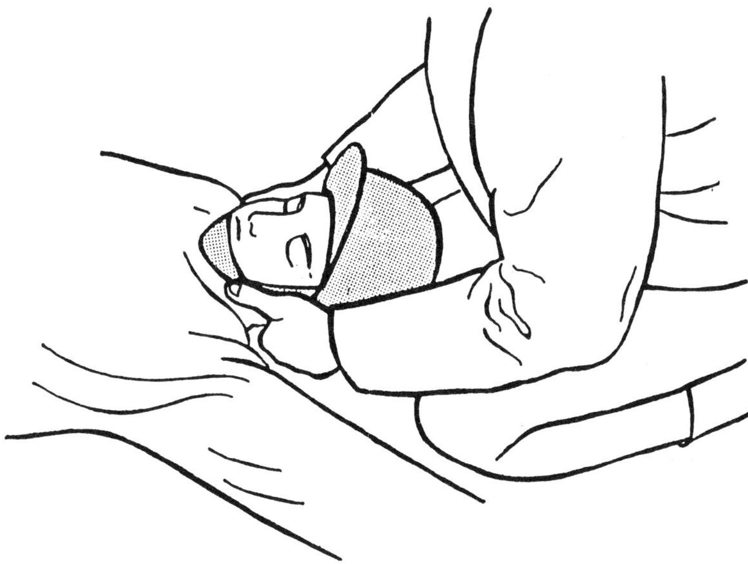

Fig. 12.4 Steadying the head.

No deficit but a possibility of instability

These patients are best treated in the same way, assuming that any movement might dislocate the spine. Both these groups must be transported as soon as possible to hospital where there is the facility for proper investigation, in this case x-rays taken both in the resting position and, if necessary, with gentle flexion and extension to show abnormal mobility. Treatment, aims to achieve reduction with stabilization in the reduced state.

Moving patients with brain or spinal injuries

When presented with an unconscious patient the attendant is understandably concerned about how to move him or her. There is a conflict of imperatives – to avoid movement which might cause dislocation and neurological damage but at the same time to get the injured person off the field of play to a place of safety. This conflict can be resolved by careful application of first-aid principles and an appreciation of priorities. As with all medical contact with ill people, there is a balance between risk and benefit. Usually the most dangerous option is to do nothing. The overwhelming imperative in such circumstances is the maintenance of adequate oxygenation of the nervous system. In practice this equates to the protection of the airway and maintenance of breathing. The next is the need to move the patient to a place of safety, generally to a medical facility where investigation and treatment can be arranged. Thus moving the patient is necessary. The fear is that by moving the patient one will cause movement of unstable bony elements, further traumatizing the spinal cord or brain. Careful consideration tends to reveal this to be a danger more apparent than real. The patient must be manoeuvred into a safe position and moved in one piece so that no relative movement occurs during transport. By and large the position of lying flat with the neck slightly extended is both safe and easy to handle, remembering that the supine position is that which protects the airway least. Thus the patient should either be prone or on the side if unable to keep his or her own airway patent. The lifting and carrying of an adult in this position require several people, with a further person to co-ordinate the process (Fig. 12.5). It is important that the task should be carried out gently and slowly with all people listening to and heeding the instructions of the non-lifting co-ordinator. When there are few

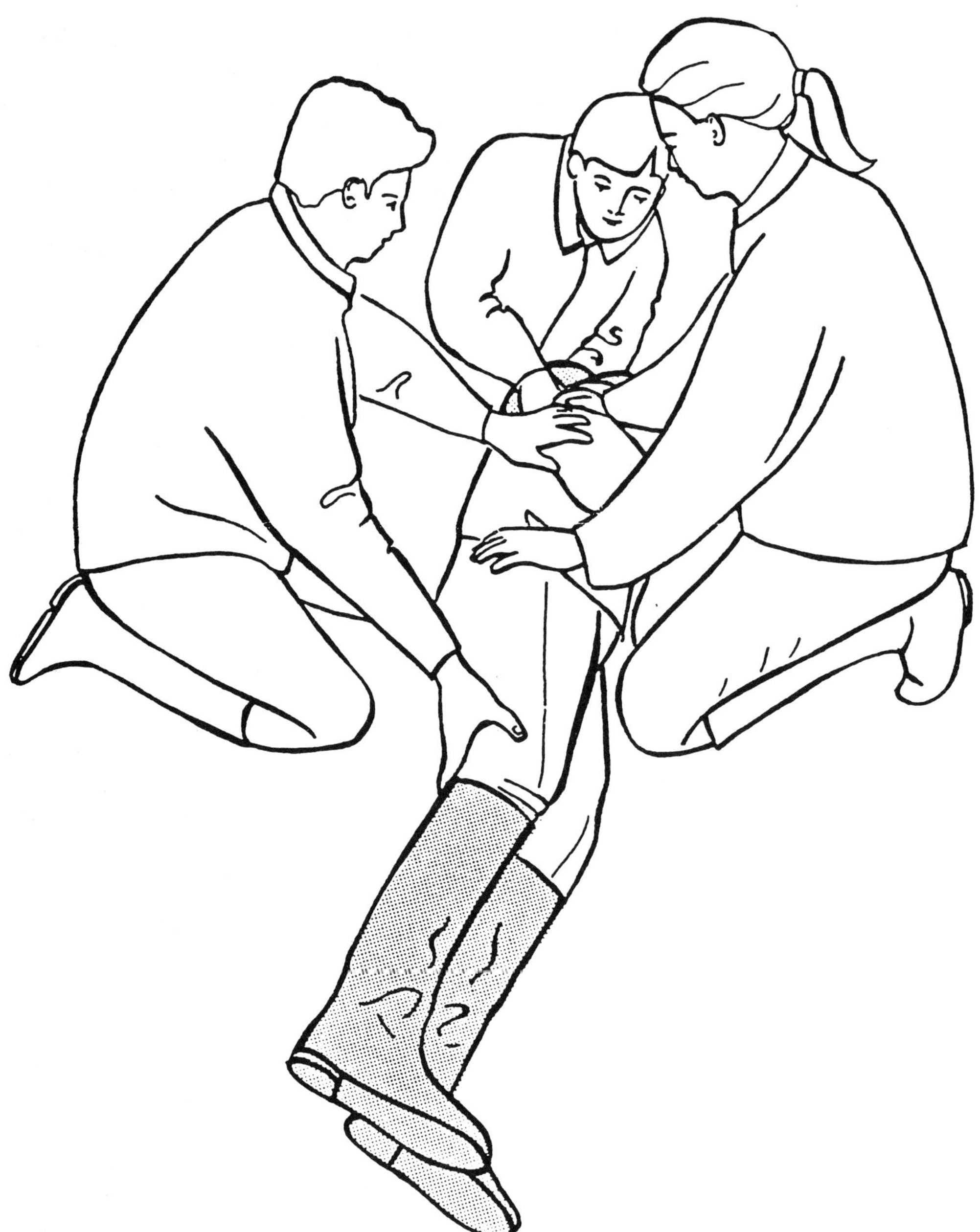

Fig. 12.5 The log roll.

people the patient may be rolled face-down on to a sheet and lifted by the corners. With care, the moving of patients is seldom a difficult matter.

Further comment should be made on the role of traction in the transport of patients with potentially unstable cervical spines. This is used in the hospital environment to aid reduction of malalignment. It is carefully controlled and generally applied through the use of skull calipers. In the emergency situation it is inevitably more crude, applied by placing both hands flat on either side over the ramus and angle of the jaw from above the patient's head. In reality the main benefit of this is to ensure that one person is giving full attention to the position of the neck, to ensure that it is in slight extension and remains in that position.

Minor injuries

The difficulty with these is that they are very hard to differentiate from those with some degree of instability. There is no absolutely certain way of recognizing this group, who in themselves do not require any treatment besides that which relieves the discomfort, usually in the form of rest either in bed or in a collar. However the presence of full, albeit painful mobility and the absence of any neurological symptoms or signs suggest that neither the basic structural integrity nor the nervous elements have been injured.

Prevention of injury in subsequent episodes

A recent injury detracts from full fitness and is therefore a risk factor. This is relevant not only in terms of a further severe injury but also in considering the cumulative effects of repeated minor and apparently inconsequential injuries.

It has been noted that those American footballers who had minor injuries were most likely to suffer further injury. It may be therefore that even minor injury interferes with the anatomical structure, weakening the defence against injury. This has worrying implications. Similarly with head injury, after apparent recovery it may be hard to believe that the patient is more likely to receive a further injury but definition and recognition of full recovery can be difficult. Psychological testing after concussive injury can show abnormalities for many months, despite the apparent full return of normality. Are these a risk factor and if not, what is the cumulative effect of a second injury some months after the first? We do not have any answers at present but first principles suggest that there is serious cause for concern (Gronwell and Wrightson, 1974, 1975).

Repeated injury has been studied in the case of boxers (Lancet, 1973) and it has been shown that it produces both clinical and radiological evidence of irreversible damage to the brain. However it is clear that the degree of damage is not directly related to the record of knock-outs. It is therefore not only those events which produce the recognized brain injury which contribute to the damage, but also the minor knocks, which are considered so benign. Footballers who have never had a head injury, as defined as loss of or clouding of consciousness have been found to have evidence of atrophy on computed tomography scanning, although no clinically evident brain damage. Fortunately most participants in sport neither suffer severe injury nor continue for long enough to be at risk from long-term damage like this. The difficulty is being sure that the long-term effects are as benign as they appear to be and, if not, agreeing what impairment is an acceptable trade for a satisfying participation in sport. More information will doubtless be provided over the coming years and it may be that this will become a serious problem in our perception of how sport is played.

Recognized syndromes

Concussion

This is a common occurrence in the field of sport. It is defined as a clinical syndrome characterized by immediate and transient post-traumatic impairment of neural function. It is generally not associated with any recognizable structural damage and leads to full recovery. It may be mild, with no loss of consciousness, moderate with loss of consciousness and retrograde amnesia, or severe with unconsciousness lasting over 5 min. There is a spectrum of severity between these grades and more serious head injuries which have a worse outcome and are with recognizable structural damage, such as contusions or brain swelling. Management must take into account the fact that all brain injury is potentially serious.

Nerve injury

This is often transient injury to a nerve, causing pain and transient deficit in its distribution. In the context of injuries to the spine it is usually in fact a nerve root rather than a nerve although the distinction is mainly semantic. It may be due to direct or indirect trauma, such as lateral flexion of the cervical spine causing compression of the root by bone in its exit foramen, or traction from shoulder depression. It is usually transient: full function returns in a few minutes and pain subsides over some hours. If the symptoms or signs persist investigation should be undertaken to exclude fracture of the lateral mass or lateral disc prolapse, which can give the same clinical picture. In players who have had this type of injury special protection against recurrence should be considered, like padding or increased exercises to strengthen the neck.

Spinal cord concussion

This is clinically analogous to cerebral concussion. There is often complete spinal cord dysfunction which is transient but recovers completely. The mechanism is not understood clearly and, like cerebral concussion, there is evidence of long-term degeneration, although acutely there may be no clinical or gross histological damage after recovery. Unlike cerebral concussion it is however less common than injury associated with structural damage. While complete recovery is usual, structural damage must be actively excluded in the normal way. As in cerebral concussion, the long-term prognosis is the subject of some debate.

Central cord syndrome

In clinical neurology this is a well-recognized syndrome resulting from damage to the centre of a segment of the cord. The symptoms and signs are related to the central grey matter and often the long tracts are unscathed. In sport this is usually associated with a fracture dislocation or disc prolapse and in its mildest manifestation presents as burning hands syndrome (Maroon, 1977). The patient will complain of painful tingling in the hands or adjacent parts of the upper limb. There are often few signs, although if sought carefully there may be loss of spinothalamic (pinprick and temperature) sensation in a small area. There are generally no long tract signs and no sphincter disturbance. Investigation often shows a swollen cord. The associated structural injury and symptoms usually settle within a few days. This is a potentially serious condition and should be treated as other structural injuries of the spine.

More serious brain and spinal cord injuries

These will be diagnosed by the persistence of neurological abnormality. Immediate transfer to hospital is indicated, and appropriate first-aid measures should be taken. Here appropriate investigations and treatment can be instituted. Neurological injury will usually be treated expectantly, although steps may be taken to reduce swelling, to decompress compressed neurological tissue or remove clots. Structural damage to the spine, malalignment or instability is treated actively with reduction and maintenance of normal position. Both the nature of the abnormality and to some extent the philosophy of the medical team will dictate whether this is done by conservative treatment, traction and maintenance, by nursing in a fixed position or by surgical intervention, involving open reduction and internal fixation. Whichever is chosen, the aim is to reduce and fix the fracture or dislocation until fusion occurs, usually within 3 months. The relative merits of these two extremes are the subject of much debate in spinal injuries circles but the purpose in each case is identical.

Other acute traumatic injuries to the head and neck

This includes the various bruises and lacerations which are fairly common in sport. These are generally entirely benign and can be treated along first-aid principles. One must remember however that lacerations will tend to be dirty, and therefore tetanus toxoid should be given to those who are unprotected. Unlike soiled cuts elsewhere, thorough cleaning can be followed immediately by primary closure. This is a reflection of the abundant blood supply to the skin of the head and neck. This also leads to quite profuse blood loss, especially from scalp wounds. Fortunately pressure on the wound edges against the skull will control this readily and suture of the galeal layer almost always arrests most of the bleeding, even if the skin itself remains unsutured. Furthermore it is always as well to remember in lacerations about the mouth how far the lips extend. Many of these apparent skin lacerations are in fact through-and-through injuries of the whole lip and require a three-layer closure – skin, subcutaneous layer and mucosa. Blunt injury to the front of the neck can rarely cause laryngeal oedema and respiratory obstruction. This should be suspected especially in head injuries. Emergency treatment for this may involve tracheostomy, although the majority will require only appropriate positioning.

Chronic injuries to the head and spine

Chronic spinal problems

These mainly consist of persistent sprains which result from repeated, often minor injury or failure of recovery of acute sprains through inadequate rest. The spine is in use in all activity except strict supine bed rest and therefore it may take some time for even relatively minor injury to recover. Painful muscle spasm to protect the injured part followed by loss of muscle bulk and strength, which leads to greater vulnerability, produces a vicious circle which can result in chronic pain in the spine. Similarly, repeated use and minor injuries can accelerate degenerative changes which may from time to time produce pain and disability. These are usually benign but long-term problems may occur. The treatment is initially symptomatic – rest, appropriate analgesia and the judicious use of non-steroidal anti-inflammatory agents – followed by measures to build up the strength of the muscles before a return to full activity is advisable.

Lumbago

By definition this term is descriptive of backache and thus is a symptom rather than a specific diagnosis. It may result from any painful back condition but usually is caused by degenerative disease, is recurrent and needs only supportive treatment. It has no specific medical meaning.

Fibrositis

This is similar, being loosely used to mean painful spasm of the neck muscles. It is associated with painful stiffness of the neck with areas of local tenderness. The spasm is a natural defence mechanism to splint an area of sprain and it is most often found after minor rotation injuries of the neck. It does not need specific treatment, although simple analgesics, muscle relaxants such as Valium, and warm compresses can give symptomatic relief. Similar pain may be found recurrently in degenerative cervical spine disease but as a clinical entity fibrositis has no exact definition, although truly inflammatory myalgia of the neck muscles can occur in certain mild viral illnesses.

Chronic neurological disease

Perhaps the most worrying problem is the possibility that, repeated, even subclinical neurological injuries may produce neural degeneration. There are good theoretical reasons for believing this to be so. For an injury to produce a change in consciousness, however mild, one can suppose fairly widespread dysfunction. Traumatized nerve cells tend to die rather than regenerate; the return of function is more a matter of recruiting back up circuits than return to health of injured pathways. If the injury is repeated this will tend in time to exhaust the reserve capacity and ultimately will produce intellectual and neurological deterioration. Furthermore the process of ageing is associ-

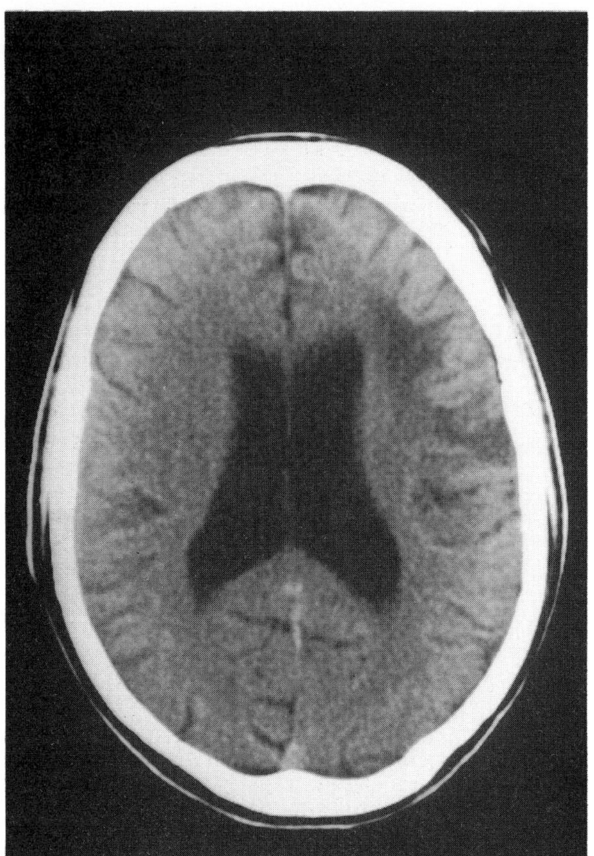

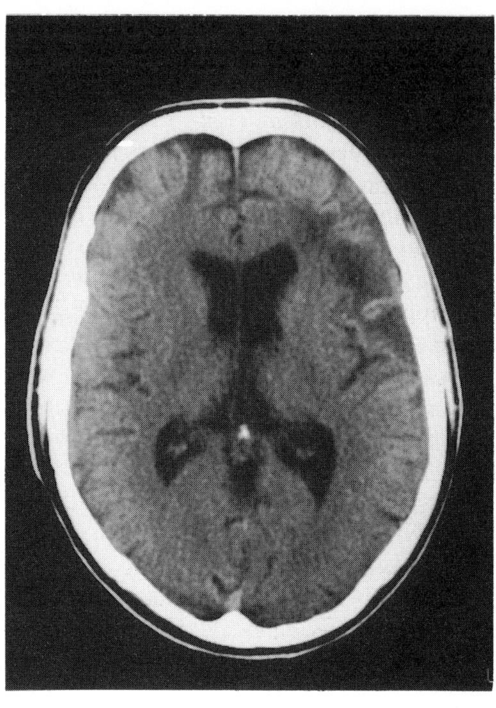

Figs. 12.6 and 12.7 Cerebral atrophy following left frontal contusions. Note the large ventricles and the low density and enlarged cortical markings in the left frontal region.

ated with the gradual eating up of neurological reserve. Thus the combination of repeated concussive episodes and increasing age would be expected to result in the earlier manifestation of neurological or intellectual changes. These include a degree of dementia, poor memory and dissociation with the realities of life, as well as more specific localized degenerative conditions such as movement disorders, spinal cord degeneration and cerebellar dysfunction. The alarming thing is that we can sometimes see the radiological features of these latter syndromes in otherwise fit sports players and as time passes, witness accelerated ageing of the nervous system. This is not an entirely theoretical complication of repeated minor neurological injury but is found in practice. It has been established in boxing (Lancet, 1973) where repeated injury has been shown to produce a progressive dementia. The radiological features are of atrophy to deep structures (Fig. 12.6 and 12.7).

Conclusion

Whether one is considering the consequences of acute craniospinal injury, or contemplating the possibility that the knocks and bangs to which sportsmen and women happily subject themselves in recreational activities might cumulatively damage the brain or spinal cord, it is clear that injuries to the head and spine are to be avoided. Severe neurological injury is devastating to the individual, horribly traumatic to those close to him or her and expensive to society in general. Failure to understand the dangers and avoid them where possible may make sport, like so many other things, a luxury we collectively cannot afford.

The role of the medical attendant is difficult. Among other things it involves deciding when the sportsman or woman ceases to be a participant and becomes a potential or actual patient. In no area does appropriate care carry such great benefit – or its absence such disastrous consequences – as in the field of neurological injury and it is always wise to be safe than sorry.

References

Adams CBT, Logue V (1971) Studies in cervical myelopathy 1. Movement of the cervical roots, dura and cord and their relation to the course of the extrathecal roots. *Brain* **94**, 557.

Addley K, Farren J (1988) Irish rugby survey: Dungannon Football Club (1986–7). *British Journal of Sports Medicine* **22**, 22.

Barber HM (1973) Horse play: survey of accidents with horses. *British Medical Journal* **3**, 532.

Burry HC, Gowland H (1981) Cervical injury in rugby football – a New Zealand survey. *British Journal of Sports Medicine* **15**, 56.

Cannon SR, James SE (1984) Back pain in athletes. *British Journal of Sports Medicine* **18**, 159.

Davies JE (1980) The spine in sport-injuries, prevention and treatment. *British Journal of Sports Medicine* **14**, 18.

Gronwall D, Wrightson P (1974) Delayed recovery of intellectual function after minor head injury. *Lancet* **ii**, 605–9.

Gronwell D, Wrightson P (1975) Cumulative effect of concussion. *Lancet* **ii**, 995–7.

Ilgren EB et al. (1984) Horse riding: a warning to the unhelmeted. *Clinical Neuropathology* **3**, 153.

Lancet (1973) Boxing brains. *Lancet* **ii**, 1064.

Lloyd RG (1987) Riding and other equestrian injuries: considerable severity. *British Journal of Sports Medicine* **21**, 22.

Maroon JC (1977) Burning hands in football spinal cord injuries. *Journal of the American Medical Association* **238**, 2049.

Maroon JC, Steele PB, Berlin R (1980) Football head and neck injuries – an update. *Clinical Neurosurgery* **27**, 414.

Sahlin Y (1988) Alpine skiing injuries. *British Journal of Sports Medicine* **23**, 241.

Schneider RC (1973) *Head and Neck Injuries in Football*. Baltimore: Williams & Wilkins.

Sortland O, Tysvaer A (1989) Brain damage in former association footballers: an evaluation by cerebral computed tomography *Neuroradiology* **31**, 44.

Sortland O, Tysvaer A, Storli O (1982) Changes in the cervical spine in association football players. *British Journal of Sports Medicine* **16**, 80.

Sparks JP (1985) Rugby football injuries 1980–1983. *British Journal of Sports Medicine* **19**, 71.

Tysvaer A, Storli O (1981) Association football injuries to the brain. *British Journal of Sports Medicine* **15**, 163.

Williams JPR, McKibbin B (1977) Cervical spine injuries in rugby union football. *British Medical Journal* **ii**, 1747.

13

Injuries to the lower limb

I. G. Stother

This chapter covers the injuries and problems in the lower limb. In most sports the knee is the most commonly injured part of the lower limb and this is reflected in the length of the section on the soft tissues around this joint. Many of the injuries of the lower limb involve the bones and these are only mentioned in passing. The chapter is organized in the following sections:

1. The groin.
2. The thigh.
3. The knee.
4. The lower leg.
5. The tendo-achilles.
6. The ankle.
7. The foot.
8. The toes.

The groin

General considerations

Pain in the area of the groin can arise from local problems with the soft tissues but also commonly arises from:

1. Problems with the lower spine, notably spondylolisthesis.
2. Problems with the hip joint, notably osteoarthritis in the older patient and slipped capital femoral epiphysis in teenagers.
3. Stress fractures of the femoral neck, notably in dancers and vegetarians.
4. Hernias.
5. Avulsion fractures from the pelvis, again notably in teenagers.
6. Gastrointestinal and urinary tract disease.

If there is no clear history of injury to the groin area and if examination reveals no obvious local pathology then these various diagnoses must be investigated.

'Groin strain' (Fig. 13.1)

The term is used to cover a number of injuries to muscle attachments around the groin area. The muscle attachments which are commonly damaged include:

1. The adductor origin from the pelvis.
2. The iliopsoas insertion into the medial femur at the lesser trochanter just below the hip joint.
3. The rectus femoris part of quadriceps femoris arising from the anterior superior iliac spine at the anterior margin of the pelvis.

Adductor strains occur with high kicks, sliding tackles and in dancers and gymnasts who do the splits awkwardly. The onset may arise from a single incident or may be insidious when the athlete gradually develops stiffness and discomfort after unusually prolonged or difficult work. The pain in the groin is almost in the midline in the skin crease. Wide separation of the legs and gripping with the knees is painful.

Examination reveals local tenderness adjacent to the symphysis pubis and extending distally along

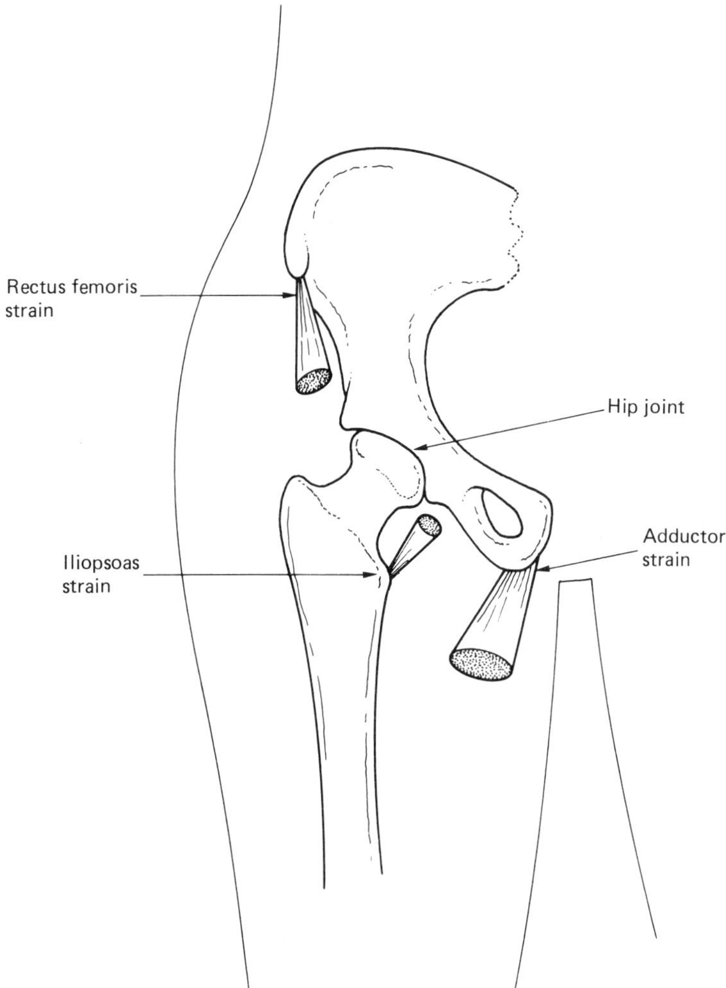

Fig. 13.1 Diagram of groin area showing the sites of damage and tenderness in different groin strains.

the bony margin. The pain and tenderness are exacerbated by pulling the knees together against resistance. It is important to compare the normal and abnormal sides as this area is tender to deep palpation in many patients, even when uninjured.

Iliopsoas insertion strains occur when the hip is flexed actively against resistance, as for example in repeated sit-ups or using a rowing machine. The athlete develops pain just below the groin crease on the inner aspect of the thigh. Tenderness is difficult to localize as the iliopsoas insertion is very deep. Flexing the hip against resistance may reproduce the pain.

Rectus femoris may be damaged at its origin just below the anterior superior iliac spine at the pelvis. This muscle, when it contracts, bends the hip and straightens the knee and may be damaged during sprint starts and in kicking, especially if the kicks are blocked. The athlete complains of pain just above the hip joint with exercise. He or she is tender over the muscle origin and this is exacerbated if the hip is flexed against resistance.

X-rays

In all patients with groin strains, but especially in young patients, X-rays should be taken to seek avulsion fractures and ectopic calcification. It may be considered appropriate to fix internally large avulsion fractures at any of these sites.

Treatment

In the absence of fractures, treatment consists of rest to allow healing. Pain may be helped by local ultrasound and the administration of oral non-steroidal anti-inflammatories. The damage to the muscle origin needs time to heal and healing takes at least 6 weeks. If the symptoms are disabling and the tenderness well-demarcated then local injection of insoluble anti-inflammatory steroid with local anaesthetic may help mobility. However, this treatment does not speed up the healing process and sound healing does not take place in less than 6 weeks.

Active and passive movement should be maintained within the limits of pain and activities gradually increased under physiotherapy supervision. Competitive sports should be avoided for about 6 weeks.

Recurrence is very common unless the activities precipitating the injury are modified and adequate time for healing is allowed.

Groin disruption

Many injuries to the groin are persistent and may not respond to conservative measures. They frequently prevent play or athletics and may in professional sportsmen and women lead to permanent unemployment. Many are disguised as pelvic instability, chronic adductor tears or osteitis pubis and treated by rest, physiotherapy or even pelvic fusion (Harris and Murray, 1974).

In recent years a syndrome of groin disruption has been recognized in male athletes rendered susceptible to the condition because of the embryonic descent of the testes. The syndrome, as described by Gilmore (1991), constitutes the following features:

1. A torn external oblique aponeurosis.
2. Torn conjoined tendon.
3. A dehiscence between the conjoined tendon and the inguinal ligament.
4. The absence of a hernia sac.

Clinical features

The condition was originally recognized in professional soccer players but may occur in athletes, ice skaters, rugby players, racket games, hockey, dancers and karateka. The onset of symptoms is gradual, with a history of a specific injury in one-third of patients. The pain experienced prevented kicking a ball and was increased by external rotation or hyperextension. Sneezing, coughing, attempting to sprint, in fact any sudden change of movement, even getting out of bed led to further pain and discomfort. At presentation the athlete could localize the pain to the inguinal, adductor or perineal region.

On examination with the little finger inverting the scrotum in males, or by direct palpation in females, the superficial inguinal ring on the affected side was dilated with tenderness and a cough impulse.

Treatment

In this syndrome surgical intervention appears to be very successful (90% return to sport). The approach is as for an inguinal hernia with the aim of restoring the anatomy to normal. The following procedures are carried out:

1. Plication of the transversalis fascia as in the Shouldice hernia repair.
2. Repair of the torn conjoined tendon.
3. Approximation of the conjoined tendon to the inguinal ligament with nylon in darn fashion.
4. Repair of the external oblique and reconstitution of the inguinal ring.

Rehabilitation

The procedure is usually performed as a day-case or overnight stay. On the first postoperative day the patient is encouraged to stand erect and during the first week to walk slowly for up to 20 min two to four times daily according to discomfort.

In the second week jogging can begin and, if tolerated, running initiated.

By the third week most can run in straight lines and do sit-ups and adductor exercises. Swimming (not breast-stroke) is a useful adjunct to rehabilitation after the first week.

By 4 or 5 weeks kicking a ball, dancing techniques or whatever movement is specific to the particular sport may be attempted.

We believe it is important to exclude inguinofemoral hernia as a cause of groin pain. A large number of symptomatic young people will have acquired hernias which may not be clinically apparent but may be demonstrated by herniography. In the absence of a hernia or pelvic instability we believe that exploration of the groin is a logical avenue to take in patients with persistent symptoms in spite of appropriate physical therapy.

The thigh

General considerations

The majority of acute injuries to the thigh are either direct contusions, muscle ruptures or both. Injuries to the front of the thigh involve the quadriceps muscle, which extends the knee, and injuries to the back of the thigh involve the hamstring muscle, which bends the knee.

Any athlete with vague thigh pain requires medical investigation as pain may arise from a number of problems:

1. The *hip joint*. Older patients may suffer from arthritis and younger patients, in their teens, may have a slipped captial femoral epiphysis. Preteenage children may have Perthes disease. Patients with hip problems will have a hip limp, usually with a Trendelenburg gait (see Chapter 10) and restriction of hip movement on examination.
2. The *femur* (thigh bone). Problems here may arise from stress fractures which can be detected by X-rays and isotope bone scan and, more rarely, by primary bone tumours which may present as constantly painful swellings. The patients often rationalize the occurrence of these swellings to episodes of trauma. Primary bone tumours can usually be diagnosed from X-rays of the femur.
3. The *spine*. Pain in the thigh may, in fact, be referred pain from pathology in the spine itself. Such pathology includes wear in the joints of the spine, as well as damage to the bone itself in spondylolisthesis and damage to the intervertebral discs ('slipped disc'). These various spinal problems can be detected by careful examination and X-rays of the lumbosacral spine.
4. Pressure or tension on the *lumbar nerve roots*. The front of the thigh is supplied by the second, third and fourth lumbar nerve roots. The most common cause of pressure on these nerve roots is a prolapsed intervertebral disc. In such cases examination of the lumbar spine will reveal loss of the normal lumbar lordosis. Examination of the thigh will reveal altered sensation, muscle wasting and a diminished or absent knee reflex jerk. In addition, the femoral nerve stretch test will be positive (with the patient lying on his or her side, extension of the hip and flexion of the knee causes marked increase in the pain in the thigh).

Quadriceps haematoma

This usually arises when the thigh is struck hard – commonly in a young, adult male playing rugby, soccer or some other contact sport and who is in collision with another player. The thigh rapidly becomes swollen and painful. Subcutaneous discoloration from bruising appears only after 2 or 3 days in most cases.

Treatment

This is initially rest, ice and oral non-steroidal anti-inflammatories. After about 48 hours gradual active mobilization can be started. Passive stretching must be avoided.

At this stage it must be ascertained that no muscle rupture has occurred. Rupture is indicated by a palpable hollow at the site of injury and a lump of muscle above the site of injury which appears when an attempt is made to lift the leg with the knee straight.

Sometimes a fluctuant haematoma develops. This should be aspirated under local anaesthetic. The needle should be inserted at the top of the haematoma so there is no leakage from the needle track. The thigh should then be firmly bandaged and mobilization should be limited to walking. Further aspirations of the haematoma are often necessary.

Symptoms persist for some weeks. Patients may easily be off physical work for about 4 weeks and off competitive games for about 8 weeks.

In a proportion of cases, especially after early and vigorous mobilization, the haematoma becomes calcified, a condition known as myositis ossificans or 'Charlie horse'.

Myositis ossificans (Charlie horse)

In this condition calcium is deposited in a thigh haematoma. It becomes hard and can be felt through the skin deep in the muscle. The muscle is tethered and movement may be restricted and painful, especially at the knee joint. The patient, who is usually being treated for a quadriceps haematoma, fails to progress.

X-rays

X-rays confirm the diagnosis with a 'cloud' of calcification in the area of the damaged muscle.

Treatment

Treatment is difficult. Usually the symptoms settle with rest and static quadriceps exercises. Passive mobilization, which is usually painful, must be avoided as this tends to cause further calcification.

Surgical excision of the abnormal calcification rarely improves the range of motion and recurrence of the calcification and tethering is common. In severe cases the symptoms may take up to a year to settle.

Quadriceps rupture

This occurs as a result of either a sudden muscle contraction or a contusion or both. History is, therefore, of a sudden onset of pain during exercise. Swelling and stiffness develop over a few hours.

It may be difficult, initially, to distinguish a contusion from a rupture because of local haematoma. However, after about 48 hours a hollow at the site of rupture with a muscle bulge above the hollow on attempted straight leg raising is usually obvious.

Treatment

Treatment may be conservative. This leaves the patient with an abnormal bulge in the upper thigh and a slight quadriceps weakness. It is unusual for more than one of the four bellies of the quadriceps muscle to be damaged in this way. Although the bulk of the power of the muscle is retained the muscle balance is altered and surgical repair of the damaged muscle is advocated for young athletes. The damaged muscle is exposed via a long incision. The haematoma is evacuated. The muscle fibres are sutured together. This may be quite difficult to achieve. The leg is then splinted with the knee straight for 6 weeks and then gradually mobilized. If the repair is sound this preserves the muscle contour and gives a stronger leg with the minimum amount of muscle scarring and minimal change in muscle balance.

Some patients may present late after a muscle rupture and present with a bulge in the upper thigh. The diagnosis can usually be suspected from a history of injury. In addition, the bulge is more prominent when the muscle contracts and at this stage there is usually minimal or no pain. In such cases it is advisable to take X-rays of the thigh to exclude any underlying bony pathology. Persisting pain which keeps the patient awake at night or calcification or bone erosion are all suspicious of more sinister pathology and some form of biopsy of the lesion is then indicated.

Quadriceps tendon rupture (Fig. 13.2)

The four bellies of the quadriceps muscle all unite in the short quadriceps tendon which inserts into the upper border of the patella. Rupture of this tendon is uncommon and it is usually an injury of those of middle age and older. A sudden quadriceps contraction, for example in a stumble or fall, usually causes rupture of the tendon. The patient complains of acute pain and inability to hold the knee straight and, therefore, inability to walk.

Examination reveals swelling just above the patella. Palpation reveals a hollow just above the patella. If the patient is asked to lift the leg in the air he or she is unable to do so.

Treatment

Treatment is by immediate surgical repair. It may be necessary to pass non-absorbable sutures

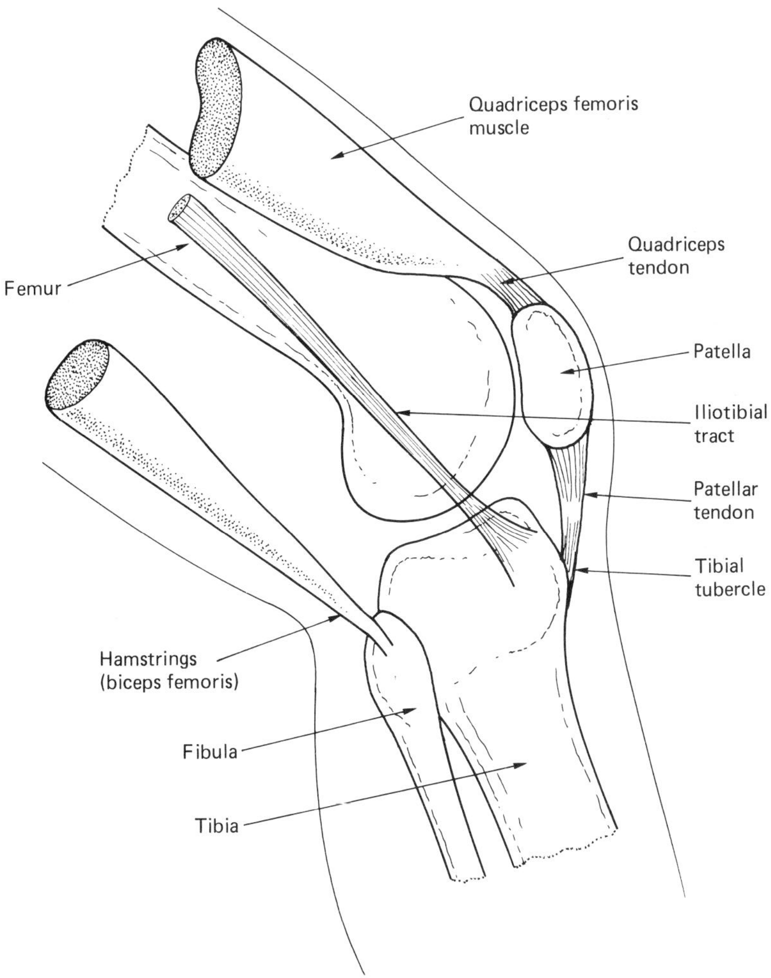

Fig. 13.2 Diagram of the knee from the lateral side showing the relations of quadriceps femoris, biceps part of hamstrings and the iliotibial tract.

through the patellar tendon and pass these through drill holes made in the patella itself. The soft tissues on either side of the patella may also require to be repaired by suturing.

Postoperatively the knee should be immobilized for 6 weeks in the extended position in a plaster cylinder or similar splint to hold the leg extended and allow healing to occur. During this time the patient should use crutches but should walk putting the injured leg to the ground rather than holding the leg with the injured foot in the air by means of quadriceps activity. On removal of the immobilization, active exercises can be started and the power of the muscle gradually built up. Once 90° of active flexion has been attained graduated loaded quadriceps exercises can be begun. Competitive sports should be avoided for at least 6 months.

Hamstring injuries (Fig. 13.2)

The hamstring muscles and tendons on the back of the thigh are typically damaged during sprinting. The athlete suddenly develops pain in the back of the thigh. The hamstrings may be damaged at their origin from the ischial tuberosity in the buttock or more distally, usually at the musculotendinous junction just above the knee joint.

The athlete complains of acute pain during the exercise. Examination usually reveals local swelling and tenderness.

Treatment

Treatment is as for quadriceps haematoma or rupture, except that the knee should be immobilized in a position of some flexion and crutches should be used to rest the leg if pain is severe. Recovery takes a similar length of time. Calcification in the damaged muscles may also occur.

In young athletes developing proximal pain in the buttock X-rays should be taken to exclude an avulsion fracture from the ischial tuberosity. This may require internal fixation.

Meralgia paraesthetica

This condition is caused by the entrapment of the lateral cutaneous nerve of the thigh as it passes through the fibres of the inguinal ligament just medial to the anterior/superior iliac spine of the pelvis. This results in abnormal sensation and numbness over the outer aspect of the thigh.

The condition is said to be common among back-packers, probably because they tend to hyperextend the hip joint.

The patient complains of discomfort and abnormal sensation over the outer aspect of the thigh.

Examination reveals sensory changes but no muscle weakness. The sensory upset is increased by extending the hip joint and by direct pressure over the lateral end of the inguinal ligament.

Treatment

Treatment may be simply by stopping the precipitating activities. If this does not help local injection of a small dose of insoluble anti-inflammatory steroid, together with some local anaesthetic into the tender area of the ligament, may help. If these measures are unsuccessful surgical decompression of the nerve in the ligament may be beneficial but the results are not consistently good and the patient should be warned of this.

The knee joint

General considerations

The knee is vulnerable in most sports. The structures most frequently damaged in the author's experience are:

1. The menisci.
2. The anterior cruciate ligament.
3. The patellofemoral joint.

The patient may present acutely with the initial injury. However, a number of patients present with chronic symptoms from their injuries to the knee.

In all patients, but especially young patients, it is important to remember that knee pain may result from damage to the hip joint.

Longitudinal tears of the medial meniscus (Fig. 13.3)

This is one of the classic knee injuries and has been well-described by Smillie. The longitudinal tear of the medial meniscus is caused by the medial femoral condyle splitting the meniscus along its length. The inner edge of the meniscus is displaced into the intercondylar notch in the middle of the knee joint.

The history is usually of a soccer player who twists on his bent knee, usually whilst sweeping a ball. There is usually no contact with any other player, nor is there any jumping or landing awkwardly. The knee is painful to walk on and will not straighten fully ('locked'). It becomes swollen over a few hours and an effusion develops.

Examination at this time reveals a knee lacking 10 or more degrees of extension, a moderate effusion and usually medial joint line tenderness.

With the knee as straight as it will go there is usually tenderness over the medial fat pad. Gentle attempts to extend the knee fully cause exacerbation of the medial pain.

If the patient is not seen for several days after the injury the displaced part of the meniscus may return to its anatomical site. This allows full extension to be regained. However, attempts to play any sport then cause further episodes of locking and the knee tends to give way as the unstable inner portion of the meniscus interposes between the joint surfaces. In these circumstances McMurray's test may be positive – rotation and extension of the knee from the flexed position produces painful clicking over the medial joint line.

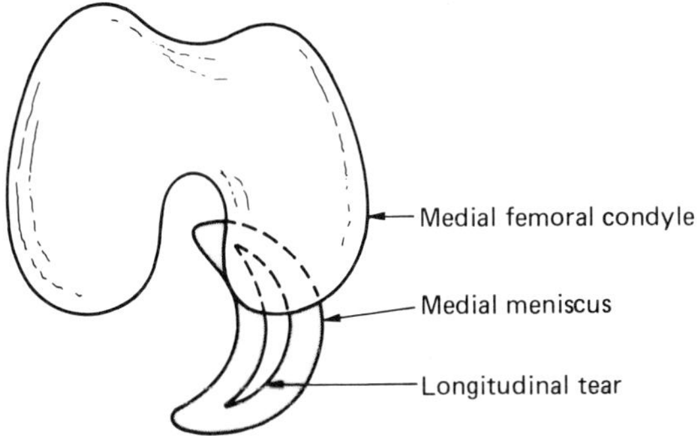

Fig. 13.3 Diagrammatic representation of the medial femoral condyle splitting the medial meniscus longitudinally.

X-rays

Plain radiographs of the knee are normal.

Further investigation

The diagnosis of a suspected meniscus tear should be confirmed by examination under anaesthesia and diagnostic arthroscopy, arthrography or nuclear magnetic resonance scanning. When this assessment is carried out it is essential to examine not only the menisci but also the knee ligaments and joint surfaces as injuries involving more than one structure are common. The presence of blood or blood staining in the joint should alert the operator to the risk of damage to structures other than the meniscus.

Treatment

In the majority of cases treatment is by excision of the torn and unstable part of the meniscus. Total meniscectomy should be avoided wherever possible because of the slower postoperative recovery and higher long-term morbidity.

In young players the tear is usually a longitudinal one which extends almost the full length of the meniscus (bucket-handle tear). In older players the tear may be a so-called cleavage tear limited to the posterior part of the meniscus.

Partial meniscectomy can be carried out arthroscopically at the same time as the diagnostic arthroscopy is performed. Removal of a full bucket-handle tear can also be carried out by open arthrotomy, which can be done under the same anaesthetic.

Posterior tears can only be treated arthroscopically if total meniscectomy is to be avoided.

In athletes who are anxious and in pain diagnostic arthroscopy and partial meniscectomy are best carried out under general anaesthetic if possible.

Rehabilitation after any form of meniscus injury is important. If the knee will not straighten fully the quadriceps muscle in the thigh, especially the vastus medialis component, wastes rapidly. Ideally, therefore, surgery of the locked knee should not be delayed for more than a few days. Even in the interim, treatment should consist of a compression bandage to support the knee together with active quadriceps exercises.

Postoperative rehabilitation consists of quadriceps and knee flexion exercises. Recovery of function is usually more rapid after arthroscopic compared with open meniscectomy. Once the patient can lift the knee straight he or she can be mobilized, partial weight-bearing, and rapidly progress to full weight-bearing. Running and jogging should be delayed for a week or so. Soccer training and similar activities are best delayed for about 2 weeks after an arthroscopic partial meniscectomy and 4–6 weeks after an open partial meniscectomy.

In teenagers with open epiphyses, consideration should be given to meniscus suture. The reason for this is that in the long term young patients do badly after meniscectomy.

Meniscus suture is most successful in peripheral tears adjacent to the meniscosynovial junction and in tears which are about 2 cm or so in length. There are various techniques described and most are about 70% successful. One of the drawbacks of meniscus suture is that postoperative recovery is slower than after partial meniscectomy. Most surgeons now recommend only a light dressing but avoidance of flexion beyond 90° for 6 weeks and avoidance of any athletic pursuits for at least 3 months.

Longitudinal tears of the lateral meniscus

These are less common than longitudinal tears of the medial meniscus but they present in the same way. Their management is identical.

Torn cystic lateral meniscus

This condition does not usually present acutely. There is a complex tear of the lateral meniscus. This is associated with a cystic swelling at the periphery of the meniscus.

The athlete usually presents with lateral knee pain made worse with any form of exercise. He or she will usually describe an aching pain which radiates up and down from the knee joint. He or she may also complain of the actual swelling of the cyst. The symptoms may be of some months' duration and may be intermittent in nature.

Examination usually reveals a cystic swelling which may be very small and just palpable or may be quite large and visible on inspection. The swelling is cystic in nature and most prominent in extension and much less obvious as the knee is flexed.

X-rays

X-rays are usually normal, although careful inspection may show the cystic swelling in the soft tissues.

Treatment

Treatment is surgical if the symptoms are disabling. The diagnosis needs to be confirmed by diagnostic arthroscopy and treatment is by excision of the torn portion of the meniscus by arthroscopic partial meniscectomy accompanied by decompressions of the cyst into the knee joint.

If the meniscus pathology is very extensive it may be necessary to carry out a total meniscectomy.

It is important that the surgery deals not only with the cyst but also the associated meniscus tear.

Rehabilitation is the same as described under longitudinal tears of the medial meniscus but is often much slower – a fact that patients need to be made aware of at the beginning of treatment.

Posterior horn tag tear of the medial meniscus (horizontal cleavage tear of the medial meniscus)

Tag tears of the posterior horn of the medial mensicus are sometimes somewhat unkindly referred to as degenerative tears. Certainly they tend to occur in older patients and the area of damage tends to be limited to the posterior horn of the meniscus. If the tags are large they interpose between the joint surfaces and cause locking and giving way. If the tags are smaller they do not cause mechanical symptoms but are associated with pain on the medial joint line behind the medial ligament. This pain tends to be more severe after exercise and troublesome at night. Symptoms from such a tear are often self-limiting and settle over a few months.

X-rays

X-rays should be taken to check that the symptoms are not due to moderate arthritic changes.

Treatment

When pain is the only symptom this may be relieved by the injection of insoluable anti-inflammatory steroid into the posterior horn area of the medial meniscus. If this is unsuccessful or if there are mechanical symptoms then a diagnostic arthroscopy or MRI scan and partial medial meniscectomy are required. In older patients arthroscopy may reveal not only meniscus pathology but also early arthritic changes in the adjacent articular surfaces. In these circumstances the conventional treatment for early osteoarthritis should be instituted. Otherwise the rehabilitation is the same as after other forms of arthroscopic meniscectomy.

Anterior cruciate ligament injuries (Figs. 13.4 and 13.5)

Damage to the anterior cruciate ligament has been brought into prominence by the more accurate

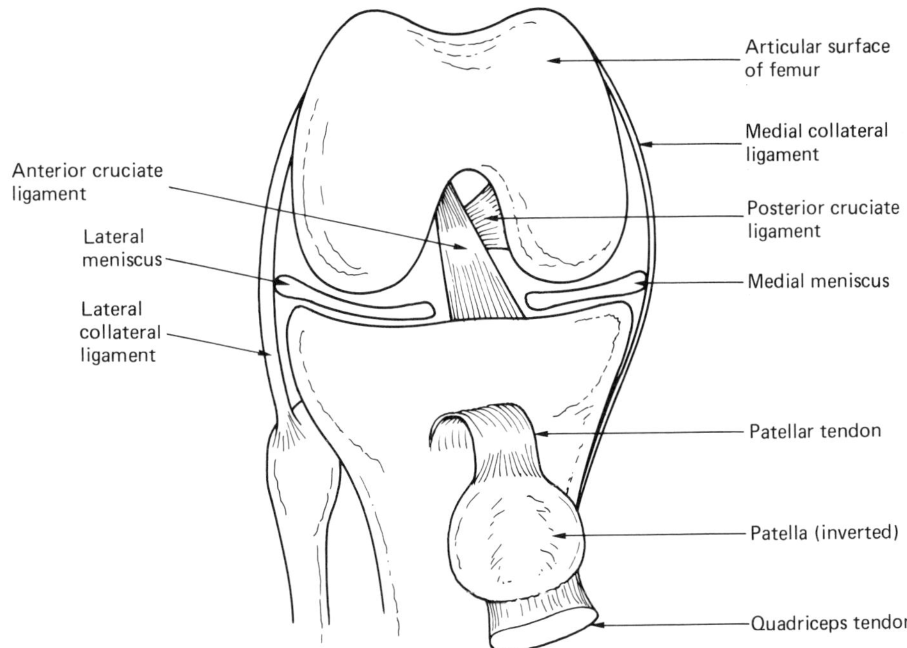

Fig. 13.4 Diagram showing the relations of the collateral and cruciate ligaments and the menisci when viewed from the front.

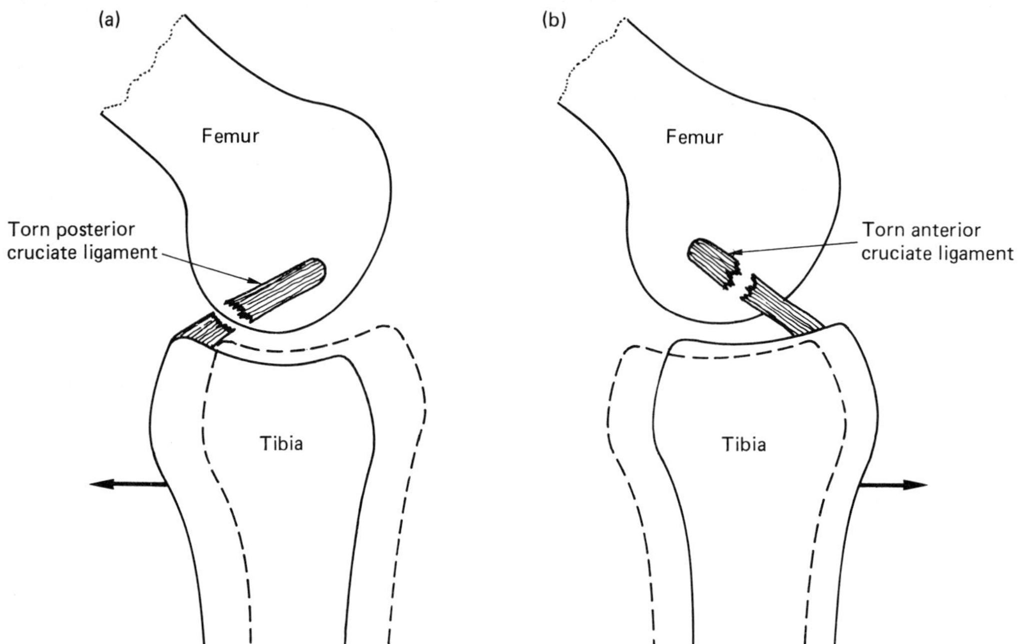

Fig. 13.5 (a) Positive posterior draw or sag sign with rupture of the posterior cruciate ligament. The tibia is displaced posteriorly relative to the femur. (b) Positive anterior draw sign – the tibia is displaced anteriorly relative to the femur. In both (a) and (b) the normal position of the tibia is shown by dashed lines.

diagnosis of acute injuries made possible over the last 25-years by the increasingly widespread use of the arthroscope. The injury occurs in contact sports, such as soccer and rugby, and in pursuits where high-speed injuries occur, e.g. skiing and ballet. In the vast majority of cases the patient will describe a sudden stop, for example landing awkwardly from a jump or a blocked tackle. More rarely he or she may describe a collision with deformity (most often into valgus) occurring at the knee joint. Many patients also report a noise, such as a pop or snap, occurring at the time of injury.

Following the injury the patient is unable to continue to run but can usually walk immediately afterwards. The damaged ligament bleeds and usually a haemarthrosis develops within an hour or so, causing a swollen, painful and sometimes throbbing joint.

Examination is superficially unremarkable. If the knee is very swollen then the quadriceps are inhibited and the knee will not extend fully. Extreme flexion beyond 90° is often painful. The anterior cruciate ligament rupture will be missed unless specifically tested for.

Examination must first check for the integrity of the posterior capsule of the knee joint. This is done with the knee fully extended when the tibia is subjected to varus and valgus strains by supporting the distal femur and pushing the foot medially and laterally. Any instability in this position indicates severe ligament damage, probably involving the posterior capsule, one of the collateral ligaments and also both cruciate ligaments.

For the anterior cruciate ligament itself three tests must be carried out. If the knee is very swollen the haemarthrosis must be aspirated first under local anaesthesia. If the knee is very painful then it may not be possible to examine the ligaments properly without general anaesthesia.

The *anterior drawer sign* is the easiest test to perform and should be done first. With the patient supine on the examination couch the knee is flexed to 90°. A visual inspection is carried out to check for a posterior sag which would indicate posterior cruciate damage. The fingers of both hands are then placed behind the upper tibia which is pulled forwards. Care must be taken to ensure the knee is not being stabilized by hamstring muscle spasm. If the tendons are tight this should be easily detected by the fingers. There is normally a few millimetres of anterior tibial glide relative to the distal femur. The examination must determine whether there is increased glide between the normal and abnormal sides and also whether the anterior glide has a definite end-point. Any increase in glide and the absence of a definite end-point is suspicious of anterior cruciate ligament damage.

The *Lachman test* is then performed. With the knee in about 30° of flexion the femur is held in one hand whilst the tibia is pulled anteriorly with the other hand. This test can be difficult in the patient who has big thighs for the examiner who has small hands. There is normally slight laxity in this position and it is important to compare the two sides.

The *pivot shift test*, which was first described by McIntosh, is the final test for the anterior cruciate ligament. The knee is very slightly flexed and the limb internally rotated by holding the heel. A valgus force is applied by the examiner placing a hand behind the upper fibula, which is lifted upwards. If the anterior cruciate ligament is torn then the upper tibia will now sublux forwards. Whilst maintaining the valgus and internal rotation forces the knee is then flexed. As flexion proceeds the tibia suddenly reduces into its normal position with a jerk. This test can be quite distressing for the patient. However, if it is positive the patient may well exclaim that this is what happens to him when his knee gives way.

A rupture of the anterior cruciate ligament has not been excluded unless all three test are negative.

In muscular athletes the results will often be equivocal and the diagnosis can only be established by examination under anaesthesia. X-rays should be taken to exclude avulsion fractures.

In ideal circumstances, where the history and initial examination lead to suspicion of anterior cruciate ligament injury, examination under anaesthesia and arthroscopy should be carried out within a few days. Where there is extensive capsular damage confirmed at examination under anaesthesia, arthroscopy should be undertaken only with extreme caution because of the risk of extravasation of irrigation fluid, which may cause a compartment syndrome in the calf.

Examination under anaesthesia examines the ligaments as outlined above. The arthroscopy serves two purposes. First, it identifies where the anterior cruciate ligament is damaged (in most cases somewhere in the mid-substance of the ligament). Secondly, it allows other damage to be identified. Posterior horn tears of one of the menisci commonly accompany up to 50% of anterior cruciate ligament tear in most series.

Treatment of acute anterior cruciate ligament injuries

Bony avulsions

The only lesions that are simply treated are the lesions where there is a bony avulsion along with an intact ligament. If the ligament has been avulsed with a piece of bone this should be reduced and internally fixed as soon as possible. Small screws are usually best for this. Care must be taken that the screw head does not impinge on the articular surface opposite in full extension. Usually the fixation needs to be protected in plaster for 4–6 weeks. Athletic training should not be undertaken for 3 months.

Tear of the ligament itself

Direct repair is almost impossible. Surgery at the time of diagnosis is only rarely indicated. It is far better to make the diagnosis at examination under anaesthesia and arthroscopy and then discuss possible treatment with the patient when he or she has recovered from the acute injury and anaesthetic. The delay this causes need be no more than 1 or 2 weeks if time is short.

Conservative treatment

The aim of conservative treatment is to re-educate the patient so that the function of the damaged anterior cruciate ligament is taken over by the hamstring muscles. Intensive physiotherapy is therefore necessary to achieve first hamstring power and second hamstring contraction when the knee is flexed 25 or 30°. Power can be developed with weights and active knee flexion against a load. Running backwards is often useful.

To get hamstrings to contract in 25 or 30° of flexion is 'unnatural'. Most patients can make their muscles contract in 90° of flexion and then the amount of flexion must be gradually reduced. Finally the patient must start running, first of all in a straight line and then turning and cutting. With such treatment many athletes return to their sport; others may return to a different sport.

Early substitution repair
The place for such procedures is not yet fully established beyond dispute. The techniques described under chronic anterior cruciate ligament instability (below) may be utilized and may be appropriate for high-grade and professional athletes.

It is important to remember that after any such procedures participation in competitive sports is not advised for a period of at least 6 months.

Chronic anterior cruciate ligament instability

Many patients who present with chronic instability with symptoms and signs of anterior cruciate deficiency have other problems which must be treated first. The whole knee joint must be assessed and the following conditions considered:

1. Persisting muscle weakness after inadequate treatment to date.
2. Meniscus tears.
3. Patellofemoral problems and other joint surface problems.

Chronic anterior cruciate ligament instability causes giving way on turning and may cause symptoms on running or even when walking. There is usually a history of a moderately severe initial injury.

Examination will reveal positive anterior drawer, Lachman and pivot shift tests. The signs of a coexisting meniscus tear should always be sought. A positive 'crunch test' is almost diagnostic of anterior cruciate laxity and a posterior horn tear of one of the menisci. The crunch test is positive if when the anterior drawer test is carried out vigorously the tibia locks momentarily in the anteriorly subluxed position as the femoral condyle displaces the inner rim of the torn meniscus forwards.

Investigation

In all patients with a chronic anterior cruciate ligament instability an arthroscopy must be performed to assess the state of the menisci. In young patients with peripheral tears of the meniscus consideration should be given to meniscus suture. Such patients probably require surgical stabilization of the anterior cruciate ligament instability at the same time if the meniscus suture is to be successful. Small tears of the menisci which can be resected to leave a peripheral rim of intact meniscus should be treated by partial meniscectomy.

Following this, conservative rehabilitation measures should be pursued vigorously (see conservative treatment of acute anterior cruciate ligament injuries, above).

If stability cannot be achieved then the patient has three alternatives:

1. To reduce the level of activity.
2. To use a derotation brace when participating in certain sports.
3. Substitution repair of the damaged ligament.

Use of a derotation brace

A derotation brace is an external appliance which substitutes for the function of the damaged ligament. To be effective the brace is quite bulky and it may not be acceptable to the patient. It is certainly not suitable for contact sports. However, intermittent use of a derotation brace may be acceptable to an older player of, for example, tennis. He or she may wear the brace when playing. Very few patients are prepared to wear a brace for more than a couple of hours at a time.

Substitution repair for chronic anterior cruciate instability

The anterior cruciate ligament has to be replaced with another material. Whatever material is used cannot replace all the functions of the natural anterior cruciate ligament which has a complex load-bearing and proprioceptive function. The patient must realize that normality is not being restored and that the procedure is not universally successful.

Substitution may be carried out using either synthetic material (such as Dacron, polypropylene, PTFE, Goretex or carbon fibre) or with autogenous material, notably fascia lata or patellar tendon. This material is inserted either in the track of the damaged anterior cruciate ligament or extra-articularly around the lateral side of the joint, roughly parallel with the original anterior cruciate ligament.

None of the synthetic materials has ideal properties and many synthetic ligaments loosen or fail over a period of 2 years or so. Their fate over a period of a life-time remains, as yet, uncertain. The author remains unconvinced that any of these synthetic ligaments stimulate the formation of a neoligament in the site of the original anterior cruciate ligament itself.

The autogenous material with the properties nearest to the natural anterior cruciate ligament is a graft made up of the middle third of the patellar tendon. Jones is credited with the early use of this material to replace the anterior cruciate. Early techniques used a long graft extending from the tibial tubercle across the patella and into the quadriceps tendon. This graft was the anchored in a bone tunnel in the tibia and passed over the lateral femoral condyle to be anchored adjacent to the lateral intermuscular septum on the lateral side of the femoral shaft.

More recently short grafts of patellar tendon with a bone plug from the patella proximally and a bone plug from the tibial tubercle distally have been used, with good early results. Fixation of the bone plugs is in bone tunnels using self-tapping headless screws. Details of one such technique have been described by Bach (1989). Cadaveric tendon grafts have recently been used with good early results.

Postoperative management does not require elaborate bracing. Crutch walking, with partial weight-bearing, can begin as soon as the patient is comfortable. The graft should be protected for 3 months, during which time walking is allowed but more vigorous activity should be avoided. Running can be commenced 3 months after insertion of the graft, by which time the bone plug should have incorporated and revascularization started. Competitive sports should be avoided for at least 6 months after any such substitution repair.

Acute medial ligament strain

This injury, which is an incomplete tear of the medial collateral ligament, characteristically occurs in skiers. The patient is often skiing on poor snow. The ski tip catches and the knee externally rotates and a valgus force strains the medial collateral ligament. Usually the skier continues to ski. If he or she stops, for example for lunch or at the end of the day, the knee becomes stiff and sore, weight-bearing is painful, skiing impossible.

Examination

Examination, usually a few hours later, reveals a knee which the patient will not extend fully by about 20° and which will not flex beyond about 80°. There is tenderness which is usually well-localized over the femoral origin of the medial collateral ligament, above the medial joint line. The ligaments are all clinically stable but stressing the medial collateral ligament causes pain.

X-ray

X-rays are normal initially. After a few weeks there may be a trace of calcification at the origin of the medial collateral ligament from the femur.

Treatment

Treatment is initially for comfort. If the patient is very sore and needs to travel home a padded support bandage and crutches may be best. Relief is often given by local infiltration of Marcain to which insoluble steroid may be added. This usually allows the knee to extend fully so that any meniscus pathology may be largely excluded on clinical grounds.

Further treatment consists of physiotherapy to mobilize the knee and local anti-inflammatory treatment. Symptoms often persist to a minor degree for several months.

Arthroscopy or MRI scanning may be useful to exclude meniscus damage and so encourage the patient to mobilize fully.

Iliotibial band sydrome – 'Runner's knee' (Fig. 13.2)

The iliotibial band runs down from the pelvis, along the lateral aspect of the thigh to insert into the lateral aspect of the tibia and Gerdy's tubercle. If the iliotibial band is well-developed and tight it may cause pressure on the knee joint synovium where it crosses the lateral femoral condyle at the joint line.

The patient experiences pain with exercise. The condition is commonest in long-distance runners with slight varus deformity of the knee and internal torsion of the lower limb.

Examination

Examination reveals localized tenderness under the iliotibial band a few fingerbreadths anterior to the hamstring tendons. Discomfort is made worse if the iliotibial band is tightened by crossing the affected leg straight over the other leg. Symptoms are diminished by abduction of the affected hip and flexion of the knee on the same side since these manoeuvres reduce the tension in the iliotibial band.

Treatment

Treatment is conservative and consists of local treatment to diminish the inflammation in the tender area, for example ice and ultrasound. Non-steroidal anti-inflammatories, given orally, may also be helpful and exercises should be given to stretch and so reduce the tension in the iliotibial band itself. It may be necessary for the athlete to modify the amount of long-distance road running.

Acute dislocation of the patella

The patella dislocates laterally. This may occur because of extreme violence, e.g. in a rugby scrum, or because the patient has an underlying tendency to dislocation. Patients who are prone to patellar dislocation are often slightly knock-kneed, have a high patella and genu recurvatum (the knee hyperextends) and may have generalized joint laxity. Many such patients are female.

Patients usually say the knee 'dislocated'. They often describe how the inner aspect of the distal femur became very prominent. This is because the patella has slid laterally. Usually the dislocation is reduced spontaneously by the patient straightening out the knee.

Examination

Examination shortly afterwards can be misleading if an accurate history is not taken. Because the patella dislocates laterally the capsular structures are torn on the medial side of the joint, causing tenderness over the medial femoral condyle and medial joint line. The tenderness, usually with some local swelling and thickening, extends well above the joint line (compared with the well-localized joint line tenderness of a torn meniscus). Any attempt to redislocate the patella by pushing it laterally with the fingers is extremely painful and causes quadriceps muscle spasm.

X-ray

X-rays should be taken, including skyline views of the patella to exclude osteochondral fractures. A small osteochondral fragment lying adjacent to the medial border of the patella is almost diagnostic of an episode of dislocation.

Treatment

Treatment is usually conservative. To allow the capsular structures to heal the knee is immobilized almost completely straight for 4–6 weeks. A padded bandage is most comfortable initially and can be replaced with either a removable splint or a padded, long-leg plaster when the initial swelling has subsided. After 4 weeks or so gradual mobilization and quadriceps exercises can be commenced in the physiotherapy department. Recovery takes at least 6 weeks.

In high-grade athletes and professional sports players arthroscopy may be indicated to assess the joint surface damage and check for other pathology. There is a recent trend towards early surgical repair of the damaged capsular structures in such patients. Rehabilitation remains as with conservative treatment.

Acute chondral and osteochondral fractures

Part of the joint surface, usually of the patella or femur, may separate, either as a chondral fracture or as an osteochrondral fracture. Such fractures occur as a result of:

1. Dislocation of the patella.
2. Overload – for example, during a sudden change of direction in squash or tennis or during weight-lifting.
3. Direct trauma – for example, a kick or motor cycle accident.

The patient experiences sudden pain. Examination reveals that there is little abnormality, except perhaps tenderness over the damaged joint surface and a trace of fluid. X-rays show no abnormality with chondral lesions but osteochondral fractures can be seen as small flakes of calcification separate from the joint surfaces. It is important to remember that large areas of articular cartilage may be associated with very small radiopaque fragments.

Diagnosis

Diagnosis is usually made at arthroscopy. Certainly the extent of any chondral damage should be assessed in this way.

Treatment

Treatment is by shaving small chondral flaps and removing small osteochondral lesions. Larger osteochondral lesions, say more than 1.5 cm in diameter, should probably be replaced in their anatomical site and internally fixed with pins or small screws such as Herbert screws. If the lesion is replaced then the knee should be immobilized in a plaster cylinder and the leg kept non-weight-bearing until the fracture has healed in 6–8 weeks. Gradual mobilization then takes a further similar period of time.

If the lesion is excised or shaved no immobilization is required. The patient should be gradually mobilized. He or she may experience some discomfort and swelling which should be treated with ultrasound, ice and non-steroidal anti-inflammatory drugs.

Patients should be warned that the joint surface will never be completely normal again and that they can expect some aching and exercise in the future.

Recurrent patellar subluxation and dislocation

Patients who suffer from episodes of recurrent subluxation of the patella usually female, have knock-kneed deformity and may have a high patella, generalized joint laxity and a poor vastus medialis part of the quadriceps muscle.

The patella subluxes laterally and the knee feels unstable and may give way when this occurs. Lateral subluxation of the right patella tends to occur when the patient turns to the left and vice-versa.

In addition, the episodes of dislocation and subluxation may damage the joint surfaces of the patellofemoral joint, causing anterior knee pain, swelling and stiffness.

Examination

Examination reveals the physical characteristics outlined above. In addition, the patient demonstrates patellar apprehension. If the knee is slightly flexed (for example, by crossing it in front of the other knee when the patient is lying on the examination couch) and the examiner then pushes the patella laterally with the fingers, the patient becomes very apprehensive as he or she fears the patella is about to dislocate. The examiner should check that attempts to push the patella medially cause less apprehension.

Treatment

Treatment initially may be conservative and is aimed to build up the vastus medialis part of the quadriceps muscle. Straight leg raising, using ankle weights, with the knee absolutely fully extended is important in achieving this.

If the problem does not resolve with these measures then surgery should be considered. The simplest surgery is a lateral release – the lateral joint capsule and retinaculum is divided from above the patella down to the joint line adjacent to the patellar tendon.

After such surgery postoperative bleeding from the lateral geniculate vessels may cause a postoperative haemarthrosis. Early knee flexion must be started after surgery to avoid the release healing back to its former position.

Further surgery in the form of a tibial tubercle transfer or medial plication of the quadriceps may be required if there is marked anatomical deformity or a lateral release is unsuccessful.

Chondromalacia patellae

This is a term which means different things to different people. It is used here to mean disorganization of the articular cartilage on the back of the patella. The patient complains of anterior knee pain during and after exercise, especially when the patellofemoral joint is loaded on ascending and descending stairs or carrying out sports where the knee is loaded in flexion, such as skiing. In addition, other symptoms include stiffness after sitting, some clicking and grating on flexion and extension and often intermittant slight swelling. The symptoms often start after unusually severe exercise and then recur with lesser activity.

Examination

Examination reveals slight quadriceps wasting. Patients are often unable to go into a full squat with the affected knee. When they do squat there is retropatellar crepitus and discomfort. The crepitus may be heard or felt, or both. In severe cases there may be diffuse, slight swelling and a small effusion in the joint.

X-ray

X-rays, including skyline views of the patellofemoral joint, are usually normal.

Treatment

Treatment is initially conservative with the use of static quadriceps exercises and the local application of ice or ultrasound, together with oral non-steroidal anti-inflammatories. Modification of activities and the use of soft-soled shoes, such as trainers, are usually also necessary.

Investigation

If these measures are not helpful then diagnostic arthroscopy should be considered to confirm the diagnosis. At arthroscopy the patellar surface and femoral groove must not only be inspected but also probed. Other causes of anterior knee pain, such as chronically displaced bucket-handle tears and fat pad trapping, must also be excluded.

Surgical treatment

Surgical treatment is unpredictable in its outcome. Local areas of abnormal articular cartilage may be shaved but often large areas of the patella are softened and the articular cartilage is unstable on probing. Often there is no obvious mechanical cause for the condition. However, if there is either recurrent subluxation, which usually damages the medial border of the patella, or evidence of excessive lateral pressure syndrome with a tight lateral retinaculum and a very stable patellofemoral joint, often with some internal torsion of the lower limb, then lateral release may be helpful.

The presence of a large area of abnormal patellar articular cartilage usually excludes participation in high-grade, competitive athletics.

'Jumper's knee' (Fig. 13.2)

This is a partial tear of the attachment of the patellar tendon to the lower pole of the patella. A jumper or sprinter develops pain over the front of the knee. This settles with rest and then recurs as activity is increased again. Maximum performance is not possible. The condition is one of an overload of the patellar tendon and its attachment to the patella; a similar condition is seen in patients with cerebral palsy who walk with a disorganized flexed-knee gait and cause overload in this area.

Examination

Examination reveals only very localized tenderness at the lower pole of the patella. A careful check should be made for symptoms and signs of chondromalacia patella and patellar subluxation.

X-ray

X-rays may show osteoporosis of the lower pole of the patella or an area of calcification just below the lower pole of the patella, when the condition may be known as Sinding–Larsen–Johansson syndrome.

Treatment

Treatment is initially by rest to allow healing. A plaster cylinder ensures this. Straight leg raising should be avoided. After 4–6 weeks the knee is gradually strengthened and mobilized.

Recurrence is common. If symptoms are troublesome surgical exploration of the tendon may be useful. The tendon should be split longitudinally. There may be an area of granulation tissue which should be excised or there may be areas of calcification which should also be excised. Recovery is slow in most cases. The knee should be splinted for 2 weeks and then gradually mobilized. Competitive sports should probably be avoided for at least 3 months.

Osgood–Schlatter syndrome (Fig. 13.2)

In teenagers with open epiphyses pain may develop over the tibial tubercle where the patellar tendon is inserted. The condition is also known as tibial apophysitis and is a type of traction apophysitis. The loads placed on the patellar tendon damage its insertion into the young patient's bone.

The patient complains of pain with exercise and sometimes also tenderness over a swollen tibial tubercle on which it is painful to kneel.

X-ray

X-rays show fragmentation of the tongue of the tibial epiphysis where the patellar tendon is attached to it.

Treatment

Treatment is by rest. Limitation of athletic pursuits may be sufficient or, if this fails, immobilization in a plaster cylinder will often settle the symptoms. Reassurance is an important part of the treatment. The majority of cases settle when the epiphysis closes.

Osgood–Schlatter ossicle

Occasionally part of the tibial tubercle affected by Osgood–Schlatter disease when the epiphysis is open fails to fuse with the tibial tubercle when the rest of the epiphysis closes. One or more small fragments of bone or ossicles persist at the attachment of the patellar tendon. Such ossicles are sometimes a cause of local pain and discomfort with exercise.

Examination

Examination reveals tenderness localized over a slightly enlarged tibial tubercle in someone whose epiphyses are closed.

X-ray

X-ray shows one or more ossicles.

Treatment

Treatment may not be needed once the cause of the symptoms has been explained to the patient. However, if disability is a problem the ossicles can be removed surgically. It may be necessary to split the patellar tendon to remove the ossicle. Some of the ossicles are within the substance of the tendon, some lie behind the tendon. Care must be taken to remove the ossicle completely and to remove all of them. Following surgery the knee is gradually mobilized but recovery is often slow and it may take 3 or 4 months to regain full activity.

The lower leg

General considerations

In the lower leg it is important always to consider not only soft tissue causes of pain but also:

1. Referred pain from the lumbosacral spine.
2. Sciatic pain from pressure or tension on the sciatic nerve, usually from a prolapsed intervertebral disc.
3. Local bone pathology – for example, stress fractures.

Compartment syndromes (Fig. 13.6; see Chapter 4)

The leg has three compartments:

1. In the anterior compartment the muscles dorsiflex the foot and toes. Damage to these

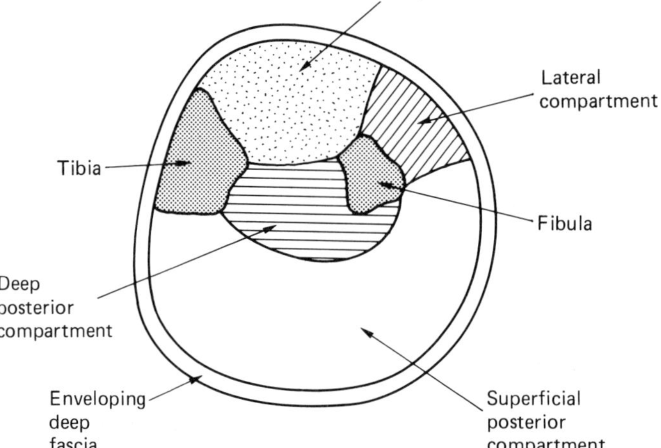

Fig. 13.6 Transverse section of the lower leg showing the anterior, lateral and deep posterior compartments separated by the intermuscular septa.

muscles causes toe scuffing and the foot slaps on the ground as the patient walks.
2. In the lateral compartment the muscles evert the foot. Damage to the muscles here may cause the ankle to invert.
3. In the posterior compartment the muscles plantarflex the foot and toes and damage to the muscles here reduces the ability to run and stand on tiptoe.

In the compartment syndromes the blood supply to the muscles in the affected compartment is embarrassed. One or more compartments may be affected. In chronic compartment syndromes the muscle in the affected compartment becomes painful and swollen and hard with exercise. The power of the muscle is reduced progressively as the exercise continues. When the exercise stops, the symptoms disappear.

In the acute condition the loss of blood supply to the muscle is virtually total. The patient, therefore, has severe ischaemic pain. The symptoms do not stop when the exercise ceases. The survival of the muscle is in jeopardy unless surgical decompression is performed as a matter of extreme urgency. The acute condition may occur *de novo* or it may follow local soft tissue trauma, a fracture, or it may develop from an established chronic compartment syndrome.

Examination

Examination reveals the hard muscle compartment after excercise. In the acute syndrome the patient is also in agony and usually cannot keep still. It is important to realize that the presence of pedal pulses distally and adequate skin circulation can coexist with a compartment syndrome.

Investigation

The diagnosis of an acute compartment syndrome is clinical. In chronic compartment syndromes the diagnosis may be more difficult. Stress fractures and referred pains must be excluded. Pressure monitoring may be useful to confirm the diagnosis.

Treatment

Treatment of any compartment syndrome is by surgical decompression, by dividing the tight, deep fascia over the affected compartment or compartments.

In acute cases a long skin incision is made. The deep fascia is divided and the muscle inspected throughout its length. In acute, severe cases primary skin closure may not be possible. Delayed closure or split-skin grafting may be necessary.

In chronic cases a subcutaneous fasciotomy through a short skin incision usually suffices.

Postoperative recovery is usually rapid provided no muscle damage has occurred. No training should be allowed until the skin is soundly healed.

The medial tibial stress syndrome (shin splints) (Fig. 13.7)

The term 'shin splints' is widely used but means different things to different people and is probably best avoided. The medial tibial stress syndrome is ill-understood but may be caused by the damage to the attachment of the muscle and deep fascia of the deep posterior compartment to the distal tibia itself. The athlete complains of pain over the distal half of the medial border of the tibia, usually following running or jumping on hard surfaces or after an increase in severity of training. The symptoms settle with rest and then recur.

Examination

Examination reveals local tenderness over the medial border of the tibia which may be slightly swollen and nodular.

X-ray

X-rays should be taken to exclude a stress fracture. Damage to the muscle and fascial attachments does not normally show on X-ray.

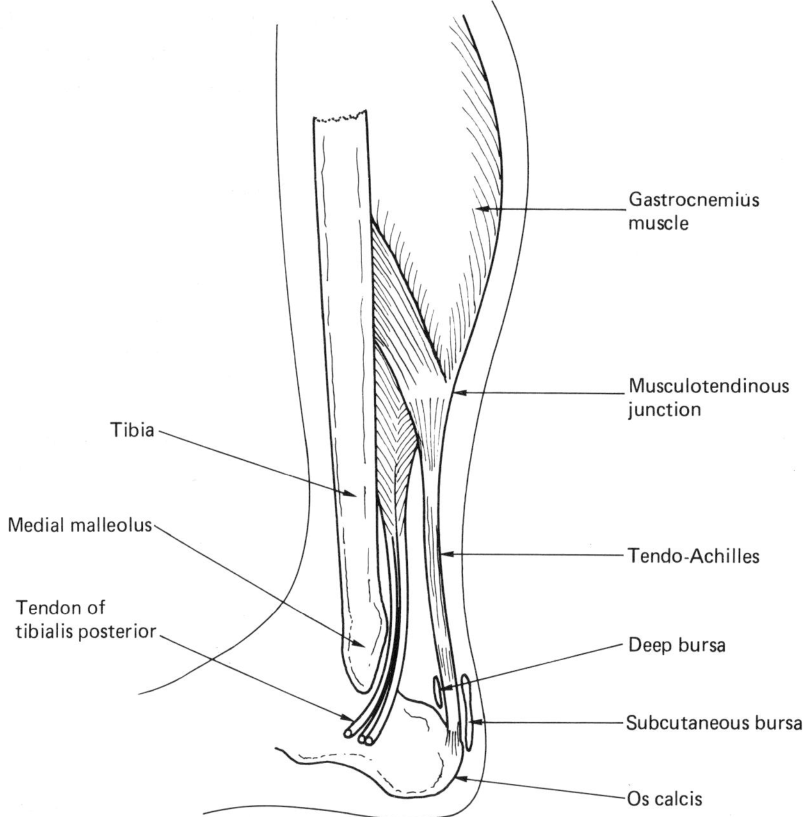

Fig. 13.7 Medial side of lower leg and ankle showing tendo-Achilles and tibialis posterior tendon.

Investigation

It may be difficult to differentiate between a deep posterior compartment syndrome and the medial tibial stress syndrome. Compartment pressure monitoring may be helpful.

Treatment

Treatment is initially conservative with rest, review of training regimes and the use of local anti-inflammatory measures, such as ice, ultrasound and oral non-steroidal anti-inflammatory drugs. If these measures fail surgical release of the deep fascia along the medial edge of the tibia may be performed but is not universally successful (such surgery also decompresses the deep posterior compartment).

The tendo-Achilles (Fig. 13.7)

General considerations

The most serious injury, which is important not to miss, is a rupture of the tendo-Achilles. Rupture must always be excluded by careful examination before any other diagnosis is entertained.

Acute rupture of the tendo-Achilles

The history is classical. The patient is running, dancing or playing sport and he or she thinks they have been struck on the back of the calf. Over the next few hours local pain and swelling occur and walking is difficult. Over a few days bruising appears around the tendon and down to the heel.

Examination

Examination can be quite misleading if the injury is seen very early. After a few hours there is local tenderness and a palpable gap where the ends of the tendon have separated.

The essential test is the so-called Thomson's test. The patient is asked to kneel with the feet hanging over the edge of the examination couch. The examiner squeezes the calf. If the tendo-Achilles is intact, the foot is plantarflexed. If the tendo-Achilles is ruptured, the foot does not move.

Active plantarflexion of the foot is not a good test for the tendo-Achilles as the long toe flexors can achieve this movement at the ankle.

Treatment

Treatment may be conservative with immobilization in an equinus plaster of Paris or surgical repair may be carried out. Either way the patient will be on crutches for 4–6 weeks in an equinus plaster. After this length of time the plaster can be changed to a below-knee walking plaster which is retained for another 4–6 weeks. When this plaster is removed the patient should use shoes with a moderate heel for a further period of 4–6 weeks.

Athletic training should not be undertaken for about 16 weeks from the time of injury and should even then be carefully graduated. Competition should be avoided for at least 6 months.

In acute ruptures the results of operative and conservative treatment appear to be very similar. In patients with varicose veins or skin damage and in older patients conservative treatment has fewer complications.

Incomplete tears of the tendo-Achilles

This is a dangerous diagnosis to make. In functional terms all tears are probably effectively complete and unless treated as such will almost certainly become complete.

Modern imaging techniques, notably magnetic resonance imaging, should make such diagnoses more objective. However, the treatment of incomplete tears remains essentially the same as the management of total rupture.

Missed and late ruptures of the tendo-Achilles

The patient often describes an incident as outlined above, and subsequently complains of difficulty walking with a normal gait. On the affected side the foot tends to slap on the ground and the patient cannot run.

Clinical examination invariably reveals a palpable gap in the tendo-Achilles. There may be bruising extending down to the heel. Thomson's test is positive.

Treatment

By 2 weeks after injury conservative treatment appears to be relatively ineffective. Surgery must, therefore, be undertaken. Because the tendon ends have separated considerable dissection and mobilization may be needed. Direct repair should be carried out, even if this means holding the ankle in considerable equinus. If this fails local tissue flaps are preferable to the insertion of avascular grafts or synthetic materials.

After such procedures the ankle must be maintained in equinus for 8–12 weeks. Wound healing may be a problem. Athletic pursuits should be delayed for about a year.

Damage to the musculotendinous junction of the tendo-Achilles

The insertion of the gastrocnemius or soleus muscles into the tendo-Achilles may be damaged during vigorous athletic pursuits. The tenderness and swelling is above the tendo-Achilles itself and extends into the bole of the calf which is often thickened swollen and tender with haematoma. The tendo-Achilles itself can always be palpated and felt to be intact throughout its length.

Dorsiflexion of the ankle and foot causes pain in

the calf and unless a careful history is taken a diagnosis of deep vein thrombosis may be made in older patients.

Treatment

Treatment is along the lines for any muscle tear with rest and local anti-inflammatory measures. Some patients may be more comfortable for 2 weeks in a padded below-knee walking plaster of Paris. Otherwise support bandaging and anti-inflammatory treatment are given. A fluctuant haematoma may require aspiration from its highest point. Very rarely in young, high-grade athletes in whom a major muscle disruption is suspected, surgical exploration to evacuate clot and appose the damaged muscles ends is indicated.

Healing always takes a minimum of 6 weeks. Athletic training should be postponed for at least this period of time and competitive sport avoided for 3 months after major tears.

Thickening and nodularity of the tendo-Achilles

Many patients present with a history of pain and discomfort in the area of the tendo-Achilles. Often there is no major injury but they describe discomfort on putting the affected foot to the ground first thing in the morning and pain and aching after exercise.

Examination

Examination reveals tenderness and thickening most commonly in the middle third of the tendo-Achilles, most obvious if compared with the asymptomatic, normal side. Occasionally active movement of the tendon will reveal crepitus or grating.

There are clinical difficulties in distinguishing thickening of the tendon itself from thickening of the surrounding paratenon – this is another area where magnetic resonance imaging may be useful if it is available.

In the absence of a definite acute injury such nodules are usually due to either degenerative tears of the tendon or inflammation of the paratenon.

Treatment

Treatment is initially conservative with rest, non-steroidal anti-inflammatories and local physiotherapy. Ice is also useful and can be self-administered at home. Such treatment may need to be continued for 2–3 months. If the condition persists the area should be explored surgically and adhesions around the tendon sheath divided and the tendon itself inspected. After such surgery early postoperative mobilization is advised. Symptoms are usually helped but recovery takes several weeks and may be incomplete.

Bursitis around the heel (Fig. 13.7)

There is a normal bursa separating the skin from the tendo-Achilles and the os calcis at the back of the heel. This may become red and inflamed with pressure from shoes. New shoes are a common cause of bursitis and blistering at this site. In the majority of cases care with footwear is all that is required to resolve the problem.

Occasionally an underlying bony ridge on the outer side of the os calcis may make the wearing of normal shoes with heels very difficult and painful. In this case the bony lump should be carefully excised at operation. Interference with the bursa itself is not helpful.

There is a second bursa lying deep to the tendo-Achilles between the tendo-Achilles and the os calcis. This bursa may become inflamed with unaccustomed exercise, especially marching uphill or mountaineering, both of which activities compress the bursa during dorsiflexion of the ankle and foot.

Examination

Examination reveals tenderness just above the insertion of the tendon and below the level of the upper border of the os calcis.

Treatment

Treatment is by rest and avoidance of hard boots and walking uphill. Rarely, a protuberance of the posterosuperior surface of the os calcis may be the cause of recurrent problems and is discovered by X-ray. If such a protuberance is discovered symptoms can be relieved by excision of a wedge of bone.

The ankle (Fig. 13.8)

General considerations

The commonest injury of the ankle is a 'sprained ankle'. Such injuries should be X-rayed to exclude fractures. If a patient develops recurrent ankle sprains the consideration must be given to the possibility of underlying neuromuscular conditions, such as nerve root compression from an intervertebral disc prolapse or Charcot–Marie–Tooth syndrome.

The acute ankle sprain

The vast majority of ankle injuries are inversion sprains. The most commonly damaged ligament is the anterior talofibular ligament running forwards from the fibula on to the hindfoot.

The injured person almost always gives a history of 'going over' on the ankle, often as a result of stepping awkwardly or slipping. They are aware of acute pain but may be able to continue walking if not running for a few hours, when the ankle becomes swollen and stiff and weight-bearing difficult.

Examination

Examination reveals swelling and tenderness just in front of the lateral malleolus over the anterior talofibular ligament. Typically the fibula itself is less tender.

The stability of the ankle should be tested using the draw sign – the heel is pulled forwards whilst the tibia is steadied. In a normal ankle there should be minimal forward glide of the heel.

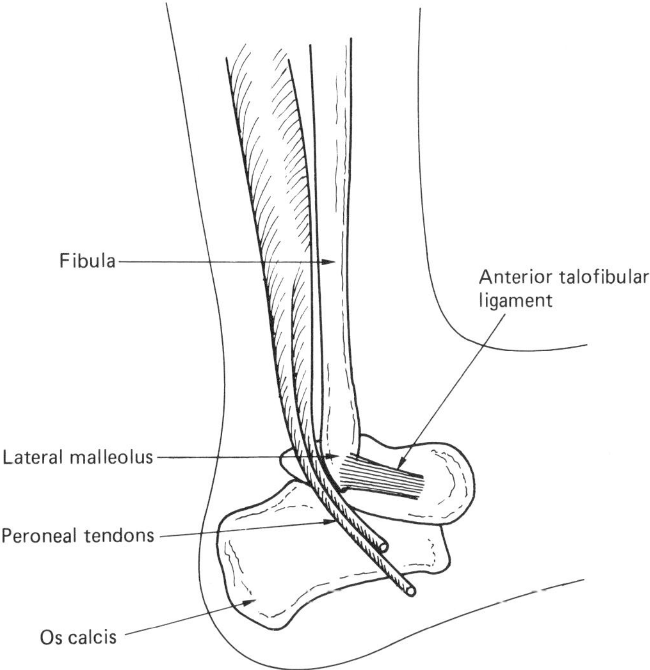

Fig. 13.8 Lateral side of ankle showing anterior talofibular ligament and peroneal tendons.

X-ray

X-rays are taken to exclude a fracture, particularly a fracture of the lateral malleolus. There is no place for stress views in an acute injury.

Treatment

The vast majority of ankle injuries can be treated conservatively. Healing of the damaged ligaments is ensured by immobilization and a light-weight below-knee walking plaster for 3–4 weeks is comfortable and allows some mobility for the patient. Such treatment is especially recommended for patients who are away from home.

Alternatively swelling and inflammation can be treated by the local application of ice and ultrasound plus oral anti-inflammatories. Treatment needs to be given daily and the ankle needs to be supported with a tubigrip bandage. Most patients will need crutches for several days.

Healing of the ligament takes about 6 weeks, whatever treatment is prescribed. Participation in contact sports before this carries considerable risk of further damage. Before any sport is undertaken the patient should have supervised physiotherapy to build up the ankle muscles, especially the evertors, and to regain ankle movement and proprioception. They should gradually progress from walking to jogging and then sprinting before sports.

Other acute ankle sprains

Rarely the medial ligament structures are damaged, notably the deltoid ligament. Features and treatment are similar to those of inversion injuries except that the medial aspect of the joint is involved.

Chronic ankle instability

Again the common chronic instability is on the lateral side of the joint. Patients usually complains of a 'weak' ankle and that they keep 'going over on it'.

Examination

Examination is often remarkably normal except that the draw test is positive. The lower limb neurology should be checked. A family history of any neuromuscular disorders should be sought.

Investigation

Stress X-rays should be taken. Anteroposterior stress views of the ankle are taken whilst the talus is tilted medially in the ankle mortise by the examiner.

Lateral stress views are taken whilst the heel is supported on a sand bag and the tibia is firmly pushed backward. It is essential to compare the normal and abnormal sides.

Ankle arthroscopy may also be useful in this condition. Ankle arthroscopy involves distracting the joint surfaces by inserting pins into the bones above and below the ankle. It allows inspection of the joint surfaces and division of adhesions.

Treatment

Treatment may initially be conservative. Physiotherapy to regain proprioceptive awareness should be attempted and should progress to wobble-board exercises.

Surgical treatment may be indicated if conservative measures fail. Essentially the damaged ligament is reconstructed using local tendon or fascia lata. Various procedures, for example the Chrisman–Snook operation or the Evans procedure, use all or part of the peroneus brevis tendon inserted through bone holes to substitute for the damaged ligament.

Postoperative rehabilitation is prolonged, with 6 weeks in plaster and a similar period of mobilization in physiotherapy before return to athletic pursuits. It is probably advisable to delay return to competitive sports for about 6 months.

Recurrent subluxation of the peroneal tendons (Fig. 13.8)

This is a rare problem. Usually there is a history of an initial single major incident when the affected foot is dorsiflexed and inverted, for example when a skier falls forward if the ski tips catch in deep snow. The patient may report something popping or snapping around the ankle joint. Pain and tenderness are localized behind the lateral malleolus where the retinaculum is torn.

If the injury does not heal soundly then the peroneal tendon subsequently subluxes over the lateral malleolus on inversion and dorsiflexion (compared with a lateral ligament problem, which is sustained and recurs with inversion and plantarflexion).

Examination

Examination shows the peroneal tendons both subluxing over the tip of the lateral malleolus.

Investigation

Recurrent inversion sprain may need to be excluded by stress views which show no talar tilt or subluxation.

Treatment

Treatment is surgical and aims to fix the tendons behind the lateral malleolus by altering the shape of the bone or reinforcing the soft-tissue tunnel or both. Following such surgery athletic pursuits should not be followed for at least 3 months.

Footballer's ankle

In this condition the patient, who has usually pursued an athletic career for some years, complains of discomfort and slight swelling around the front of the ankle, especially after exercise involving marked plantarflexion or dorsiflexion.

Examination reveals diffuse tenderness over the front of the ankle joint and slight limitation at the extremes of both dorsiflexion and plantarflexion. There is no instability.

X-ray

X-rays reveal calcified material around the joint margins anteriorly. These are minor avulsions and calcified areas in the capsule, often with marginal osteophytes.

Treatment

Treatment is initially conservative with local anti-inflammatory measures. If the condition is persistently symptomatic then surgery to excise the osteophytes may be helpful, although they do tend to recur.

Arthroscopy of the ankle joint and arthroscopic division of adhesions and shaving of the osteophytes may be efficacious and allow a rapid recovery.

Tibialis posterior syndrome

This condition, which is strictly a chronic tenosynovitis of the tibialis posterior tendon at the lower end of the tibia and behind the medial malleolus, presents as pain, tenderness and swelling over the inner aspect of the shin and ankle. It is common in road runners, especially if they have a tendency towards flat feet.

Examination

Examination in acute cases may reveal a lot of local swelling just behind the medial malleolus. Movement of the ankle is restricted and may cause palpable local crepitus.

X-ray

X-rays of the ankle are normal in the majority of cases, although new bone formation just above the medial malleolus has been described.

Treatment

Treatment initially is by rest and anti-inflammatories. This may be for 3 or 4 weeks in a well-padded below-knee walking plaster or by the local application of ice and ultrasound. Oral non-steroidal anti-inflammatory tablets are also useful.

Once the condition has settled consideration should be given to modifying the footwear by the use of a moderate heel and possibly also a valgus insole (longitudinal arch support). Some form of insole may be necessary for return to road-running.

If the condition recurs or fails to settle then the existence of systemic conditions, especially rheumatoid arthritis, should be considered. Once these have been excluded persisting problems can be treated by surgical decompression of the tendon sheath. A synovial biopsy should be taken at this time.

Even after surgery the athlete may need to modify his or her activities to prevent recurrence.

Rupture of the tibialis posterior tendon

In younger patients, the tendon may be lacerated if the foot is cut on glass or other sharp material. Spontaneous rupture of this tendon may occur in middle age. The patient presents with the local features of tenosynovitis of the tendon, behind the medial malleolus but in addition, has a unilateral flat-foot deformity. The heel is in valgus and the forefoot is pronated. The patient cannot stand on the affected foot and rise from the heel on to tiptoe.

Treatment

Treatment is by surgical exploration of the tendon sheath which most often shows attrition or complete rupture of the tendon. Ruptured tendons require substitution repair. Decompression may be adequate where there is marked synovitis and the tendon shows attrition but is still intact.

Following such surgery the athlete must be warned that he or she will have to modify his or her activities if recurrence is to be prevented.

The foot (Fig. 13.9)

General considerations

There is a wide range of normal foot posture. However, several problems are associated with the extremes which are:

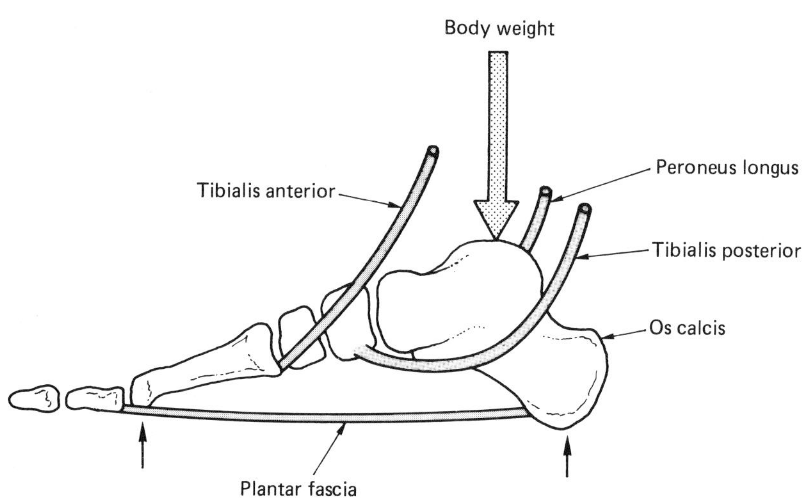

Fig. 13.9 Longitudinal arch of the foot viewed from the medial side. The plantar fascia ties together the anterior and posterior pillars of the arch. The tendons shown are important for the active maintenance of the arch.

1. Pes plano-valgus – a very flat foot with a low, longitudinal arch, valgus heel and supinated forefoot.
2. Pes cavus – a foot with a very high arch, varus heel and pronated forefoot.

Whenever patients with foot problems are seen they should always be asked to bring along the footwear which is associated with their symptoms.

Examination should include assessment not only of the ankle, subtalar, mid tarsal, forefoot and toe joints, but also of the calf muscle bulk and lower limb neurology and circulation.

Pes plano-valgus

Pes plano-valgus may be either congenital or may develop in middle age. In middle age many patients develop spread of the foot with loss of the longitudinal arch, loss of the transverse metatarsal arch at the base of the toes, together with increased width of the forefoot and increased valgus of the heel. The patient may complain of the increased width of the forefoot which makes it difficult to get shoes that fit. In addition, the loss of the transverse metatarsal arch may cause pain in the forefoot on walking or running. Often the patient who was able to walk or run in different shoes with impunity finds that certain shoes cause discomfort in the forefoot, under the metatarsal heads. It is important to emphasize to such patients that they will need to take care with their shoes and make sure they are appropriate.

Examination

Examination of the foot usually reveals a broad foot with convexity of the platar surface under the metatarsal heads. The apex of the convexity may be tender to touch. Occasionally there is a local tender spot with numbness of the adjacent parts of two of the toes (Morton's metatarsalgia).

X-ray

Any patient presenting with forefoot pain after exercise should have X-rays taken to exclude a stress fracture of the metatarsals. Changes in the metatarsophalangeal joint, such as arthritis in older patients and osteochondritis in younger patients, can also be excluded.

Treatment

Treatment initially should be conservative and aimed to restore the foot posture. Improved intrinsic foot muscle tone may help and may be achieved with physiotherapy, including faradic footbaths. External support in the form of insoles, incorporating dome metatarsal pads and sometimes valgus insoles under the longitudinal arch, may also relieve symptoms. In younger patients the use of shoes with a moderate heel may improve foot posture considerably.

Tibialis posterior syndrome

The valgus posture of the heel and loss of longitudinal arch in pes plano-valgus may predispose the patient to the tibialis posterior syndrome (see ankle problems, above).

Pes cavus

Pes cavus is usually congenital. Extreme forms may be associated with neurological conditions, such as spine bifida occulta or Friedreich's ataxia.

In the patient with exaggerated arches the weight is taken on a relatively small area of the sole of the foot under the metatarsal heads and heel. In the forefoot the skin under the metatarsal heads is very thickened. The metatarsal heads may be very prominent and tender (metatarsalgia). In addition the plantar fascia running between the metatarsal heads and the heel may be heavily loaded and stretched, giving rise to pain, usually at the attachment of the fascia to the heel (plantar fasciitis).

Metatarsalgia with pes cavus

The patient complains of tenderness under the metatarsal heads. This occurs when the patient is walking or running and often he or she will say it feels like running on glass or stones. They may also complain of thick skin or callosities under the metatarsal heads themselves.

Examination

Examination reveals a high arched foot with callosities under the metatarsal heads which are themselves very tender. In severe cases the toes are often curly and contribute relatively little to weight-bearing, thus increasing the pressure on the metatarsal heads. In assessing such feet it is important to evaluate the mobility of the hindfoot and midfoot and also of the toes, especially the big toe.

It is necessary to assess the foot with the heel held in the neutral position to see if there is fixed deformity of the forefoot (usually pronation with the first metatarsal head lying below the level of the fifth metatarsal head).

Treatment

Treatment of metatarsalgia in pes cavus is difficult. Only patients with relatively little fixed deformity will be helped by moulded insoles which allow the forefoot to be slightly pronated whilst the heel is straight. Such insoles allow the weight to be taken on a wider area of the sole of the foot. Roomy shoes and possibly even surgical shoes may be necessary to accommodate such an insole.

Chiropody to pare down existing callosities may also be useful.

In young patients soft tissue operations may reduce the cavus deformity and allow weight-bearing over a wider area of the sole of the foot. The high longitudinal arch may be lowered by a Steindler release – the plantar fascia, abductor hallucis, flexor digitorum brevis, quadratus planti and abductor digiti minimi are all released off the plantar surface of the os calcis. The foot is immobilized in plaster for 4 weeks after the procedure and then mobilized with physiotherapy.

Again in young patients the claw deformities of the toes may be corrected by flexor extensor transfers or flexor tenotomies. Where the big toe is markedly flexed at the interphalangeal joint this may be corrected by fusion and the long flexor tendon transferred and sutured to the metatarsal head. These manoeuvres increase the weight-bearing area of the sole of the foot.

In older patients with rigid deformities bony correction may be the only effective treatment. Such operations as triple arthrodesis are indicated for difficulty in walking and are certainly not of use for enabling sufferers to return to competitive athletic pursuits.

Metatarsalgia and forefoot pain in the absence of pes cavus

In these circumstances various pathologies should be excluded. Clinical examination should exclude: verrucae and foreign bodies (always check the shoes). X-rays should exclude stress fractures, sesamoiditis under the big toe and osteochondritis of the metatarsal heads. Serology should exclude early rheumatoid arthritis (especially in female patients).

Plantar fasciitis

This usually occurs in patients of middle age and above who complain of pain along the inner border of the heel. The pain is especially bad when the foot is put on the ground first thing in the morning. It then gradually eases but usually prevents walking for pleasure and running. One or both heels may be involved.

Examination

Examination reveals tenderness on the sole of the foot just in front of the malleoli where the plantar fascia inserts into the os calcis, which can usually be palpated through the skin. This pain and tenderness is made worse by dorsiflexion of the ankle and toes. Often the tender plantar fascia can be palpated as a tight band in the sole of the foot.

X-ray

X-rays of a lateral view of the os calcis may show a heal spur but this is of very doubtful significance.

Treatment

Treatment may be conservative initially. The load stretching the plantar fascia may be reduced by heel pads with cut-outs over the tender area. The local inflammation may be treated by rest, local ultrasound, oral non-steroidal anti-inflammatory drugs and, if these are ineffective, by injection of insoluble steroid with local anaesthetic into the tender area in the hindfoot. The injection should be carried out through the medial border of the foot and not the sole of the foot. If the athlete has marked varus of the heel and pronation of the forefoot special moulded insoles to correct for these deformities may be useful in enabling athletic activities to be pursued.

The condition tends to recur. Steroid injections, if useful, may be repeated, probably not more often than three times at intervals of at least 6 weeks.

The toes (Fig. 13.10)

General considerations

Toe problems may be acute, arising as the result of a single major incident. Conditions which arise in this way include:

1. Nail damage.
2. Hyperflexion or hyperextension injuries.

Other problems may arise without any single precipitating incident and such problems include:

1. Infection of nails and skin.
2. Deformities of the big toe – notably bunions, hallux valgus and hallux rigidus.
3. Deformities of the small toes – notably claw toes and hammer toes.

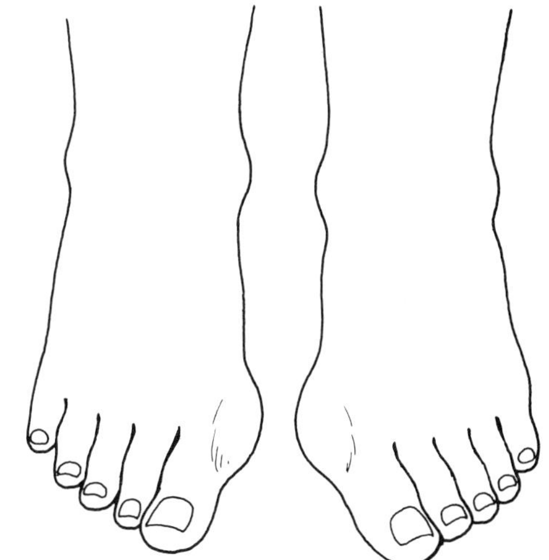

Fig. 13.10 Bilateral hallux valgus with bunions (see text).

Nail damage: subungual haematoma

Previously normal nails may be damaged in certain activities. Shoes which are too tight may cause bruising under the toe nails if the patient walks downhill for long distances and the nail is banged against the front of the shoe. Sportsmen or women who kick awkwardly or get trodden on may similarly get bruising under the toe nail.

Patients may be alarmed by the appearance of the toe which looks black with the blood underneath it. Sometimes this blood is under pressure and then the toe throbs.

If the only complaint is of the appearance patients should be reassured and advised to modify their footwear. They should also be warned that the toe nail will probably fall off over the next few months as the new nail grows underneath.

If the affected toe is throbbing, relief can be given by draining the blood by gently piercing the nail over the centre of the black area. This may be done with a red-hot paperclip. Care should be taken not to press on the nail so the tip of the paper clip does not damage the underlying nail bed. The procedure produces a lot of smoke and a spurt of blood, followed rapidly by relief of pain. Following this a light dressing should be applied and once more the patient should be warned that he or she may lose the nail.

Nail damage in claw toes

If the small toes are clawed the nail may come into contact with the sole of the shoe so that the end of the nail takes weight. The patient usually complains of pain at the tip of the affected toe.

Examination

Examination shows a claw toe with thickening of the nail and the skin where the nail is in contact with the inner of the shoe. Palpation of this area is very tender.

Treatment

Treatment is by first checking the shoe to make sure that the shoe is not too short and that there is no irregularity damaging the toe. If the shoe is satisfactory passive stretching to uncurl the toe may help, as may exercises to improve the intrinsic muscles of the foot. However, in most adults the toe is rigidly curled with fixed-flexion deformities in the interphalangeal joints. In such cases the only effective long-term treatment is surgery to arthrodese these joints in a straight position.

Young patients may be helped by either flexor extensor tendon transfers or flexor tendon tenotomies to uncurl the toes (see section on claw toes and hammer toes, below).

Hyperflexion and hyperextension injuries

These usually involve the big toe which is forced upwards – hyperextension – or curled downwards – hyperflexion – as a result of a sudden major injury. The patient knows that he or she has injured the toe immediately. There is pain and swelling over the injured joint, either the interphalangeal joint or the metatarsophalangeal joint at the base of the toe.

Examination

Examination reveals local swelling and tenderness and later bruising. Active flexion and extension should be checked to ensure there is no tendon rupture.

X-ray

X-rays should be taken to exclude any bony injury.

Treatment

Treatment is for the capsular and ligament damage – ice, ultrasound and rest for 2 or 3 weeks, followed by protected mobilization. The capsular healing takes approximately 6 weeks and competitive sports are best avoided for this period if possible.

Bunions, hallux valgus and hallux rigidus

These conditions are essentially bone and joint deformities and detailed discussion of them is outside the scope of this chapter. However, in view of their common occurrence they are included briefly for completeness.

A bunion – a swelling at the base of the big toe without deformity of the toe itself – is often due to footwear being too narrow or the front of the shoe being too pointed. Any patient presenting with a bunion without toe deformity should be advised to use wider shoes as the first line of treatment.

Hallux valgus – a big toe pointing towards the lateral side – may present in teenagers as well as in middle age. Essentially the younger the patient, the greater the indication for corrective surgery to preserve the metatarsophalangeal joint at the base of the toe. Surgery which excises the affected joint, for example Keller's arthroplasty, or fuses the joint should be avoided wherever possible in athletes who wish to continue their activities.

Hallux rigidus – a stiff joint at the base of the big

toe – may occur with a bunion, with hallux valgus deformity or on its own. The stiffness in the joint causes pain in the base of the toe on running and inability to wear shoes with a high heel or to stand on tiptoe. Because of this stiffness the patient may transfer the weight over to the lateral side of the foot whenever he or she runs, with subsequent risk of metatarsal pain and ankle inversion injuries.

Examination

Examination of a patient with hallux rigidus reveals limited dorsiflexion of the big toe, usually with pain. In most patients it is difficult to improve hallux rigidus sufficiently to enable them to continue to participate in sports involving running and jumping.

Claw toes and hammer toes

Claw toes (curly toes) cause pain under the nail, as described above, and hammer toes cause pain on the dorsum of the toe and under the metatarsophalangeal joint. In adults examination of claw toes and hammer toes usually reveals fixed deformities of the joints of the affected toe. These deformities can usually be corrected by fusion into a straight position. Most athletes are able to return to active participation in their sports after such surgery, although recovery may easily take 6 months.

In children and teenagers the deformities of the toes may be mobile and soft tissue correction in the form of capsulotomies, tenotomies and tendon transfers may correct the deformities adequately and permanently.

Further reading

The groin

Gilmore OJA (1991) Ten years' experience of groin disruption – a previously unsolved problem in sportsmen. Sports Medicine Symposium. Pfizer Institute Edinburgh (March)

Harris NH, Murray RO (1974) Lesions of the symphysis in athletes. *British Medical Journal* **4**, 211–14.

The thigh

Jackson DW, Feagin JA (1973) Quadriceps contusions in young adults. *Journal of Bone and Joint Surgery* **55A**, 95.

MacEachern AG, Plewes JL (1984) Bilateral simultaneous spontaneous rupture of the quadriceps tendon. *Journal of Bone and Joint Surgery* **66B**, 81–3.

Rothwell AG, Walton M (1980) The quadriceps haematoma – a clinical and experimental study. *Journal of Bone and Joint Surgery* **62B**, 270–1.

The knee

Aichroth PM (1984) Dislocation of the patella. In: Jackson JP, Waugh W (eds) *Surgery of the Knee Joint*. Chapman and Hall Medical, pp 192–209.

Bach BR (1989) Arthroscopy assisted patellar tendon substitution of anterior cruciate ligament insufficiency. *American Journal of Knee Surgery* **2**, 4–20.

Chen SC, Ramanathan EBS (1984) Treatment of patellar instability by lateral release. *Journal of Bone and Joint Surgery* **66B**, 334–48.

Dandy DJ (1984) *Arthroscopic Management of the Knee* 2nd edn. Churchill Livingstone, Edinburgh.

DeFondren FB, Goldner JL, Bassett FH (1985) Recurrent dislocation of the patella treated by the modified goldthwait procedure. *Journal of Bone and Joint Surgery* **66A**, 993–1005.

Goodfellow J (1984) Chondromalacia patellae. In: Jackson JP, Waugh W (eds) *Surgery of the Knee Joint*. Chapman and Hall, pp 210–33.

Goodfellow J, Hungerford DS, Woods C (1976) Patello-femoral joint mechanics and pathology (1+2). *Journal of Bone and Joint Surgery* **58B**, 287–99.

Haven K (1985) Meniscus repair in the athlete. *Clinical Orthopaedics* **198**, 31–5.

Hubbard MJS (1987) Arthroscopic surgery for chondral flaps in the knee. *Journal of Bone and Joint Surgery* **69B**, 794–6.

Insall I (1982) Patellar pain – current concepts review. *Journal of Bone and Joint Surgery* **64A**, 147–52.

Ireland J, Trickey EL, Stocka DJ (1980) Arthroscopy and arthrography of the knee. *Journal of Bone and Joint Surgery* **62B**, 3.

Jones KG (1963) Reconstruction of the anterior cruciate ligament using the central third of the patellar ligament. *Journal of Bone and Joint Surgery* **45A**, 925–32.

Mital MA, Matza RA, Cohen J (1980) The so called unresolved Osgood–Schlatter's lesion. *Journal of Bone and Joint Surgery* **62A**, 732–9.

Noyes FR, McGinness GH (1985) Controversy about treatment of the knee with anterior cruciate ligament laxity. *Clinical Orthopaedics* **198**, 61–76.

Odensten M, Hamberg P, Nordin M, Lysholm J, Gillquist J (1985) Surgical or conservative treatment of acutely torn anterior cruciate ligament. *Clinical Orthopaedics* **198**, 87–93.

Ogilvie-Harris DA, Jackson RW (1984) The arthroscopic treatment of chondromalacia patellae. *Journal of Bone and Joint Surgery* **66B** 660–5.

Rosenthal RK, Levine DB (1977) Fragmentation of the distal pole of the patella in spastic cerebral palsy. *Journal of Bone and Joint Surgery* **59A**, 934–9.

Smillie IS (1978) *Injuries of the Knee Joint*. Churchill Livingstone, Edinburgh, pp 83–112.

Stother IG (1990) Arthroscopy. *Injury* **21**, 263–6.

Tapper EN, Hoover NW (1969) Late results after meniscectomy. *Journal of Bone and Joint Surgery* **51A**, 517.

The lower leg

Bourne RB, Rorabeck CH (1989) Compartment syndromes of the lower leg. *Clinical Orthopaedics* **240**, 97–104.

Rorabeck CH, Bourne RB, Fowler PJ (1983) The surgical treatment of exertional compartment syndromes in athletes. *Journal of Bone and Joint Surgery* **65A**, 1245–51.

Wallensten R (1983) Results of fasciotomy in patients with medial tibial syndrome or chronic anterior com partment syndromes. *Journal of Bone and Joint Surgery* **65A**, 1252–5.

The tendo-Achilles

Carden DG, Noble J, Chalmers J, Lunn P, Ellis J (1987) Rupture of the calcaneal tendon. *Journal of Bone and Joint Surgery* **69B**, 416–20.

Thompson C, Doherty JH (1953) Spontaneous rupture of the tendon of Achilles – a new clinical diagnostic test. *Journal of Trauma* **19**, 514–22.

The ankle

Bjorkenhen JM, Sandelin J, Santavirta S (1988) The Evans procedure and the treatment of chronic instability of the ankle. *Injury* **19**, 70–2.

Evans DL (1953) Recurrent instability of the ankle and method of surgical treatment. *Proceedings of the Royal Society of Medicine* **46**, 343–4.

Evans G, Hardcastle P, Frenyo AD (1984) Acute rupture of the lateral ligament of the ankle: to suture or not to suture. *Journal of Bone and Joint Surgery* **66B**, 209–12.

Ferkel RD, Fischer SP (1989) Progress in ankle arthroscopy. *Clinical Orthopaedics* **240**, 210–20.

Glasgow MM, Jackson A, Jamieson AM (1986) Instability of the ankle after injury to the lateral ligament. *Journal of Bone and Joint Surgery* **62B**, 196–200.

Norris SH, Mankin HJ (1978) Chronic tenosynovitis of the posterior tibial tendons with new bone formation. *Journal of Bone and Joint Surgery* **60B**, 523–6.

Snook GA, Chrisman OD, Wilson TC (1985) Longterm results of the Chrisman-Snook operation for reconstruction of the lateral ligament of the ankle. *Journal of Bone and Joint Surgery* **67B**, 1–7.

Stother IG (1974) Incidence of minor fractures in twisting injuries of the ankle. *Injury* **5**, 213–14.

Zoellner J, Clancy W (1979) Recurrent dislocation of peroneal tendon. *Journal of Bone and Joint Surgery* **61A** 292–4.

The foot

Funk DA, Cass JR, Johnson KA (1986) Acquired adult flat-foot secondary to posterior tibial tendon pathology. *Journal of Bone and Joint Surgery* **68A**, 95–102.

Guiloff RJ, Scadding JW, Klenerman L (1984) Morton's metatarsalgia. *Journal of Bone and Joint Surgery* **66B**, 586–91.

McCluskey WP, Lovell WW, Cummings RJ (1989) The cavo-varus foot deformity: aetiology and management. *Clinical Orthopaedics* **247**, 27–37.

Ross ERS, Menelaus MB (1984) Open flexor tenotomy for hammer toes and curly toes in childhood. *Journal of Bone and Joint Surgery* **66B**, 770–1.

Scranton PE (1983) Principles in bunion surgery – current concepts review. *Journal of Bone and Joint Surgery* **65A**, 1026–8.

14

Injuries to the upper limb

J. Chase
K. Carnine

Treatment of shoulder injuries

Anatomy of the shoulder

The anatomy of the shoulder is complex. The underlying bony framework of the humerus, clavicle, scapula, thorax and sternum is supported by specialized soft tissue structures. Bones articulate at the acromioclavicular, sternoclavicular, glenohumeral and scapulothoracic articulations. They are connected by coracoclavicular, coracoacromial, acromioclavicular, sternoclavicular and glenohumeral ligaments. The latter three ligament complexes blend into the sternoclavicular, acromioclavicular and glenohumeral joint capsules as integral parts of those structures. The joint surfaces of the glenohumeral articulation are covered with hyaline articular cartilage while the sternoclavicular and acromioclavicular joints are fibrocartilaginous and contain intra-articular menisci. The glenoid labrum of the anteromedial aspect of the glenohumeral capsule is another specialized anatomical structure of the shoulder area which deepens the socket, augments anterior stability and helps to contain the humeral head.

The shoulder is the most mobile and least stable major joint of the body. The glenoid fossa is only slightly concave and shallow and its surface area is only one-quarter of the surface area of the humeral head. Gravity, instead of helping to stabilize the joint such as in the knee or hip, instead exerts a downward force on the joint through the weight of the arm. The bony structures of the shoulder provide little stability and the capsular and other soft tissue structures are loose and flexible to provide maximum range of motion. They offer little impediment to forces that tend to destabilize the joint.

Static stabilizers of the joint include the glenohumeral ligaments. The superior and middle glenohumeral ligaments are specialized thickenings of the anterior capsule originating from the upper glenoid and extending horizontally to their insertion into the anterior aspect of the humerus. The inferior glenohumeral ligament is the thickest part of the anterior capsule extending laterally and caudally to insert on to the anatomical neck of the humerus. Recurrent instability of the shoulder may be associated with a deficiency between the superior and middle glenohumeral ligaments, or with congenital absence of the inferior glenohumeral ligament, the latter appearing to have the most important role in stabilizing the shoulder joint in abduction and external rotation. When the arm is dependent, the superior glenohumeral ligament suspends the humerus in combination with the deltoid and supraspinatus muscles, the coracohumeral ligament, the tendon of the long head of the biceps and the slope of the glenoid. The intra-articular portion of the long head of the biceps has a particular role in suspension of the humeral head, as well as in humeral head depression while attempting forward flexion or abduction. The long head of the triceps originates from the inferior aspect of the glenoid and crosses both the shoulder and elbow joints posteriorly. The inferior portion of the shoulder capsule is lax with a dependent fold, which allows the extremes of motion of the shoulder. The capsule blends into the supraspinatus superiorly and infraspinatus posteriorly. The subacromial/subdeltoid bursa infrequently communicates with the shoulder joint, but may communicate with the subscapular bursa and/or the infraspinatus bursa posteriorly. The tendon of the long head of biceps exits from the shoulder through the synovial sheath and crosses under the transverse humeral ligament which may be a site of impingement. The glenohumeral joint is supplied by the suprascapular, upper subscapular, and circumflex (axillary) nerves.

Dynamic glenohumeral stability is maintained by the long head of the biceps and the muscles of the rotator cuff, including the subscapularis, supraspinatus, infraspinatus and teres minor. These muscles are rotators of the humerus and pull the humeral head into the glenoid fossa, locking it into position and stabilizing the scapulohumeral link for upper extremity function. Selectively, they can resist displacing forces resulting from contraction of larger shoulder muscles. When a patient is completely relaxed, the humerus can be pushed forward and backward in the joint through a fairly significant range. But when muscles are contracted, this excursion is almost completely obliterated. Patients with capsular laxity can improve glenohumeral stability by strengthening the small rotator muscles.

The rotator cuff is a complex of tendons that attach to the humeral head by blending into the superior, anterior and posterior aspects of the shoulder capsule. Anteriorly, subscapularis internally rotates the humerus. Superiorly, supraspinatus abducts and posteriorly the infraspinatus and teres minor externally rotate the arm. The subacromial bursa separates the rotator cuff from the acromion and facilitates shoulder motion by creating a gliding phenomenon between the cuff and the bony overhang of the acromion. Other bursae in the shoulder also function by providing motion with the minimum of friction. They are in intimate relationship with the tendons and the shoulder capsule.

A knowledge of the anatomy of the shoulder is important in understanding symptoms and clinical findings in shoulder problems.

Physical examination of the shoulder

To provide appropriate and successful treatment to any shoulder joint condition, an accurate diagnosis must be made. A careful history of the onset and course of the patient's symptoms, mechanism of injury, and assessment of disability are extremely important. Dynamic tests such as plain X-rays, arthrograms, ultrasound studies, computed tomography arthrograms, magnetic resonance imaging, cine radiography, and electromyographic tests may all be helping in confirming a clinical diagnosis. At times these sophisticated tests may identify lesions which are not easy to appreciate clinically. Nothing is more important, however, than a careful and knowledgeable physical examination by a clinician who understands the anatomy and biomechanics of the shoulder and is aware of the pathophysiology of the many conditions which may affect the shoulder.

Inspection

The most valuable assessment of a shoulder problem may be at the time of first presentation. The age of the patient, physical condition and level of activity will vary. One must observe the manner in which the patient holds the shoulder and arm, its gross appearance and other conditions which may contribute to the shoulder condition of which the patient complains. Mechanics of motion of the arm during gait, the manner in which she or he disrobes and shakes hands, and the general appearance of the patient are all important.

Knowledge of the unique anatomy of the shoulder girdle allows systematic inspection of the area. The shoulder can be evaluated from the anterior, lateral, posterior and superior aspects. Contour, symmetry, temperature, discoloration, wasting, deformity and mechanic of motion must be evaluated. Abnormal bony prominences suggest subluxation or dislocation. A protective posture of the shoulder or arm implies pain and/or apprehension. This may occur following trauma or when there are other painful conditions, such as acute calcific tendonitis. Neurological deficiencies such as Erb's or Klumpke's birth palsies have characteristically abnormal attitudes of the shoulder and arm. A high-riding or sagging shoulder suggests muscle spasm or weakness respectively.

Normal symmetry and posture rule out many abnormalities. Swelling may be difficult to appreciate in the shoulder, but its presence suggests an active inflammatory process or other abnormal conditions such as a benign tumour, or neoplastic process. Discoloration can occur post-trauma or with inflammation. Increased warmth may indicate inflammation, or muscle wasting is consistent with a primary muscle or secondary neurological abnormality. Generalized wasting implies disuse. Specific wasting indicates the need for evaluation of the spinal canal, cervical spine and peripheral nerves and muscles. A full-thickness rotator cuff tear of some duration will be associated with a supraspinatus or infraspinatus atrophy.

Palpation

Anatomical knowledge is also critical for appreciation of abnormalities on palpation. Positioning the arm allows palpation of structures not normally exposed. The location of tenderness, soft tissue or bony defects implies specific structural abnormality.

Movement

After inspection and palpation, range and mechanics of motion must be evaluated. The shoulder is the most mobile joint in the body. Motion occurs in a combination of planes. Almost 360° of movement is possible by virtue of contributions from the sternoclavicular, acromioclavicular, glenohumeral and scapulothoracic articulations. By far the biggest contribution occurs at the glenohumeral and scapulothoracic joints. The glenohumeral joint accounts for approximately two-thirds of the overall motion and the remaining one-third is accounted for by the scapulothoracic mechanism. When documenting range of motion, true glenohumeral movement can be estimated by fixing the scapula against the thorax. Scapular thoracic movement increases as the arm is elevated. When frozen shoulder or significant glenohumeral osteoarthritis or rheumatoid arthritis is present, shoulder motion may be almost entirely scapulothoracic. Both active and passive range of movement are important. Passive testing is necessary when active range of motion is voluntarily or structurally limited. When active range of motion is not restricted, then passive ranges need not be measured. While motion of the shoulder is occurring, it is important to evaluate the patient for pain (e.g. impingement sign and/or other manifestations of pain), mechanics of movement, crepitus and apprehension (which may imply instability).

The most important motions of the shoulder are forward flexion, abduction, extension and rotation. A patient cannot put his or her hand behind the back if extension is seriously limited. The normal range of movement is as given in Table 14.1.

Neuromuscular examination

Following the evaluation and measurement of range of motion, neurological function and strength of the shoulder girdle must be ascertained. Testing the arm in different positions isolates a particular muscle or group of muscles. It is important to test strength at 0° of abduction and

Table 14.1 Normal range of movement of the shoulder

Motion of the shoulder	Range
Abduction	0–180°
Forward flexion	0–180°
External rotation (with arm at side)	0–90°
Internal rotation (with arm at side)	0–90° (may be less in the dominant arm of active individuals)
External rotation in abduction	0 90°
Internal rotation in abduction	0–90°
Extension	0–45°
Adduction	0–45°

at 90° of abduction with the arm in neutral, internal and external rotation. This tests specific parts of the rotator cuff as well as deltoid and other shoulder muscles. When weakness or wasting is present, the neurological system should be tested to determine whether a deficiency exists. Sensory patterns, reflexes, strength and bulk of the muscles and examination of the neck are all important. Strength in the non-dominant arm is normally less than in the dominant arm. Detection of neurological involvement of the suprascapular, axillary, median and ulnar nerves is relatively straightforward. The long thoracic nerve, the accessory nerve, the musculocutaneous nerve, the thoracodorsal and the anterior thoracic nerves are all important.

Joint stability

Deformity, mobility and stability of all the shoulder girdle joints should be assessed. Subcutaneous joints such as the sternoclavicular and acromioclavicular are easier to evaluate than the glenohumeral and scapulothoracic articulations. The patient should be examined in a relaxed position. Pain, guarding and/or apprehension with passive stressing suggest instability. In some cases, examination under anaesthetic may be necessary to evaluate joint stability adequately.

Vascularity

The vascular supply to the shoulder and arm must also be examined. Normal pulses do not necessarily indicate normal vascularity. Skin texture, colour, temperature, sensation, hair growth, sweating and capillary filling also help to evaluate the vascular supply. Ulcerations or other skin lesions may indicate arterial or venous abnormalities. There are special tests to evaluate the status of the thoracic outlet where neurological and vascular structures can be compromised (Brown, 1983).

After a careful history and a thorough physical examination have been completed, additional specialized tests may be necessary for further assessment or to confirm a clinical impression or diagnosis.

Shoulder impingement syndrome

The shoulder plays a key role in many activities of daily life, work and athletics. The shoulder possesses a high degree of mobility that contributes to function. There is a delicate balance between mobility and stability. Because many activities require maximum range of movement, stability may be jeopardized. Often, more is demanded of the shoulder than it can tolerate on a repetitive or sometimes singular basis. Overhead or overhand activities are particularly prone to producing difficulty.

Occupations such as painting, wallpapering, carpentry and housework place great demands upon the shoulder. Athletics such as swimming, football, baseball and tennis that involve overhead use of the arm likewise create stresses on the shoulder which may result in painful overuse conditions of the shoulder, collectively known as the impingement syndrome. This is an inflammatory process of shoulder rotator cuff and biceps tendon tissues that probably accounts for the largest percentage of patients with shoulder pain. There are many aetiologies and varying presentations. The pathophysiology is basically a specific or cumulative injury that results in swelling of some part of the rotator cuff causing pinching of the inflamed and painful tissue against the acromion or some other part of the subacromial arch as the shoulder is raised overhead. This pinching is the aetiology of the impingement syndrome and demonstration of the point at which pain is elicited – usually 80–110° of abduction and/or forward flexion – is the clinical impingement sign.

Anatomical factors responsible for the development of shoulder impingement syndrome

1. The anterior aspect of the scapular acromion process, the coracoacromial ligament, and the undersurface of the acromioclavicular joint

make up the subacromial arch where impingement on the rotator cuff and biceps tendon tissues occurs. It has been shown by Neer that the functional arc of shoulder elevation is in the sagittal rather than in the coronal plane. With internal rotation of the shoulder, the greater tuberosity of the humerus is brought under the acromion and coracoacromial ligament. Further impingement occurs in wider abduction as the tuberosity moves under the lateral acromion and acromioclavicular joint.

2. The shape of the acromion may influence the development of rotator cuff abnormality. An increased anterior slope of the acromion, especially a hooked configuration, can predispose to rotator cuff pathology. The supraspinatus outlet projection on X-ray may help to assess the inferior aspect of the acromion. This view is taken as a lateral scapular X-ray with the beam slanted 10° caudally.
3. The blood supply to the rotator cuff has also been implicated. The lateral aspect of the supraspinatus and the intra-articular portion of the biceps tendon are relatively avascular (Rathbun and MacNab, 1970). This may explain why the majority of rotator cuff and biceps lesions are in these areas. Chronic irritation of the avascular leads to inflammatory tendinitis followed by wear and attrition, leading eventually to partial or complete-thickness rotator cuff or tendon tears. When these tissues become worn, their stabilizing effect on the humeral head in the glenoid during abduction and forward flexion of the arm is impaired. The deltoid, which normally functions around a fixed humeral head, begins to cause proximal humeral migration and to pull the head up against the undersurface of the acromion. This causes further impingement and degenerative change.

Rotator cuff tears

Rotator cuff tears may result from progressive pathology or may occur acutely in young patients due to trauma. It is accepted that there are three stages of progressive shoulder cuff pathology.

Stage I: Oedema and haemorrhage (any age).
Stage II: Fibrosis and tendinitis (usually less than 25 years of age).
Stage III: Tendon degeneration, bony sclerosis and spur formation, and tendon ruptures (greater than 40 years of age).

The three stages of pathology, which may also involve the biceps tendon, subacromial bursa and acromioclavicular joint, create a great variety of symptoms and clinical findings. These vary in degree from mild tendinitis with minimal pain and no loss of motion, to marked inflammatory symptoms, disabling pain, and some variable loss of movement. The final stage of rotator cuff tear presents as weakness, pain and loss or significant impairment of voluntary movement.

Stage I lesions may occur at any age but are common in younger people, especially those who work overhead or athletes who throw or swim. The cuff becomes oedematous and haemorrhagic. It is usually a reversible condition whose diagnosis is relatively straightforward. Aching discomfort is noticed during or after activity. The shoulder is often uncomfortable at night. Pain may radiate down the arm. There is often specific tenderness over the greater tuberosity insertion of the supraspinatus and at the anterior edge of the acromion where impingement occurs in forward flexion and elevation of the arm. The arc of movement is painful, especially at 90° where the impingement site occurs. Pain is often increased by resistance to motion. When the biceps tendon is involved, as it often is, there will be local tenderness over the tendon anterior to the humeral head and there may be pain on resisted forward flexion of the humerus or resisted supination of the forearm. An injection of local anaesthetic beneath the anterior acromion or into the biceps tendon sheath may relieve symptoms and signs, and is a useful diagnostic test.

Stage II lesions develop with repeated insults to the shoulder cuff mechanism of supraspinatus tendon, biceps tendon and subacromial bursa. The tendons become fibrotic and the subacromial bursa thickens. The common age group is 25–40 years. The shoulder joint is often stiff and there may be acromioclavicular joint pain in addition to signs similar to those of a stage I lesion. There may be an unusual painful 'catching' sensation in the shoulder as the arm is brought down from the elevated position. This is thought to be due to scar tissue being caught under the acromion. By the time this develops, simple avoidance of the activity that causes the pain is not enough to resolve the lesion, as is the case in stage I disease. There may be biceps tendon pain radiating down the arm, which is characteristic of stage II impingement. Tests for biceps involvement are local tenderness over the tendon, pain with resisted forward flexion of the arm with the elbow extended and the forearm supinated (Speed's test) and proximal biceps tendon pain with resisted forearm supination with the elbow flexed (Yeagerson's test).

Stage III pathology rarely presents before age 40 and is usually associated with a long history of pre-existing symptoms. Tendon degeneration, bony changes and tendon rupture result from the attrition process. Partial rotator cuff tears with increasing pain, stiffness, weakness and disability limit or prohibit activities and work capability. Pain is often worse and more noticeable at night. A relatively minor insult can cause extension to a full-thickness tear with resultant sudden shoulder weakness and variably diminished ability to elevate the arm effectively. If an injection of local anaesthetic into the subacromial space relieves the pain but does not improve strength or range of active abduction, the diagnosis of a complete tear is likely. Specific weakness is abduction and external rotation is also consistent with a tear to the superior and posterior aspects of the cuff where tears most commonly occur. The diagnosis can be confirmed by arthrography, ultrasound, or magnetic resonance imaging.

Acute rotator cuff tears

Full-thickness tears may occur in young patients without pre-existing abnormality. The most common mechanism is a heavy fall on to the outstretched arm, as may happen in a sporting event or work injury. The sudden force along the length of the arm avulses the attachment of the supraspinatus and other tendons from the humerus, these tendons being taut while attempting to break the fall. It is important to recognize the injury as more than a severe sprain. Careful clinical examination and the use of local anaesthetic to eliminate pain and demonstrate true mechanical weakness is critical in making the diagnosis. Appropriate imaging studies may be obtained for confirmation.

Treatment of the acute rotator cuff tear

Acute tears of the rotator cuff in younger individuals are best dealt with by surgical repair. This is particularly true when the injury is to the dominant arm or the patient is an athlete or labourer who requires overhead use of the arm. Cuff tears are treated by open surgery. The earlier the surgical intervention, the easier the repair, and the better the prospect of recovery of function. In addition to repair of the rotator cuff, it is often necessary to decompress the subacromial space because the repaired cuff is thickened and therefore may predispose to the development of impingement symptoms.

Treatment of shoulder impingement syndrome

Shoulder impingement syndrome of whatever cause may respond to rest, modification of activity and locally applied anti-inflammatory gel, or oral anti-inflammatory medication.

Physiotherapy techniques such as ice, friction massage, contrast baths, whirlpool, ultrasound and iontophoresis (ultrasound used to encourage penetration of topical corticosteroids or other anti-inflammatory gel into the soft tissues) may reduce pain and inflammation and speed recovery.

The judicious use of a local depot corticosteroid into a bursal space, tendon sheath or into the joint may be very effective. This medication must be administered by sterile technique and the patient must be informed of possible risks of its use, which may be minimized by avoiding repeat injections. The injections should not be directly into the substance of the tendon, ligament or capsule. A temporary increase in inflammation and pain may occur immediately after injection, and symptoms may be lessened by simultaneous injection of a local anaesthetic. Thereafter there should be rapid relief of, or at least improvement in symptoms, which may be short-lived, but often lasts for a considerable time.

For those cases where no significant relief of severe symptoms can be achieved by these conservative methods, surgical intervention may occasionally be justified, although the success rate is not high. Subacromial decompression may be performed by open surgery or arthroscopically. This procedure consists of resection of the subacromial bursa, section of the coracoacromical ligament and bevelling of the anterolateral corner of the acromion. The rotator cuff itself may require debridement, and if the inferior aspect of the acromioclavicular joint is prominent because of osteophytes, they should be resected (Neer, 1972).

The painful shoulder: differential diagnoses

Instability from overuse

Athletic individuals may make excessive demands on their shoulders and this leads to abnormal stress on the rotator cuff mechanism and shoulder capsule. Uneven or eccentric shoulder loading is caused by the extreme external rotation and short sharp force involved in the repetitive actions of overhand sports. These forces stretch ligamentous, capsular and muscular tissues, leading to the stretching and breakdown of static stabilizers of the shoulder, such as glenohumeral ligaments, anterior glenoid labrum, and the anterior and posterior capsular structures, and shoulder pain results. Chronic repetitive activities that consistently reproduce these stresses lead to a gradual development of shoulder instability. Functional mobility and stability are disrupted and this causes a chain reaction of unco-ordinated muscle activity leading to silent subluxation and impingement. Although these problems are not commonly seen in the average population, they do occur in a significant number of athletes. This condition may be difficult to distinguish from more common forms of impingement.

Instability and subluxation

Instability of the shoulder may be painful if, in attempting to maintain the humeral head within the glenoid, these patients put an excessive demand on their rotator cuff tendons. Tendinitis results. Examination demonstrates generalized tenderness of the rotator cuff and impingement sign may be present.

Subacromial bursitis and calcific tendinitis

Acute bursitis may occur from trauma with resultant bleeding and inflammation, or it may be due to a chemical irritation associated with an ischaemic process in which calcium phosphate is deposited in the bursae or other soft tissues. Acute calcific tendinitis is a severe form which develops over a matter of days and may be preceded by shoulder strain or other unaccustomed activity. The treatment of acute calcific tendinitis is a local infiltration of a steroid preparation, but it is sometimes necessary to decompress the collection of calcific deposit surgically to relieve the severe symptoms. Acute tendinitis can occur without obvious calcific deposits, or calcium may be present in the absence of symptoms. These changes encroach on the subacromial space and produce impingement. Supraspinatus tendinitis and bicipital tendinitis are often associated with degenerative changes in the tendon tissue, which may lead eventually to rupture.

Referred pain

Patients with neck injury or other abnormalities of the cervical spine may present with symptoms in the area of the shoulder or arm. Degeneration of an intervertebral disc and associated nerve root impingement results in pain referred along the distribution of the nerve. Cervical spine imaging and electrodiagnostic studies can be helpful in differential diagnosis.

Frozen shoulder

Impingement syndrome or other inflammatory problems about the shoulder can produce adhesive capsulitis or frozen shoulder.

Shoulder–hand syndrome

Shoulder–hand syndrome is a painful shoulder disability associated with pain and swelling in the hand of the same arm. There may be changes consistent with Sudeck's atrophy and reflex sympathetic dystrophy. The condition may follow myocardial infarction, pleurisy or other intrathoracic lesions, cerebral vascular accidents and neck disease. Patients tend to keep their shoulder immobile with the arm held close to the side and the hand in a characteristic position of metacarpophalangeal joint extension. Venous and lymphatic abnormalities may play a role. Patients are generally past middle age.

Neuropraxia

The shoulder area is supplied by the suprascapular, infrascapular and axillary nerves, amongst others. Trauma to the suprascapular nerve can mimic a rotator cuff tear with involvement of the supraspinatus and infraspinatus muscles. Patients present with a history of trauma to the shoulder and often posterior pain. Muscle atrophy may be present and there is weakness in abduction and external rotation. Impingement sign is negative. Diagnosis is by electromyography. Most lesions are neuropraxias and recover spontaneously.

Bicipital tenosynovitis

The biceps tendon is an important component in the aetiology of the shoulder impingement syndrome. It is important to understand its role as a depressor of the humeral head, flexor and abductor of the shoulder. Bicipital tenosynovitis is a frequent cause of shoulder pain and is often seen in athletes and heavy labourers. The bicipital groove of the humerus may be too shallow or the supporting fibrous structures which hold the tendon in the groove may have been torn or stretched. The resulting tendon instability leads to chronic inflammation and pain. There may also be impingement symptoms. Pain may develop gradually or be precipitated by excess activity. It may radiate into the upper arm or forearm. Alternatively the pain may be localized around the deltoid insertion into the humerus. Characteristically, patients have discomfort when the hand is placed behind the back or behind the head, and the tendon is exquisitely tender on palpation. An X-ray taken with the beam directed tangentially may demonstrate the lack of depth of the groove or perhaps marginal osteophytes. Surgical stabilization of the tendon within the groove may be necessary and may be combined with excision of the intra-articular portion of the tendon.

This clinical condition, when chronic and recurrent, may lead to spontaneous rupture of the biceps tendon due to attrition, which is treated conservatively, leaving an inevitable cosmetic deformity but minimal weakness (Neer *et al.*, 1977).

Acromioclavicular osteoarthritis

The acromioclavicular joint may also be critically involved in the impingement process by virtue of painful degenerative joint disease, inferior osteophyte formation, and intra-articular soft tissue abnormality. Acromioclavicular changes commonly present late in the disease process.

Classification and terminology of shoulder instability

Shoulder subluxation is an excessive translation of the humeral head on the glenoid that may produce symptoms or disability which are usually transient and short-lasting. Conversely, dislocation is a complete disruption of the glenohumeral articulation where immediate spontaneous relocation does not take place. Recurrent instability may present as either dislocation or subluxation.

Anterior (subcoracoid) dislocation

The great majority of acute traumatic shoulder dislocations are anterior (or subcoracoid). Patients who describe the shoulder as having been out of joint and who required someone else to 'put it back in' have almost certainly suffered an anterior dislocation. Appropriate X-rays should be made with the shoulder in the dislocated position to document direction and position of instability. Anteroposterior and axillary views are the most useful and easy to interpret. A lateral scapular view may be of value. The acute episode frequently leads to chronic recurrent instability. The axillary nerve is at risk because of its proximity to the joint. The Bankart lesion of labral and capsular detachment from the glenoid is frequently present. There may be combinations of upper and/or lower capsular, labral and glenohumeral ligament detachments. Regardless of pathology, the trauma creates a pocket into which the humeral head dislocates. Along with capsular and ligamentous injury, there is stretching of the subscapularis muscle and enlargement of the subscapularis bursa. After anterior dislocation of the humeral head, a bony defect in the posterior aspect of the head is frequently created, caused by impaction of the humeral head against the anterior glenoid (the Hill–Sachs lesion). This lesion is on the posterolateral aspect at the margin of the articular cartilage. When the defect is large, it plays a significant part in the development of recurrent instability. Recurrent anterior dislocation is the most common form of shoulder instability.

Treatment and prognosis of acute glenohumeral dislocation

Extreme pain accompanies an acute dislocation, and the spasm of the powerful muscles of the anterior and posterior axillary folds increases as the pain increases. Therefore, first-aid attempts to reduce an acute dislocation in a strong healthy subject usually fail, and are in fact dangerous because of the increased risk of axillary nerve damage and fracture. It is usually necessary (and advisable) to ensure a degree of relaxation either by intravenous sedation or even by administering a general anaesthetic. Failure to reduce the joint may be due to interposition of soft tissue or a fracture fragment from the glenoid rim, humeral head or tuberosity and therefore it is essential to obtain an X-ray to identify any such fracture before attempting reduction. Whichever manoeuvre is employed – several have been described – it must be gradual and controlled to minimize the risk of further damage.

The treatment programme post-reduction is usually considered to have a major influence on the likelihood of recurrent instability. Also, paradoxically, the degree of trauma causing the initial dislocation appears to be inversely proportional to the likelihood of recurrent dislocation (Rowe, 1962).

The arm should be immobilized in internal rotation and with the forearm across the chest for a minimum of 4 weeks, followed by a gradual return to normal activity by the end of 3 months. Nevertheless, the incidence of recurrent instability is high. Younger patients are particularly likely to suffer recurrent dislocation (Rowe and Sakellarides, 1961) found that 90% or more of patients under 20 and 60% of patients between 20 and 40 are likely to suffer further dislocation, but only 15% of patients over 40, who may also have an associated rotator cuff defect. This strict programme of immobilization followed by gentle rehabilitation is usually attempted by most orthopaedic surgeons but a study from Sweden (Hovelius, 1987) of the progress of young adults after acute dislocation of the shoulder demonstrated that the high rate of redislocation was unaffected by shorter or longer initial periods of immobilization.

When recurrent dislocation occurs despite appropriate initial treatment and rehabilitation, then a surgical repair must be considered. Many surgical procedures have been described for the treatment of recurrent anterior glenohumeral dislocation. They are designed to address specific components of the anterior instability. The Putti–Platt and Magnuson–Stack procedures involved tightening and/or realignment of the capsule and subscapularis tendon while the Bankart repair consists of the re-attachment of the avulsed glenoid labrum. These techniques have the disadvantage of limiting subsequent full external rotation and the Bristow operation is popular for patients proposing to return to their sport. It involves transferring the coracoid process to the anteroinferior surface of the neck of the glenoid, with its attached muscles, coracobrachialis and the short head of biceps, providing a dynamic sling under the humeral head in abduction and external rotation.

Postoperative rehabilitation of any of these repairs includes 3–6 months of supervised therapy to regain full range of movement and strength. Patients should not be encouraged to return to normal activities or sport until they have achieved maximum recovery and have developed strength in that joint at least equivalent to the contralateral normal joint. A good indication of readiness to return to contact sport is to ensure that the player has regained the ability to bench-press his or her weight.

Posterior dislocation

Posterior shoulder instability is uncommon. It is usually attributable to violent trauma and the diagnosis is often missed. A fracture of the anterior humeral head, known as a reverse Hill–Sachs lesion, often occurs where the head is impacted against the posterior glenoid. A missed acute injury may be recognized later as a chronic established condition. Posterior shoulder dislocations often occur in patients who experience grand mal seizures.

The posterior labrum of the shoulder joint is not as supportive as the anterior structure and there are no significant posterior ligaments to reinforce the capsule. The inferior glenohumeral ligament may offer some degree of posterior stability. The infraspinatus and teres minor tendons do not confer as much support posteriorly as the subscapularis tendon does anteriorly. Recurrent posterior instability, reverse Bankart lesions and posterior glenoid erosions are infrequently identified. Posterior instability may represent only subluxation rather than the frank dislocation. Once posterior dislocation has occurred, significant laxity of the posterior capsule of the joint may occur, leading to recurrent episodes of instability. Posterior subluxation or dislocation may be habitual and possibly associated with psychiatric problems. Surgical treatment is frequently unsuccessful in these patients and is therefore inappropriate.

Patients with posterior instability may not suffer a recognizable initial episode of trauma requiring manipulative reduction. The condition may develop gradually and as time passes patients may learn to avoid positions in which the shoulder is unstable. It is very important to attempt to establish the mechanism and direction of shoulder instability by physical examination and imaging techniques. While many patients may not be able to demonstrate their instability, it is often not possible for the examiner to appreciate it either. A positive apprehension test is an important guide to the direction of instability. Examination under anaesthetic with X-ray screening may be the only reliable method of diagnosis.

The treatment of recurrent posterior dislocation is surgical, and several techniques have been described, including osteotomy of the neck of the scapula, posterior bone block, transfer of the biceps tendon and other soft tissue repairs.

Inferior glenohumeral instability

This condition is rarely a dislocation but is frequently subluxation. It may occur as a result of laxity following injury, surgical reconstruction or may follow an infection. Although the humeral head commonly rides superiorly with rotated cuff pathology, it may in certain situations sublux inferiorly. Inferior subluxation and instability are associated with multidirectional laxity due to generalized capsular abnormality and demand careful evaluation. The basic abnormalities are poor support below the joint and poor suspension superiorly. Glenoid and humeral head lesions are uncommon. Trauma may serve as a precipitating factor in bringing the condition to the attention of the patient. The episode commonly occurs while lifting an object with the arm abducted. The instability is often bilateral and frequently symptomatic on only one side, rather than both. At times, patients will be able to demonstrate instability with their arms in full abduction overhead. Inferior dislocation in this direction is known as luxatio erecta.

Patients with inferior instability often have a negative apprehension test. The instability may be demonstrated by pulling vertically downwards on the arm with the patient in the seated position or by pushing downwards along the axis of the humerus with the arm abducted. Apprehension may be demonstrated if the patient experiences pain associated with the instability. A course of strengthening exercises for the deltoids, supraspinatus and other rotator cuff muscles will often preclude the need for more invasive treatment.

Multidirection instability

This condition is becoming more widely recognized and better understood. Combinations of anterior or posterior and inferior instability pose a challenge to both diagnosis and treatment. Instability may occur anteriorly and inferiorly, posteriorly and inferiorly, or in all three directions. Labral, humeral head and capsular defects secondary to trauma are not usually present. When one of the more classic lesions is identified, it may signify the predominant direction of the instability, but does not rule out a multidirectional component. The development of symptoms may be the result of the patient's level of activity combined with inherent shoulder capsular laxity and the condition may be bilateral. Multidirectional instability may result from a traumatic episode but few present with frank dislocation. Not all patients find instability disabling, and many can perform actively in athletics. Diagnosis may be difficult, with the list of differential diagnosis including impingement syndrome, tendinitis and rotator cuff abnormality. Patients may complain of symptoms related to work overhead or with the arms at the sides. They may state that the shoulder 'comes out' with certain positions or activities.

Careful examination is paramount in understanding the type of instability present and may include fluoroscopy and other imaging techniques. Examination under anaesthetic may offer additional significant information or may indeed be the only way to appreciate the underlying situation. The predominant direction of symptomatic instability must be documented. When clinical history and findings are not consistent with unidirectional instability, the diagnosis of multidirectional instability must be considered. The key to resolution of this condition appears to be reduction of the inferior capsular redundancy with a capsular shift procedure such as that described by Neer and Foster (1980). Conservative means of activity modification and muscle strengthening may be sufficient forms of treatment. Associated problems of impingement syndrome, acromioclavicular joint disease, or rotator cuff or biceps tendon pathology must also be dealt with.

Subluxation of the glenohumeral joint

This condition has not received a great deal of attention in the literature. As already stated, there is a small degree of normal translation of the glenohumeral joint, particularly in the relaxed or anaesthetized patient, and if excessive glenohumeral movement occurs and creates symptoms, they are usually short-lived but painful. The condition may also be known as apprehension shoulder. Subluxation may occur as a result of trauma but not necessarily dislocation. When dislocation has not occurred, the condition may be more subtle and difficult to recognize. At times, the patient will describe an episode of numbness in the arm after a traction injury. She or he may complain of a 'catching' in the joint or a fear that the shoulder will 'come out' with particular activities or in certain positions. There may be associated pain and numbness with the episodes of subluxation followed by symptoms of aching discomfort. The apprehension sign is usually positive. As mentioned above, subluxation of the shoulder may be habitual and performed at will as a 'party piece' or may be a symptom of a psychiatric disorder.

The patient should be examined in the sitting position with the arm placed in various degrees of abduction and external rotation. The examiner, standing behind the patient, pushes the humeral head forward on the glenoid to demonstrate a positive apprehension test. In patients with posterior laxity, examination may be performed in the sitting or supine position. X-ray in the axillary projection may reveal changes on the antero-inferior rim of the glenoid.

Other injuries associated with glenohumeral dislocation

A previously normal and stable shoulder cannot be dislocated unless a significant force is applied. When this occurs, tissues in the neck, shoulder, arm and chest may also be injured. Fractures may occur with or without significant soft tissue components. An avulsion fracture of the greater tuberosity may idicate a significant rotator cuff disruption. Fractures of the humerus or glenoid may result in instability or impingement if allowed to heal in a displaced or inadequately reduced position. Open reduction may be indicated.

Neurological injuries

The brachial plexus and the axillary nerve are closely related anteriorly, inferiorly and medially to the glenohumeral joint. These structures may be injured in anterior glenohumeral dislocations. Axillary nerve is the neurological structure most frequently involved but the musculocutaneous, suprascapular, infrascapular and long thoracic nerve may also be injured. Parts or all of the brachial plexus may be involved. Patients who are slow to recover from shoulder injuries should have their neurological status fully evaluated. Electromyographic testing is helpful in diagnosis. Most nerve injuries heal spontaneously within a 6-month period but in many instances recovery may be frustratingly slow.

Vascular injuries

Vascular injuries may result when glenohumeral dislocation occurs or at the time of reduction. The axillary artery is not particularly mobile where it passes beneath the pectoralis major and injuries often involve this portion of the artery, either beneath the muscle or distal to it. Intimal tear, occlusion, laceration, avulsion of a branch or complete rupture have been recorded. These injuries are more common in older patients, particularly when attempts are made to reduce a chronically dislocated joint. Excessive pain, expanding swelling and diminishing peripheral pulses should alert the examiner to the possibility of vascular injury. Arteriography is the best tool for diagnosis of type and location of injury.

Rotator cuff injuries

Rotator cuff tears may occur in association with glenohumeral dislocations and fracture dislocations. The incidence is greater in patients over 40 and increases dramatically after the age of 60. A rotator cuff tear should be suspected when there is pain or weakness or limitation of active abduction, forward flexion and external rotation. Ultrasonography or arthrography, magnetic resonance imaging and other studies can identify rotator cuff defects. Repair of the acute lesion is frequently indicated in the younger patient.

Acromioclavicular and strenoclavicular dislocations

The anatomy of the clavicular joints

The clavicle acts as a strut and moves in complex unison with the scapula in the scapulothoracic component of shoulder movement. The lateral end moves by elevation and depression during shoulder girdle movement and the clavicle also rotates around its own long axis. The fibrous joints at either end rely for their stability on a series of strong ligaments, and both joints contain a fibrocartilaginous meniscus which strengthens them further.

The coracoclavicular ligament consists of two parts the conoid and the trapezoid, which act as a fulcrum around which the clavical moves.

The sternoclavicular joint

The sternoclavicular joint is seldom significantly displaced but posterior dislocation of the clavicle can be dangerous. When the shoulder sustains significant trauma, the sternoclavicular joint ligaments may tear and the joint becomes displaced. This mechanism of injury usually results in anterior displacement of the medial end of the clavicle. Pressure on the sternoclavicular joint from the front or a blow to an abducted shoulder may create a posterior dislocation. This injury can compress neurovascular structures or the trachea, creating an emergency situation requiring immediate reduction by manipulation or more likely by open surgery. Pain from the more common anterior dislocation may be referred to the shoulder, making this injury difficult to diagnose at times. In the acute anterior dislocation, an attempt should be made to relocate the joint by manipulation, but may be unsuccessful. Only when chronic instability is painful is it necessary to consider surgical stabilization or resection of the medial clavicle, but the vast majority of cases are treated successfully by conservative means.

The acromioclavicular joint

Injuries to the acromioclavicular joint are also usually managed successfully by conservative measures. These injuries are often graded I to VI: grade I injury is a simple sprain; grade II injury is a partial displacement; grade III injury is a complete dislocation; grade IV injury is a posterior dislocation of the distal end of the clavicle; grade V injury is a more severe version of grade III injury; and grade VI injury is an inferior dislocation of the distal clavicle. Grade I and II injuries, even though they may result in some prominence of the distal clavicle, rarely cause lasting symptoms that require treatment. Even grade II separations can often be treated conservatively with great success. Patients who do not do well with conservative management may be relieved of most of their symptoms by excision of the distal clavicle if degenerative joint disease is the cause of the pain. Grade III injuries, where the coracoclavicular and acromioclavicular ligaments are disrupted, and if the dominant arm of a throwing athlete is involved, are cases in which surgical intervention may be appropriate. The coracoclavicular ligaments should be reconstructed, in addition to relocation and stabilization of the acromioclavicular joint and associated soft tissues. Even with operative treatment, pain due to later degenerative changes of the acromioclavicular joint may necessitate excision of the distal clavicle (Mumford, 1941).

Acute rupture of the tendon of the long head of biceps

The tendon may rupture without any predisposing pathology, in circumstances similar to those described for acute rotator cuff tears. The other mechanism which may cause the tendon to rupture is a sudden extending force acting across the elbow during active flexion, such as in weight-lifting.

Treatment of acute rupture of the tendon of the long head of biceps

In the young, athletic or otherwise active person, surgical repair of the acute rupture should be considered. End-to-end anastomosis of the tendon may be possible, or alternatively the distal end may be inserted into a drill hole in the humerus after establishing the non-contracted length of the muscle.

Acute injuries of glenoid labrum

The glenoid labrum is an important structure. Injury to this structure anteriorly or posteriorly can occur in throwing events, wrestling, boxing, racket sports and in heavy labour, or after trauma. Failure to respond to rest, physiotherapy and other conservative measures should alert the examiner to the possibility of damage to the labrum being the cause of protracted shoulder pain. Imaging studies such as arthrography and magnetic resonance may identify a labrum tear, and arthroscopic techniques have been described for resection or reattachment of the damaged portion. If there is associated shoulder instability an open procedure may be necessary to repair the labrum as part of a stabilization procedure.

Adhesive capsulitis (frozen shoulder)

Aetiology

This condition, also known as scapulohumeral periarthritis, was originally thought to occur as a result of obliteration of the subdeltoid bursa. Later it was felt that a breakdown of intra-articular biceps tendon tissue led to the problem (De Palma, 1949). It is now recognized that the condition develops following rotator cuff tendinitis, usually in the area of the supraspinatus, with gross contracture of the rotator cuff and shoulder capsule, and adhesion between the opposing walls of the dependent inferior capsular fold. Frozen shoulder may also be secondary to other causes such as a heart attack or fracture of the forearm or hand, or other injury or underuse of the limb.

Pathological changes

The primary pathology in the rotator cuff extends to involve capsular and then coracohumeral ligament contracture. In early stages, there is increased blood supply to the synovium, followed by hypertrophy. Synovial folds may become adherent and extensions behind the subscapularis and around the biceps tendon become obliterated. The biceps tendon commonly demonstrates advanced degenerative change related to interference with its blood supply as it courses over the humeral head. These changes are secondary to the diffuse rotator cuff tendinitis. Degenerative changes in the cuff are first noted in the relatively avascular zone over the humeral head, described as the ‘critical zone’ by Codman. Microscopic specimens reveal separation of collagen fascicles and accellularity, and later fragmentation. It is thought that pressure on the cuff from the underlying convexity of the humeral head gives rise to long-standing diminished vascularity followed by sequential degenerative changes. Tissue cell death causes an inflammatory reaction of tendinitis. A cellular immune response may follow which invokes an antibody reaction. The tendinous material becomes infiltrated with lymphoid cells. This seems to play a part in the production of the overall clinical syndrome.

Clinical presentation

Adhesive capsulitis may begin with dull, aching pain, frequently without antecedent trauma. It is more common in women and is unusual in younger patients. Movement of the shoulder aggravates the pain and later the inflammatory reaction leads to the production of adhesions and further limitation of movement. This chronic cycle results in persistent pain, limitation of motion and disability. The final stage of the condition is characterized by rotator cuff and capsular contraction limiting all directions of movement. This late stage is aptly called frozen shoulder and pain may be less severe than during the developing stages.

The position of the humerus after contractions have occurred complicates the problem. Contracture of the subscapularis and coracohumeral ligaments results in marked limitation of external rotation. This causes impingement of the greater tuberosity of the humerus against the acromion on attempted abduction. The inferior capsular fold is obliterated, which causes further restriction of glenohumeral movement, and the arm can be abducted away from the body only by scapulothoracic movement. This leads to stress on the acromioclavicular joint, causing degenerative change which may further inhibit rehabilitation. Movement of the scapula around the chest wall may cause traction on the suprascapular nerve, particularly as it is restricted by the suprascapular ligament as it goes through the suprascapular notch. This increases pain and wasting.

During the later stages of the disease process, scapulothoracic motion may also be restricted. X-rays may identify osteoporosis resulting from disuse and may demonstrate superior migration of the head of the humerus, as is often seen with large rotator cuff tears. Arthrography characteristically demonstrates obliteration of synovial pouches. The glenohumeral joint space is maintained.

Prognosis and treatment of frozen shoulder

The condition appears to be self-limiting and runs a course of from 6 to 18 months. It may simultaneously resolve with resolution of pain and restoration of movement, but many patients suffer protracted disability. This latter group of patients appears to be characterized by increased levels of pain during the process, and they may have difficulty co-operating with or participating in a supervised programme of rehabilitation. In patients who do not respond to conservative methods of management, including subacromial steroid injection and intensive physiotherapy, closed hydraulic distension or manipulation under general anaesthetic may be beneficial. Surgical release of contracted structures and release of the suprascapular nerve may rarely be indicated.

Aids to diagnosis of shoulder problems

Plain X-ray examination of the shoulder has been the most frequently utilized diagnostic tool. Unfortunately, X-rays do not identify many soft tissue problems, or in some cases do not suggest soft tissue pathology until degenerative bone, joint and soft tissue changes have become established. Until recently, the only other diagnostic aid commonly employed was arthrography. This study, in which radiopaque contrast material is injected into the joint, allows some interpretation of soft tissue abnormality, but is not very specific. False-negative and false-positive findings may be encountered. Cine radiography offers an opportunity to assess certain forms of instability, and bursography, although frequently used in North America, also provides information about certain soft tissues.

There have been great advances in the ability to diagnose pathology of the shoulder joint. These include ultrasonography, in which non-invasive ultrasound provides information about soft tissues, especially in the rotator cuff, and detects fluid collections in the soft tissues. Computed tomography is a valuable tool for skeletal diagnosis and its diagnostic acumen can be further enhanced by its use in combination with intra-articular contrast medium, i.e. computed tomography arthrography. The greatest sensitivity and most detailed information however is being demonstrated with increasing experience and technical ability in the indications for and interpretation of magnetic resonance imaging. This sophisticated diagnostic tool, which is non-invasive and does not involve ionizing radiation, has been a major advance in the diagnosis of soft tissue pathology. Certain skeletal abnormalities can also be demonstrated with this technique. Electromyographic testing and nerve conduction studies give information about the muscular and neurological tissues. Arteriography, lymphangiography and venography may also be useful at times.

Another extremely valuable diagnostic tool is the arthroscopic evaluation of the shoulder joint and the subacromial space (Andrews *et al.*, 1984). Arthroscopy is not only a very sensitive diagnostic tool, but also arthroscopic surgical treatment of certain conditions is being developed.

A careful and complete history, an observant physical examination and the appropriate use of diagnostic testing should lead to the accurate diagnosis of most shoulder pathology. With correct diagnosis an optimal treatment plan can be developed.

The upper extremity

Anatomy of the upper arm

The bulkiness of the upper arm is due to the prominence of several large muscles – the deltoid over the point of the shoulder and lateral upper arm, both heads of biceps anteriorly, and the three heads of triceps posteriorly.

The posterior axillary fold is made up of the spiralling tendon of latissimus dorsi and teres major, and the anterior axillary fold is the inferior border of pectoralis major. Anteriorly, the latter muscle lies beside the medial border of deltoid – the deltopectoral groove between them is a useful approach for surgical access to the shoulder joint. In the groove lies the cephalic vein, and the groove is extended distally between the biceps tendon and the insertion of the deltoid muscle, providing a useful approach for surgery to the proximal humeral shaft.

A further prominent landmark is the distal end of the biceps and the lacertus fibrosus, which is a palpable tight band in the antecubital fossa. Other muscles in the lower half of the upper arm are the coracobrachialis, brachioradialis and brachialis.

The brachial artery and median nerve leave the axilla and course through the upper arm under cover of the coracobrachialis, and are applied closely to the humeral shaft along with the musculocutaneous nerve. The ulnar nerve lies behind these structures. The radial nerve passes behind the humeral shaft in the proximal arm and spirals round the lateral border of the humerus, at which point it is vulnerable to injury. It eventually comes to lie anterior to the elbow under cover of the brachioradialis muscle.

General discussion

Upper arm pain may be from the neck in cervical radiculopathy or may be due to radiation of pain into the arm from intrinsic shoulder problems. In addition, neurological lesions, for example carpal tunnel syndrome in the wrist and other nerve entrapment syndromes, may present as upper arm pain, although there is no intrinsic problem in the upper arm itself. Reflex sympathetic dystrophy may also result in upper arm pain and malfunction.

Tumours

Tumours may and do occur in the arm. Benign lesions such as lipomata can be quite sizeable. If myositis ossificans develops it is usually as a result of trauma (see Chapter 4). Metastatic lesions are not uncommon in the proximal humerus. Computed tomography, isotope bone scanning and magnetic resonance imaging are all useful techniques in the evaluation of soft tissue swellings around the shoulder.

Contusions

The shoulder and upper arm are commonly subjected to direct violence in falls, accidents or in contact sports. Contusions are managed conservatively, as outlined in Chapter 4. Severe injury to the flexor mass on the front of the elbow may develop myositis ossificans.

Tendinitis

Tendinitis is a frequent upper arm condition seen in all age groups and most commonly involves the long head of the biceps tendon at this level (see above). A rarer form of tendinitis in the upper arm is at the insertion of the deltoid muscle into the lateral humeral shaft. Deltoid tendinitis may be treated similarly to bicipital tendinitis but does not present the same potential for spontaneous tendon rupture.

Tendon rupture

Rupture of the proximal end of the long head of the biceps has been dealt with in the section on the shoulder (above).

Rarely, the biceps tendon ruptures from its insertion into the lacertus fibrosus and radial tubercle in the proximal forearm. When this occurs, there is severe pain in the antecubital fossa. This is usually caused by more violent physical activities involving extremely forceful flexion of the arm. It is rarely associated with the more degenerative type of rupture, which occurs in the tendon of the long head of the biceps. Pain relief is usually achieved by immobilization for a period of 1–2 weeks and symptomatic management, including the use of non-steroidal anti-inflammatory medications, analgesics, ice, etc., and rarely is surgical repair required. Frequently with this injury patients do seem to require physiotherapy to achieve full elbow flexion and supination.

Occasionally, direct trauma may result in injury to or rupture of the triceps tendon, but generally this is in association with a fracture of the olecranon. Rupture of the coracobrachialis and the short head of the biceps tendon may occur with trauma, and in some cases may result in avulsion of the tip of the coracoid process. This latter injury may be managed by reattachment with a single surgical screw. The majority of other tendon ruptures may be treated conservatively in most cases.

Muscle tears

Almost all tears of the deltoid muscle are proximal. These tears involve the origin of the muscle in the shoulder area and rarely involve distal deltoid muscle tissue. Muscle substance tears may occur in the biceps, brachialis, triceps, brachioradialis, pectoralis major muscles, etc. All are managed symptomatically with rest, compression, ice, immobilization, non-steroidal anti-inflammatory medications, analgesics, physiotherapy and rehabilitation.

Nerve injuries

The radial nerve is occasionally injured in association with a fracture of the mid-shaft of the humerus. The nerve usually recovers without surgical repair. However, if surgery is indicated for internal fixation of the fracture, the nerve should be explored at the same time. Prolonged observation may be required before there is evidence of reinnervation of both sensory and motor branches. It is extremely important during the period of observation to maintain daily passive range of motion of all joints of the wrist and hand and arm affected by the radial nerve palsy, to avoid permanent joint stiffness which would impair extremity function, even if there is eventually complete radial nerve recovery. If there is no evidence of radial nerve recovery either clinically or by electromyogram studies performed at 6 weeks and repeated a few weeks later, surgical exploration of the nerve may become necessary (Ackroyd and Stainforth, 1987). At the time of surgery, the nerve is frequently found to be bound down in the healing bone callus and surrounding bone fragments. This can be managed by gently freeing the nerve from its bony entrapment and there can be a reasonable expectation of recovery. Rarely, the nerve may be found to have been transected. This will require microsurgical re-anastomosis and has a poorer prognosis.

A temporary radial nerve palsy may occur with prolonged pressure on the radial nerve as it courses around the posterior humeral shaft and is frequently referred to as 'Saturday-night palsy'. This may occur in the individual who has been sitting backwards in a chair for a prolonged period of time with the arms over the back of the chair, resulting in direct pressure to the radial nerve. This presents as loss of radial nerve sensory distribution to the hand and forearm and absence of active radial motor function. In particular, the distal radial nerve motor functions of extension of the wrist and fingers of the hand are lost. Slow recovery can be anticipated in almost all cases.

Occasionally other nerve injuries can occur, usually in association with penetrating wounds, for example, a gunshot or stab wound to the inner arms might cause injury to the musculocutanous nerve and result in biceps muscle paralysis. Penetrating wounds resulting in neurovascular injury require direct surgical approach and repair. Treatment depends on the specific aetiology of the injury as well as the level of injury. For example, gunshot wounds causing nerve damage usually result in nerve tissue loss and a gap in the nerve. This requires a complex surgical repair to bridge the gap in the nerve, whereas in a direct or penetrating stab wound nerve endings are sharply transected. Microscopic nerve repair is strongly recommended for re-anastomosis of any major peripheral nerve transection, regardless of the cause of the injury. Ulnar nerve lesions are more common in relation to the elbow joint and will be discussed further in relation to the elbow joint.

Anatomy of the forearm

Prominent anatomical features in the forearm are the medial flexor muscle mass and the lateral common extensor muscle mass. The radial head may be palpated as it rotates in its groove during supination and pronation of the forearm. The ulna is subcutaneous throughout its entire length from the olecranon proximally to the distal ulnar styloid. Both bones are maintained in their position by strong supporting ligaments. The annular or orbicular ligament secures the radius to the ulna proximally, as does the lateral collateral ligament. The proximal ulna has some inherent stability by virtue of its articulation with the humerus and joint capsule attachments. Distally, the ulna is stabilized at the radioulnar joint by a strong ligamentous band between the radius and ulna. There is a small meniscus-like cartilaginous structure between the distal radius and ulna. The interosseous mebrane between the radius and ulna is also a strong stabilizing structure. This membrane essentially creates a separation of the forearm soft tissues into anterior or volar and posterior or dorsal compartments.

There are three layers in the flexor muscle mass. The muscles in the superficial layer from lateral to medial are the pronator teres, flexor carpi radialis, palmaris longus and flexor carpi ulnaris muscles. The intermediate layer consists of the flexor digitorum superficialis muscle. The deep layer is composed of the flexor digitorum profundus and flexor pollicis muscles. Distally in the anterior compartment of the forearm is the pronator quadratus muscle.

The extensor muscles in the dorsal compartment of the forearm are divided into superficial and deep layers. The muscles of the superficial layer from lateral to medial are the brachioradialis, extensor carpi radialis longus and brevis, extensor digitorum, extensor digiti minimi and extensor carpi ulnaris. The deep layer consists of the supinator, extensor pollicis longus, extensor pollicis brevis, abductor pollicis longus, and extensor indicis muscles. At the wrist the extensor muscles are tendinous structures and they are stabilized by the dorsal carpal ligaments.

The brachial artery divides into the radial and ulnar arteries. The radial artery in the proximal forearm lies deep to the brachioradialis muscle and becomes subcutaneous at the level of the wrist. The ulnar artery lies deep to the pronator teres muscle in the proximal forearm. A branch of the ulnar artery is the common interosseous artery which then divides into the anterior and posterior interosseous arteries which supply the dorsal and volar compartments of the forearm respectively. The main branch of the ulnar artery travels with the ulnar nerve into the distal forearm beneath the flexor digitorum superficialis muscle and enters Guyon's canal in the hand.

The radial nerve divides proximal to the forearm into the posterior interosseous nerve and the radial sensory nerve. The sensory nerve travels with the radial artery deep to the brachioradialis into the distal forearm. The posterior interosseous nerve passes between the two heads of supinator and lies on the posterior surface of the interosseous membrane with the posterior interosseous artery and innervates most of the extensor group of muscles.

The median nerve enters the forearm between the two heads of the pronator teres muscle and supplies motor innervation to a majority of the flexors of the wrist and hand. The main branch of the median nerve is the anterior interosseous nerve, which lies on the anterior interosseous membrane. The main trunk of the median nerve then passes distally into the forearm, lying superficial to flexor digitorum profundus, and enters the wrist through the carpal tunnel.

The ulnar nerve emerges from its groove on the dorsum of the medial epicondyle of the humerus and enters the forearm between the two heads of flexor carpi ulnaris and reaches the wrist lying on flexor digitorum profundus, to lie medially and close to the ulnar artery. The motor branches which originate at the level of the elbow supply the flexor carpi ulnaris and medial half of the flexor digitorum profundus.

Communicating branches between the median and ulnar nerves in the forearm are common.

The spatial relationship between the shafts of the radius and ulna, maintained by the superior and inferior radioulnar joints and by the fibres of the interosseous ligament, is complex, and allows pronation and supination. Any deformity of radius or ulna resulting from injury will compromise this complex arrangement and can interfere with the ability to pronate and supinate.

General discussion

Cervical spine lesions with cervical radiculopathy, proximal or distal nerve entrapment syndromes, reflex sympathetic dystrophy, intrinsic shoulder and upper arm or hand conditions all may have a profound effect on forearm function. Therefore, abnormal forearm function may not always be a reflection of intrinsic abnormalities in the forearm itself.

Tumours

Tumours, both benign and malignant, may occur in the forearm and are managed as tumorous conditions elsewhere in the body. Metastatic malignant conditions rarely occur in the forearm.

Contusions

Superficial contusions to the forearm are not unusual and are not a problem in terms of long-lasting disability. Contusions are only a problem in clinical management when they involve the deeper structures, including muscle tissue and the periosteum. The ulna, being subcutaneous virtually throughout its entire length, is particularly subject to periosteal injury. These contusions usually are effectively managed with rest, ice, elevation, and occasional immobilization. The more severe contusions may require treatment with non-steroidal anti-inflammatory medications, infiltration of a corticosteroid, or aspiration if a fluid haematoma occurs, followed by local compression. Outpatient physiotherapy measures to decrease local pain and swelling and improve muscle function may be helpful.

Myositis ossificans may occur following a deeper, more severe contusion of the forearm muscles, but generally is not as common as myositis in the upper arm or elbow. The management of myositis ossificans is similar to that discussed in Chapter 4.

Tenosynovitis

Chronic tenosynovitis of the forearm tendons is a common and often quite disabling condition. It may involved the tendons of either the flexor muscles or the extensor muscles. Generally, it seems to be slightly more common in the extensor tendons of the wrist and hand. Occasionally, tenosynovitis may occur following a direct blow or trauma to the tendon or tendon sheath, but more commonly it is associated with repetitive movement and falls into the category of overuse syndromes.

De Quervain's tenovaginitis affects the abductor pollicis longus and extensor pollicis brevis tendons as they pass over the distal radial styloid. This is frequently associated with marked local tenderness in the area of the tendons at the base of the thumb and distal forearm. There may also be palpable nodular thickening of the tendon sheath and on auscultation crepitus may be heard as the tendons move through the sheath. The patient may experience a 'catching' or 'snapping' sensation on moving the thumb. There is weakness of grip and pain on resisted extension of the thumb and wrist or resisted radial deviation of the wrist. This condition may be slightly more common in women. The patient may also report a generalized feeling of weakness in the forearm and hand secondary to the pain and frequently will drop objects because of the severity of pain.

Acutely, this condition may be managed by conservative measures, including, ice, rest and elevation. The more chronic cases of de Quervain's tenovaginitis may respond to corticosteroid injection into the tendon sheath, avoiding injecting into the substance of the tendon since this may result in tendon necrosis. The use of non-steroidal anti-inflammatory medication is also helpful, as well as physiotherapy measures, including iontophoresis, local heat, ultrasound, and other pain-relieving and muscle-strengthening modalities. Wrist and thumb splints may also prove helpful in the more chronic forms of tenosynovitis.

Occasionally, with a chronic refractory de Quervain's tenovaginitis, surgical release of the tendon sheaths may be required. This surgical procedure, although technically relatively easy, may, unless extreme care is taken, result in damage to the superficial branches of the radial nerve, with decreased skin sensation distally and hypersensitivity of the scar (Faithfull and Lamb, 1971). Following surgical release, a period of immobilization is required which may vary, depending on which authority is quoted, but may extend for a period of 1–6 weeks. Outpatient physiotherapy and rehabilitation may be required postoperatively following surgery for de Quervain's tenovaginitis.

Forearm flexor tenosynovitis is another type of overuse syndrome and frequently is seen in individuals performing repetitive gripping or manipulative motions, as occurs in factory assembly-line work, racket sports, etc. Flexor tenosynovitis may also be associated with some swelling in the anterior forearm. There is both local pain and generalized weakness in grip and wrist flexion. Flexor tenosynovitis may also occur in association with carpal tunnel syndrome with appropriate symptoms of that condition. Management is similar to that mentioned for de Quervain's tenosynovitis. Acute management includes local ice, rest, and compressive support and is followed by nonsteroidal anti-inflammatory drugs, splints, outpatient physiotherapy, and occasional complete immobilization in a cast. Surgery is rarely indicated for this condition unless in association with carpal tunnel syndrome. Acute trauma may occasionally result in tenosynovitis but it is more commonly an indication of overuse and may necessitate a change in vocational or sporting activities or, in racket sports, attention to the shape and size of grip.

Compartment syndromes (see Chapter 4)

The aetiology of forearm compartment syndrome is as varied as in other areas of the body. This syndrome may occur with fracture of the forearm, muscle swelling with extreme exercise, prolonged external pressure from a cast or splint, the unconscious patient lying on his or her arm, injections of drugs or other materials into the forearm muscles, bleeding from trauma or bleeding disorders, snake or insect bites, severe local infections, etc.

The signs and symptoms of the volar forearm compartment syndrome are weakness of finger and wrist flexion, severe forearm pain, local forearm swelling, marked tenderness on palpation of the muscles and fascia of the forearm, decreased sensation of the volar aspect of the fingers and hand, particularly in the median nerve distribution, and severe pain on passive extension of the fingers and wrist. The pain is invariably severe and out of proportion to the degree of trauma or injury which has occurred. Distal pulses may be diminished, but it should be noted that a full-blown compartment syndrome may occur in the forearm with apparently normal radial and ulnar pulses. Therefore, the presence of distal pulses in the wrist does not confirm the adequacy of circulation to the muscles and vital structures of the forearm. The use of Doppler signals for detecting pulses may also be misleading since signals may occasionally be detected even when there is severely compromised compartment function.

In the more severe cases of anterior forearm compartmental syndrome, the fingers are held in flexion and the thumb is abducted and extended. If an established compartment syndrome of the forearm is not treated in a timely manner, there will be muscle necrosis of both the superficial and deep compartments of the anterior forearm. Nerve damage to the median and ulnar nerves occurs as well. This ultimately results in a markedly atrophic forearm with fingers held in a claw position with the thumb extended and abducted. This is Volkmann's ischaemic contracture, as classically described in children in association with a supracondylar fracture of the humerus and damage to the brachial artery. The symptoms of acute brachial artery occlusion, whether from embolus, spasm or an intimal flap, are virtually identical to the symptoms of a forearm compartment syndrome. Both exhibit symptoms of forearm compartment ischaemia and neurovascular compromise, and both conditions may occur in the same patient. If arterial compromise is demonstrated by arteriography, surgical repair of the artery is necessary. It is generally wise to perform a fasciotomy of the forearm at the same time. Fasciotomy of the forearm is easily performed by a longitudinal ulnar incision and should be combined with a release of the transverse carpal ligament at the wrist.

Recurrent chronic compartment syndromes may also occur in the upper extremity, but are generally more frequent in the lower extremity related to excessive muscle exercise and associated muscle swelling. This sometimes may cause a somewhat confusing clinical picture, since similar types of symptom may also occur with chronic tendinitis, fatigue fractures, etc. Frequently the treatment is to modify the patient's activities to avoid the intensive exercises which bring on the severe forearm pain and compartment syndrome. In the recalcitrant patient a subcutaneous fasciotomy may rarely be required.

Nerve entrapment syndromes

Whilst nerve entrapment syndromes are rare in the forearm, ulnar nerve entrapment at the elbow and median nerve entrapment at the wrist are the most common examples in the upper extremity. The posterior interosseous branch of the radial nerve may occasionally become entrapped by a fibrous tissue band in the arcade of Frohse. Fractures or fracture dislocations about the elbow may result in increased pressure on the nerve. This may occasionally be confused with tennis elbow because of the chronic proximal lateral forearm pain. The difference is that the nerve entrapment will have demonstrable weakness or loss of motor function of the posterior interosseous innervated extensor muscles of the forearm. This may be documented with electromyogram and nerve conduction studies and presents with pain more localized to the anterior aspect of the elbow, as well as pain on resisted supination of the forearm. Occasionally these symptoms may develop after vigorous physical activity and may be difficult to differentiate from a compartment syndrome. Surgical exploration of the posterior interosseous nerve and freeing of the entrapment may occasionally become necessary for the refractory case that does not respond to conservative measures.

Superficial or sensory branches of the radial nerve may also be entrapped in the forearm by scar tissue, tight cuffs or a watch strap or bracelet. This usually results in specific tenderness in the area of radial nerve entrapment and diminished skin sensation distal to the point of nerve entrapment. Superficial branches of the radial nerve may also be injured in lacerations or surgical incisions, as seen with surgical release for chronic de Quervain's tenovaginitis.

Nerve entrapments involving the median or ulnar nerve in the forearm are uncommon. Injury to these nerves may occur with penetrating wounds or fractures. The associated motor and sensory deficit in the forearm and hand depends on the level of injury. Primary repair of any major peripheral nerve transection is recommended. In the forearm the injury with the best prognosis for recovery is to the radial nerve, which is primarily a sensory nerve at this level and does not involve motor function of the hand. Lacerations of the median and ulnar nerves in the forearm may result in extremely disabling injuries with loss of gross and fine motor function in the hand, and have a much worse prognosis for recovery. When closed fractures result in nerve injury in the forearm, recovery of the nerve can usually be anticipated. With these injuries, observation for reinnervation is recommended and avoidance of early surgical exploration. However, if the nerve injury develops after a closed manipulation for a fracture or a dislocation, early exploration of the nerve is recommended. If open reduction and internal fixation are planned, nerve exploration is also recommended.

The radial nerve is the one most commonly injured in the upper extremity. The ulnar nerve is less commonly injured and the median nerve least of all. Approximately 40% of peripheral nerve injuries follow bone and joint trauma, an additional 40% resulting from lacerating or penetrating wounds caused by sharp objects or weapons. The techniques of surgical repair for each peripheral nerve will not be discussed here and are quite specific for each nerve at each level and vary according the degree of damage. Microscopic re-anastomosis of peripheral nerve lacerations requires an extremely experienced and skilled surgeon for the best prognosis for recovery.

Anatomy of the elbow joint

The medial and lateral epicondyles serve as the origin for important muscle groups affecting the function of the elbow joint and forearm. The medial epicondyle is the origin of the common flexor muscles of the forearm. The lateral epicondyle is the origin of the common extensor muscles for the forearm. The muscles of pronator teres, flexor carpi radialis, palmaris longus, flexor carpi ulnaris and flexor digitorum superficialis all originate from the medial epicondyle and join the flexor digitorum profundus and flexor pollicis longus to comprise the common flexor muscle mass of the proximal medial forearm. These muscles provide flexion of the elbow, wrist and hand, as well as pronation of the forearm. The muscles of brachioradialis, extensor digitorum, extensor digiti minimi, extensor carpi radialis longus and brevis, extensor carpi ulnaris, supinator and anconeus all originate from the lateral epicondyle and comprise the common extensor muscle mass of the proximal lateral forearm. These muscles provide extension of the elbow, wrist and hand as well as flexion of the elbow. The other elbow flexors are the biceps, brachialis and pronator teres muscles. Biceps also contribute to supination. The space between the flexor and extensor muscle groups contains a number of vital structures travelling into the forearm and is called the antecubital fossa. Its borders are the pronator teres muscle medially, and the brachioradialis laterally. The biceps tendon and aponeurosis divide the antecubital fossa into medial and lateral compartments.

The neurovascular bundle in the medial compartment contains the brachial artery and vein and the median nerve. The brachial artery divides distally in the antecubital fossa into the radial artery and ulnar artery. The radial artery passes distally under the brachioradialis muscle to lie beside the radial nerve in the lateral compartment. The ulnar artery passes underneath the pronator teres muscle medially, joining the ulnar nerve. The ulnar nerve passes from behind the medial epicondyle and is now anterior in the forearm underneath the flexor muscle mass of the forearm. The median nerve passes deeply in the antecubital space and remains in the deep compartment of the forearm on the surface of the flexor digitorum profundus muscle. Proximally in the antecubital space, the radial nerve lies in the interval between the brachioradialis and brachialis muscle and divides into the posterior interosseous nerve and the dorsal radial sensory nerve. The posterior interosseous nerve is the motor nerve to the extensor muscles of the forearm, and it extends dorsally into the forearm after winding around the radial neck laterally. The superficial or sensory branch of the radial nerve joins the radial artery underneath the brachioradialis muscle in the forearm. The brachial artery also supplies recurrent branches to both the radial and ulnar sides of the elbow joint in the antecubital fossa. These recurrent branches are of significance in collateral circulation about the elbow joint. There are two main bursae of the elbow joint, one lying between the common triceps tendon and the bone and the other lying between the triceps tendon and the subcutaneous tissues in the posterior surface of the elbow – the olecranon bursa.

The main ligaments of the elbow joint are the medial or ulnar collateral ligament and the lateral or radial collateral ligament. The medial collateral ligment arises from the medial epicondyle and inserts into the proximal ulnar shaft. The lateral ligament arises from the lateral epicondyle and inserts in the proximal radial shaft and orbicular ligament. These ligaments are the main varus and valgus stabilizers of the elbow joint. The annular or orbicular ligament encircles the radial neck, thus stabilizing the radial head in its groove in the ulna. The capsular attachments of the elbow joint also contribute to stability. The anterior capsule is frequently injured in hyperextension injuries of the elbow joint.

General discussion

Ligamentous injuries about the elbow joint, injuries to the musculotendinous origins about the elbow joint and intra-articular problems of the elbow joint must be considered.

Tumours

Tumours, both benign and malignant, may involve the elbow joint. Malignant tumours about the elbow joint of non-osseous origin are rare. Benign tumours such as lipomata, ganglion cysts and bursitis may occur about the elbow joint.

Intra-articular problems

Intra-articular problems of loose bodies, arthritic conditions, infective synovitis and gouty arthritis must be considered. In the investigation of acute swelling of the elbow an accurate history, examination, aspiration, X-rays and laboratory studies should be done. Occasionally other studies may be used, including isotope bone scan, arthrography, computed tomography scan, magnetic resonance imaging and elbow arthroscopy.

Vascular injury

Vascular injuries about the elbow joint are, fortunately, relatively uncommon and are almost always associated with fractures and damage to or occlusion of the brachial artery. This is presented in more detail under the discussion of compartmental syndromes, above.

Other injuries

Fractures, fracture dislocations, and intra-articular bone injuries of the elbow joint will not be discussed here but are important injuries and sources of disability about the elbow joint. Specific ligamentous and musculotendinous conditions commonly occurring in the elbow joint will be discussed below.

Ulnar nerve injury

The ulnar nerve is fairly superficial as it transverses the ulnar groove posterior to the medial epicondyle of the elbow. The ulnar nerve at this point is vulnerable to injury from a direct blow, as well as traction injury due to repeated valgus strain at the elbow in throwing events. This may result in an acute ulnar nerve injury or a chronic ulnar neuritis at the elbow joint. Angular deformity of the elbow may result from a previous fracture or developmental abnormality with increased carrying angle (cubitus valgus). This increased carrying angle may place the ulnar nerve under tension and result in injury as it courses through the ulnar groove.

Ulnar neuritis may occur following childhood fracture. The onset of ulnar nerve problems occurs in adult life in association with this valgus deformity – thus the term ‘tardy ulnar palsy’. Scarring may occur from repetitive trauma or entrapment from previous fractures of the medial epicondyle.

The ulnar nerve may also become unstable in its soft tissue attachments in the ulnar groove. When this occurs, the patient will report repetitive snapping at the medial aspect of the elbow which may actually be the ulnar nerve snapping back and forth over the medial epicondyle.

The symptoms of ulnar neuritis are pain in the medial aspect of the elbow and some radiating pain along the ulnar side of the forearm. This is usually associated with paraesthesia in the little and ring fingers of the hand and occasionally in the forearm also. As is the case in all nerve entrapment syndromes, the pain seems to be worse at night. Symptoms may be aggravated by the position of the patient’s arm when sleeping due to direct pressure on the nerve. The ulnar nerve symptoms can also be aggravated by increased activities, possibly resulting from swelling of the nerve. If the nerve is unstable in the ulnar groove and snapping occurs on motion of the elbow joint, particularly into flexion, this will obviously cause increased ulnar nerve symptoms. Occasionally, there may also be some ulnar intrinsic motor weakness and atrophy in the hand in association with ulnar nerve dysfunction. A positive Tinel’s sign at the elbow on tapping the ulnar nerve may also be found if the nerve is irritated or injured.

Treatment is usually rest and non-steroidal anti-inflammatory medication and avoidance of those activities which tend to aggravate the symptoms. Occasionally a period of physiotherapy will be helpful. Training or re-education of muscles and instruction in proper body mechanics will be helpful if ulnar neuritis is associated with throwing sports. Occasionally a posterior splint or cast is used if other simpler conservative measures are not successful. An injection of corticosteroid into the area of the ulnar nerve at the elbow (but not into the ulnar nerve) may be helpful. If all else fails, surgical intervention may become necessary. Surgery involves freeing the nerve and its fascial investments, both proximally and distally, to allow adequate mobilization of the nerve to its new position transposed anterior to the medial epicondyle. This method is generally successful in relieving ulnar entrapment syndrome, but it may not be necessary in every case.

Acute and chronic elbow sprains

Sprains of either medial or lateral collateral ligaments or hyperextension injuries to the elbow are not infrequent. They are usually associated with sporting activities but can occur with other forms of trauma as well. When acute, these injuries are quite painful but are adequately managed with compression, ice, elevation, rest, tape splinting, analgesics, non-steroidal anti-inflammatory medications, posterior splinting or bracing. The elbow is essentially a stable joint and it is virtually impossible to sprain it by excessive flexion. Therefore, a majority of injuries are caused by hyperextension and/or varus or valgus forces about the joint.

The most frequently injured collateral ligament in hyperextension of the elbow is the medical collateral. Varus or valgus instability is difficult to test in the elbow joint and frequently cannot be demonstrated if there is also associated bony instability of the joint. Rarely is surgical repair required for an acute ligamentous injury of the elbow.

Physical findings will be of acute pain in the area of ligament injury either at its bony attachment or in the substance of the ligament. Worsening of the pain by applying either varus or valgus stress will be demonstrable depending on which ligament is injured. Moving the elbow into extension may produce the pain in the damaged ligament, since hyperextension injuries may also involve injury to one or both of the collateral ligaments.

Chronic sprains of the elbow joint frequently occur with sports involving repetitive throwing where there is extreme valgus stress at the point of release. This injures the medial collateral ligament of the elbow and causes a lateral compressive force at the elbow joint. Chronic medial collateral ligament sprain of the elbow joint has been occasionally called 'thrower's elbow'. This condition particularly occurs in individuals who fail to warm up or stretch before exercising and in individuals with poor throwing mechanics and techniques.

Another condition causing medial elbow pain in the child or adolescent is 'little league elbow' (see Chapter 21). This also involves the medial structures of the elbow with chronic medial pain due to repeated valgus stress on the medial collateral ligament. In the growing child this causes a chronic stress at the epiphyseal plate of the medial epicondyle. Early in this condition, the X-rays of the elbow may be entirely normal. As the condition progresses without treatment, it may eventually result in separation and avulsion of the medial epicondyle. If the medial epicondyle is widely separated, it may require surgical replacement and pinning, with care being taken not to injure the ulnar nerve in the process.

In the more chronic stages of these conditions of elbow sprain, a chronic lateral compression injury to the elbow joint surface occurs with breakdown of articular cartilage and separation of osteochrondral fragments, resulting in loose bodies, as well as osteochrondritis dissecans of the capitulum. Eventually severe osteoarthritis, ulnar neuritis and chronic elbow pain may occur. Chronic elbow sprains are managed by correcting improper throwing mechanics, muscle strengthening, and anti-inflammatory drugs; local corticosteroid injections and bracing may be helpful. Surgical intervention is occasionally necessary and might involve reconstruction of the medial collateral ligament of the elbow, ulnar nerve transposition or open arthrotomy. Intra-articular problems may now be managed by arthroscopic surgery. Arthroscopic techniques have been shown to be applicable in the elbow joint (Sisk, 1987) and include arthroscopic debridement, synovectomy, removal of loose bodies, lysis of joint adhesions and debridement of osteochondral lesions. This may be done relatively safely on an outpatient basis without much trauma or morbidity to the patient and should become an increasingly popular technique in the management of intra-articular problems of the elbow.

Lateral epicondylitis

One of the most common problems occurring in the elbow involving soft tissues is lateral epicondylitis or tennis elbow (Coonrad and Hooper, 1973). This manifests as an acute or chronic pain in the area of the lateral epicondyle of the elbow. There may be pain also in the common extensor origin or the lateral side of the joint or on the radial head. The exact aetiology of this condition is not known; there are a large number of theories or opinions as to the cause. The condition definitely occurs with repetitive motion of the forearm and hand in gripping and turning activities. Lateral epicondylitis may occur in office workers, as well as heavy physical labourers, and in some individuals may represent a type of overuse syndrome. However, on some occasions, lateral epicondylitis appears spontaneously without any apparent explanation for the onset of the symptoms. The most significant physical finding of lateral epicondylitis is severe tenderness in the area of the lateral epicondyle of the elbow. Occasionally some swelling is present. There is also marked pain at the extremes of supination and pronation of the forearm as well as sharp pain at the lateral epicondyle and in the proximal extensor muscle mass on extension of the wrist and hand against resistance. There may be pain in the lateral joint capsule and radial head also. The patient frequently complains of weakness or inability to perform repetitive forearm rotations or to grip forcefully. X-ray findings are usually normal but occasionally may show some soft tissue calcification in the area of the lateral epicondyle.

Treatment consists of symptomatic management, usually including ice, rest, non-steroidal anti-inflammatory medication, Velcro forearm bands, injection of corticosteroids, outpatient physiotherapy, and occasionally posterior arm splints or a cast. In racket sports it may be possible to implicate the size and shape of the handle grip, and experimentation with grips of different thickness may achieve dramatic relief of symptoms. In extremely refractory cases, surgery may be required. Surgical release of the common extensor mechanism from the lateral epicondyle is the most commonly performed procedure. A variety of other procedures have been advocated for this chronic condition. Chronic pain seems to wax and wane and may spontaneously disappear as mysteriously as it appears.

Lateral elbow pain is not always due to tennis elbow or lateral epicondylitis, and a large number of other conditions have been reported to cause similar symptoms. These include bursitis of the radial humeral head, mucinous degeneration of various of the tendons comprising the common extensor mechanism, entrapment of the posterior interosseous nerve, synovitis of the radiohumeral joint, and chronic lateral collateral ligament sprain. Lateral epicondylitis may occur alone or in conjunction with these other conditions. In treating lateral epicondylitis, it is important to consider these other diagnoses as well. This is especially so if standard conservative methods of treatment have proven unsuccessful and surgical intervention is being considered.

Medial epicondylitis

Medial epicondylitis of the elbow is occasionally seen, although much less frequently than lateral epicondylitis (Coonrad and Hooper, 1973). Periostitis of the musculotendinous origin of the flexor muscle mass on the medial epicondyle and medial collateral ligament injuries often present with a similar clinical picture. Both conditions may occur in the same patient. Both present with medial elbow pain tenderness on examination. Both conditions tend to be made worse with activities such as throwing. In medial epicondylitis, the pain frequently is reproduced or worsened by forced palmar flexion of the wrist against resistance or forced pronation of the forearm. Medial collateral ligament pain may be worsened with valgus stress at the elbow or full extension of the elbow joint. X-rays are helpful only in the adolescent or child in differentiating avulsion fractures from medial epicondylitis or medial collateral ligament sprain.

The treatment of medial epicondylitis is virtually identical to that recommended for lateral epicondylitis, and consists of rest, immobilization, physiotherapy, training of proper muscle mechanics and throwing techniques, corticosteroid injections and non-steroidal anti-inflammatory medications. Occasionally, surgical release of the common flexor muscle origin from the medial epicondyle is required. As described under the treatment of lateral epicondylitis, in sports involving gripping a racket or club, symptoms may respond to alteration of the size and shape of the grip.

Olecranon bursitis

Another soft tissue condition commonly occurring in the elbow is olecranon bursitis, in which there is swelling of the olecranon bursa, as well as local tenderness about the bursa. The condition may be caused by repetitive pressure on the olecranon such as the office worker's elbow resting on a desk surface for prolonged periods. Other sources of repetitive minor trauma to the posterior elbow joint can lead to bursitis. This may occasionally occur with acute trauma as well and is also seen as an acute septic process or in allergic reactions to insect stings. The olecranon bursa may also be swollen due to gout or other inflammatory or allergic processes. X-ray examination of the elbow in olecranon bursitis is usually normal except for soft tissue swelling. There may occasionally be an associated olecranon spur at the tip of the elbow. This is usually further evidence of chronic and repetitive trauma to the olecranon.

The treatment of choice for olecranon bursitis is local direct pressure on the swollen bursa, either by an Ace bandage and Ace elbow sleeve, or by direct compression and avoidance of further trauma to the swollen bursa. Occasionally posterior splint immobilization is necessary to avoid further motion or trauma to the swollen bursa. In the non-injected case of olecranon bursitis, non-steroidal anti-inflammatory medication or local corticosteroid injections may sometimes prove effective. If an infection is suspected because of erythema swelling of the olecranon bursa, a carefully done sterile needle aspiration for culture and sensitivity may be performed. Needle punctures seem to have a tendency to cause infections if not done under sterile conditions in this area and may result in complications worse than the original process. Occasionally for chronic suppurative olecranon bursitis, an open incision, drainage and debridement are required.

Radial head subluxation

Radial head subluxation is a condition that occurs in infants and young children. It is also frequently referred to as 'nursemaid's elbow' or 'pulled elbow'. This usually occurs when a child is forcefully pulled or jerked by the arm with the arm in extension. The result is an acute radial head subluxation with the child experiencing sudden, severe elbow pain. When the occurs, the child will usually refuse to move the elbow, which is held in a slightly pronated and somewhat flexed position. X-rays are of little benefit, even when comparison views of the opposite elbow are used. The diagnosis is usually made by a combination of history and limitation of motion, especially the absence of supination and flexion of the elbow. Treatment for this is mild sedation and gentle manipulation of the arm into full supination and flexion of the elbow joint. Usually this results in a quick reduction of the radial head and no further treatment is needed. Occasionally an arm sling or posterior splint may be used for a few days if the elbow is slightly painful after reduction.

Acute and chronic elbow dislocation

Acute dislocations of the elbow without fracture do occur, especially in contact sports or other non-sports-related trauma. Usually the proximal ulna and radius dislocate posteriorly on the distal humerus with the elbow in hyperextension. This injury occurs with a fall on to the extended arm, driving the end of the humerus over the coronoid process of the ulna and tearing the anterior capsule of the joint. This may also result in a tear of the collateral ligaments of the elbow, usually the medial collateral. Momentary subluxations without true dislocation may occur and may be of a chronic recurring nature. The instability of subluxation is difficult to demonstrate or reproduce during the examination. Subluxation almost always spontaneously reduces prior to the patient being seen. Dislocations may also be complicated by fractures in the elbow joint. Because of this possibility an X-ray is recommended prior to attempted reduction and another X-ray post-reduction.

Chronic recurrent dislocations usually result from an unrecognized bony fragment in the joint or from inadequate immobilization of the elbow, preventing adequate soft tissue healing. Acute dislocations should be immobilized for at least 3 weeks after reduction to allow soft tissue healing of the collateral ligaments, joint capsule and muscles. Recovery of joint motion and arm strength following acute elbow dislocations is generally quite slow and may require the assistance of a physiotherapist or trainer. Chronic recurrent dislocation of the elbow may be treated with elbow restraints or braces to prevent hyperextension or collateral instability. Rarely does this require surgical reconstruction of the supporting soft tissues of the elbow joint. Other directions of dislocation may occur, for example, medial, laterial or anterior, but are much rarer and almost always there is a fracture or bony avulsion. In children, the equivalent fracture and avulsions frequently involve the epicondyles and the epiphyseal plates. Dislocations involving bony injuries will not be dealt with here other than to mention that they do occur and represent serious injuries to the elbow joint.

A chronic unreduced dislocation of the elbow is a rare finding. This is usually associated with fairly marked ectopic ossification about the elbow joint and myositis ossificans. Achieving reduction of these dislocations is extremely difficult, even with open surgical techniques. The prognosis is likely to be incomplete recovery of joint motion and there is a high probability of permanent elbow stiffness.

Distal biceps tendinitis and rupture

Biceps tendinitis at the elbow may occur in either or both of the lacertus fibrosus or the biceps tendon as it inserts into the bicipital tubercle of the radius. Distal biceps tendinitis presents as a chronic, insidious, painful condition. This is frequently associated with repetitive physical activities and should be treated as a type of overuse syndrome rather than an acute injury. By contrast, rupture of the biceps tendon occurs as a result of extremely forceful flexion of the elbow against strong resistance or in very heavy lifting with the elbow in a flexed position. When rupture of the tendon occurs, the individual usually experiences a sudden, painful snap in the front of the elbow joint. There is immediate weakness of active flexion of the elbow as well as weakness of supination. In comparison, the pain of distal bicipital tendinitis is usually gradual and insidious in onset, and is much less severe than with acute tendon rupture. In both conditions there is tenderness and swelling in the distal antecubital fossa in the area of the biceps tendon and lacertus fibrosus. However, the soft tissue swelling and ecchymosis is usually much more pronounced with acute tendon rupture.

Treatment for both conditions is by elevation, immobilization, ice and other measures of symptomatic management. The elbow is immobilized in 90° of flexion by a posterior splint for a period of 7–10 days. Tendon rupture may occasionally be associated with avulsion of the bicipital tuberosity from the proximal radius. This avulsion may include a fragment of bone which may be surgically reattached. Rupture or avulsion of the bicipital tendon may be incomplete and will respond to conservative measures of rest, ice, compression and eventual strengthening and therapy in the recuperative period. Long-term disability is unusual after this injury.

Myositis ossificans

Myositis ossificans may occur about the elbow joint as a result of trauma, even without dislocation or subluxation of the joint (see Chapter 4). However, surgical excision of mature myositis ossificans is more likely to be required in the elbow than in other sites, either because of direct pressure on neurovascular structures or because of marked restriction of elbow joint motion.

References

The shoulder

Andrews JR, Carson WG, Ortega K (1984) Arthroscopy of the shoulder: technique and normal anatomy. *American Journal of Sports Medicine* **12**, 1.

Brown C (1983) Compressive invasive referred pain to the shoulder. *Clinical Orthopaedics and Related Research* **173**, 55.

Codman AE (1937) Rupture of the supraspinatus 1834–194. *Journal of Bone and Joint Surgery* **19A**, 643.

De Palma AF, Gallery C, Bennet C (1949) Anatomy and degenerative lesions of the shoulder joint. *American Academy of Orthopedic Surgery Instructional Lectures* **VI**. Ann Arbor: JW Edwards.

Hovelius L (1987) Anterior dislocation of the shoulder in teenagers and young adults. Five year prognosis. *Journal of Bone and Joint Surgery* **69A**, 393–9.

Mumford EB (1941) Acromioclavicular dislocation: a new operative treatment. *Journal of Bone and Joint Surgery* **23**, 799.

Neer CS II (1972) Anterior acromioplasty for the chronic impingement syndrome in the shoulder. *Journal of Bone and Joint Surgery* **54A**, 41.

Neer CS II (1983) Rotator cuff arthropathy. *Journal of Bone and Joint Surgery* **65A**, 1232.

Neer CS II, Foster (1990) Inferior capsular shift for involuntary inferior and multidirectional instability of the shoulder. *Journal of Bone and Joint Surgery* **62A**, 897.

Neer CS II, Bigliani LV, Hawkins RJ (1977) Rupture of the long head of the biceps related to subacromial impingement. *Orthopaedic Transactions* **1**, 111.

Rathbun JB, McNab I (1970) The microvascular pattern of the rotator cuff. *Journal of Bone and Joint Surgery* **52B**, 540.

Rowe CR (1962) Acute and recurrent dislocations of the shoulder. *Journal of Bone and Joint Surgery* **44A**, 998–1008.

Rowe CR, Sakellarides HT (1961) Factors related to recurrences of anterior dislocation of the shoulder. *Clinical Orthopaedics and Related Research* **20**, 40.

The upper extremity

Ackroyd CE, Staniforth F (1987) In: Ed. Hughes, Benson, Colton *Orthopaedic* Edinburgh: Churchill Livingstone, p 876.

Coonrad RW, Hooper WR (1973) Tennis elbow: its course, natural history, conservative and surgical management. *Journal of Bone and Joint Surgery* **55A**, 1177.

Faithfull DK, Lamb DW (1971) De Quervain's disease – a clinical review. *The Hand* **3**, 23–33.

Further reading

Carson WG Jr (1988) *Arthroscopy of the elbow*. Instructional Course Lecturer, American Academy of Orthopedic Surgeons, **37**, 195–201.

D'Ambrosia RD (1977) *Musculoskeletal Disorders: Regional Examination and Differential Diagnosis*. Philadelphia: JB Lippincott.

Dhillon KS Sengupta S, Singh BJ (1988) *Acta Orthopaedica Scandinavica* **29**, 419–24.

Edmonson AS, Crenshaw AH (1980) *Campbell's Operative Orthopedics* vols 1 and 2. St Louis: CV Mosby Company.

Gainor BJ, Olson S (1990) Combined entrapment of median and anterior interosseous nerve in a pediatric. Both bones of the forearm fracture. *Orthopaedic Trauma* **4**, 197–9.

Gartland JJ (1965) *Fundamentals of Orthopedics*. Philadelphia: WB Saunders.

Henry AK (1973) *Extensile Exposure*. London: Churchill Livingstone.

Madsen FA (1980) *Compartmental Syndromes*. New York: Grune & Stratton.

Mirovsky Y, Hendel D, Halperin N (1988) Anterior interosseous nerve palsy following closed fracture of the proximal ulna. Case report and review of the literature. *Archives of Orthopaedic Trauma and Surgery* **107**, 61–4.

O'Donoghue D (1976) *Treatment of Injuries to Athletes*. Philadelphia: WB Saunders.

Poehling GG, Whipple TL, Sisco L (1989) Elbow arthroscopy: A new technique. *Arthroscopy* **5**, 222–4.

Quiring DP, Warfel JH (1960) *The Extremities*. Philadelphia: Lea & Febiger.

Rang M (1974) *Children's Fractures*. Philadelphia: JB Lippincott.

Schweitzer G (1988) Bilateral avulsion fractures of olecranon apophyses. *Archives of Orthopaedic Trauma Surgery* **107**, 181–2.

Turek SL (1977) *Orthopedics Principles and Their Application*. Philadelphia: JB Lippincott.

White SH, Goodfellow JW, Mowat A (1988) Posterior interosseous nerve palsy in rheumatoid arthritis. *Journal of Bone and Joint Surgery* **70**, 468–71.

15

Injuries to the eye

C. J. MacEwen

Introduction and epidemiology

Eye trauma remains one of the leading causes of ocular morbidity and visual impairment in modern ophthalmic practice. The assessment and treatment of eye injuries constitute a significant and increasing proportion of the workload in all hospital eye departments. An estimated 2.5 million eye injuries occur in the USA each year and over 1 million Americans suffer from visual impairment as a result of trauma (National Society to Prevent Blindness, 1980). Although no accurate figures are available for the UK, it can be assumed that eye injuries are at least as common in this country.

The majority of injuries occur in males under 25 years of age – women and the elderly are the least affected. Most cases are superficial and can be treated on an outpatient basis. However, because such injuries are most common in the active, working population they have enormous economic implications in terms of cost to the country as a whole due to time lost from work (Schein *et al.*, 1988). The more serious injuries involve long periods of inpatient care, multiple surgical procedures and often the ultimate loss of sight. For these reasons preventative measures are being evaluated and introduced in areas that pose a threat to the eye through injury.

Epidemiology

The epidemiology of serious eye trauma has changed significantly during the course of this century. Between 1908 and 1913 over 70% of a total of 1000 eye injuries which required hospital admission were due to accidents at work (Garrow, 1923). Most of these injuries occurred in high-risk occupations, such as metal workers and miners, and were due to penetrating trauma. The introduction of protective goggles and headwear and their enforced use by legislation successfully resulted in the reduction of serious work-related injuries. Sight-threatening injuries and secondary infection from foreign body penetration are now much less frequent. Although the workplace remains the commonest place for eye injuries to occur, the majority now are superficial and less than 1% require inpatient care. They are usually due to failure to comply with the eye protection regulations (MacEwen, 1989).

Road traffic accidents (RTAs) replaced industry as the most common source of serious injury in the 1960s and 1970s due to the increased volume of traffic and road use (Mackay, 1975). The injuries were usually penetrating and bilateral due to the face hitting the broken fragments of windscreen glass. This source of trauma was controlled, again by legislation, when the seat belt law came into effect in 1983. This resulted in a rapid reduction in RTA-related eye injuries (Vernon and Yorston, 1984) and this source of injuries has now almost completely disappeared.

The reduction in work- and RTA-related injuries in association with more time available for leisure activities has meant that sport is currently the major cause of eye injuries which are sufficiently serious to require hospital admission

(MacEwen, 1989). The strong regional variation in sporting popularity means that quite different patterns of injury and responsible sports have become evident. In Ireland, for example, hurling is the commonest cause of sporting eye injury (Canavan *et al.*, 1980) whereas baseball is implicated in the USA (Vinger, 1981). Soccer is a favourite pastime in the UK and therefore is responsible for the majority of eye injuries in sport in this country (Jones, 1987; MacEwen, 1986). Different sports, however, carry different risks; the combat sports pose the greatest threat to sight. Any sport, however, which uses rapidly moving balls, employs sticks and rackets or involves any degree of body contact carries a relatively high risk of injury.

Sport and all domestic recreational activities taken together account for 75% of eye injuries requiring hospital admission. Many domestic accidents involve the same type of activities that are found in the work environment, such as hammering, painting and drilling. Leisure-time activities or accidents in and around the home are the commonest causes of eye injury in women and children. Unfortunately, proportionately, more of the injuries that occur in children are sight-threatening compared with the adult population. This is particularly so in toddlers who have immature motor skills and insufficient experience to protect themselves from the hazards around the home. Another feature of injuries to children, which has only recently become recognized, is that of non-accidental injury and this should be considered in all cases, especially those with a poor or improbable history.

In addition to the above, assaults still form a significant proportion of serious injury, usually in certain inner-city areas and often in deprived groups of the population.

Most information available on eye injuries involves methods of management and eventual outcome. More emphasis needs to be placed on the cause of the injury so that prevention can be directed to the appropriate areas.

Aetiology

The basic mechanisms of eye injury can be classified as follows:

1. Blunt injuries.
2. Injuries caused by large, sharp objects.
3. Injuries caused by small flying particles.
4. Chemical burns.
5. Physical burns.

Each of these mechanisms produces a different spectrum of injury. They will therefore be described separately.

Blunt trauma

Blunt or contusional injuries are caused by a direct blow to the eye and surrounding tissues by an object such as a fist or a ball. No penetration takes place, although in severe cases rupture of the periorbital skin or eyeball may occur. This is the commonest type of trauma occurring in sport because the vast majority of sport-associated eye injuries are caused by the ball and most of the remainder by direct body contact. The size of the ball has been thought to influence the amount of resultant ocular damage (Editorial, 1973); small balls are considered able to enter the bony orbital aperture easily and strike the globe directly, whereas larger ones (considered as those with a diameter of 10 cm or more) dissipate most of their force to the periorbital tissues. Squash therefore attracted attention as a potentially dangerous sport; however, it has become evident that the larger, heavier balls can cause as much ocular damage as the smaller balls. This is because their increased momentum makes a significant injury more likely and also because their larger surface area increases the likelihood of potential eye contact. Fists are responsible for most other blunt injuries, both on and off the sports field.

Periocular tissues

The surrounding tissues absorb a proportion of the force and the ensuing periorbital bruising may be marked due to the thin, elastic tissues overlying this highly vascular area (Fig. 15.1). Extensive bruising often makes examination of the underlying globe difficult due to the tense swelling of the lids. There may be associated facial fractures of the malar complex or orbital blow-out fractures.

Blow-out fracture

A blow-out fracture is caused by an acute rise in intraorbital pressure during a blunt blow to the eye. The weakest part of the orbit fractures, usually the floor or the medial wall, characteristically leaving the orbital margins intact (Fig. 15.2). As the forces return to normal some of the orbital contents become entrapped in the fracture site, causing mechanical limitation of eye movement. This leads to the classic features of blow-out fracture – enophthalmos (expanded orbital cavity, with some contents herniating into the maxillary or ethmoid sinuses), double vision with limitation of eye movements and infraorbital anaesthesia (Fig. 15.2).

Ocular damage

A direct blow to the eye itself results in well-recognized changes in shape. The globe becomes flattened in its anteroposterior diameter and expands in its equatorial direction (Fig. 15.3). The flattening forces cause direct damage and contrecoup concussional injuries from shock waves set up at the site of impact. The expansile forces cause tearing of structures in the stretched equatorial plane. The extent of these changes depends on the amount of force with which the eye is hit and from which direction the blow comes.

Direct and flattening forces

In minimal cases superficial ocular damage such as subconjunctival haemorrhage may have a

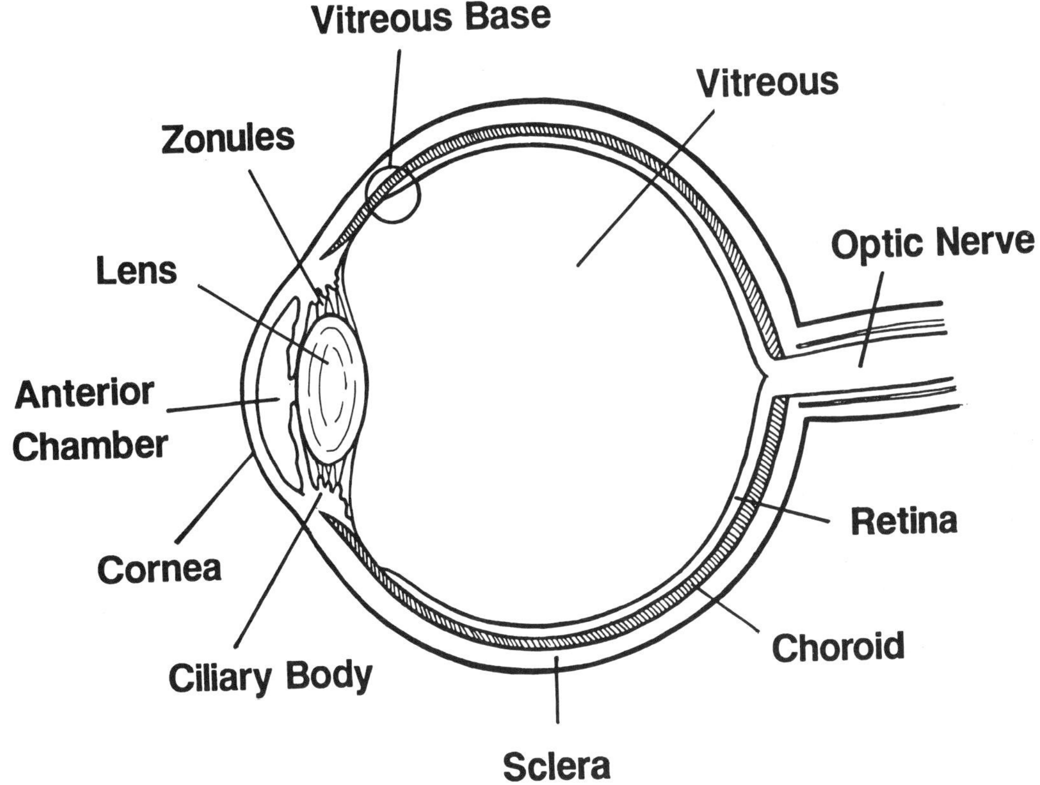

Fig. 15.1 The anatomy of the normal eye in sagittal section.

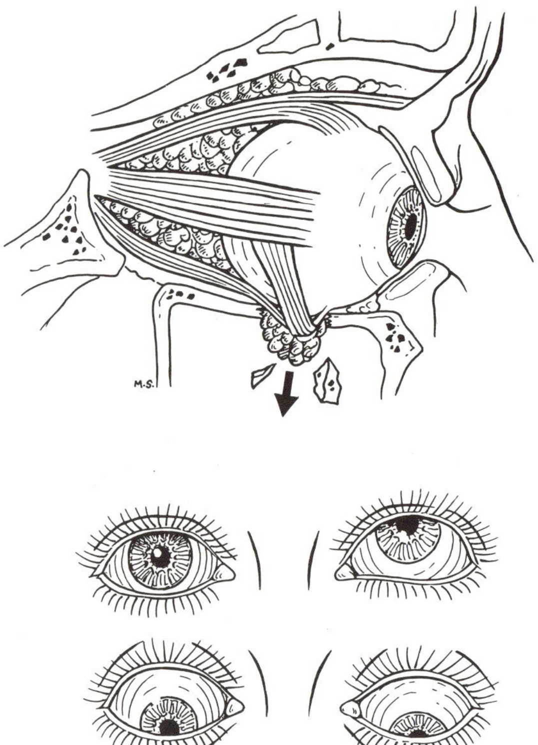

Fig. 15.2 The effect of a blow-out fracture on the vertical eye movements. The right eye cannot look up or down adequately because it is mechanically limited due to entrapped orbital tissues in the fracture site.

dramatic appearance but is usually minor and rarely signifies serious damage. However it is important to realize that it may be associated with other more significant injuries and may conceal deeper injury of the sclera.

Corneal epithelial loss may occur at the site of direct impact with a resultant corneal abrasion. The repair of the epithelium is usually rapid and complete, although in some cases poor healing and inadequate bonding to the basement membrane result in a recurrent corneal erosion which may persist for many months.

Anterior segment

The forces flattening the eye may be sufficient to cause contact of the cornea with the iris and the lens (Fig. 15.3). The whole iris lens diaphragm becomes temporarily displaced, which may cause traumatic anterior uveitis and bleeding into the anterior chamber (see section on hyphaema, below) from small tears in the iris sphincter around the pupil (Fig. 15.3a). The outcome is permanent contusional iris anomalies which result in an irregular, persistently enlarged, poorly reacting pupil. This prevents appropriate focusing and control of light entering the eye.

Contusional lens opacities are usually situated under the capsule of the lens and progress into the cortex with further lenticular growth. The metabolism may be sufficiently disturbed to produce a rapidly progressive cataract requiring surgical removal.

The aqueous humour present in the anterior chamber is forced rapidly backwards through the pupil and drainage angle when the cornea is pushed backwards. This can cause damage to the angle and partial detachment of the ciliary body (Fig. 15.3b). This injury is often accompanied by an acute rise in intraocular pressure and predisposes to the development of glaucoma (Kaufman and Tolpin, 1974).

Posterior segment

Contrecoup injury causes retinal oedema (commotio retinae) or retinal haemorrhages [(Fig. 15.3 (1 and 2) and 15.4 (1 and 2)]. These changes are usually transient but the photoreceptors may be permanently functionally damaged, causing field defects or reduction in vision. The most serious form of this injury is macular oedema which may result in the development of a cyst with subsequent macular hole formation, causing a permanent reduction in central vision.

Expanding forces

The expanding forces damage a variety of structures inside the eye; in the most severe cases the sclera itself ruptures. When this occurs, it usually does so at one of the weaker areas – at the corneoscleral limbus, under one of the extraocular muscle insertions or around the insertion of the optic nerve.

As the eye expands equatorially, circumferential intraocular structures (iris, lens, ciliary body

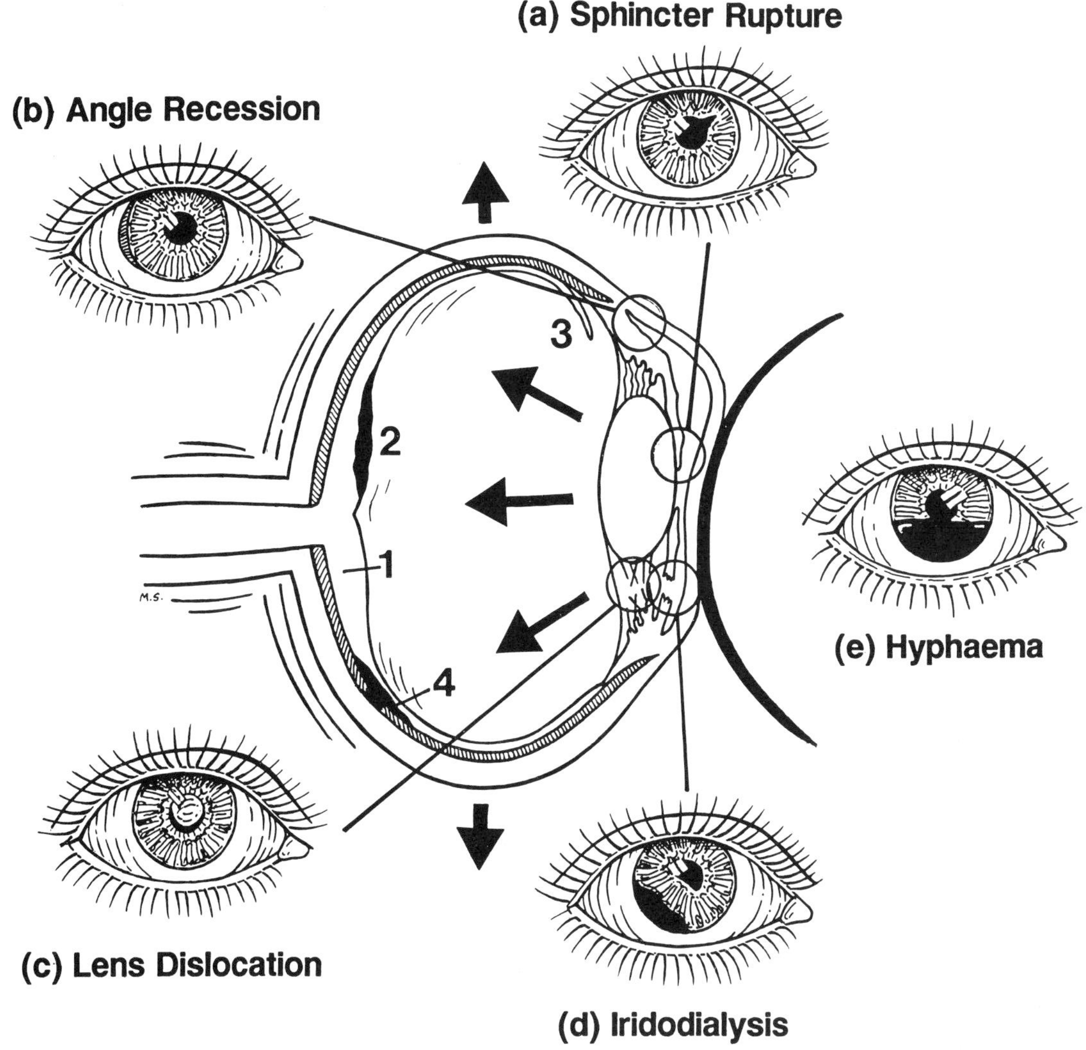

Fig. 15.3 The effect of blunt truama on the globe. The eye becomes flattened in its anteroposterior diameter and expands equatorially. This produces tearing and contusional damage within the eye. Inserts demonstrate more clearly the effects at various locations in the eye. 1=Retinal oedema; 2=retinal haemorrhage; 3=retinal dialysis; 4=choroidal rupture with haemorrhage.

and vitreous) are rapidly stretched and may become disinserted from their origins. Damage to the zonules which support the lens results in subluxation or dislocation of the lens. The lens may partially or totally disinsert from its zonular attachments (Fig. 15.3c), become unstable and in some circumstances completely dislocate either forwards into the anterior chamber or backwards into the vitreous cavity. The fragile periphery of the iris tends to tear or become disinserted at the iris root, causing an iridodialysis (Fig. 15.3d). In the acute phase the vascular iris bleeds into the anterior chamber and the resultant hyphaema prevents a detailed examination of the extent of the anterior segment damage.

Hyphaema

Bleeding into the anterior chamber or hyphaema (Fig. 15.3e) is usually the result of damage to the highly vascular iris or ciliary body. Its presence

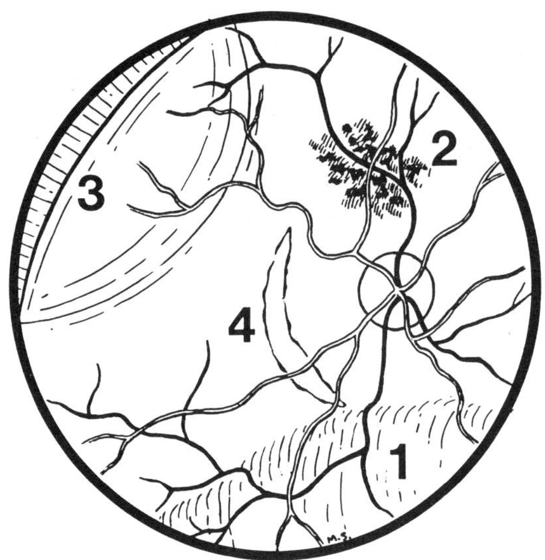

Fig. 15.4 Blunt trauma affects the posterior segment, as seen with an ophthalmoscope. 1=Peripheral retinal oedema; 2=retinal haemorrhage; 3=retinal dialysis with associated retinal detachment; 4=choroidal rupture.

indicates that a significant contusional injury has taken place and that a thorough examination of the eye is necessary to look for treatable effects of blunt trauma and the source of the bleeding. The blood generally reabsorbs over the next 4–5 days. The main concern is that a more substantial, secondary haemorrhage develops. This occurs in approximately 25% of those affected with large hyphaema (Read and Goldberg, 1974) and causes a significant and rapid elevation in the intraocular pressure such that the optic nerve function is threatened and the final visual outcome is poorer.

Posterior segment

The vitreous gel is densely adherent to the retina at the vitreous base and therefore as the vitreous expands equatorially, the retina tends to tear in this peripheral area [Figs 15.3(3) and 15.4(3)]. This is often complicated by the development of vitreous haemorrhage and retinal hole or dialysis formation. Untreated, this will lead to retinal detachment.

The vascular choroid, unlike the more elastic retina and sclera, ruptures easily when stretched. This choroidal rupture causes subretinal haemorrhage and the ultimate development of a pale atrophic scar. The commonest site for such ruptures is, unfortunately, at the posterior pole directly under the macular region and results in a characteristic crescent-shaped scar with significant reduction in visual acuity [Figs 15.3(4) and 15.4(4)].

Optic nerve

Optic atrophy may follow any significant blunt injury. This can be due to a number of different mechanisms: firstly, from compression or interruption of the blood supply to the nerve; secondly, from complete or partial mechanical avulsion of the nerve from its insertion to the globe; thirdly, because of increased intraocular pressure and lastly, secondary to extensive retinal damage.

Localized blunt trauma

There is a specific type of blunt injury which is caused by high-velocity particles (usually airgun pellets) hitting the eye and skidding alongside the eyeball and passing onwards into the orbit. These objects do not have sufficient momentum to enter the eye itself but cause significant intraocular disruption because of the intense force at a localized point on the scleral surface. Vitreous haemorrhage, retinal detachment, macular scarring and serious disruption of the intraocular contents all occur, with resultant poor visual acuity.

Large sharp objects

Large objects such as children's fingers, pieces of paper or twigs commonly scratch the ocular surface and the injuries caused are frequent sources of corneal abrasions and conjunctival lacerations. Together these account for more than 25% of all acute eye injuries attending Accident and Emergency departments.

Injuries which penetrate the ocular surface are much rarer. A large proportion of these, unfortunately, affect children, who are often struck by or fall on to potentially penetrating objects such as pens or toys.

RTAs were previously the cause of many bilateral penetrations but are now infrequent. In the adult age group assaults are responsible for nearly all penetrating injuries seen now.

Superficial damage

Large sharp objects which hit the eye at low velocity usually cause superficial conjunctival lacerations or corneal abrasions.

Intraocular damage

Objects travelling at higher speed cause corneal perforations. Small ones are usually self-sealing, especially if they are oblique, but larger lacerations tend to leak aqueous with subsequent flattening of the anterior chamber. The iris becomes incarcerated in the wound with a resultant irregular, peaked pupil (Fig. 15.5). This plugging of the wound may prevent complete loss of the anterior chamber contents, although larger lacerations cannot spontaneously close. Deeper penetrations involve the iris, lens and anterior vitreous cavity (Fig. 15.6). Penetration of the lens capsule inevitably results in cataract formation which is often associated with intense intraocular inflammation secondary to the leakage of lens proteins.

Reflex protective lid closure usually ensures that the lids are struck before the eye. They may dissipate some of the force, but do not prevent ocular involvement. Objects travelling at high speed lacerate the lid and often also penetrate the globe. Penetrations through the upper or lower lid which pass directly through sclera cause a combination of anterior and posterior structure damage which is not always obvious as the penetration may be concealed due to its posterior location (Fig. 15.6). The intraocular contents may prolapse through such wounds with loss of the lens, uveal tissue, vitreous and retina. Intraocular haemorrhage is almost inevitable with blood from the damaged choroid and ciliary body. This mixture of blood, vitreous and lens material causes organization and scarring within the eye which can prevent the restoration of any useful vision.

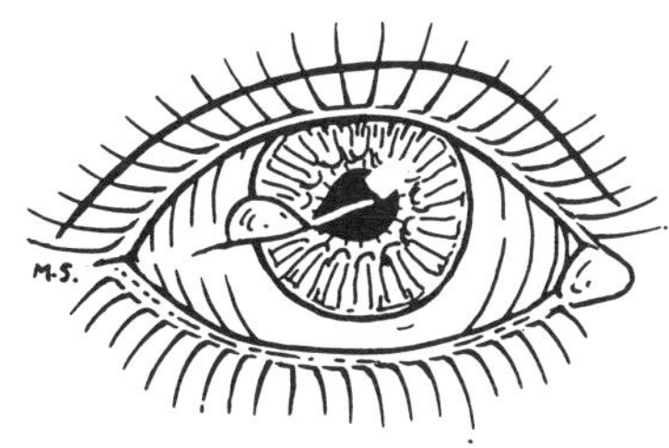

Fig. 15.5 A small corneal laceration. A knuckle of iris is prolapsing through the wound, causing an irregular pupil.

Small foreign bodies

Patients with corneal and subtarsal foreign bodies represent more than 50% of the cases with acute ocular trauma presenting to casualty departments. This type of injury usually occurs when working in a dusty atmosphere or under a car.

Intraocular foreign bodies (IOFBs) are more unusual, although they used to be a common industrial injury. The heads of hammers tend to become brittle with use and small pieces fly off during hammering. These small fragments are characteristically sharp and easily able to penetrate the eye. This used to be a frequent industrial injury but is now more common in people carrying out do-it-yourself work at home. Small pieces of shattered spectacle glass can become embedded in the cornea or enter the eye when glasses are broken, especially during sport.

Superficial damage

Small pieces of dust or debris being blown or falling on to the surface of the eye cause the majority of superficial eye injuries. These small objects can become attached to the back of the upper lid (subtarsal foreign bodies) and rub up and down over the cornea as the eye opens and closes, causing a painful corneal abrasion. As the cornea is richly innervated this superficial injury is extremely painful.

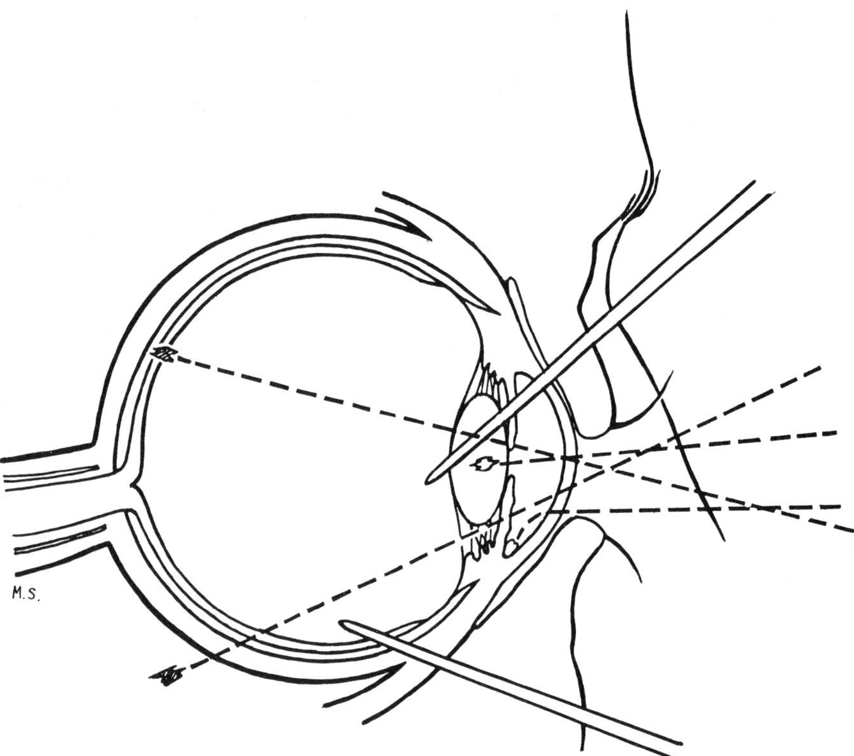

Fig. 15.6 The outcome of penetrating trauma depends on the extent of penetration, the tissue affected and the type of material that penetrates.

Intraocular foreign bodies

If the object is travelling fast enough and is reasonably sharp it may enter the eye to become an IOFB. The smaller and slower-moving objects will decelerate into the anterior chamber and remain there, and are sometimes easily seen attached to the iris. Most, however, are not visible with the naked eye and others drop downwards, under the influence of gravity, into the drainage angle of the anterior chamber and therefore out of direct view (Fig. 15.6).

Faster-moving objects pass into the lens and whilst some remain there many pass on into the posterior segment. Once in the vitreous they may remain there or settle on the retina with an associated localized haemorrhage or hole formation. Through-and-through injuries, in which an object passes directly through the eye, are rare. They carry a very poor prognosis, because they set up associated destructive shock waves.

The potential damaging effects of the foreign body depend on its composition. Non-toxic, inert, sterile materials such as glass or plastic are well-tolerated if they do not produce much structural damage on their pathway through the eye. They cause minimal long-term effects if they are not recognized, and often become encapsulated in fibrous tissue if left alone. The commonest materials to enter the eye, however, are metals and they oxidize to cause inflamation and metallosis. Copper is particularly toxic, causing a severe inflammatory response and frequently loss of the eye if the particle is not promptly removed. Iron-containing foreign bodies are common and the deposition of ferric ions results in siderosis. The symptoms of this chronic condition are night blindness, constriction of visual fields and eventual blindness.

Organic or vegetable materials are usually involved as part of a more extensive injury and cause rapid suppuration. Once the surface of the eye has been breached the danger of intraocular infection increases. Established endophthalmitis, even with very low-grade pathogens, carries a very poor prognosis for any visual recovery.

Chemical burns

Chemical burns are amongst the most urgent emergencies in ophthalmological practice, and the rapidity with which treatment is initiated considerably affects the prognosis. Chemical burns may occur in industrial or agricultural accidents, strong acids and alkalis being necessary in the manufacture of other compounds and for industrial cleaning. Multiple household agents – ammonia, disinfectants, detergents and bleaches – are also capable of causing significant burns. Acid burns from explosions of car batteries are increasing in frequency.

In sports, chemical burns can occur from chlorine in swimming pools or lime burns from the line markings on football and rugby pitches.

Burns caused by acids and alkalis are potentially very serious. In general, alkalis are more damaging than acids. Strong alkalis damage cell membranes and therefore rapidly penetrate tissues. Acids on the other hand coagulate structural proteins and therefore tend to limit their own spread, making the injury less extensive.

Superficial damage

The lids are commonly the only tissues damaged as the rapidity of the blink reflex effectively prevents any ocular contact. The lids may suffer a superficial burn but more extensive damage with stronger chemicals leads to permanent scarring which may prevent adequate closure and therefore exposure of the globe.

If the lids do not close rapidly enough the lower conjunctiva or cornea is most likely to be burned, as the eye rolls upwards under the upper lid in response to attack (Bell's phenomenon), leaving these areas most vulnerable. The weaker acids and alkalis cause epithelial loss only with surrounding hyperaemia.

Deeper damage

More extensive burns penetrate the collagen and structural proteins of the cornea and sclera. They are evident as haziness of an otherwise clear cornea and scleral vascular damage. The resultant scleral ischaemia gives the eye a white non-inflamed appearance which on closer inspection is seen to be due to complete destruction of the vascular elements. This results in secondary necrosis and destruction of the outer layers of the eye. The most severe burns are less painful than the superficial ones because of complete corneal anaesthesia. The conjunctival epithelium and glandular structures are irreversibly destroyed, leading to an abnormal ocular surface and tear film which ultimately may be the limiting factor in reconstruction of badly burned eyes.

If the anterior chamber is entered then shrinkage and scarring of intraocular tissues take place with increased intraocular pressure which is resistant to treatment and secondary cataract formation.

Physical burns

Ocular thermal damage is usually associated with more extensive head and neck burns, often due to house fires or explosions. Loss of lashes and brows is most frequent with surrunding hyperaemia of the skin and lids. Small particles of molten metal which strike the cornea can cause localized deep burns with resultant stromal scarring, but otherwise the eye is rarely involved.

Various elements of the electromagnetic spectrum are absorbed by the different structures of the eye. Ultraviolet radiation is absorbed by the DNA of the cornea, preventing normal epithelial turnover. This causes superficial corneal damage 4–6 hours after exposure. Flash burns in welders are a very common presentation of this type of injury, and burns of sunray lamp users are becoming more frequent. Snow blindness, seen in skiers and climbers, is also due to corneal ultraviolet toxicity. A more serious effect is solar retinopathy when the development of macular burns threatens vision.

Chronic exposure to the infrared end of the spectrum has been recognized as causing cataracts in the form of exfoliation of the lens capsule. These became known as glass-blower's cataracts as this occupation was subjected to this type of radiation. Microwaves have similarly been implicated in the development of early lens opacities, but modern microwave ovens now have strict shielding regulations.

Iatrogenic radiation damage from the treatment of head and neck cancer is becoming less frequent with the availability of adequate screening techniques. Cataract and radiation retinopathy however are recognized complications several years after the completion of treatment.

Lasers have a therapeutic role in the management of a variety of ocular diseases but accidental damage, both in industry and medical practice, has been reported.

Examination and management

Prompt assessment and early treatment of eye injuries are of the utmost importance as these prevent or minimize further damage.

Examination

Immediate/touchline assessment

Injuries tend to occur in situations which are far from ideal, making detailed examination of the eye at the sight of the injury virtually impossible. In these adverse circumstances, the role of the attending doctor without any specialized equipment is simply to exclude or confirm serious eye injury and to transfer the patient to the local hospital as safely and as soon as possible.

An evaluation should always be carried out bearing in mind the nature (blunt, sharp, etc.) of the injury. A good light should be used, if possible. It may be difficult to open the eyelids because of periorbital swelling and bruising, but an attempt should be made to ease them apart gently. If this is not possible pressure should not be exerted as an underlying ocular rupture may be present. An initial assessment of visual acuity is important and this can be performed by firstly asking the patient if he or she is aware of any subjective change in vision. The ability to count fingers or to identify facial details should then be tested for in each eye separately.

It is very important to identify the source of any bleeding to determine whether it is coming from the eye itself or, less seriously, from the periorbital tissues. Foreign material on the cornea may be visible, but no attempt should be made to remove it in case of causing a further damage. The depth of the anterior chamber should be compared to that on the other side and the presence of any blood within the chamber noted. An evaluation of the pupillary size, shape and reactions is also important.

Suspicious findings indicating the need for further examination include severe pain; poor visual acuity, especially if the patient indicates a subjective reduction in vision; conjunctival swelling; irregular pupil; afferent pupillary defect; blood in the anterior chamber, and hazy view of iris and pupil. All chemical burns should be washed out without delay and suspected perforations or IOFBs should be referred immediately to the nearest hospital. If a rupture or penetration is suspected a pad should be gently applied to the eye before transfer.

The most important consideration however for the doctor on the touchline, concerned with the initial management of a patient with an eye injury, is that if there is any doubt at all about the extent or severity of the injury urgent hospital referral is indicated.

Casualty assessment

A more detailed examination should be possible in the Accident and Emergency department with the assistance of brighter lighting, better equipment and the availability of local anaesthetic, fluorescein and cycloplegic drops.

Superficial injuries such as corneal abrasions and lid lacerations can be treated within the Casualty department and the patient allowed home with appropriate advice and recommendations for follow-up.

History
Clear details of the nature of the injury must be determined in order that an appropriate examination may be performed. The exact circumstances at the time of the incident and the nature of the object causing the injury should be described in detail. The type of eye protection in use at the time should also be ascertained as this can alter the effects of an injury. If an IOFB is suspected from the history then X-ray examination is mandatory, e.g. if a patient has been using a hammer or drilling, an IOFB must be assumed to be present until proved otherwise. If the injury was the result of a chemical burn it is essential to determine the agent which caused the burn, although seeking this information should not delay irrigation of the eye; this should be carried out immediately.

Examination
Examination of the eye should be carried out using the best source of illumination possible. Both eyes should be examined in a systematic manner, firstly by evaluating visual function and then by examining the eyes themselves. Visual function is determined by assessing the visual acuity, visual fields and extraocular movements. Acuity should be measured using a standard Snellen chart with the patient wearing spectacles if required. If the patient's glasses were broken at the time of the injury, a pinhole will provide a good estimation of the corrected vision. If no charts are available a gross assessment of visual acuity can be measured by testing the ability to count fingers or read newsprint. Visual fields are best tested by the confrontation method. The full range of horizontal and vertical eye movements is observed while asking the patient if double vision is experienced in any direction of gaze.

Examination of the eyes and surrounding tissue takes place in a logical sequence by examining from the front to the back. The lids, orbital margins and facial bones are inspected and palpated for fractures followed by assessment of the eye itself. The cornea should be examined for abrasions or foreign bodies. Instillation of topical anaesthesia may assist examination by reducing the pain sufficiently to allow full opening of the eye. The depth of the anterior chamber should be assessed while noting the presence or absence of blood with the chamber. Direct and consensual pupillary responses are recorded in addition to noting whether the pupils are equal and of regular or irregular dimensions. All this can be carried out using direct illumination with no additional equipment, although magnification using the slit lamp provides more detail.

The fundi are examined with a direct ophthalmoscope, particular attention being paid to the clarity of the ocular media and any haemorrhages or oedema present in the retinal surface. Fundal examination should be attempted in all cases as soon as possible as intraocular haemorrhage or cataract formation may prevent an adequate view later. It is important to dilate the pupils in order to perform this examination properly; however, if significant head trauma is suspected or a hyphaema is present then this should be avoided. If there is any suspicion of penetration or rupture, such as extensive subconjunctival haemorrhage, conjunctival swelling, full-thickness lid lacerations or obvious intraocular haemorrhage in association with reduced vision, then examination under anaesthetic is mandatory.

In most cases a clinical assessment should be sufficient to determine the extent and severity of injury. However it is essential to remember the possibility of an IOFB which is not always readily visible. A plain X-ray is therefore required for all patients with suspected IOFBs.

Specialist assessment

If the patient has sustained a significant eye injury or there is any doubt about the severity of the injury he or she should be referred to an ophthalmologist.

There are several pieces of equipment which can and should be used to provide more information about the injured eye. The anterior segment should be fully examined using a slit lamp. This may demonstrate lesions such as small entry wounds or foreign bodies, uveitis, corneal swelling or haziness which are not visible by the naked eye. Indirect ophthalmoscopy provides a good overall view of the fundus, enabling search for foreign bodies or retinal tears. A tonometer allows accurate measurement of intraocular pressure, which is essential for treatment. Specialized lenses for the examination of the drainage angle and the fundus are also available.

Even with all this equipment it is not possible in some cases to make a complete assessment of an injured eye. In this event, it is necessary to carry out an examination of the eye under general anaesthetic, including an exploration of the subconjunctival space for scleral perforations. General anaesthesia may also be required for unco-operative patients, whether due to excess alcohol or very young age.

Computed tomography scanning and magnetic resonance imaging are useful for the identification and localization of IOFBs. Ultrasonography should be carried out in cases of vitreous haemorrhage which persist and indeed may be the only method of adequately assessing the posterior segment.

Presentation and management

Blunt injuries

Periorbital

Periorbital bruising is very common and usually settles spontaneously within days or weeks and requires simple lid-cleansing to prevent build-up of conjunctival secretions. If the bruising is severe, adequate assessment of the eye may be difficult because swelling of the lids prevents opening. Bruising may be associated with bursting injuries of the lid skin, these require careful exploration and suturing.

Blow-out fracture

Severe periorbital bruising associated with diplopia, enophthalmos and infraorbital anaesthesia is pathognomonic of a blow-out fracture. In the early period this may not be evident because of eye closure due to excessive bruising. As this settles clinical features suggestive of the blow-out become obvious. Indications for surgical intervention to elevate the fracture are; diplopia in the primary position, significant enophthalmos or persistent infraorbital anaesthesia 10–14 days after the injury. Most cases do not require surgery.

Superficial damage

The conjunctiva needs careful examination in all injured eyes as it may conceal a more serious underlying rupture of the globe. Any significant swelling or haemorrhage associated with poor vision requires further investigation. Subconjunctival heamorrhage is easily recognized and is often associated with periorbital bruising. This spontaneously disappears within days to weeks. Corneal abrasions may not be obvious until stained with fluorescein, which highlights the epithelial loss. These should be treated with topical broad-spectrum antibiotic ointment, a cycloplegic drop and a firm pad and bandage for 24 hours. It is essential that the eye is closed under the pad and the patient should be given adequate analgesia.

Hyphaema

Severe blunt trauma is usually associated with hyphaema due to tearing of the anterior segment structures (Fig. 15.3e). A blood level may be obvious or diffuse red blood cells in the anterior chamber may simply obscure the details of the pupil and iris. The patient complains of reduced or blurred vision. The amount of pain usually depends upon the extent of the surrounding injury, but severe pain suggests an associated rise in intraocular pressure. This may be accompanied by nausea and, if so, antiemetics should be given in addition to analgesia. The prognosis of an uncomplicated hyphaema is good (the majority absorb spontaneously in 2–6 days) and is mainly dependent on the amount of associated blunt damage to the intraocular structures at the time of injury.

The development of a secondary haemorrhage is the main concern in patients with hyphaema. This usually occurs between 2 and 5 days after the injury. The size of hyphaema does not influence the rate of secondary haemorrhage. The re-bleed is more substantial than the primary hyphaema and this is associated with increased intraocular pressure. This can cause optic nerve damage and corneal blood staining. The management of hyphaema is therefore aimed at reducing the incidence of secondary bleeding. The best way to achieve this remains controversial and the most appropriate management requires clarification. Mydriatics, antibotics, steroids, bed rest and occlusive padding may all have a role in the prevention of secondary bleeds. Oral antifibrinolytics are also now being used more widely in this regard (McGetrick *et al.*, 1983). If a secondary hyphaema does occur, treatment is directed at medical reduction of increased intraocular pressure, although in some cases surgical removal of the clot is required.

Once the blood has cleared a good view of the intraocular structures can be obtained under magnification and it is usually possible to determine the source of the bleeding. A small tear at the pupil margin is common and the pupil may be traumatically enlarged or irregular and relatively immobile due to iris sphincter damage. These injuries are of no prognostic significance and require no treatment. Of more importance are injuries such as disinsertion of the iris from its root (iridodialysis; Fig. 15.3d), which may require surgical repair. The drainage angle should always be examined with a gonioscopy lens to determine the presence and degree of angle recession. The risk of subsequent glaucoma is higher in those with extensive angle damage and they require regular review for early detection and treatment of the condition (Kaufman and Tolpin, 1974). In all cases of hyphaema therefore it is essential to examine the eye in detail to determine the cause of the bleed so that prophylactic measures can be undertaken, if necessary.

Lens

Rapidly progressive lens opacities require surgical removal of the cataract to allow a clear view of the posterior pole and to prevent the complications of hypermaturity. Lens subluxation requires observation to ensure that if the lens dislocates it moves backwards into the vitreous cavity and does not fall forwards to lie in the anterior chamber, which may lead to corneal decompensation and raised intraocular pressure. If this occurs then removal of the lens is required, but otherwise a subluxated or dislocated lens should be left untreated.

Posterior damage

Although the posterior segment should be fully examined in all cases of blunt trauma, it may be necessary to postpone this for some days after the initial injury because full dilation of the pupil may precipitate further haemorrhage from an iris sphincter tear.

Retinal oedema [Figs. 15.3(1) and 15.4(1)] is evident as a greyish-white sheen from the retina which may be associated with superficial retinal haemorrhages [Figs. 15.3(2) and 15.4(2)]. This settles without treatment but may precipitate the development of a macular hole at the posterior pole with associated reduction in vision and also pigmentary scarring. Unfortunately, no treatment is of any benefit.

It is important to look closely for a peripheral retinal dialysis [Figs. 15.3(3) and 15.4(3)] as this will progress to retinal detachment if left untreated. The presence of an intravitreal haemorrhage overlying the vitreous base should alert one to a retinal dialysis. Careful examination using an indirect ophthalmoscope with indentation of the eye to allow a good view of the anterior retina is required. If a dialysis is found it must be treated with cryotherapy or laser to promote an adhesive scar between the retina and the choroid to prevent the development of retinal detachment.

Choroidal ruptures (Figs. 15.3(4) and 15.4(4)] are recognized by subretinal blood, usually at the posterior pole, with associated reduction in vision. In time these form a scar. No treatment is of any benefit and a central blind spot remains.

Ruptures

Rupture of the globe should always be suspected in patients who have had significant blunt injuries. These are usually recognized by poor visual acuity associated with conjunctival haemorrhage or swelling and intraocular bleeding preventing a clear view of the posterior pole. In addition the intraocular pressure is usually reduced. Management consists of a full examination of the sclera under general anaesthetic. The rupture is likely to take place at the corneoscleral limbus and may radiate backwards to the equatorial region, or under the insertion of one of the rectus muscles. Any prolapsed ocular contents should be excised and the scleral wound closed using interrupted non-absorbable nylon sutures. The prognosis for such severely damaged eyes is poor. If there is no prospect of any visual recovery in a cosmetically damaged eye then enucleation should be considered.

Penetrating injuries

Lids

Lid lacerations, as with any facial wounds, require careful closure for good cosmetic results. If the lid margin is involved, this requires particular attention as accurate alignment of the edges is of the utmost importance to prevent an irregular notch with associated functional and cosmetic implications. Treatment may be carried out in Casualty, with the following instructions (Fig. 15.8):

1. The grey line must be opposed first (with a non-absorbable suture), as the accurate placement of this will prevent malalignment of the lid margin.
2. The anterior lid margin is sutured.
3. Deep bites of catgut are used to close the tarsal plate.
4. The skin is closed with a non-absorbable suture.

Full-thickness lid lacerations should be regarded as potential globe lacerations until proved otherwise. Any laceration at the medial

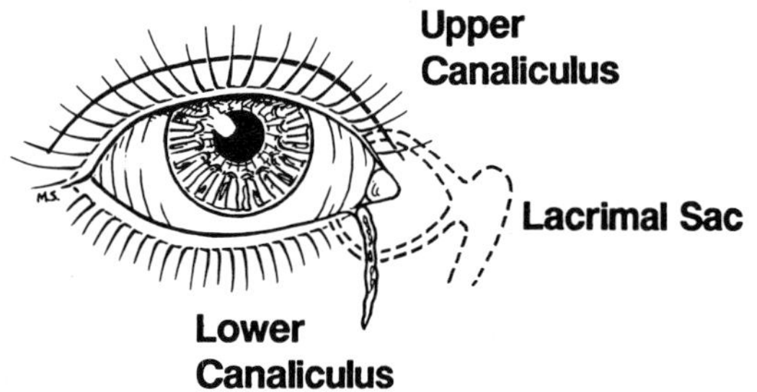

Fig. 15.7 The canalicular apparatus is frequently damaged in lacerations at the medial canthal region.

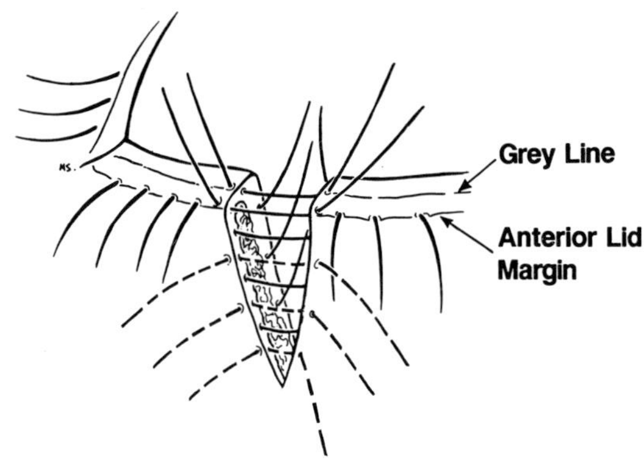

Fig. 15.8 Lacerations of the lid require careful suturing. The grey line must be opposed accurately and the lid is closed in layers to prevent notching of the lid margin.

aspect of the lid may involve the lacrimal drainage apparatus (Fig. 15.7). This requires specialist attention as reconstruction of the canalicular anatomy may be required to prevent persistent watering and intubation of the system is often necessary.

Superficial damage

Conjunctival lacerations are usually self-closing but may require exploration to ensure that there is no underlying perforation of the sclera. If the injury is extensive it may require cleansing, debridement and suture. Topical antibiotic treatment should be instilled to prevent secondary infection.

Corneal abrasions are very common. The patient presents with a painful, photophobic red eye and complains of watering and difficulty in opening the eye. This is extremely painful and may make ocular examination difficult due to blepharospasm. Local anaesthetic drops will assist in the assessment of patients with corneal abrasions as this will allow them to open their eyes for examination. Staining and fluorescein drops clearly indicates an area of bare epithelium. However topical anaesthesia should not be used as a method of analgesia as this inhibits epithelial healing. The best management is to keep the eye firmly closed with a pad and bandage, to relieve any discomfort. Any loose epithelial tags should be removed under magnification and instillation of antibiotic ointment and cycloplegic drops relieve ciliary spasm for patient comfort. These abrasions usually heal within 24–48 hours, although incomplete or abnormal bonding between the epithelium and the underlying basement membrane may result in recurrent corneal erosions. These are recognized by repeated symptoms of corneal abrasion with no history of further trauma.

Ocular penetration

Small oblique corneal lacerations may pass unnoticed as they are self-sealing and the anterior chamber depth is maintained. However larger lacerations are usually recognized by incarceration of iris within the wound, causing an irregularly shaped pupil and also a flat anterior chamber. Any prolapsed tissue should be removed, or replaced if still considered viable. Loss of the lens and vitreous can occur through larger wounds. Closure of the wound should take place with the operating microscope using a monofilament suture, burying the knots to prevent irritation and subsequent vascularization of the cornea.

Penetrating injuries which involve the anterior capsule of the lens will require early surgical removal of the lens. Those which involve the posterior segment should be treated in the same manner as bursting injuries. Examination determines the extent of the injury and any prolapsing tissue should be removed. Accurate repair using the operating microscope is essential. The sclera should be closed with a non-absorbable suture to prevent secondary inflammation. The aim of surgery is to restore the ocular anatomy while removing any disorganized tissue. Lacerations involving both the anterior and posterior segments carry the worst prognosis. A combination of vitreous blood and soft lens matter causes significant scarring and the majority recover no useful vision.

Sympathetic ophthalmitis

Sympathetic ophthalmitis is a bilateral granulomatous inflammation affecting both eyes in response to a rupture or penetrating injury of one eye. The condition is thought to be an autoimmune response to a previously hidden soluble retinal antigen which becomes exposed at the time of the injury. The injured eye is known as the 'exciting' eye and the other eye is the 'sympathising' eye. The incidence after injury is fortunately very low (Allen, 1969), but the effects can be so devastating that it must always be considered as a possibility when dealing with a patient who has a severely damaged eye. Removal of the injured, potentially exciting eye prevents the development of sympathetic ophthalmitis, but once established the conditions progresses independently in each eye. There is therefore no point in removing the exciting eye after the sympathetic response has begun. In fact, the uninjured, sympathising eye may well end up as the poorer eye due to the severe inflammation. Since sympathetic ophthalmitis does not occur within the first 7–10 days of injury there is always time available to evaluate the prognosis of the injured eye after the primary repair has been performed. Enucleation should, therefore, never be carried out as an initial procedure.

Sympathetic ophthalmitis can occur any time after a penetrating injury, but most commonly within the first 2 months. The more severe the injury, the higher the chances of developing sympathetic. However, more important factors include delay in presentation and poor medical or surgical management. Rapid microsurgical repair with neat apposition of the wound edges and removal of any devitalized prolapsed tissues has reduced the incidence of this previously more frequent complication. The appropriate use of antibiotics and steroids has also helped enormously. This once inevitably blinding condition became treatable with the development of steroids and cytotoxic agents. Once established, the condition follows a relapsing course and exacerbations must be treated vigorously with topical and systemic steroids.

A severely injured eye should only be enucleated for pain and/or poor cosmesis when it has no potential for any useful vision. The threat of sympathetic ophthalmitis should not, on its own, be an indication for enucleation and the possible value of a retained eye must be weighed against the very low risks of developing sympathetic.

Small foreign bodies

Superficial foreign bodies

Patients with small corneal or subtarsal foreign bodies present with a painful, watering, photophobic eye. The particle sitting on the corneal surface can be more easily visualized using fluorescein staining. Vertical linear staining of the superior cornea suggests an underlying subtarsal foreign body which can only be visualized after everting the upper lid with a cotton bud. After instillation of topical anaesthesia the foreign body can be removed using a hypodermic needle or a cotton bud. This usually produces a rapid resolution of symptoms. Topical antibiotic ointment should be instilled and a pad applied for 24 hours to promote epithelial healing and protect the anaesthetized cornea.

The prognosis is excellent as long as the injury is superficial and secondary infection does not cause a corneal ulcer.

Intraocular foreign bodies

The presentation of patients with IOFBs varies from minimal external signs to more obvious intraocular disruption. All have a history of being involved in an incident in which a rapidly moving small particle has struck the eye.

Examination should be directed towards finding the entry wound. This is often small and only detectable under magnification. If the entry wound is not readily seen the foreign body itself may be visible in the anterior chamber. However the intraocular material is often sitting hidden in the drainage angle or embedded in the lens, ciliary body or retina. Careful examination may reveal the IOFB but X-ray examination should be carried out to determine the exact nature and site of the object. In this respect the nature of the foreign body is very important as glass or vegetable matter is usually radiolucent. Computed tomography scanning is essential to localize the material accurately prior to surgical removal, although magnetic resonance imaging should be avoided in those with metal IOFBs.

Foreign bodies present within the anterior segment can be removed directly, either with forceps or using a magnet. The lens should be removed if it has been ruptured or in combination with any foreign body which has remained inside it. Foreign bodies within the posterior segment should be removed during the course of a vitrectomy. If the facilities for this procedure are not available, magnetic material may be removed using a magnet and any secondary repairs carried out at a later date. It is essential that the location is accurately determined before this is carried out as movement of a magnetic foreign body may cause further intraocular damage.

The prognosis depends on the nature of the foreign body, the site of impaction and extent of damage to other intraocular structures.

Chemical burns

Rapid irrigation of any eye which has suffered a chemical burn may make the difference between retention or loss of any useful vision. Copious amounts of water or saline should be used to irrigate the conjunctival sac and any lumps of particulate material should be removed with forceps. Irrigation should ideally take place until litmus paper shows neutral; however this may not be possible and 30 min should be sufficient.

Superficial burns

Both acid and alkali can produce superficial burns to the skin of the lids and loss of corneal and conjunctival epithelium, most readily evident by staining with fluorescein. The skin is best left dry and topical antibiotic ointment should be applied to areas of corneal and conjunctival loss.

Deeper burns

The presence of limbal ischaemia or corneal clouding indicates very severe burns with the likelihood of corneal and scleral melting and subsequent perforation of the globe. Such patients need hospital admission and may require treatment for raised intraocular pressure as well as topical antibiotics to prevent secondary infection and cycloplegics for patient comfort. Ascorbic acid reduces further damage by its free radical scavenging activity and topical steroids limit further inflammation in the immediate post-injury period. In the following weeks the ocular surface may fail to re-epithelialize, with resultant repeated ulceration which may even proceed to perforation.

The long-term results are often disappointing because of generalized collagen shrinkage and scleral scarring. The loss of conjuctival epithelial glandular elements results in a poorly functioning surface mucous membrane which allows drying of the ocular surface. In addition the lid cover may be inadequate because of scarring and the lid may become adherent to the surface of the eye.

Physical burns

Superficial damage

Rapid reflex lid closure often limits thermal burns to the lashes, brows and eyelids. Small pieces of molten metal which come into contact with the cornea are more likely to cause injuries that result in permanent stromal scarring. These should be removed as soon as possible and topical antibiotics applied to prevent any infection and subsequent corneal ulceration. The area of corneal scarring is usually small and does not interfere with vision.

Ultraviolet radiation damages the corneal and conjunctival epithelium. Pain, watering and hazy vision usually begin 4–6 hours following exposure. This is usually seen in welders (flash burns), sunbed users or skiers. The cornea may appear slightly hazy to the naked eye and fluorescein drops demonstrate superficial punctate staining. Often the patients cannot open their eyes for examination because of the pain. Treatment consists of topical antibiotic ointment for lubrication and comfort in addition to cycloplegic drops and a firm pad and bandage. Systemic analgesia may also be required.

The role of advanced medical and surgical treatment

The introduction of microsurgery and vitrectomy was a major advance in the treatment of eye injuries and these were paralleled by pharmacological innovations such as the introduction of steroids and antibiotics. The operating microscope was first used in ophthalmology in the 1960s and in combination with the development of refined microsurgical instruments, delicate needles and non-reactive suture materials, greatly improved the prognosis for eye injuries. Magnification using binocular viewing allows better alignment of lacerations, clean removal of prolapsed and devitalized tissues or foreign material and accurate reformation of the damaged globe. This improved surgical approach has reduced all complications of ocular trauma including sympathetic, intraocular scarring, endophthalmitis and retinal detachment. It also ensures better management of the complications that do arise such as corneal scarring, cataract and glaucoma.

Further advances in surgery were introduced in 1970 when closed vitrectomy was developed by Machemer (1971). This microsurgical technique employs the introduction of three identical 20-gauge instruments through the pars plana of the ciliary body (Fig. 15.9). They consist of an infusion line, a cutting/suction instrument and an intraocular light pipe. In addition similar-gauge forceps, scissors and magnets may be introduced to the eye instead of the cutting device, maintaining a closed chamber to cut and remove large foreign objects. The vitreous is removed in association with any haemorrhage or organized scar tissue, while maintaining a formed globe. This allows clear visualization of the retina so that retinal holes or tears can be identified and treated. IOFBs are removed in this way and in addition the damaged lens can be broken up and aspirated through these small surgical wounds. The vitreous is replaced by isoto-

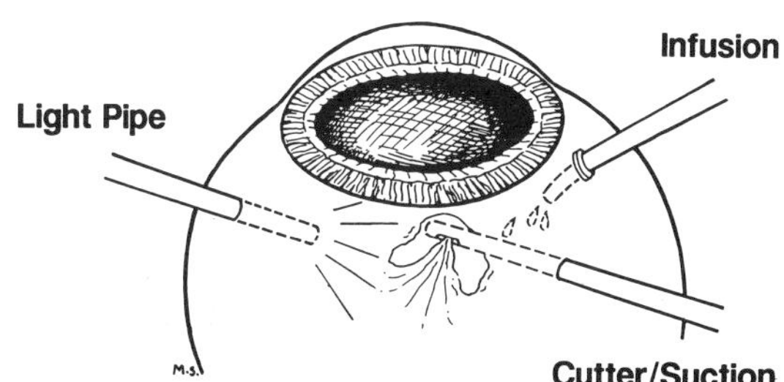

Fig. 15.9 Vitrectomy is performed via the pars plana of the ciliary body, using three common-gauge instruments to remove vitreous and/or foreign material, with endoillumination and an infusion line.

nic saline; however, in some cases of complex retinal detachment this may be replaced by gases or silicone oil to improve chorioretinal adhesions.

Adequate, non-toxic levels of intraocular antibiotics have reduced the incidence of and improved the prognosis for cases of post-traumatic endophthalmitis.

The post-traumatic inflammatory and reparative responses are responsible for scarring, opacification of the media and ultimate visual loss. Topical and systemic steroids have successfully reduced these and improved the ocular morbidity.

Rehabilitation

The time taken to recover from serious eye injury and the completeness of that recovery are extremely variable. Rehabilitation and return to normal activities are dependent on the type and severity of injury sustained and the degree of visual loss. It is helpful to consider the patients in one of the following groups:

1. No significant visual loss in either eye.
2. Reduction of visual acuity in one eye only or partial visual field loss.
3. Significant loss of acuity or field in both eyes.

No significant visual loss in either eye

In this group of patients the major determinant of their future management is the type and extent of injury. For example, corneal abrasions simply require first aid and patients can return to their usual lifestyle as soon as their symptoms allow. Similarly, patients with blunt injuries who have developed hyphaema, but minimal structural damage, usually recover fully with little effect on visual function (assuming that retinal tears, detachments or significant angle damage have been excluded). They can return to normal activities approximately 2 weeks after the incident. In contrast, a penetrating wound probably leaves an area of permanent weakness in the sclera or cornea (caused either by the injury itself or by the surgical repair). No strenuous exercise or even bending over, which increases intraocular pressure, should be allowed for at least 6 weeks and the patient should be advised that the eye is permanently susceptible to further injury. Return to work or participation in any sporting activities should be disallowed during the early period, and the affected patient should always wear protective devices when participating in sport. Fortunately these injuries often serve as a stimulus for patients to wear the appropriate protective devices when carrying out future 'at-risk' activities. Retinal detachment repair *per se* need not preclude a return to normal activities as the surgically induced chorioretinal adhesions should be as strong as before the injury and no limitations are required.

Loss of visual acuity in one eye or partial field loss

Rehabilitation in this group of patients is not so dependent on the type of injury. Having lost vision in one eye they rely more on the remaining eye. For most purposes they should be able to see adequately and resume a completely normal life. However, they are faced with the problems associated with loss of binocular vision and subsequent loss of three-dimensional depth perception which lead to misjudgement of distances. This may make them more vulnerable to injury of the other eye, especially when playing ball games. The patient should be advised to be particularly protective of the affected side. As the patient is now effectively 'one-eyed', consideration must be given to the wisdom, or otherwise, of continuing participation in sports. If they do return to their sport they should always wear maximum eye protection and if glasses or contact lenses are required, these should be worn under a pair of polycarbonate goggles.

Significant loss or reduction of vision in both eyes

Most injuries are fortunately superficial and unilateral. However occasionally patients may lose the vision in their only useful eye or in both eyes due to injury. Bilateral injuries are usually due to penetrating trauma sustained as a result of assault of RTA. It is unusual to suffer a blunt injury which affects both eyes, although blunt head trauma may cause cerebral damage which results in bilateral visual field loss. In patients with bilateral ocular damage the aim of rehabilitation is to maximize any potential visual function by surgical techniques such as removal of vitreous haemorrhage or cataract, if this is possible. Unfortunately however, despite surgical intervention, the end-result may be that the patient is left with little visual function. In that event all rehabilitation is geared towards the best form of optical correction such as spectacles, contact lenses or magnifying aids and to maximize any vision present. Contact lenses have the advantage of providing a smooth anterior surface to the eye. They may take the form of cosmetic contact lenses which may effectively reduce pupil size for those with iris damage. If a patient is 'so blind as to be unable to perform any work for which eyesight is essential', then the patient should be registered as blind, with the resultant benefits of Social Department back-up. They may require retraining for employment. If the patient is a very keen sportsperson he or she should be encouraged to take part in the expanding group of enthusiasts involved in sports for the visually handicapped.

Prevention of eye injuries

The loss of visual function for whatever reason is always a tragedy. This is particularly so when it occurs as a result of trauma. It has been estimated that more than 90% of all eye injuries are preventable (NSPB). In some situations, for example in industry, the concept and practice of eye protection are well-established and it has been shown that the use of adequate and appropriate protection reduces the number and severity of injuries. However eye injuries are still extremely common during domestic and leisure-time activities and have major implications not only for the affected individual but in economic terms for the country as a whole. Prevention has therefore assumed great importance.

There are two main ways in which a strategy for prevention of eye injuries could be implemented: firstly by avoiding or modifying activities that are known to be associated with a particular risk of eye injury and secondly by using eye protection during these activities. For example, Canadian ice hockey has successfully combined both these methods of prevention by firstly introducing the high sticks law, in which it became illegal for players to raise the stick above shoulder height during play, and secondly by making the use of face masks compulsory at high-school-level matches. This has prevented an estimated 70 000 eye injuries (see Chapter 21) (Parver, 1986).

Protection at work

The most recent protective legislation in the workplace is the Health and Safety at Work Act 1974. This holds employers, employees, designers and manufacturers responsible for safety at work. It defines the processes for which protection is required and indicates the best methods for achieving this. Different tasks demand different levels of protection, from standard spectacles with toughened polycarbonate lenses which provide minimal protection to more enclosed goggles or visors which are needed for hammering, grinding or protection against chemical injuries. The British Standard 2092 polycarbonate protector provides 'general purpose protection' but is not intended for specific tasks such as working with chemicals or molten metal for which special grades are available.

In order for this form of legislation to be effective there must be rigorous checks on its implementation. Factory inspectors are therefore appointed to ensure observance of the Act, to give advice on how to remedy any breaches in the law and finally, if necessary, to initiate any legal proceedings against individuals or companies who continue to contravene the regulations. These inspectors also have the authority to close down a workplace if it is considered unsafe. Despite these measures, eye injuries at work continue to occur, although at a reduced rate. However the introduction of this legislation and the wearing of eye protection mean that most of these injuries are now superficial, and due to non-compliance with the regulations (MacEwen, 1989).

Protection in the home

It is strange that although people are now used to wearing protective goggles or glasses at work they often do not wear protection when carrying out similar tasks, such as hammering or drilling, at home. It is obviously not feasible to legislate for the compulsory use of eye protection in the home. However, protective glasses are widely available in do-it-yourself shops and perhaps the retailers should be obliged to give more safety advice on the tools they sell. In addition to this the public must be made more aware of the risk of eye injury in the home, through campaigns such as the Royal National Institute for the Blind year of prevention 'be wise, protect your eyes' campaign 1990.

Protection for road traffic accidents

The reduction of RTA-related eye injury is, along with work-related eye injuries, one of the success stories in terms of prevention of eye injuries. Better car design has improved their overall safety and the introduction of laminated windscreens has reduced the risk of penetrating eye injuries. However the major advance was, of course, the introduction of the seat belt legislation in 1983 which produced a reduction of up to 77% of RTA-related eye injuries (Hall *et al.*, 1985; Cole *et al.*, 1987) almost overnight.

Protection during sport

Sporting injuries, previously described as the 'preventable epidemic' (Vinger, 1981), have now emerged as the main challenge for eye protection. Twelve per cent of all eye injuries reported in the USA and 43% of all eye injuries requiring hospital admission in the UK occur during sporting activities (National Society to Prevent Blindness, 1980; MacEwen, 1989).

Injuries occur in all types of sport; many are severe and cause permanent loss of vision. As discussed earlier, the risk of injury is related to the type of sport, which can be classified as low, medium, high and very high-risk sport. This classification is useful in considering preventive strategies. In the low-risk sports, such as jogging, cycling and aerobics which do not employ balls, implements or body contact, no eye protection is usually required. However it is important to recognize that the eyes may also need protection against injuries caused by mechanisms other than blunt trauma. For example, skiers and mountaineers should always wear sunglasses as protection against the hazards of ultraviolet radiation, and swimmers should wear goggles to prevent chlorine burns of the cornea.

The use of goggles, face masks or other protective devices is usually recommended for the medium and high-risk sports such as those involving fast-moving balls or pucks and the use of sticks, bats or rackets. Ordinary spectacles do not provide any protection. Indeed they may actually do more harm than good if the glass splinters or hinges break and fragments enter the eye, converting a potentially blunt injury into a penetrating one (Easterbrook, 1978; Feigelman *et al.*, 1983). The open, lenseless eye guards with rim protection only (Fig. 15.10) are also hazardous as they can funnel the mouldable squash ball directly on to the globe, causing more damage than they prevent. Contact lenses also provide no protection, but can be worn under goggles to correct refractive errors.

The main problems in terms of eye protection in sport are in the high and very high-risk activities, such as the contact and combat sports. By the very nature of these sports it is difficult to design eye protection which would not interfere with the sport itself. Helmets such as those worn in American Football probably have no place on a rugby or football pitch as it might be expected that they protected the eyes at the risk of causing more severe injuries to the rest of the body. However amateur boxing has successfully introduced

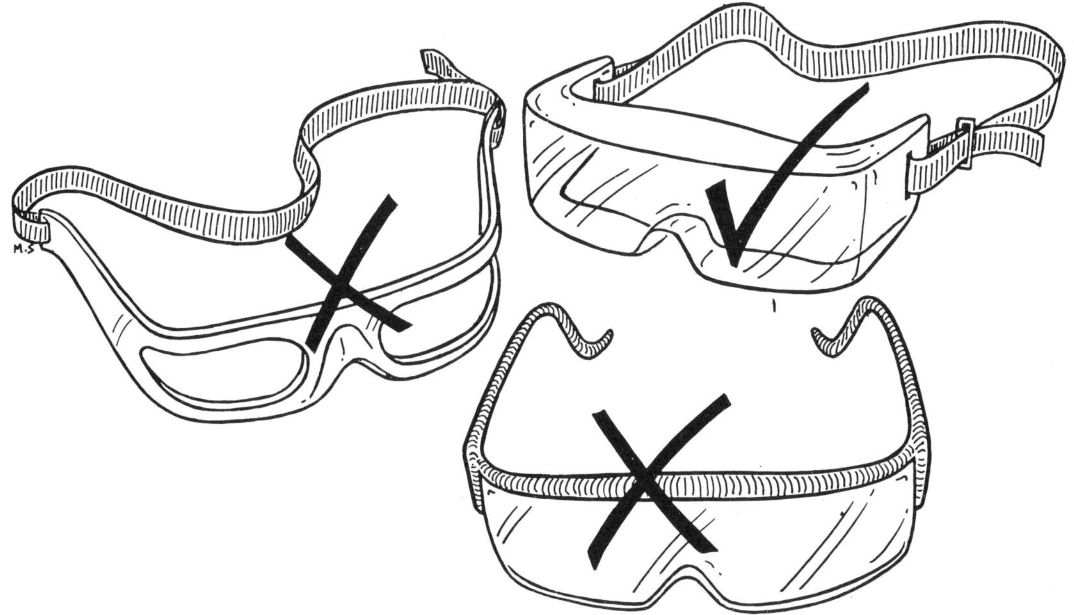

Fig. 15.10 Eyeguards of various descriptions are available for use in sport. The one-piece complete polycarbonate pair protects the eyes appropriately, but the others do not provide adequate protection.

leather head protectors which should also be used by professional boxers during sparring and the authorities are considering the introduction of thumbless boxing gloves to reduce the number of eye injuries in the ring from 'thumbing'. In view of the high risk it is essential that combat sports participants are screened before each match to ensure that they do not already have significant eye problems. The rules of the sport should include the requirement for regular ocular examinations and well-defined minimal levels of visual acuity and field of vision before participation is allowed. Unfortunately the present screening standards may not be adequate. A recent study found that 58% of boxers had sight-threatening pathology, despite a recent medical examination which had passed them as fit for continuation of their boxing licence (Giovinazzo *et al.*, 1987).

Eye protection devices

Unfortunately the range of devices for eye protection during sport is extremely limited at present. Many are not well-designed, having been based on industrial glasses which were developed for a completely different purpose. The ideal device for eye protection should be moulded in one piece, with no hinges (Fig. 15.10). It should be made of 3 mm polycarbonate, which is a long chain polymer that deforms permanently before breaking. This material is lighter and thinner than standard glass or plastic and has been successfully used for military and industrial safety glasses for many years. Eye protection devices should be comfortable and convenient, optically clear with a wide field of vision, anti-scratch and anti-fog and have high-impact resistance (Fig. 15.10). It should also be possible to incorporate a refractive correction into the lenses, if required. Unfortunately there is still no guidance in the form of a British Standard for sports eye protection and the first objective therefore must be to define this. Secondly, the public must be provided with information about the risk of eye injury during sport and encouraged to use eye protection. Legislation was effective in reducing ocular morbidity in industry and on the road; therefore it should also work in the sports arena, but this has been avoided so far.

Eye trauma is one of the leading causes of loss of

sight in this country and therefore every effort must be directed towards effective prevention.

References

Allen JC (1969) Sympathetic ophthalmia. A disappearing disease. *Journal of the American Medical Association* **209**, 1090–2.

Canavan YM, O'Flaherty MJ, Archer DB, Elwood JH (1980) A 10 year survey of eye injuries in Northern Ireland. 1967–1976. *British Journal of Ophthalmology* **64**, 618–25.

Cole MD, Clearkin L, Dabbs T et al. (1987) The seat belt law and after. *British Journal of Ophthalmology* **71**, 436–40.

Easterbrook M (1978) Eye injuries in squash, a preventible disease. *Canadian Medical Association Journal* **118**, 298–305.

Editorial (1973) A ball in the eye. *British Medical Journal* **ii**, 195–6.

Feigelman MJ, Sugar J, Jednock N et al. (1983) Assessment of ocular protection for racquet ball. *Journal of the American Medical Association* **250**, 3305–9.

Garrow A (1923) A statistical enquiry into a thousand cases of eye injury. *British Journal of Ophthalmology* **7**, 65–80.

Giovinazzo VJ, Yannuzzi LA, Sorenson JA et al. (1987) The ocular complications of boxing. *Ophthalmology* **94**, 589–96.

Hall NF, Denning AM, Elkington AR (1985) The eye and the seat belt in Wessex. *British Journal of Ophthalmology* **69**, 317–19.

Jones NP (1987) Eye injuries in sport: an increasing problem. *British Journal of Sports Medicine* **71**, 701–5.

Kaufman JH, Tolpin DW (1974) Glaucoma after traumatic angle recession. A ten year prospective study. *American Journal of Ophthalmology* **78**, 648–54.

MacEwen CJ (1986) Sport associated eye injuries: a casualty department survey. *British Journal of Ophthalmology* **71**, 701–5.

MacEwen CJ (1989) Eye injuries: a prospective survey of 5671 cases. *British Journal of Ophthalmology* **73**, 888–94.

McGetrick JJ, Jampol LM, Goldberg MF et al. (1983) Aminocaproic acid decreases secondary haemorrhage after traumatic hyphaema. *Archives of Ophthalmology* **101**, 1031–5.

Machemer R, Buettner H, Norton EWD, Parel JM (1971) Vitrectomy: a pars plana approach. *Transactions of the American Academy of Ophthalmology and Otolaryngology* **75**, 813–20.

Mackay GN (1975) Incidence of trauma to the eyes in car occupants. *Transactions of the Ophthalmological Society of UK* **95**, 311–14.

National Society to Prevent Blindness (1980) *Fact Sheet*. New York: National Society to Prevent Blindness.

Parver LM (1986) Eye trauma; the neglected disorder. *Archives of Ophthalmology* **104**, 1452–3.

Read JE, Goldberg MF (1974) Traumatic hyphaema: comparison of medical treatment. *Transactions of the American Academy of Ophthalmology and Otolaryngology* **78**, 799–803.

Schein OD, Hibberd PL, Shingleton BJ et al. (1988) The spectrum and burden of ocular injury. *Ophthalmology* **95**, 300–5.

Vernon SA, Yorston DB (1984) Incidence of ocular injuries from road traffic accidents after the introduction of the seat belt law. *Journal of the Society of Medicine* **77**, 198–200.

Vinger PF (1981) Eye injuries. In: Vinger PF, Hoerner EF (eds) *Sports Injuries; The Unthwarted Epidemic*. Littleton: PSG Publishing.

16

Soft tissue pains in the growing child

D. A. Sherlock

Introduction

The management of a child with musculoskeletal pain presents difficulties over and above management of similar problems in an adult. Children, especially infants and babies, cannot clearly localize or express their symptoms, thereby denying the clinician the benefit of a history. Examination of an unco-operative child may be uninformative. Children are subject to different disease patterns than adults, some of which may be obscure. Add parental anxiety to this diagnostic morass and it is all too easy to understand the unease with which many doctors regard children's orthopaedic problems. To compound matters, textbooks of children's orthopaedics tend to concentrate on 'real' pathology and ignore the numerous benign aches and pains with which children present. Further confusion arises from differing interpretations as to the boundary between normal variants and pathology.

Part of this chapter, therefore, will be devoted to benign and normal variants as well as covering more recognized pathologies. Given that wide variation exists between doctors and cultures in interpreting what is normal or pathological, the views expressed below must be somewhat idiosyncratic, though most are accepted by a significant body of opinion in the UK and some are backed by scientific evidence. Due to the wide spectrum of childhood musculoskeletal disease some subjects will necessarily be covered only superficially or omitted. References are provided for readers who wish to investigate specific topics more fully.

Growing pains

Sharrard contends that normal growth is never painful, but the term 'growing pains' is readily understood and accepted by most parents, suggesting that benign musculoskeletal pains are a genuine phenomenon. 'Night cramps', or better, 'benign leg pains' (BLPs) are now probably more acceptable descriptions. Two patterns of BLPs are commonly seen. Both occur in children, aged usually between 2 and 8 years, who are otherwise healthy and very active. The pains tend to occur more frequently following periods of increased physical activity but may occur at any time.

In the more common pattern, the child awakes crying from sleep and may limp into its parents' bedroom. The pain, which is quite severe, is poorly localized in the leg and may affect either side at different times, though one side may predominate. With reassurance, rubbing and occasionally paracetamol, the pain subsides such that by 20–40 min it has gone. Children who suffer these pains often sleep heavily with their legs folded up under themselves. The most likely cause of these symptoms is muscular cramps, which explains the severity and rapid resolution of the pain.

Less frequently, a child complains of poorly localized bilateral or unilateral leg pains towards the end of the day or after walking long distances. There is no limp but the gait may become somewhat untidy. The pain is longer lasting than for night cramps but with rest, reassurance and occasional analgesia the child settles off to sleep without problem. It is probable that these symptoms represent fatigue discomfort of joints or muscles which have been overused.

The diagnosis of BLP is one of exclusion so other pathologies must first be eliminated. The history of short-lived, poorly localized, mobile pains in a child who is otherwise very active and healthy and who has no family history of neuromuscular disease suggests BLP. Clinical examination should confirm that all lower limb joints move freely and symmetrically and that there is no localized bony tenderness or evidence of neuromuscular disease.

Further investigation by blood tests is rarely indicated unless there are features of muscle weakness to suggest a muscular dystrophy, when a creatinine phosphokinase estimation may be diagnostic. Similarly, X-rays are only necessary when the pains are frequently localized to one joint. Management is symptomatic with reassurance, rubbing the affected area and simple analgesics if required. Most children grow out of these pains by age 8. The frequency of night cramps may be diminished by the parents untangling the child's limbs when they go to bed.

Gait problems

An abnormality of gait is the reason for referral in almost a quarter of children seen in a typical children's orthopaedic clinic. Intoeing or a pigeon-toed gait is the most common complaint, but out-toeing or a splay-foot gait is also seen. The degree of toeing out or in is often asymmetrical. Thus Scrutton and Robson (1968) found that 18% of 50 unselected and otherwise normal children intoed unilaterally. McSweeney (1971) noted intoeing in 13.2% and out-toeing in 0.5% of 1320 children seen for reasons other than gait problems. One-third of his intoers corrected by age 7, but whether their intoeing corrected or not, two-thirds (8.8%) of these children had radiological evidence of persisting femoral anteversion. Conversely, one-third showed a persistent intoeing gait without evidence of a femoral torsional abnormality.

These observations raise three questions. Firstly, is there a relation between intoeing/out-toeing and femoral torsional abnormalities? Secondly, are these gait patterns merely a normal variant (such as blue eyes and left-handedness), or are they pathological and likely to give rise to osteoarthritis of the hips? Thirdly, can we modify the condition by treatment?

In answer to the first question, Fabry *et al.* (1973) using X-rays and Moulton and Upadhyay (1982) using ultrasound demonstrated that children with unilateral intoeing had a consistent increase in femoral anteversion (i.e. the angle between the femoral neck axis and the transcondylar plane) on the affected side. However, femoral anteversion is physiological, being about 60° at 30 weeks' gestation (Somerville, 1957), 40° at birth and reducing to 16° by age 16 (Kling and Hensinger, 1983). It is paradoxical that internal rotation of the hips is minimal at birth and increases up to age 2 years while femoral anteversion is simultaneously decreasing. The paradox is explained by recognizing that the *in utero* position produces flexion (hence the 'sway-back' of normal toddlers) and external rotation hip contractures which stretch out over the first 2 years of life. Thus the external rotation contracture initially masks the underlying femoral anteversion, which is revealed as the contracture decreases (Coon *et al.*, 1975).

The second question is more difficult to answer. On theoretical grounds Somerville (1977) suggested that persistent femoral anteversion (PFA) could give rise to osteoarthritis of the hip, knee and foot. Studies by Kling and Hensinger (1983) and Wedge and Wasylenko (1978) revealed no association between PFA and osteoarthritis of the hip, but Reikeras *et al.* (1983) did find such an association. Probably the most cogent evidence against a significant link between PFA and osteoarthritis is the knowledge that hip arthritis not secondary to recognized causes (Perthes disease, trauma, skeletal dysplasias, etc.) is rare in the under-60 age group and clearly does not approach the 9% of the population with PFA noted by McSweeney (1971).

In answer to the third question, Fabry *et al.* (1973), Staheli *et al.* (1977) and Kling and Hensinger (1983) have shown that conservative measures such as twisters, Denis Brown splints and shoe modifications are ineffective in correcting PFA. Thus derotation osteotomy of the femur is the only certain way of rectifying PFA. The consequences in terms of complications and resources of performing such major surgery on 9% of the population for a condition which has not been shown to be harmful would be horrific. Surgical correction is, however, occasionally indicated when marked anteversion persists after age 7, and is associated with hip pain and unsightly squinting of the knees.

In dealing with the intoeing child, parents complain less about the cosmetic effect than that the child is always falling, which is attributed to it tripping over its own feet. While this may be so, these children are often clumsy in other ways as well. Clinical examination is necessary to exclude neuromuscular causes of their clumsiness, but such abnormality is rarely found. What is notable is that many of these children, in addition to having a greater range of internal compared with external rotation at the hip, have significant joint laxity with hyperextendable knees, elbows, metacarpophalangeal joints and thumbs. It is reasonable to postulate that their clumsiness may relate in part to inefficient proprioceptive input since lax joint structures allow excessive movement before becoming tight and firing their stretch receptors.

Joint laxity may also explain PFA. When the foot is fixed, as in weight-bearing, hip extension normally produces tension in the anterior hip capsule and ligaments, thereby inducing a retroversion force and encouraging the anteverted femoral neck to remodel. If the hip capsule is lax these corrective forces are reduced so that remodelling is slower and less complete.

Despite this early clumsiness, Staheli *et al.* (1977) found no evidence that PFA in a child affected later athletic performance. Indeed it is part of folklore that intoers tend to be good athletes, though this may be more a reflection of suppleness (i.e. joint laxity) than the PFA.

Since it is clear that treatment of femoral anteversion is either ineffective or excessive, the condition is best managed by explanation and reassurance. It is traditional to encourage the child to walk with the feet pointing forwards, to entrain a more acceptable gait habit. Splay-legged sitting should be discouraged since it causes a continuing anteverting force to bear on the femoral neck. Furthermore in this position the child commonly sits on the externally rotated foot, which may produce an ugly-looking external tibial torsion. Advice to get the child dancing or playing football may increase confidence and help motor education.

Out-toeing is much less a problem. Its relative rarity and tendency to improve visibly over a reasonable period of time and the lack of association with clumsiness make reassurance more readily acceptable than for intoeing. Occasionally anxiety is raised by the child just beginning to walk who has a markedly out-toed gait and may appear to drag one leg by walking slightly sideways. This is partly explained by the external rotation hip contractures mentioned previously. An external rotation gait widens the walking base and improves stability and balance, as also does the crabwise gait, which places the feet at right angles to each other – an undoubted advantage when you are still new to walking. As the child gains confidence these patterns of walking disappear.

Bow legs and knock knees

Bow legs (genu varum) or knock knees (genu valgum) in a child frequently cause anxiety to parents, yet they are usually physiological. Salenius and Vankka (1975) in a radiological study of 979 children referred for unrelated reasons, found that it is normal to have genu varum under age 2 and for genu valgum subsequently to develop. Initially the degree of valgus may be quite extreme but it gradually diminishes to the normal angle of valgus by age 7. Similarly, Morley (1957) noted an intermalleolar distance of more than 2.5 cm in 74% and more than 5 cm in 22% of otherwise normal children aged 3–3½ years. The degree of varus and valgus is increased by lax ligaments, especially in the heavier child. The deformities are exaggerated by the external rotation posture of the hip in the child under 2 which produces an apparent bow leg while a knock knee is simulated by an internal rotation posture at the hip in the child aged 2–7. Bulky calf muscles, especially in association with an internal rotation posture, further accentuate the appearance of valgus.

Accurate measurement is, therefore, essential to determine the true amount of varus or valgus and is best done with the child lying with both patellae pointing forwards. For genu varum the medial malleoli are pressed together whilst the distance between the femoral condyles is measured. Similarly genu valgum is measured by the intermalleolar distance while the medial femoral condyles are held together.

If the deformity is inappropriate for the child's age or is persistently unilateral or more than 10 cm radiological assessment is essential. Blount's disease, Schmidt's-type metaphyseal dysostosis or rickets are causes for bow legs persisting beyond age 2 years. Blount's disease and Schmidt's dysostosis can be treated by medial periosteal release, lateral epiphyseal stapling or valgus osteotomy while rickets usually responds to correction of the biochemical abnormalities. Progressive genu valgum is best treated by medial epiphyseal stapling of tibia and/or femur at the knee or by supracondylar femoral varus osteotomy. Varus tibial osteotomy is not recommended since to protect the proximal epiphyseal plate it must be done quite distally, with the risk of producing an anterior compartment syndrome.

Flat feet

Infant feet are chubby and give the appearance of flat feet. This perhaps explains why Morley (1957) found that 97% of otherwise normal children under 18 months, assessed by clinical examination and footprint records, had flat feet. Since only 4% of children remain flat-footed by age 10 the condition can be seen to be largely self-resolving.

Examination is required however to exclude fixed deformity or genu valgum which may exaggerate the appearance of flat-footedness. Inspection of the shoes will show if there is excessive wear on the medial aspect of the sole and heel since normally wear occurs over the centre or outer aspect of the heel. Benign flat feet are symmetrical and asymptomatic. They correct to produce a varus heel and a satisfactory medial longitudinal arch when the child stands on tiptoe or if the great toe is dorsiflexed at the metatarsophalangeal joint. Movements of the ankle, subtalar and midtarsal joints are full and painless. The presence of a swelling in the medial longitudinal arch, which does not correct with tiptoe standing, and loss of heel prominence suggest a degree of congenital pes valgus, the most extreme form of which is the very rare congenital vertical talus.

Radiographic examination is only indicated if pain or limited movement has been elicited and may reveal a tarsal coalition or congenital vertical talus.

Treatment of asymptomatic flat feet requires only reassurance. If the child complains of discomfort or examination reveals distortion of the shoe or excessive medial wear, the use of sturdy shoes with heels that flare out, rather than being undercut, is recommended. As the heel wears the damaged area should be excised and new rubber or metal segments inserted to prevent the shoe from tipping over medially with consequent accelerated wear and distortion. In severe cases shoes with a medial arch support such as Startrite Inneraze or prescription of a plastic longitudinal arch support insert will help.

The painful condition of peroneal spastic flat foot, where the foot is pulled into valgus by peroneal muscle spasm, results from a tarsal coalition which comprises an abnormal bony bar or synchrondrosis between any two tarsal bones. Such bars probably represent failure of complete segmentation of the primitive hindfoot mesenchyme. The most common bars are medial talocalcaneal and calcaneonavicular. Other family members may also have a tarsal coalition, not necessarily of the same type, suggesting a degree of inheritance. The pain commonly starts in an adolescent following a minor injury to the foot.

Examination reveals a rigid valgus hindfoot with varus movements resisted by peroneal muscle spasm. Radiographs confirm the presence of a coalition, though visualization is difficult in the rare case presenting under 8 years when the bar is still largely cartilaginous. Later, secondary degenerative changes occur in the adjacent tarsal joints.

Conservative treatment often produces satisfactory resolution and comprises rest, non-steroidal analgesics, or occasionally a period of immobilization in a below-knee plaster. If this fails and secondary changes are absent, excision of a calcaneonavicular bar through a dorsolateral incision often provides satisfactory pain relief. Excision of a medial talocalcaneal bar is much less successful. Once secondary changes are present only a triple arthrodesis will relieve intractable symptoms.

Congenital flat foot and congenital vertical talus are rare. They are often associated with congenital defects such as arthrogryposis or spina bifida. Their aetiology is unclear since they do not always occur in association with paralytic disorders. Clinically the tendons of tibialis anterior, the toe extensors, the peronei and the tendo-Achilles are contracted while tibialis posterior is thin and elongated. Congenital vertical talus is differentiated from postural calcaneovalgus in that the heel, rather than being prominent, is small due to being fixed in equinus. Radiographs show the talus pointing vertically rather than horizontally with the calcaneum in some equinus and no longer parallel with the talus. When the navicular ossifies at age 2 years, it is seen to be dislocated to lie along the dorsal surface of the talar neck.

In milder forms, with treatment started soon after birth, it is sometimes possible to realign the navicular on the talus by applying serial long leg plasters with the foot maximally plantarflexed. Subsequently the hindfoot equinus is corrected by surgical posteromedial release with lengthening of the tendo-Achilles. More commonly, the position is fixed. In these cases surgery is required to realign the talus, either excising the navicular as described by Colton (1973) or preserving it and using a two-stage procedure as proposed by Sharrard (1979).

Toe deformities

Parents not infrequently seek advice regarding toe deformities in their children. They may suggest that these deformities are the cause of gait abnormalities or a child's reluctance to walk. Since toe deformities rarely cause pain, other sources of discomfort should be excluded before accepting that the foot is the culprit.

It is common in the infant for there to be some over-riding of the second on the third toe. This probably results from the shorter interdigital cleft between the second and third toes and is further accentuated by the chubbiness of the infant foot. As the foot becomes slimmer and spreads with weight-bearing and growth the deformity disappears. Treatment with strapping or surgery is rarely necessary. A degree of syndactyly between the second and third toes is occasionally seen but is asymptomatic and requires no treatment.

Other common toes problems include congenital curly toes, congenital over-riding fifth toes, metatarsus varus and adolescent hallux valgus and rigidus.

Congenital curly toes

This condition is often familial and may involve one or more toes, most commonly the fourth. Failure of normal development of the intrinsic muscles to the toe results in a flexion and usually external rotation deformity which mainly affects the distal interphalangeal joint. If a parent has the condition and is asymptomatic it is likely that the child will behave similarly. Where significant under-riding causes rubbing or painful contact of the toenail with the sole of the shoe, surgery provides the only effective treatment. Often division of the flexor profundus tendon at the level of the distal interphalangeal joint is sufficient, though correction of the deformity may take some months. More severe deformities warrant transfer of the flexor profundus tendon into the lateral aspect of the extensor expansion where it acts as an intrinsic muscle to flex the metatarsophalangeal joint while extending the interphalangeal joints. Fixed deformities require arthrodesis of the affected joint, which is best left until toe growth ceases at age 10.

Congenital over-riding fifth toes

In this condition, which may be unilateral or bilateral, the fifth toe lies proximally and dorsally, overlapping the fourth toe. Surprisingly it is rarely symptomatic. Surgery offers the only effective treatment. Satisfactory results have been reported after V–Y plasty or Z-plasty of the tight dorsal structures, Butler's procedure (Cockin, 1968) and even amputation.

Metatarsus varus

This common condition is one cause of intoeing. It comprises adduction and supination of the forefoot on the hindfoot and varies from a minimal deformity, visible only on active contraction of abductor hallucis, to marked 'hooking' of the forefoot associated with a deep skin crease on the medial side of the foot.

The condition is usually self-correcting. Thus Rushforth (1978) found that of 130 untreated feet followed up for 7 years, only 4% showed a persisting stiff deformity with a further 10% having a mild asymptomatic persisting forefoot adduction. He could not predict under the age of 3 years which feet would not resolve, which makes advice on treatment difficult.

Probably it is best to treat those feet which can be corrected beyond neutral with regular parental manipulative correction and the use of shoes with a stiff medial last. More severe cases warrant the use of serial plasters, preferably before the child's first birthday. Treatment for 8–10 weeks with three to five changes was advised by Ponsetti and Becker (1966), the plasters being applied with the heel in equinus and varus and the forefoot abducted and pronated. They treated only one in nine cases of metatarsus varus with such plasters and only two out of 379 feet required surgery.

Where correction has not been achieved by age 3, surgical release of abductor hallucis and the first metatarsocuneiform joint, then 6 weeks in plaster (Bleck, 1967), is usually enough, though the anomalous insertion of tibialis posterior described by Browne and Paton (1979) should be sought and dealt with if found. Relapses and older children up to age 7 respond well to a full medial tarsometatarsal release (Heyman *et al.*, 1958). Children over 6 years with symptomatic metatarsus varus probably require multiple basal metatarsal osteotomies, as described by Berman and Gartland (1971).

Kite (1967) describes a very rare familial type of metatarsus varus where the foot is rigid and serpentine is shape, often associated with a ball-and-socket ankle joint (Lloyd-Roberts and Clark, 1973). Correction of these deformities is virtually impossible. Attempts to do so usually make matters worse by increasing stiffness, suggesting that provision of suitable footwear is the best approach.

Adolescent hallux valgus and rigidus

Hallux valgus in the adolescent may be brought to the attention of the doctor because of pain or deformity at the first metatarsophalangeal joint. Parents often worry that poorly fitted shoes have been the cause. It is almost impossible to find modern fashion shoes which fit these children, who usually have broad feet but in most cases there is a strong family history of hallux valgus which suggests that at most shoes are only a contributory factor. Medial deviation of the first metatarsal (metatarsus primus varus), defined as a first intermetatarsal angle of more than 9 or 10° is frequently associated with hallux valgus, though which is the primary abnormality is unclear. Piggott (1960) observed that if the amount of first metatarsophalangeal valgus (as measured on an anteroposterior radiograph) exceeded 25° progressive hallux valgus was inevitable, while angles between 20 and 25° warranted careful watching.

Surgery is the only effective treatment for hallux valgus. According to Helal *et al.* (1974) the best results follow correction of the metatarsus primus varus by Wilson's osteotomy (1963). This involves an oblique osteotomy of the first metatarsal neck with lateral, plantar and proximal displacement and varus realignment of the metatarsal head. Growth may cause recurrence of the metatarsus primus varus so operation is best postponed till skeletal maturity at age 13–14. It is noticeable that in many cases of adolescent hallux valgus full dorsiflexion of the first metatarsophalangeal joint in the dorsiflexed foot is prevented by an easily palpated tight band of the medial plantar aponeurosis. In some cases division of this band produces resolution of the hallux valgus. Indeed it may be that part of the success of the realignment operations (which involve shortening the first ray) comes from detensioning of this band.

Where there is clear evidence that muscle imbalance is the cause of severe hallux valgus, as in spina bifida and cerebral palsy, division of the tendon of adductor hallucis combined with a basal osteotomy is necessary to correct the deformity.

Hallux rigidus in children and adolescents occurs equally in males and females, unlike in adults where males predominate. There is often a family history (Bonney and McNab, 1952). Trauma is suspected as the cause giving rise to an osteochondritis of the first metatarsal head (Goodfellow, 1966; McMaster, 1978). Pain and flexor spasm at the first metatarsophalangeal joint cause the patient to walk on a supinated foot.

Initial treatment should comprise a period of rest in a below-knee plaster of Paris cast or a shoe with a stiffened sole and metatarsal rocker. If these are ineffective and there is a sufficient range of plantar flexion (30°), a dorsal wedge extension osteotomy of the proximal phalanx (Kessel and Bonney, 1958) or the first metatarsal neck usually produces enough relief of symptoms until skeletal maturity when arthrodesis of the first metatarsophalangeal joint becomes feasible.

The osteochondritides

These are a disparate collection of conditions with the common link that they involve 'a non-inflammatory, non-infectious derangement of normal bony growth occurring at various ossification centres at the time of their greatest developmental activity' (Buchman, 1929).

The aetiology of the osteochondritides is largely unknown, though vascular disturbance, trauma and genetic factors assume varying degrees of importance depending upon the site of the disease.

It is helpful to subdivide the osteochondritides into three groups:

1. Traction apophysites.
2. Avascular osteochondritides.
3. Osteochondritides dissecans.

Traction apophysites

These occur at an epiphysis into which a powerful muscle tendon inserts. The underlying aetiology is probably largely trauma, which may be either acute or, more commonly, chronic, though there is also a genetic element. The conditions in this group are:

1. Osgood–Schlatter's disease.
2. Johansson–Larsen syndrome.
3. Sever's disease.
4. Epiphysitis of the fifth metatarsal base.
5. Greater trochanteric epiphysitis.
6. Ischiopubic osteochondritis.

Osgood–Schlatter's disease

This condition occurs most commonly in boys, usually between the ages of 9 and 13. It presents as pain and swelling over the tibial tubercle, aggravated by activity and eased by rest. A lateral radiograph shows characteristic fragmentation of the tibial tubercle (Fig. 16.1). Since the problem appears to result from overuse, treatment is directed towards restriction of activity to a level which makes the symptoms tolerable. Where a child will not co-operate, a plaster of Paris cylinder may be used to enforce rest. Hamstring stretching exercises may be helpful if they are found to be tight. When symptoms persist despite these mea-

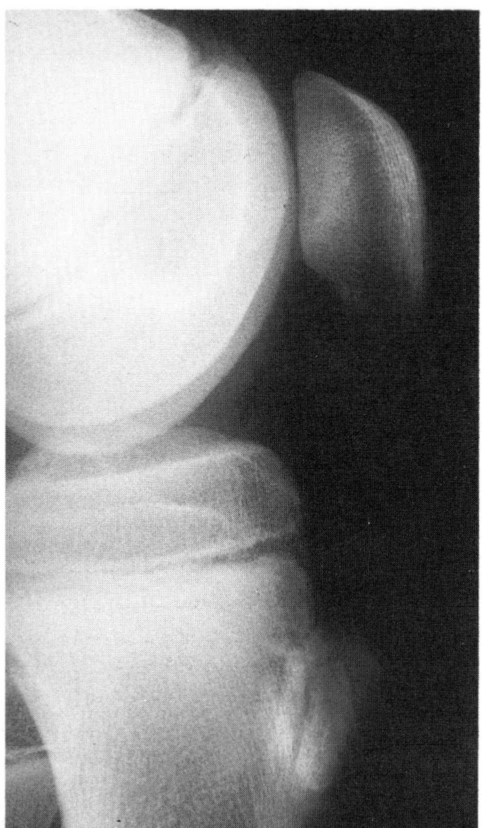

Fig. 16.1 Osgood–Schlatter's disease. There is fragmentation of the tibial tubercle.

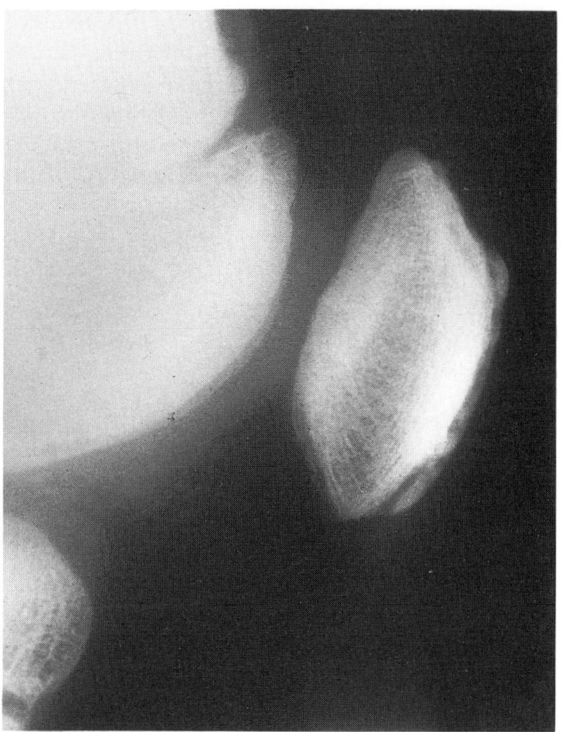

Fig. 16.2 Johansson–Larsen syndrome. There is fragmentation of the anterior and inferior surfaces of the patella.

sures it is common to see on a lateral radiograph a nodule of bone which has separated completely from the tibial tubercle. Exploration of the tibial tubercle via a tendon-spitting incision reveals the nodule lying within a lake of bursal fluid deep to the patellar tendon. Excision of the nodule brings rapid relief of the symptoms. All other forms of operative intervention should be avoided since they may damage growth of the tibial tubercle, producing a back-knee deformity.

Johannson–Larsen syndrome

This closely resembles Osgood–Schlatter's disease but the pain and radiographic changes are localized to the lower pole of the patella (Fig. 16.2) rather than the tibial tubercle. Treatment is as for Osgood–Schlatter's disease.

Sever's disease

This condition comprises an acute or chronic traction injury of the tendo-Achilles where it inserts into the secondary centre of ossification of the os calcis. It presents as heel pain in a child aged 9–12. Palpation of the tendo-Achilles insertion is locally tender. A lateral radiograph excludes other causes of heel pain. The presence of fragmentation and sclerosis of the epiphysis is of questionable significance, since similar changes are seen in normal feet. Indeed, it is possible that the symptoms arise from inflammation of the bursa lying behind the tendo-Achilles rather than the os calcis. In any case, treatment involves reduction in activity, if necessary by a below-knee plaster of Paris, and heel raises which may act either by defunctioning partly the calf muscles or by realigning the tendo-Achilles.

Epiphysitis of the fifth metatarsal base

Pain and prominence of the fifth metatarsal base presenting in a child, usually female, aged 12 or 13, suggests a traction apophysitis of the epiphysis at the base of the fifth metatarsal by peroneus brevis. A radiograph shows the epiphysis displaced slightly laterally from its normal position. Restriction of activity is usually sufficient treatment, though rarely a period in a below-knee plaster of Paris is needed.

Greater trochanteric epiphysitis

Hall (1958) describes this rare osteochondritis of the greater trochanteric epiphysis which occurs in overweight immature boys. It represents a traction apophysitis of the insertion of the hip abductors.

Ischiopubic osteochondritis

This condition represents with pain in the groin of a child aged 9–12 years. Radiographs show irregularity and cystic changes at the point of maximum tenderness over the ischiopubic synchondrosis (Fig. 16.3). This probably represents a traction apophysitis of the insertion of the hip adductors or extensors.

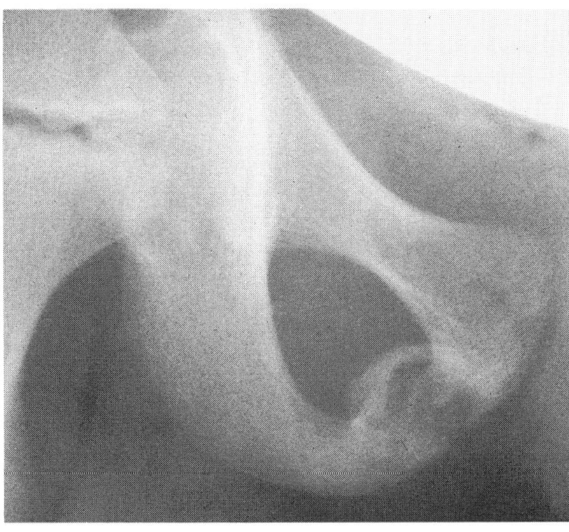

Fig. 16.3 Ischiopubic osteochondritis. There is an apparent lytic lesion of the ischiopubic synchondrosis.

Avascular osteochondritides

This important group includes avascular necrosis of the:

1. Femoral head (Legge–Calvé–Perthes disease).
2. Navicular (Köhler's disease).
3. Second or third metatarsal head (Freiberg's disease).

A number of other uncommon osteochondritides have been reported in which pain is associated with sclerosis on a radiograph of the affected epiphysis. Histological proof of ischaemia is not always available but the pattern of sclerosis progressing through fragmentation to recovery is very similar to Perthes disease. Such osteochondritides include the capitulum (Smith, 1964), base of first metatarsal or base of great toe proximal phalanx (Sharrard, 1979), proximal tibial (Boldero and Mitchell, 1954) and distal tibial (Siffert and Arkin, 1950) epiphysis. Calvé's (vertebral) epiphysitis resembles an avascular osteochondritis but appears to be secondary to eosinophilic granuloma in most cases (Compere *et al.*, 1954). The granulomatous disease may, however, cause an ischaemic collapse of the vertebral body.

Perthes disease

This fascinating condition is of unknown aetiology, though geographical and environmental factors are clearly important, with affected children tending to come from families of lower socioeconomic status. Associated growth abnormalities with short distal limbs, hands and feet and delayed bone age are common, as are genitourinary abnormalities and inguinal herniae. Boys are affected four times as often as girls over an age range of 2–18 years, though 80% of cases occur between 4 and 9 years. Fifteen per cent of children have bilateral involvement.

The pathological process is that of a single or

multiple episodes of acute ischaemic necrosis involving part or all of the proximal femoral epiphysis (Fig. 16.4). Commonly a subchondral fracture, which may be visible radiologically, results in flattening of the epiphysis. The necrotic bone initially appears sclerotic on radiographs due to a combination of compaction, calcification of necrotic marrow and surrounding osteoporosis. In time the dead bone is phagocytosed and replaced with fibrocartilage, giving the radiological appearance of fragmentation of the necrotic bone. Enchondral ossification of this cartilage heals the defect but ossification in the thickened areas of cartilage anteriorly and laterally caused by flattening results in an increasingly oval-shaped head and widening of the femoral neck. As the acetabulum remodels to maintain congruency with this oval head, sliding of the head within the socket on abduction is gradually limited by impingement laterally of the head against the acetabular margin – a process known as hinge abduction. Clinically this is revealed by progressive loss of rotation, with hip movement occurring only from adduction in extension to abduction in flexion.

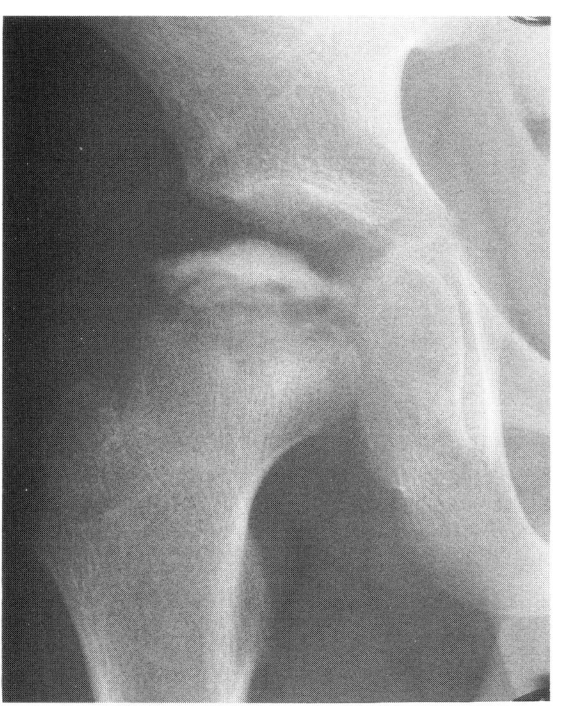

Fig. 16.4 Perthes disease of the right hip. This is Catterall grade 4 with lateral subluxation, lateral calcification, Gage's sign and a horizontal epiphysis.

The appearance of Perthes disease can be simulated by other conditions. In bilateral cases these include spondyloepiphyseal and multiple epiphyseal dysplasias and hypothyroidism while infection, eosinophilic granuloma, lymphoma, haemophilia and Gaucher's disease may imitate unilateral cases.

Long-term results suggest that 86% of patients will suffer from osteoarthritis of the hip by age 65, though most will not develop symptoms until their 50s or 60s (Catterall, 1987). Nearly 10%, however, develop severe arthritis before age 35.

Ideally treatment would comprise prevention of the ischaemic episodes but this is not feasible at present, even if we could identify the children at risk. Thus we must concentrate on trying to minimize deformity of the femoral head since marked deformity is associated with a poor outcome (Stulberg *et al.*, 1981; Catterall *et al.*, 1982). Given the above facts and the knowledge that 60% of children will do well even without treatment, there is sadly much nihilism about the treatment of Perthes disease. However, in 40% of cases we can improve the result by intervention and our aim is to identify these children. To this end Catterall describes four prognostic factors:

1. *Age and sex*. The younger the child at the onset of the disease, the less likely is severe damage to the epiphysis and the longer is the period for remodelling. Girls seem to have more serious forms of the disease and so tend to do worse than boys.
2. *The stage of disease at diagnosis*. The chronology of the disease process is marked by five stages – onset, sclerosis, fragmentation, healing and the final result. Once healing has commenced no further deterioration in the end-result occurs.

   There is thus little point in treating cases who have reached this stage unless an arthrogram demonstrates hinge abduction, which can be treated by a valgus extension osteotomy of the femoral neck to realign the leg to a neutral

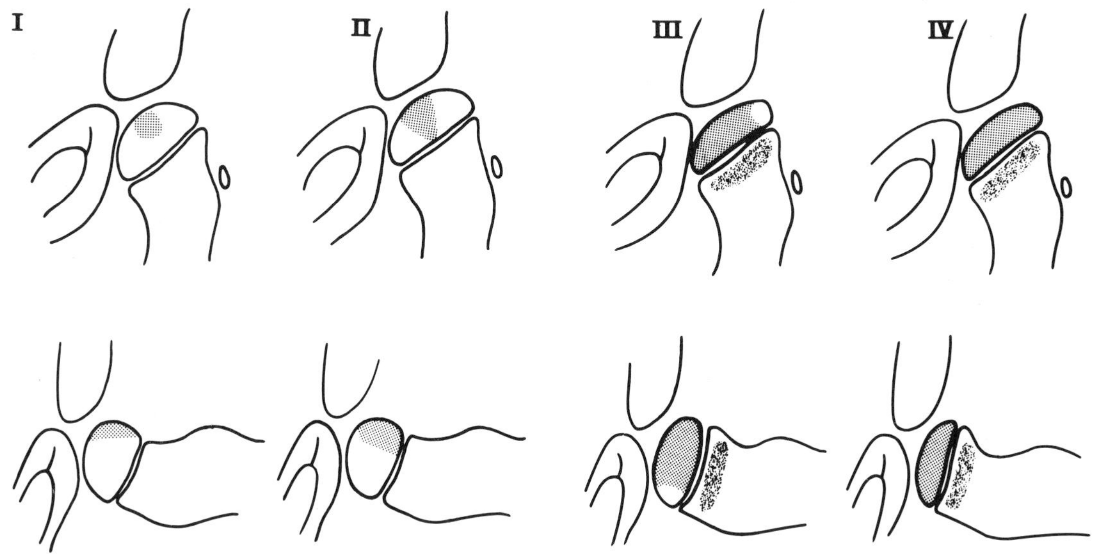

Fig. 16.5 Catterall groups. Diagrammatic anteroposterior and lateral views of a left hip to demonstrate the site and extent of necrosis in the four groups.

position while maintaining maximum hip congruency (Quain and Catterall, 1986).

3. *Group.* Catterall (1971) described four radiologically defined groups depending on the degree of head infarction. These are illustrated in Figure 16.5. In 92% of untreated cases groups I and II did well while 91% of groups III and IV had a poor outcome.
4. *At-risk signs.* A poor prognosis was also noted by Catterall for cases which demonstrated certain 'at-risk' signs. Clinical at-risk signs are progressive stiffness of the hip, an increasing adduction contracture and a heavy child. Radiological at-risk signs comprise Gage's sign, calcification lateral to the epiphysis, lateral subluxation, a horizontal growth plate and diffuse metaphyseal changes. These are illustrated diagrammatically in Figure 16.6.

Treatment indications for early-stage disease can thus be defined as follows:

Under 7
No treatment – groups I–III without at risk signs.
Treatment – groups II–IV with at risk signs.
Over 7
No treatment – group I.

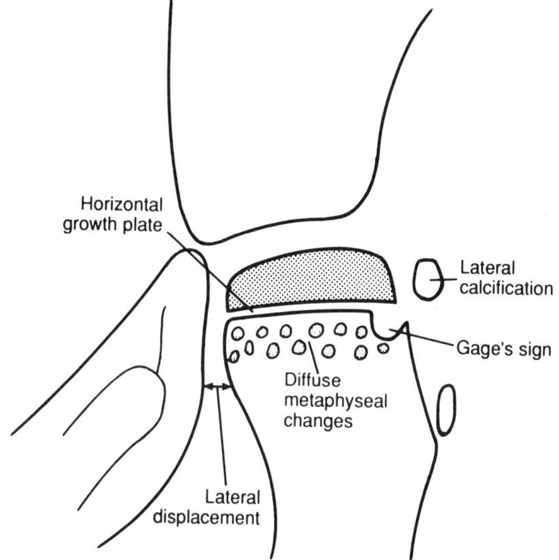

Fig. 16.6 Diagrammatic representation of a left hip showing the five signs of the 'at-risk' hip. Not all would necessarily present in one case.

Treatment – groups II–IV with or without at risk signs.

Even those children who do not require treatment should probably be advised to restrict their more vigorous activities so as to reduce the risk of further trauma-induced ischaemia or deformity. When advised, the aims of treatment are containment, maintenance of movement to encourage remodelling and reduction of forces through the hip to diminish the risks of further deformity or ischaemia. Abduction of the hip achieves this by placing the softened head deep within the confines of the acetabulum and reducing forces through the hip (Heikkinen and Puranen, 1980). This is best done by first assessing the hip by an arthrogram performed under the relaxation of a general anaesthetic to demonstrate the position of maximum containment of the head. A Batchelor plaster is then applied, initially with an adjustable bar, so that the legs can be adjusted daily without causing discomfort while retaining hip movement until the position of maximum congruency demonstrated by the arthrogram is reached. Once this position is attained it can be maintained in plaster with a definitive bar until healing commences (usually about a year, though in older children it can be as long as 2–4 years).

The same result can also be achieved surgically by realigning the leg to neutral while maintaining maximum hip congruence by a subtrochanteric osteotomy. This has the advantage of a shorter time in plaster and accelerates the onset of healing, especially in the older child. For the child aged over 8, however, the usual varus of the osteotomy does not remodel as in younger children, which leaves a short, bowed leg on the affected side. A corrective valgus osteotomy is then required once healing has finished. In these children, therefore, some form of primary shelf or pelvic osteotomy may be more appropriate since it obviates the need for a second operative procedure.

Köhler's disease

This condition, which is commonest in boys aged 3–5 years, presents with mid-foot pain and tenderness and a limp or refusal to weight-bear. Radiographs of the foot show sclerosis and flattening of the navicular (Fig. 16.7a) followed over a period of 2 years by fragmentation and full reconstitution of the navicular (Fig. 16.7b). Treatment is symptomatic with rest in a below-knee plaster of Paris for 4 weeks and subsequently a medial longitudinal arch support when necessary.

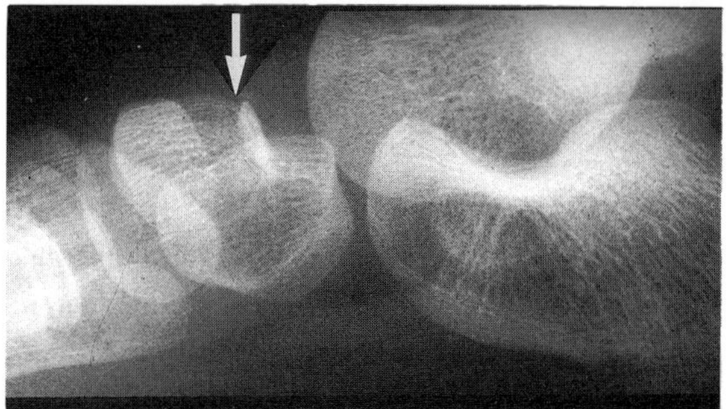

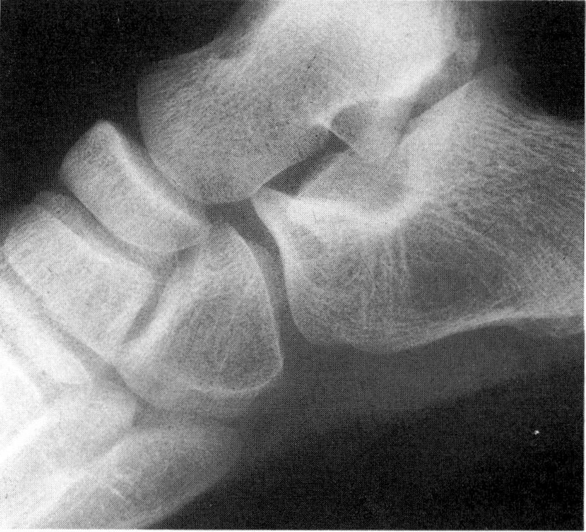

Fig. 16.7 Köhler's disease. (a) Collapse with sclerosis of the navicular (arrow); (b) fully healed 2 years later.

Freiberg's disease

This presents with metatarsalgia and tenderness localized to the second or third metatarsophalangeal joint. Radiographs of the foot show widening of the distal metaphysis with a concave depression and collapse of the metatarsal head. There is usually either a history of trauma or the second toe is found to be longer than the first, which predisposes the metatarsal head to repeated minor trauma. Treatment is symptomatic through use of a stiffened sole or a metatarsal bar. Secondary degenerative changes are common and in the adult can be relieved by excision of the metatarsal head.

Osteochondritis dissecans

In this condition a small piece of articular cartilage and underlying bone separates from a joint surface. The fragment usually remains *in situ* but eventually may separate as a loose body. Its aetiology is known though, as with the other osteochondritides, a combination of ischaemic, traumatic and genetic factors is implicated. The knee is most commonly involved but the elbow, ankle and hip may also be affected.

The knee

Osteochondritis dissecans of the knee most commonly affects the lateral aspect of the medial femoral condyle inferiorly (Fig. 16.8) or posteriorly, though it occurs occasionally over the anterior part of the condyle. It presents predominantly in boys over a wide range of ages (7–25 years) with a peak aged 15–16. Because symptoms are vague, usually discomfort on activity and episodes of swelling and giving way, radiographs are essential in most cases of knee pain in order not to miss the occasional case of osteochondritis dissecans amongst the large numbers with anterior knee pain. The patella is also rarely affected with osteochondritis dissecans, presenting as for anterior knee pain.

Clinical examination reveals only quadriceps wasting and possibly localized tenderness over the medial femoral condyle or patella.

Where osteochondritis dissecans is suspected, four-view radiographs of the knee (anteroposterior, lateral, skyline patellar and tunnel views) should be taken. If osteochondritis dissecans is found in one knee the other should also be radiographed.

Treatment should be conservative with marked restriction of activity or occasionally use of a weight-relieving splint for severe symptoms. If the fragment has already separated the loose body is removed arthroscopically. In these circumstances the crater is usually well-healed with fibrocartilage but if the edges of the crater are seen to be unstable they should be trimmed back while any raw bone should have multiple fine drill holes made to encourage growth of fibrocartilage. Persisting symptoms and lack of evidence of healing over 1–2 years on radiographs warrants arthroscopic examination. If the fragment can be flipped in and out of place, removal of fibrous tissue to reveal bone on both surfaces, insertion of cancellous bone graft and fixation of the replaced fragment with a Herbert screw or Smillie pins may allow healing to proceed. An area of depressed discoloured articular cartilage which is otherwise intact can be treated with multiple fine drill holes

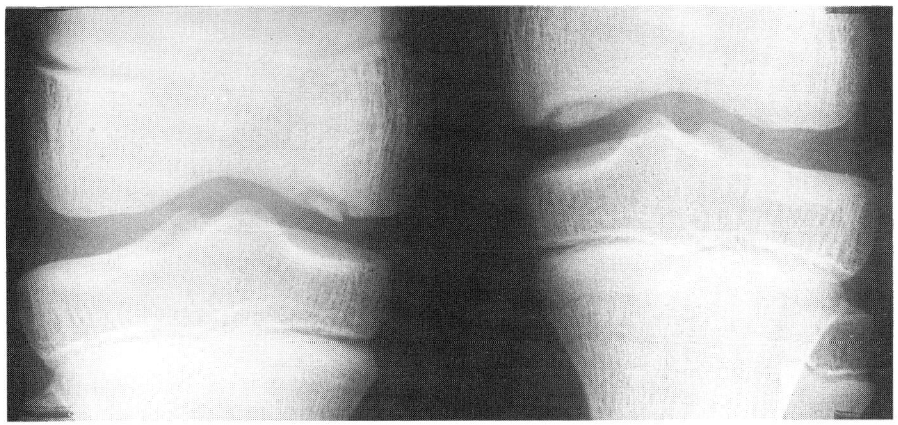

Fig. 16.8 Osteochondritis dissecans of the knees. The inferolateral aspects of both medial femoral condyles are affected.

to encourage revascularization. Osteochondritis dissecans of the patella requires only removal of any loose bodies and drilling of the defect.

The elbow

Osteochondritis dissecans of the elbow is rare and involves the capitulum. It presents usually in boys aged 10–20 years with symptoms of pain, clicking, locking and loss of extension in the elbow. There may be a relationship with trauma, especially racket games and karate, but since both elbows are frequently involved the significance of such trauma is unclear.

Removal of any loose bodies is the only treatment required.

The ankle

Osteochondritis dissecans of the ankle occurs at the medial corner of the apex of the dome of the talus (Fig. 16.9). It presents with pain, swelling and clicking of the ankle. Treatment is primarily conservative with restricted activity or occasionally a below-knee plaster. Persisting symptoms require removal or reattachment of the fragment but since the surgical approach involves a medial malleolar osteotomy, it must await closure of the distal tibial epiphysis.

The hip

This rare condition presents between 10 and 14 years with hip pain and a limp. Radiographs reveal a translucent area with a central avascular fragment in the weight-bearing zone of the femoral head. Treatment initially is by bed rest and relief from weight-bearing by crutches or a calliper, but if symptoms persist exploration through a posterior approach to remove or drill the fragment may be required.

Transient synovitis

Transient synovitis is a common condition. It usually affects the hip though other joints, such as the knee or ankle, may rarely suffer short-lived episodes of pain and swelling mimicking transient synovitis of the hip. It presents between the ages

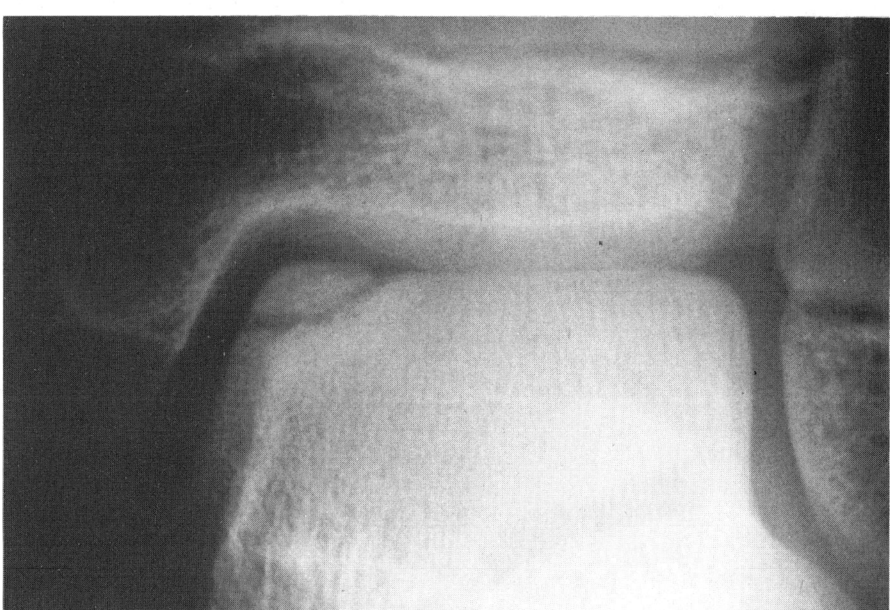

Fig. 16.9 Osteochondritis dissecans of the talus. The medial corner of the superior talar surface is affected.

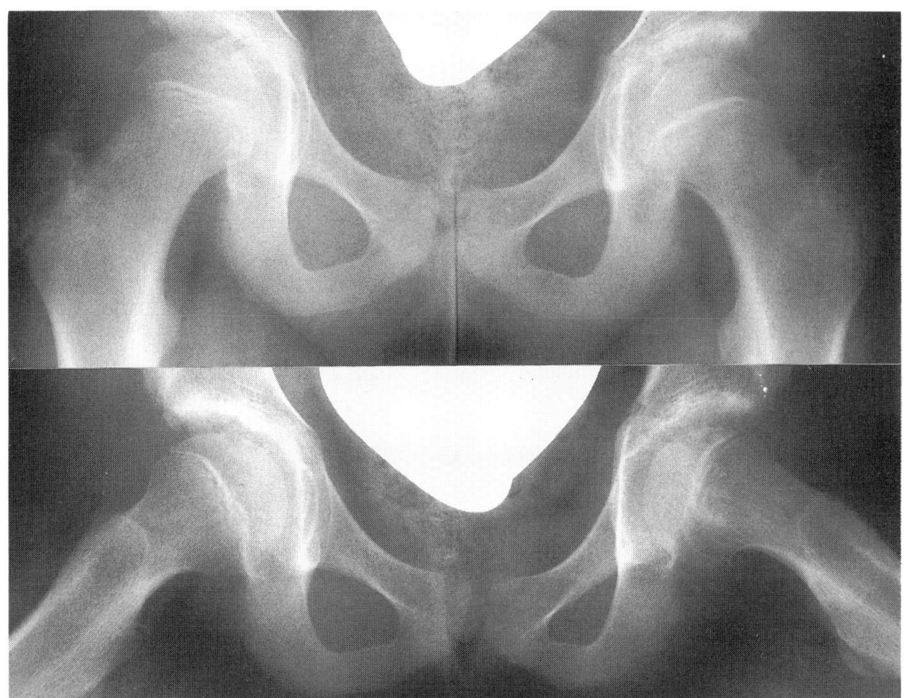

Fig. 16.10 Slipping capital femoral epiphysis. *Top*: Anteroposterior view, which appears normal. *Bottom*: Lateral view, showing a mild chronic slip of the left hip.

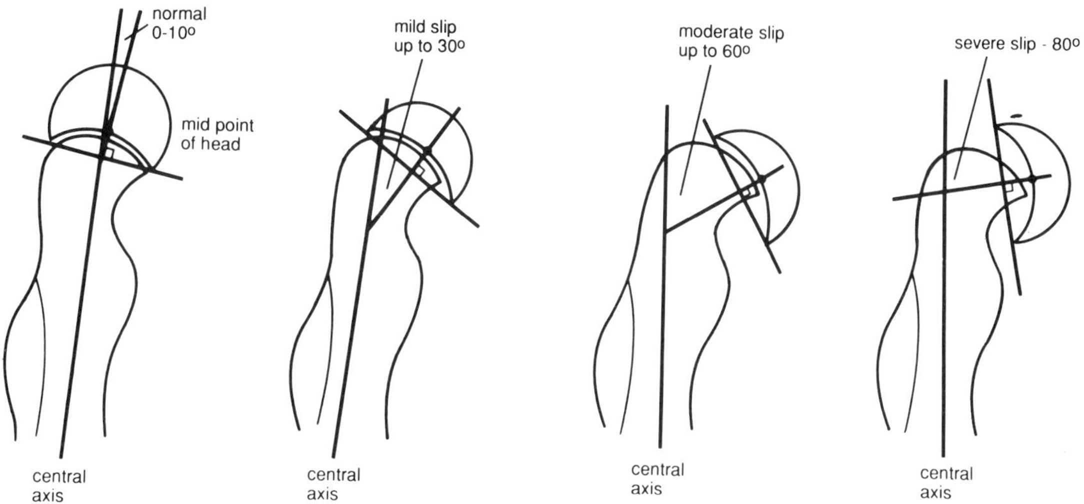

Fig. 16.11 Measurement of the degree of slip. The angle between a line drawn at 90° to the margins of the head and the femoral shaft axis gives a measure of the degree of slip.

Operative technique

The anaesthetized child is placed on a fracture table with the affected leg in slight abduction and neutral or slight internal rotation. The other leg is fully abducted and flexed to allow image intensifier screening of the hip in the anteroposterior and lateral planes. A lateral incision is made over the greater trochanter and with X-ray guidance two or three pins of the appropriate length are introduced via the lateral cortex across the physis into the femoral head.

The procedure becomes progressively more difficult as the degree of slip increases. By placing the entry point anteriorly on the trochanter or even on the base of the femoral neck anteriorly it is usually possible to achieve a satisfactory disposition of the pins. It is important not to transgress the joint space. Screening the pins while moving the C-arm of the intensifier through 90° allows them to be withdrawn sightly if necessary. Unfortunately it is often difficult to visualize the joint space well in obese patients and the use of plain X-rays or the finding of free hip movement without grating may be required to confirm proper pin placement. After closure of the wound the patient is nursed free in bed. Mobilization on crutches can be commenced at 48 hours, increasing from partial to full weight-bearing as symptoms allow. Radiographs of both hips should then be taken at intervals of 3–4 months to detect slip of the other hip or 'growing off' the pins of the affected hip. The pins should be removed once the growth plate has closed.

The treatment of severe degrees of slip and moderate slips where little remodelling can be expected is more difficult. Correction of the deformity at its site of origin is associated with an appreciable risk of avascular necrosis of the femoral head. On the other hand leaving the deformity by fixing the head *in situ* or attempting correction by subtrochanteric or intertrochanteric osteotomy leaves unchanged the intra-articular incongruity. The result is inevitably early osteoarthritis, whose treatment by total hip replacement may be compromised by the deformities produced by more distal osteotomies. The modification of cervical osteotomy described by Clarke and Wilkinson (1990) is claimed by the authors to produce good correction with an acceptably low rate of avascular complications.

Where the risks of complication are considered excessive or if the physis is already closed, the range of hip movement can be usefully increased by excising the anterosuperiorly projecting 'knob' of femoral neck (Heyman *et al.*, 1957).

Anterior knee pain or chondromalacia patellae

Chondromalacia patellae occurs in adolescents between 13 and 19 years with the characteristics of anterior knee pain and crepitus aggravated by prolonged sitting or holding the knee in flexion. Approximately 7% of schoolboys and 19% of schoolgirls complain of such symptoms (MacKechnie–Jarvis and Boobbyer, 1984). These authors noted an association between chondromalacia patellae and persistent femoral anteversion which was not confirmed by Fairbank *et al.* (1984), who found only that those with chondromalacia patellae enjoyed sport more than asymptomatic children. Sport may be the significant factor since it was mentioned earlier that many children with persistent femoral anteversion are good at and enjoy sport.

Goodfellow (1984) considers chondromalacia patellae a misleading term because 'surface degeneration of the patellar cartilage, particularly of its medial facet, is a common disorder, even in youth' and 'progresses, in extent and in severity, throughout life and is almost universal in old age'. Furthermore arthroscopy of patients with chondromalacia patellae demonstrates normal articular cartilage in about half the knees with only minor changes in the rest, suggesting that these changes are incidental rather than causative. The term 'anterior knee pain' is therefore preferable and will be used henceforth.

Anterior knee pain can be divided broadly into two groups: the majority, with normal articular cartillage, who are probably exceeding their patella's capacity to resist the forces applied to the knee through overuse; and the rest who have some underlying abnormality such as lateral subluxation, a flexion contracture or tight hamstrings. The former require no more than careful clinical examination and standard radiographs before being advised of the benign nature of the condition. Thus Goodfellow (1984) found that, of a group of patients with anterior knee pain followed up for 5–8 years, 94% still had pain but 45% had less pain and only 13% required analgesics. Most only had pain once or twice a week. Surgical treatment of this type of anterior knee pain has no rationale and may make matters worse. The following advice helps to minimize symptoms:

1. *Static quadriceps exercises.* These help by reducing the risk of a fall, which will further aggravate anterior knee pain since giving way of the knee is a common symptom with anterior knee pain. Muscle wasting and weakness secondary to the pain may give rise to aching in the muscles, which in turn produces further wasting and weakness and can be overcome by increasing quadriceps muscle bulk and power.
2. *Straight leg sitting to relax the patellofemoral joint.* The question as to why one knee is more painful that the other is often raised. Possible explanations include leg dominance, minor differences in the anatomy of the two knees or the direction in which the legs are crossed. Whatever the explanation it is clear that the degree of patellofemoral contact and forces are minimized by the legs-extended position.
3. *Avoidance of activities which cause most pain.* These commonly include squatting, kneeling, climbing and descending stairs, hill-walking and jogging. However, joints are designed to move and require exercise for proper development and nourishment. Pain is protective and limits activity, thereby preventing damage to the joint. I, therefore, encourage children to undertake any activity they wish so long as they can tolerate the pain and the balance of pleasure to pain is positive.
4. *Weight reduction where applicable.* Because of the anatomy of the knee, the patellofemoral joint is subject to forces many times body weight during vigorous activity. Minimizing body weight will obviously minimize these forces.
5. *Analgesia.* Since pain will occur despite the above advice, parents should have a supply of simple analgesics or mild non-steroidal anti-inflammatory drugs (e.g. ibuprofen) available for use when the pain is severe or before undertaking an activity which usually brings on the pain (e.g. a long car journey).

For the group of patients whose anterior knee pain is secondary to an underlying abnormality, treatment is of the underlying problem. Thus patellar subluxation requires vastus medialis exercises, or lateral release and/or medial plication with medial transfer of the lateral half of the patellar tendon as appropriate. Flexion contractures of the knee or hip will respond to stretching exercises or appropriate tendon-lengthening surgery.

Popliteal cysts

Popliteal cysts are common in children, with a male preponderance. Most arise before age 7 in the region of the semimembranosus/gastrocnemius or semitendinosus tendons. They comprise simple cysts of synovial tissue containing viscous synovial fluid. Most are painless and present as a noticeable lump in the popliteal region just distal to the transverse skin crease. The swelling is often more prominent after exercise and shrinks with rest. Dinham (1975) found that 51 of 70 popliteal cysts treated conservatively disappeared within an average of 20 months. Of 50 cysts treated surgically, 21 recurred, some more than once. It seems sensible, therefore, to offer no treatment, expecting natural resolution of most popliteal cysts. Where there are significant symptoms, the cyst may be excised but patients should be warned of the high risk of recurrence.

Mensical injuries

Symptomatic meniscal injuries are rare in children. When they occur the greater vascularity of a child's meniscus, especially in its peripheral third, makes repair of the structure more likely to succeed. Since meniscectomy may result in persisting symptoms in 58% of children and produce radiographic changes in as many as 73% (Zaman and Leonard, 1978), every effort should be made to preserve a meniscus damaged by trauma.

Meniscal symptoms may also arise from a

discoid lateral meniscus. This rare entity was thought by Smillie (1948) to represent persistence of the disc-shaped meniscus present at birth, but Kaplan's explanation (1957) that these menisci merely have abnormal peripheral attachments now seems more acceptable. Two types of discoid meniscus exist: one type has a peripheral attachment to the capsule and the other is attached only via Wrisberg's ligament. Discoid menisci are also thickened and thus lack suppleness, which makes them more prone to tears. Treatment of a discoid meniscus is by partial or total lateral meniscectomy.

Juvenile chronic arthritis

The childhood inflammatory arthropathies have become increasingly complex as additional subgroups are identified. The differing clinical presentations, immunology and epidemiology of these subgroups suggest more than one aetiology for juvenile chronic arthritis (JCA), though none has been fully elucidated. JCA can also be stimulated by numerous other conditions which include transient synovitis, bone and joint sepsis, leukaemia and the rheumatic disorders of systemic lupus erythematosus, rheumatic fever, dermatomyositis, scleroderma and mixed connective tissue disease.

Schaller (1984) suggests a classification for JCA which has five distinct subgroups. These are listed below with their percentage incidence.

Systemic-onset disease	20%
Rheumatoid factor negative polyarticular JCA	25%
Rheumatoid factor positive polyarticular JCA	5%
Pauciarticular JCA type 1	30–35%
Pauciarticular JCA type 2	10–15%

Systemic-onset disease

This can present at any age in childhood equally in males and females, with intermittent fevers occurring once or twice daily over several weeks. The fevers are usually accompanied by a rash of 1 cm pale red maculae occurring anywhere on the body. There are associated hepatosplenomegaly and lymphadenopathy and pleuritis, pericarditis and myocarditis which are usually mild. Mesenteric adenitis may give rise to abdominal pain. Joint and muscle pains are initially only present during the fevers but gradually symmetrical multijoint arthritis develops. Iridocyclitis does not occur. Investigations almost invariably demonstrate a leukocytosis and anaemia, which may be marked. The systemic symptoms remit after several months but half the children will have later recurrences. In a quarter of cases the polyarthritis persists after remission of the systemic symptoms.

Rheumatoid factor negative polyarticular JCA

This type occurs predominantly in girls, presenting often very young, though it can occur at any age. There is a symmetrical polyarthritis, classically involving the small joints of the hands, though any joint except possibly the thoracolumbar spine may become affected. There may be mild systemic features of a low-grade pyrexia, growth retardation and a minor degree of hepatosplenomegaly and lymphadenopathy during periods of active joint disease. Iridocyclitis and pericarditis are uncommon. Investigations reveal a mild anaemia but are negative for rheumatoid factor. The majority of these children do well but in 10–15% there is severe joint destruction.

Rheumatoid factor positive polyarticular JCA

This usually occurs later in childhood in girls and mimics classical adult rheumatoid arthritis with a symmetrical polyarthritis, rheumatoid nodules, rheumatoid vasculitis, splenomegaly and leukopenia, rheumatoid lung disease and a positive rheumatoid factor on serological testing. Iridocyclitis does not occur. Over half progress to severe joint destruction.

Pauciarticular JCA type 1

Type 1 disease is seen most commonly in girls under 5 years of age. Affected joints tend to suffer little damage despite a prolonged time course. Only a few (= *pauci*) joints are involved but the hip, sacroiliac joints and spine are spared, even on long-term follow-up. However, iridocyclitis, which is usually asymptomatic, occurs in 30–35% of children and may cause permanent problems with cataract formation, secondary glaucoma or partial or total blindness. Antinuclear antibodies are present in virtually all cases with iridocyclitis. Three-monthly slit lamp examinations over the initial years of the disease are necessary to allow early diagnosis and treatment of this serious complication.

Pauciarticular JCA type 2

Type 2 disease occurs predominantly in boys older than 8 years and usually involves a small number of joints in the lower limbs, especially the hip and sacroiliac joints. In 5–10% of cases there is an acute iridocyclitis, as is seen in ankylosing spondylitis or Reiter's syndrome. A positive family history for spondyloarthropathy is common but not all these children progress to ankylosing spondylitis or other arthropathies. Possibly 10–15% of children with apparent JCA have in reality a spondyloarthritic condition such as ankylosing spondylitis, Reiter's syndrome, reactive arthritis, the arthritis of inflammatory bowel disease, psoriatic arthritis or enthesopathy (inflammation of ligament and tendon insertions with or without an associated transient arthritis) which declares itself with time.

Non-steroidal anti-inflammatory drugs such as naproxen or ibuprofen remain the mainstay of treatment for JCA. Salicylates are no longer used because of the risk of Reye's syndrome. Failure of response to adequate doses of non-steroidal anti-inflammatory drugs is an indication for use of second-line drugs such as penicillamine, antimalarials or gold. Systemic corticosteroids are sometimes necessary, especially for systemic symptoms, but should be avoided if possible for joint symptoms since they do not prevent joint destruction and have many undesirable side-effects. However, injection of triamcinolone into affected joints was found by Allen *et al.* (1986) to produce sometimes marked remission of symptoms, often for prolonged periods. The same group (Sparling *et al.*, 1990) noted no evidence that such injections caused long-term joint damage – except possibly in the case of the hip – even when multiple injections had been used. This mirrors our own experience. Iridocyclitis requires treatment with dilating agents and topical, or rarely, systemic steroids.

Physiotherapy is vital to maintain muscle bulk and joint movement and may require hospital admission for intensive treatment in severe disease. Exercises may be supplemented by night splints to help control increasing joint contractures.

Surgery has little part to play in the majority of these children, though rarely synovectomy or release of fixed joint contractures can be helpful. Severe joint destruction, particularly of the hip, occasionally warrants joint arthroplasty despite the dubious long-term prognosis of such implants. Arthrodesis of joints such as the ankle or hindfoot should be withheld until growth ceases, if possible.

Stress fractures

Stress fractures are not uncommon in children. They occur at any age. The most common site is the junction of the proximal and middle thirds of the tibia (Fig. 16.12), but the fibula, femur, pars interarticularis, metatarsals, navicular, ulna, humerus, patella, first rib, medial sesamoid and pelvis are also affected. Clinically stress fractures present with gradually increasing pain aggravated by exercise. There is tenderness localized to the affected area, accompanied on occasions by local redness and swelling.

Initially radiographs are normal since a fracture line is not often visible. At this stage diagnosis may be aided by running an ultrasound probe along the affected bone to produce typical pain as the probe

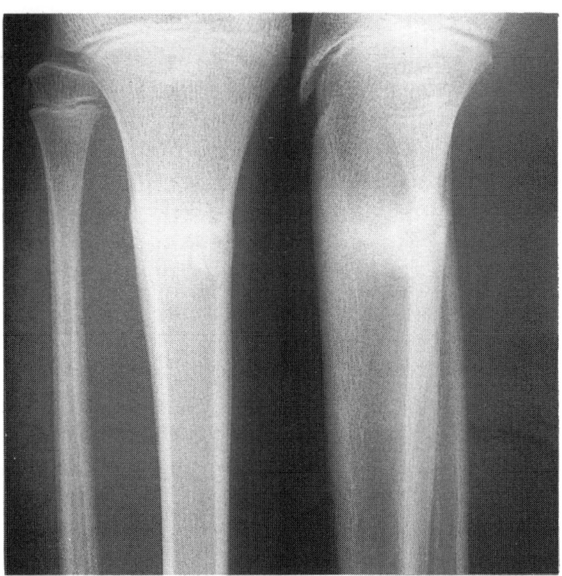

Fig. 16.12 Stress fracture of the tibia. A line of sclerosis with periosteal reaction is visible in the proximal third of a right tibia.

crosses the fracture site. Alternatively a technetium bone scan will show increased uptake in the region of the fracture. In time subperiosteal new bone forms; this may be quite florid in young children, simulating an osteogenic or Ewing's sarcoma. Since a biopsy will show active cell replication and new bone formation this may further reinforce the impression of a sarcoma in the unwary, hence the importance of recognizing the lesion for what it is.

Specific sports may be associated with particular sites of stress fracture. Thus running has produced stress fracture of the tibia, tarsal navicular and distal femur. Gymnastics and American football commonly cause stress fractures of the pars interarticularis of the lumbar spine. Distal fibular stress fractures occur in association with ice skating and ulnar fractures with tennis and volleyball. Basketball has resulted in tibial and navicular stress fractures while breast-stroke swimming has also caused a tibial stress fracture. One case of a patellar stress fracture has been reported in a soccer player. Baseball has produced stress fractures of the tibia and humerus (Yngve, 1990).

Restriction of activity is usually sufficient treatment till healing is complete, though occasionally plaster splintage is required.

Joint and bone sepsis

In Glasgow over the last 30 years the incidence of acute haematogenous osteitis of long bones has more than halved, while the frequency of infection of cancellous bones and joints has remained fairly stable. The presenting features of bone and joint sepsis seem also to be changing. Both changes probably reflect an improvement in resistance to infection as a result of better nutrition, housing and standards of hygiene.

Staphylococcus aureus remains the most commonly implicated organism for both joint and bone sepsis, though substantial numbers of cases result from *Haemophilus* (especially in neonates), pneumococcus and *Escherichia coli*.

Despite the falling incidence of long bone sepsis, osteitis still most commonly occurs in long bones with the distal femur, proximal tibia, upper end of humerus or lower end of radius being the preferred sites. There is often a history of prior minor trauma, though this is of questionable relevance, given the frequency of such trauma in children and the fact that infection of closed fractures is extremely rare. The slowing of blood flow in the sinusoidal vessels of the metaphyseal region and the presence at the junction between epiphysis and metaphysis of developing arterioles which are easily damaged by trauma may explain the predilection for bacterial emboli to cause sepsis in the metaphyseal region of long bones. Haematogenous joint sepsis may arise primarily in the joint or be secondary to spread from adjacent osteitis, especially where the metaphysis is partly intracapsular, as is the case for the proximal humeral metaphysis, all the metaphyses at the elbow, the proximal and distal femoral metaphyses and the distal ulnar metaphysis. Unless osteitis is aborted by early treatment, pus forms and finds its way through the cortex to collect subperiosteally before eventually bursting into the surrounding soft tissues and tracking to the skin to drain. The cortex, deprived of its intramedullary blood supply by pressure-induced thrombosis and of its periosteal supply by the periosteal stripping, dies and gradually separates from the surrounding living bone to produce a sequestrum. New bone laid down under the stripped off periosteum forms the involucrum. The sepsis may progress to chronic osteitis with thickened abnormal bone honeycombed with multiple small abscesses discharging through sinuses to the skin. Alternatively the sequestrum may be discharged or resorbed with complete healing. Complications of acute osteitis include septicaemia and infection of other structures or even death, or growth plate damage resulting in progressive deformity or shortening of the affected bone.

Septic arthritis, whether primary or secondary, results in production of intra-articular pus. Unless treated, this pus destroys the articular cartilage to produce fibrous or bony ankylosis.

Acute sepsis classically presents with severe pain, often of sudden onset, in the limb of a child. There is an associated pyrexia. Examination reveals swelling and reddening over the affected bone or joint. In osteitis there is exquisite tenderness over the bone while septic arthritis is identified by marked restriction of joint movement. Unfortunately, classical cases are less common these days. Often sepsis presents insidiously with poorly localized pain, refusal to walk and a low-grade pyrexia. Localization of osteitis may be difficult and on occasions requires a technetium bone scan to identify the site. In septic arthritis the degree of restriction of joint movement may not be marked. Recent administration of antibiotics for upper respiratory tract infection is not uncommon.

Investigations should include a white cell count, erythrocyte sedimentation rate, blood cultures and joint aspiration where appropriate. C-reactive protein measurements are useful when available since they begin to fall within 12–24 hours if antibiotic treatment is effective. Radiographs should be obtained to exclude other pathologies such as fracture, chronic sepsis or tumour but will be normal for the first 2 or 3 weeks in acute sepsis, apart from soft tissue swelling.

Treatment of all acute infections is by high-dose intravenous antibiotic and bed rest. Initially the antibiotic will need to be given on a 'best-guess' basis but can be changed in response to clinical progress or sensitivity results from cultures of blood or joint aspirate. If the infection has been caught before there is appreciable pus formation, this treatment may be sufficient. Where there are significant amounts of pus additional measures such as repeated joint aspiration or incision and drainage of the pus will be necessary. As pain and swelling resolve the child can be allowed to mobilize.

Antibiotics should be continued for at least 3 weeks or longer if there has been considerable bony damage. The child should not return to sport until a satisfactory range of painfree movement of the affected limb has been attained, though swimming can be encouraged from an early stage.

References

Normal variants

Coon V, Donald G, Houser C, Bleck EE (1975) Normal ranges of hip motion in infants between 3 months and 6 months of age. *Clinical Orthopaedics and Related Research* **110**, 256–60.

Fabry G, MacEwan GD, Shands AR (1973) Torsion of the femur. A follow up study in normal and abnormal conditions. *Journal of Bone and Joint Surgery* **55A**, 1726–38.

Kling TF, Hensinger RN (1983) Angular and torsional deformities of the lower limbs in children. *Clinical Orthopaedics and Related Research* **176**, 136–42.

McSweeney A (1971) A study of femoral torsion in children. *Journal of Bone and Joint Surgery* **53B**, 90–5.

Moulton A, Upadhyay SS (1982) A direct method of measuring femoral anteversion using ultrasound. *Journal of Bone and Joint Surgery* **64B**, 469–72.

Reikeras O, Bjerkreim I, Kolbenstvedt A (1983) Anteversion of the acetabulum and femoral neck in normals and in patients with osteoarthritis of the hip. *Acta Orthopaedica Scandinavica* **54**, 18–23.

Salenius P, Vankka E (1975) The development of the tibio femoral angle in children. *Journal of Bone and Joint Surgery* **57A**, 259–61.

Scrutton D, Robson P (1968) The gait of 50 normal children. *Physiotherapy* **54**, 363–8.

Sommerville E (1957) Persistent foetal alignment of the hip. *Journal of Bone and Joint Surgery* **39B**, 106–13.

Sommerville E (1977) Persistent foetal alignment of the hip. Treatment. *Acta Orthopaedica Belgica* **43**, 552–6.

Staheli LT, Lippert F, Denotter P (1977) Femoral anteversion and physical performance in adolescent and adult life. *Clinical Orthopaedics and Related Research* **129**, 213–16.

Wedge JH, Wasylenko MJ (1978) The natural history of congenital dislocation of the hip: a critical review. *Clinical Orthopaedics and Related Research* **137**, 154–62.

Feet

Berman A, Gartland JJ (1971) Metatarsal osteotomy for the correction of adduction of the fore part of the foot in children. *Journal of Bone and Joint Surgery* **53A**, 498–506.

Bleck EE (1967) Spastic abductor hallucis. *Developmental Medicine and Child Neurology* **9**, 602–8.

Bonney G, McNab I (1952) Hallux valgus and hallux rigidus. A critical survey of operative results. *Journal of Bone and Joint Surgery* **34B**, 366–85.

Browne RS, Paton DF (1979) Anomalous insertion of the tibialis posterior tendon in congenital metatarsus varus. *Journal of Bone and Joint Surgery* **61B**, 74–6.

Cockin J (1968) Butler's operation for an overriding fifth toe. *Journal of Bone and Joint Surgery* **50B**, 78–81.

Colton CL (1973) The surgical management of congenital vertical talus. *Journal of Bone and Joint Surgery* **55B**, 566–74.

Goodfellow JW (1966) Aetiology of hallux rigidus. *Proceedings of the Royal Society of Medicine* **59**, 821–4.

Helal B, Gupta SK, Gojaseni T (1974) Surgery for adolescent hallux valgus. *Acta Orthopaedica Scandinavica* **45**, 271–95.

Heyman CH, Herndon CH, Strong JM (1958) Mobilization of the tarsometatarsal and intermetatarsal joints for the correction of resistant adduction of the fore part of the foot in congenital metatarsus varus. *Journal of Bone and Joint Surgery* **40A**, 299–310.

Kessel L, Bonney G (1958) Hallux rigidus in the adolescent. *Journal of Bone and Joint Surgery* **40B**, 668–73.

Kite JH (1967) Congenital metatarsus varus. *Journal of Bone and Joint Surgery* **49A**, 388–97.

Lloyd-Roberts GC, Clark RC (1973) Ball and socket ankle joint in metatarsus adductus varus. *Journal of Bone and Joint Surgery* **55B**, 193–6.

McMaster MJ (1978) The pathogenesis of hallux rigidus. *Journal of Bone and Joint Surgery* **60B**, 82–7.

Morley AJM (1957) Knock-knee in children. *British Medical Journal* **2**, 976–9.

Piggott H (1960) Natural history of hallux valgus in adolescence and early adult life. *Journal of Bone and Joint Surgery* **42B**, 749–60.

Ponsetti IV, Becker JR (1966) Congenital metatarsus adductus: the results of treatment. *Journal of Bone and Joint Surgery* **48A**, 702–11.

Rushforth GF (1978) The natural history of hooked forefoot. *Journal of Bone and Joint Surgery* **60B**, 530–2.

Sharrard WJH (1979) *Paediatric Orthopaedics and Fractures* 2nd edn. Oxford: Blackwell Scientific Publications.

Wilson JN (1963) Oblique displacement osteotomy for hallux valgus. *Journal of Bone and Joint Surgery* **45B** 552–6.

Osteochondritis

Boldero JL, Mitchell GP (1954) Osteochondritis of the superior tibial epiphysis. *Journal of Bone and Joint Surgery* **36B**, 114–5.

Buchman J (1929) Résumé of the osteochondritides. *Surgery, Gynecology and Obstetrics* **49**, 447.

Catterall A (1971) The natural history of Perthes' disease. *Journal of Bone and Joint Surgery* **53B**, 37–53.

Catterall A (1987) Perthes' disease. In: Bennet GC (ed) *Paediatric Hip Disorders*. Oxford: Blackwell Scientific Publications, pp 141–58.

Catterall A, Pringle J, Byers PD, Fulford GE, Kemp HBS (1982) Perthes' disease: is the epiphysial infarction complete? *Journal of Bone and Joint Surgery* **64B**, 276–81.

Compere EL, Johnson WE, Coventry MB (1954) Vertebra plana (Calvé's disease) due to eosinophilic granuloma. *Journal of Bone and Joint Surgery* **36A**, 969–80.

Hall TD (1958) Osteochondritis of the greater trochanteric epiphysis. *Journal of Bone and Joint Surgery* **40A**, 644–6.

Heikkinen E, Puranen J (1980) Evaluation of femoral osteotomy in the treatment of Legg-Calvé–Perthes' disease. *Clinical Orthopaedics and Related Research* **150**, 60–8.

Quain S, Catterall A (1986) Hinge abduction of the hip. Diagnosis and treatment. *Journal of Bone and Joint Surgery* **68B**, 61–4.

Sharrard WJH (1979) *Paediatric Orthopaedics and Fractures* 2nd edn. Oxford: Blackwell Scientific Publications.

Siffert RS, Arkin AM (1950) Post-traumatic aseptic necrosis of the distal tibial epiphysis. *Journal of Bone and Joint Surgery* **32A**, 691–4.

Smith MGH (1964) Osteochondritis of the humeral capitulum. *Journal of Bone and Joint Surgery* **46B**, 50–4.

Stulberg SD, Cooperman DR, Wallensten R (1981) The natural history of Legg-Calvé-Perthes' disease. *Journal of Bone and Joint Surgery* **63A**, 1095–108.

Transient synovitis

Blockey NJ, Porter B (1968) Transient synovitis of the hip. A virological investigation. *British Medical Journal* **4**, 557–8.

Fernandez de Valderrama JA (1963) The 'observation hip' syndrome and its late sequelae. *Journal of Bone and Joint Surgery* **45B**, 462–70.

Hardinge K (1970) The etiology of transient synovitis of the hip in childhood. *Journal of Bone and Joint Surgery* **52B**, 100–7.

Kallio PE (1988) Coxa magna following transient synovitis of the hip. *Clinical Orthopaedics and Related Research* **228**, 49–56.

Svalastoga E, Kiaer T, Jensen PE (1989) The effect of intracapsular pressure and extension of the hip on oxygenation of the juvenile femoral epiphysis. A study in the goat. *Journal of Bone and Joint Surgery* **71B**, 222–6.

Slipping capital femoral epiphysis

Clarke HJ, Wilkinson JA (1990) Surgical treatment for severe slipping of the upper femoral epiphysis. *Journal of Bone and Joint Surgery* **72B**, 854–8.

Gelberman RH, Cohen MS, Shaw BA, Kasser JR, Griffin PP, Wilkinson RH (1986) The association of femoral retroversion with slipped capital femoral epiphysis. *Journal of Bone and Joint Surgery* **68A**, 1000–7.

Heyman CH, Herndon CH, Strong JM (1957) Slipped femoral epiphysis with severe displacement: a conservative operative technique. *Journal of Bone and Joint Surgery* **39A**, 293–303.

Jones JR, Paterson DC, Hillier TM, Foster BK (1990) Remodelling after pinning for slipped capital femoral epiphysis. *Journal of Bone and Joint Surgery* **72B**, 568–73.

Knees

Dinham JM (1975) Popliteal cysts in children. The case against surgery. *Journal of Bone and Joint Surgery* **57B**, 69–71.

Fairbank JCT, Pynsent PB, Van Poortvleit J, Phillips H (1984) Mechanical factors in the incidence of adolescent patello-femoral pain. *Journal of Bone and Joint Surgery* **66B**, 279–80.

Goodfellow JW (1984) Chondromalacia patellae: a mythical disease? *Journal of Bone and Joint Surgery* **66B**, 455–6.

Kaplan EB (1957) Discoid lateral meniscus of the knee joint: nature, mechanism and operative treatment. *Journal of Bone and Joint Surgery* **39A**, 77–87.

MacKechnie-Jarvis A, Boobbyer GN (1984) Chondromalacia in adolescents: its relationship to limb maltorsion in 692 knees. *Journal of Bone and Joint Surgery* **66B**, 279.

Smillie IS (1948) The congenital discoid meniscus. *Journal of Bone and Joint Surgery* **30B**, 671–82.

Zaman N, Leonard MA (1978) Meniscectomy in children: a study of 59 knees. *Journal of Bone and Joint Surgery* **60B**, 436–7.

Juvenile rheumatoid arthritis stress fractures

Allen RC, Gross KR, Laxer RM, Malleson PN, Beauchamp RD, Petty RE (1986) Intra-articular triamcinolone hexacetonide in the management of chronic arthritis in children. *Arthritis and Rheumatism* **29**, 997–1001.

Schaller JG (1984) Chronic arthritis in children. *Clinical Orthopaedics and Related Research* **182**, 79–89.

Sparling M, Malleson P, Woods B, Petty RE (1990) Radiographic follow up of joints injected with triamcinolone hexacetonide for the management of childhood arthritis. *Arthritis and Rheumatism* **33**, 821–6.

Yngve DA (1990) Stress fractures in the pediatric athlete. In: Sullivan JA, Grana WA (eds) *The Paedriatric Athlete*. American Academy of Orthopaedic Surgeons Seminar pp 235–40.

17

Rehabilitation

H. C. Burry

Definition

Rehabilitation can be considered to be the restoration of the damaged individual to the fullest functional status that can be attained taking into account the extent of the disease or trauma that has caused the damage. It is important to distinguish *impairment*, which is the loss of physical, physiological, cognitive or psychological function from *disability*, the loss of ability to perform an activity and *handicap* which is the loss of ability to perform a role or roles in society. Thus a concert pianist may have a finger amputated (impairment), is consequently unable to produce the rapid depression of piano keys and combinations of keys required in expert performance (disability), and is therefore unable to continue a career as a concert performer (handicap).

Rehabilitation is the process of containment of the impairment which leads to disability, or in a case of established impairment, the limitation of consequent disability.

It is important to realize that medical and surgical care cannot be neatly separated from rehabilitation either conceptually or practically. Thus the process of rehabilitation must commence on the first day of treatment. It must encompass not only the physical but also the psychosocial and vocational aspects of the problem. Therefore rehabilitation is not merely the management of the injured part – it is the management and ultimate restoration of the whole person.

Rehabilitation – the process

It is important to bear in mind the fact that the rehabilitation process commonly requires a number of persons to work together to solve a multi-faceted problem. Thus there are three essential principles of rehabilitation to bear in mind. They are communication, co-ordination and co-operation. If communication is not excellent between the various professionals, if their efforts are not co-ordinated by some defined mechanism and if any of the persons involved fails to co-operate with the others then a fourth 'C' will prevail – chaos!

The process demands normal management principles:

1. Evaluation of the problem – what is wrong?
2. Identification of realistic objectives – what needs to be done?
3. Construction and adoption of strategic plan – how to reach the goal?
4. Implementation of the plan.

Rehabilitation – the players

As noted above, rehabilitation commences properly with the acute management of the illness or injury. The acute physician or surgeon may well involve a rehabilitation consultant at an early stage and may require assistance also from other medical specialists. Depending upon the nature of the case various health professionals may become involved e.g. nurses, physiotherapists, occupational therapists, speech pathologists, psychologists, psychiatrists, podiatrists, prosthetists and social workers. Frequently in complicated cases, particularly where there are complex social and vocational issues, a person who can act as 'fixer' or 'facilitator' will be an invaluable member of the team.

The important role of X-ray and other imaging techniques in diagnosis and assessment of progress is described in Chapter 8.

Rehabilitation – the instruments

A full discussion of all the pharmaceutical, physical and psychological agents and techniques that might be employed in the rehabilitation of persons with soft tissue lesions is not appropriate in this text and only a few particularly important aspects will be touched upon.

Pharmaceutical compounds

Non-steroidal anti-inflammatory drugs (NSAIDs)

Painful soft tissue lesions usually present an element of inflammation. The inflammation may be unhelpful in the healing process, e.g. excessive or causing considerable pain which limits functional use of the part. Such inflammation may obstruct appropriate exercise regimes from being instituted. A large number of NSAIDs are available. They have some variation in therapeutic effect and mode of administration. Some are short-acting and must be given three or four times daily to achieve adequate tissue concentration levels but others are very slowly cleared from the body and may be administered once daily. The chief advantage of the slow-acting drugs is greater compliance but this must be balanced against the theoretical enhanced risk of toxic reactions, since it will be some time after the onset of the toxic reaction before the drug is cleared from the system. NSAIDs have a role in the management of acute sprains, tenosynovitis, enthesopathies, painful low back and neck syndromes and occasionally in the management of diffuse painful conditions such as fibromyalgia syndrome.

The use of NSAIDs may be associated with side-effects and toxic reactions. Most common amongst these are irritation of the gastrointestinal tract with the prospect of gastrointestinal bleeding and ulcerogenesis, skin rashes and rarely renal complications. They are also hazardous when used to treat persons who suffer from asthma and in other situations where concomitant use of other drugs may lead to competition for serum protein binding sites, e.g. anticoagulants. Thus the decision to prescribe NSAIDs should be made in consultation with the patient, and only after careful consideration of the likely benefits as opposed to the possible dangers.

Psychotropic agents

Drugs such as diazepam which produce muscle relaxation are used occasionally in conditions associated with acute spasm and more commonly to treat disorders akin to the fibromyalgia syndrome. It is likely that their action in these disorders is more due to a central sedative action than to direct effects on muscle motor units. Small doses of antidepressants are sometimes prescribed in a single evening dose in an attempt to improve sleep patterns in sufferers from fibromyalgia.

The use of corticosteroids

Corticosteroids are the most potent anti-inflammatory agents available. Used systematically in high dose they produce a large spectrum of clinical effects, not all of which are advantageous to the subject.

It is unusual for soft tissue disorders to necessitate the use of systemic corticosteroids. One exception might be the early inflammatory phase of adhesive capsulitis of the glenohumeral joint (frozen shoulder). Injections of corticosteroid accurately placed into localized lesions such as inflammatory enthesopathies (e.g. epicondylitis, plantar fasciitis), tendon synovial sheaths, bursae, trigger points and in some circumstances persistently inflamed joints may produce a dramatic reduction in inflammation with consequent relief of pain and restoration of function.

It is known that local corticosteroid injections have some actual or potential harmful effects, e.g. local skin atrophy and tissue necrosis at the site of injection. There is a substantial risk of tendon rupture after intratendinous injection. For this reason, corticosteroid should never be injected into tendons, but may be used by injection into the space between the parietal and visceral layers of a tendon sheath. The risk of introduction of infection is a further hazard. It has been suggested that intra-articular corticosteroid injection leads to loss of articular cartilage and osteonecrosis but a controlled study in primate joints did not support this contention (Gibson *et al.*, 1976).

When local infiltrations are carried out, a high concentration of corticosteroid can be delivered to the site of injury, providing a dramatic effect. As noted above, the effect however is not only to suppress inflammation; local necrosis can also be expected. This must be borne in mind when consideration is being given to using this form of therapy. In some cases where recovery is being delayed by the persistence of a small, painful, well-defined focus in a damaged muscle, ligament or tendon attachment, and local massage and remedial exercises have not been able to overcome the problem, progress may well be accelerated by an accurate local infiltration. If localization is precise, tenderness and pain will be abolished. The main advantage of using local anaesthetic as a diluent is that it provides a check on the accuracy of both the diagnosis and the injection placement.

Nerve blocks and epidural injections

Regional pain syndromes and pain associated with nerve root compression are often managed with various types of injection therapy. Many techniques have been described (Cousins and Bridenbaugh, 1988). The objective may be reduction of inflammation by injection of corticosteroid, temporary nerve block by use of local anaesthetic or nerve ablation by use of phenol or other toxic substance. Epidural injections of corticosteroid have been shown to be effective in the management of sciatica syndrome but recently concern has been expressed at a possible connection between a long-acting corticosteroid preparation and arachnoiditis with or without paralysis and other hazards (Nelson, 1989). Other injections have been aimed at the zygapophyseal joints and their nerve supply. Because of the proximity of vital structures it is essential that any manoeuvre involving the use of toxic substances should be carried out under X-ray control.

Apart from therapeutic effects, local anaesthetic injections into ligaments and small joints of the spine can be a useful aid in diagnosing the source of obscure pain.

Rubifacients

Various types of emollient and counterirritant have been used for many years in the management of rheumatic complaints. Old favourites include oil of wintergreen (methyl salicylate), turpentine and capsicum but more recently corticosteroids and NSAIDs have been advocated. A use has also been suggested for thrombolytic agents. Although there is little evidence that the topical use of these agents has any beneficial pharmacological effect, and good reason to suppose that they could not exert any local effect except on the skin and subcutaneous tissue, nevertheless such applications frequently seem to induce consumer satisfaction and almost certainly do no harm.

Physical therapy

Exercise

Therapeutic exercise – particularly hydrotherapy – are the mainstays of the management of soft tissue injury. Exercises may be designed to enhance muscular strength, endurance, elasticity or speed of contraction. Various types of exercise can be employed, including isometric (contraction without movement), isotonic (constant load throughout movement) and isokinetic (equal velocity of displacement throughout). Both concentric (muscle shortens during contraction) and eccentric (muscle lengthens during contraction) exercise schedules can be employed. Eccentric exercises are associated with greater power production but are known to cause significant degrees of muscle damage in some cases (Friden *et al.*, 1983). Different effects can be obtained by varying the load or resistance, the number of repetitions, the velocity of movement and the arc through which the joint moves. It is also possible to identify weakness of a particular muscle and prescribe specific exercises to rectify the imbalance (Saal, 1988).

Hydrotherapy is particularly effective in encouraging increased range of movement in the presence of stiffness and pain.

The opposite to exercise therapy – relaxation therapy – also has a place in the management of soft tissue syndromes, most particularly fibromyalgia. The Alexander technique and Feldenkrais are two regimes currently in vogue. Biofeedback may be a useful adjunct to relaxation therapy.

Manipulation and mobilization

Manipulation was first employed in the times of Hippocrates. Modern manipulative techniques became more well-known in the latter part of the 19th century and chiropractic, osteopathy and more recently physiotherapeutic techniques are now widely employed not only for the management of spinal disorders but also for the treatment of peripheral joints and soft tissues (Maitland and Corrigan, 1983).

The precise genesis of back pain remains shrouded in mystery in the majority of patients. It is not surprising therefore that it has been hard to discern which patients will derive benefit from mobilizing or manipulative techniques. Evidence of efficacy and definition of the group of patients most likely to benefit have proved elusive (Moritz, 1979).

Electrotherapy

A large number of devices and techniques have been described and many are still used. The biological effects of ultrasound are better known than most other physical modalities of therapy (see Chapter 8). It remains a matter for conjecture whether many of the modalities actually improve the rate of healing either due to inherent biological effects or by placebo. More work is needed to provide validation of these expensive therapeutic techniques.

Splints and supports

A number of different materials and appliances are available for providing support to soft tissues and joints. Unfortunately, splints decrease mobility and immobility may be an important factor in the genesis of reflex sympathetic dystrophy. Therefore immobilizing splints should be avoided in persons suffering from regional pain syndromes. Players and athletes apparently derive benefit from elastic supports, e.g. applied to the muscle of the forearm in the case of lateral epicondylitis or to the calf or thigh in the case of lower limb muscle strains and tears. It is not clear whether this support is physiological or psychological.

Podiatry has produced many benefits for the sufferer from pain in the foot and leg. Over the ages there has been a tendency to neglect the feet, particularly postural aspects of foot function. However, it is now clear that conditions such as the pronated forefoot, valgus and varus hind-foot, short first metatarsal and tarsal bars are the cause of much discomfort and may be associated with stress fractures. Interest in the subject and improved knowledge have been inadvertently accelerated by the endurance runners who may place each foot on the ground 50 000 times in a single week in the course of their training! Consideration of technique in athletes and swimmers is essential to an understanding of the nature and pathogenesis of soft tissue pain in these at-risk groups, in which even a trivial fault will be multiplied by overuse.

Psychology and psychiatry

Across the whole spectrum of disorders of the soft tissues lies the shadow of psychological and psychiatric disturbances. The word 'shadow' is used advisedly because the interface between psyche and soma is poorly understood and the cause of much difference of opinion and dispute. Some situations are easy to understand; for example, the anxiety of an élite athlete struck down with an injury during a period of intense build-up, or the child athlete suffering from the 'ugly parent syndrome'. Other clinical situations associated with chronic pain syndromes commonly obscured by issues of compensability are a morass and will be considered further later in the chapter. Suffice to say, failure to recognize pain as a somaticization disorder leads to many ill-conceived physical and surgical interventions and horrendous long-term results.

Ergonomics

Poor posture is increasingly recognized as a cause of chronic pain. Poor posture may be inherent in the individual or forced upon him or her by the nature of a work activity or station, by poorly designed seating and even by unsatisfactory beds. It is now known that maintenance of a posture by static contraction of muscle groups may at first lead to discomfort and later to pain which may not resolve when the strain is relieved.

Injury prevention

Stemming from a knowledge of the ergonomics of an activity is the opportunity to study the workplace furniture and sporting techniques to uncover initiatives that can be taken to prevent injury. Unfortunately there is a tendency for the population to regard safety as boring, leading to a general disinclination to be involved in either funding or participating in safety programmes.

The spectrum of soft tissue disorders

Disorders of the soft tissues encompass such a large number of conditions ranging from acute injury to chronic pain syndromes that it is not practicable to describe rehabilitation programmes for all in this text. In planning a programme there are four major considerations.

1. The physical status of the patient – age and physical fitness.
2. The psychological status.
3. The hopes and aspirations – for instance, a world-class marathon runner restored to within 1% of normal functioning will none the less be approximately a quarter of a mile behind his or her expected position at the finish of the race. Thus 99% is not good enough. On the other hand, an older recreational player may well be delighted to be restored to within 1% of normal functioning. Such consideration must always be taken into account when the treatment plan and objectives are under consideration.
4. The nature of the tissue. Muscle has good blood supply, can be actively exercised and heals quickly, but tendons have poor blood supply with consequent uncertain healing capacity. Effort should be directed to increasing blood flow by suitable exercises, but increased tension, which decreases blood flow in tendon, should be minimized.

It should also be borne in mind that fractures are accompanied by disruption of the soft tissues, and it is the latter that are often the site of persistent pain and dysfunction following union of the fracture.

Examples of rehabilitation programmes

In order to illustrate the principles of rehabilitation two examples have been chosen. The first outlines the procedures adopted in the management of an acute traumatic event, the second the approach to the more complex problem of a regional pain syndrome.

Example 1 – Acute trauma

A player has received a blow on the anterior aspect of the thigh. He is assisted off the field. Induration is already present in the quadriceps muscle, knee flexion is limited to 90° by pain and there is difficulty in active extension of the knee joint because of pain and weakness. Partial rupture of the quadriceps muscle is diagnosed and management in the acute stage is instituted as described in Chapter 3. It is important to realize that the rehabilitation phase will be greatly affected by the success of the management of the acute phase and in particular the attempts to limit the size of the haematoma.

Treatment plan

Objectives

1. Reduce pain.
2. Reduce muscle spasm.
3. Limit haematoma.
4. Accelerate haematoma resorption.
5. Assist and control scar tissue formation and remodelling, attempting to avoid the known complications listed in Table 17.1 (Burry, 1978).
6. Restore range of movement in hip and knee joints.
7. Restore all aspects of muscle function – strength, endurance, elasticity and speed.
8. Maintain cardiorespiratory fitness.
9. Maintain morale.
10. Restore skills.

Table 17.1 Complications of soft tissue injury

Failure of healing process
Excessive fibrosis
Adhesions
Encysted haematoma
Organized haematoma
Calcification
Ossification
Infection
Necrosis (anterior compartment syndrome)
Compression neuropathy

Strategies

(Management of the acute phase is described in Chapter 3)

Management of the restorative phase

Exercise

Active exercises are the key to success. Exercise has a positive effect on the healing process by increasing blood flow and ensuring that as connective tissue is laid down to repair the damaged muscle, remodelling occurs. To ensure that no adhesions form to surrounding structures and that the muscle retains its normal functional length, it must be borne in mind that the maturation of fibrous connective tissue leads to an overall shortening. This could lead to restriction of the elasticity of the muscle tendon complex, predisposing to further tears when the muscle is exposed to eccentric action, particularly in the uncontrolled situation of competition. Muscles acting over two joints, such as rectus femoris, are particularly vulnerable. Exercise during the restorative phase will also prevent the loss of strength and endurance that inevitably accompany disuse. Early in the recovery process muscle contraction and lengthening will be painful. The assurance must be provided that this pain does not indicate more damage, and can be expected.

In the early phase hydrotherapy may be particularly beneficial. Heat has a sedative effect on pain receptors and reduces muscle spasm. The support of hydrostatic pressure and relief of pain and spasm enable movements to be increased in range and speed with little discomfort. In addition, exercises in the pool can be used to maintain overall fitness. While one limb is out of action the other three can be strenuously exercised either in the pool or in the gymnasium so that return to competition can be accelerated. It is essential that no sudden passive stretch is applied to the healing muscle as violent disturbance of the healing tissues may lead to the formation of myositis ossificans traumatica. This is particularly likely to occur when the muscle avulsion involves or is in close proximity to the muscle attachment to the subjacent bone.

As healing proceeds and the strength and elasticity of the damaged muscle improve, level-surface running can be commenced with speed and duration of exercise being slowly increased. During this phase it is essential that any exercise period be preceded by adequate warm-up and active stretching programmes. Only when full range of movement has been restored will it be safe to commence exercise programmes designed to enhance the velocity of contraction and eccentric power.

Other therapy
Various forms of heat-generating equipment, electrical field stimulation, ultrasound and cryotherapy can be used in the hope of accelerating resorption of haematoma and oedema, reducing inflammation, easing pain and spasm and assisting connective tissue repair. Such treatment should be seen as adjunctive rather than specific or definitive. During this phase attention must be paid also to maintenance of morale and restoration of confidence. Lack of confidence leads to inappropriate and stilted movements which in competitive play leave the player vulnerable to new injuries.

Residual small localized foci of tenderness causing pain on movement may sometimes be resolved by accurate local injection of corticosteroid and local anaesthetic. There is sometimes strong pressure on a team doctor to provide pain-relieving local anaesthetic infiltrations to enable a player to short-cut the appropriate rehabilitation phase and return to competition. The use of local anaesthetic in these circumstances is unethical and exposes the player to the risk of further damage. Such injections should never be carried out.

Accident prevention
It is important to bear in mind the possibility that an athlete has a technical fault which predisposes to injury. If this fault can be identified and eliminated by practice, repeated injuries may be avoided. A further possible cause of injury which should be considered in prophylaxis is the use of inappropriate equipment, e.g. footwear providing too little or too much adhesion to the playing surface or too little support to the ankle and foot joints.

Objective measurement of progress

Over recent years interest in muscle testing has increased with the development of technology which enables objective assessment of muscle action. The use of isokinetic dynamometry provides reproducible measurement of the power of a muscle or group of muscles expressed as torque. Units such as KinCom are capable of assessing both concentric and eccentric strength. It is therefore possible to test both the power generated by the agonist concerned in the movement as well as the eccentric function of the antagonist. Estimates can be made of the balance between strength of agonists and antagonists. Imbalance is thought to be of importance in the genesis of muscle tears.

The muscle can also be tested for endurance by setting up tasks which involve varying both numbers of repetitions and resistance loads.

Velocity of contraction can be assessed by measuring time lapse between initiation stimulus and completion of a movement. Elasticity is more difficult to assess but has a bearing on velocity.

Testing should also include an assessment of the range of movement of the joint or joints over which the muscle acts. Thus for a lesion of rectus femoris it would be appropriate to measure the range of hip extension and knee flexion together and compare the injured side with the normal. A player should not be allowed to return to competition until a full range of movement is restored.

Function should be thoroughly tested on the playing field including the following components:

1. Endurance.
2. Speed.
3. Acceleration.
4. Ability to change direction.
5. Standing jump height.
6. Ability to work against resistance, e.g. kicking a ball.

A simple test programme might include a 12 minute run, shuttle runs, standing jump test and work with a ball.

An added advantage of the fitness assessment is the boost to the confidence of the player when the test is successfully completed. This elimination of anxiety about possible break-down during the next competitive event will undoubtedly enhance performance.

Example 2 – Regional pain syndrome

A female process worker aged 39 developed pain in the right side of the neck and shoulder 6 months previously, apparently after making a sudden movement. She ceased work 1 week after the incident, returning to work 1 month later. Her condition relapsed on the first day when she resumed her normal duties. Since that time she has experienced diffuse pain mainly in the right trapezius region and her right arm feels heavy and weak. There are several tender areas in the trapezius muscle. Rotation of the cervical spine to the left is restricted by pain in the right shoulder. There are no neurological abnormalities. An X-ray of the cervical spine shows minor degenerative changes in the mid cervical region. Treatment consisting of sessions of ultrasonic therapy with massage and traction has been carried out three times weekly since the injury and she has also received treatment with several NSAIDs.

A diagnosis has been made of regional pain syndrome. Other alternative terms which might have been used are occupational overuse syndrome or repetitive strain injury. The latter term, which was coined to identify an epidemic of disability particularly amongst keyboard operators in Australia, is an unfortunate misnomer as it includes the notion of repetitive movement, strain and injury, all of which may be either absent or difficult to define. Regional pain syndrome is preferable, as it prejudges neither cause nor pathology.

Management planning

The team approach

Two very important factors must be borne in mind. The first is that duration of time of incapacity to work has an inverse relationship with the percentage chance of ever returning to the work force. Even at 6 months the chance of successful case management with resolution of symptoms and return to the workforce is as low as 20% in some systems. The need for early, efficient and effective intervention to avoid chronicity is obvious.

The second is that although many injuries resolve swiftly and with minimal intervention, it is essential to ensure adequate communication between the treating doctor, any other health professionals involved, the employer, the employee and possibly an employee's representative. If these persons do not work as a team, maintaining appropriate interchange of information and with the same goals, failure is almost inevitable.

Steps in management are as follows:

1. Define the pathophysiology of the condition.
2. Examine the psychological, social and vocational aspects of the case.
3. Define achievable goals.
4. Determine what interventions must be undertaken in order to resolve the identified problems.
5. Implement the plan.
6. Re-evaluate the situation to assess progress and, if necessary, revise long-term goals.
7. Put in place any feasible strategies which will reduce the risk of recurrence.

1. In the hypothetical case outlined above there is a lack of concordance between the nature of the trauma, the minimal physical signs of tissue damage and the degree of incapacity.

2. This discrepancy suggests that psychosocial or vocational factors are involved in the pathophysiology of the condition. The programme already undertaken has not addressed any issues other than a vague notion that the symptoms are due to primary cervical spinal dysfunction and secondary muscle involvement. A team approach is now required to analyse the case, looking for physical and emotional factors within the workplace and in the home environment that may have a bearing on the genesis of the symptoms. An assessment of the work site, to include the organization of the work station and work practices, together with organizational factors and attitudes, is essential. Commonly the precipitant to this type of regional pain syndrome is an unsatisfactory work station which requires the worker to maintain a posture involving rotation and/or side-flexion of the spine for long periods of time. The static load imposed upon the relevant muscle groups may lead to the development of diffuse or localized muscle pain, presumably of myofascial origin and possibly resulting from spasm associated with minimal damage to muscle fibres resulting from overuse.

Negotiation may be necessary with the organization to allow for improvement of the work station or work practices to eliminate postural strains and if this is not possible, work rotation may be organized. It is not uncommon for employer's representatives to fail to understand the employee's situation and misinterpret the syndrome as one of 'compensationitis'. The hostility thus engendered is countered by anger, resentment and a desire for vindication on the part of the worker. Skilled counselling by a psychologist with a thorough understanding of occupational diseases is now necessary to heal the rift between the two parties. Not uncommonly, anxiety regarding the diagnosis, the prognosis (imagined or actual), hostility of work mates, financial and compensation issues and eroded self-esteem lead to reactive depression and a psychiatric assessment may be necessary. In addition causes of anxiety and depression may be present in the non-work environment which have actually predisposed to development of problems in the workplace.

3. Realistic objectives with respect to relief of pain, restoration of movement and return to the workforce are now identified in consultation with the patient and the employer.

4. Initiatives can now be planned to achieve these objectives. They will include (a) careful explanation to the patient of the problem and the plan and appropriate physical therapy together with negotiation with the employer regarding return to work.

5. The process is commenced with all interested parties fully aware of the agreed plan.

General approach to therapy

1. Minimize passive forms of treatment, particularly those of an invasive nature. Treatment by surgical procedures or local injections or drug therapy should be delivered only to treat clearly defined and identified lesions. Well-intentioned but ill-considered surgery, such as resection of cervical ribs, release of carpal tunnel and incision of entheses, may all produce catastrophic results, reinforcing the patient's fears of an untreatable mysterious underlying pathology and leading on to other problems such as reflex sympathetic dystrophy.
2. Bear in mind that the perseverance of symptoms does not necessarily mean that the initiating pathological lesion remains.
3. Shift the responsibility for management of the pain to the patient with the therapeutic team merely providing assistance as required.
4. Ensure continuity of management by avoiding involvement of rival clinicians in a competitive situation. In general, inappropriate surgery, successive referrals and consultations providing conflicting views and opinions merely serve to heighten the patient's confusion, reduce the confidence in the competence of the professions and induce anxiety.
5. Remember that a person who has been away from the workplace for a number of months will have difficulty at first coping with a full day of physically or intellectually demanding work and a work-hardening process may be necessary before return to work takes place.

Specific treatments

Physical therapy

Exercises – exercises may be designed to provide stretching of functionally shortened muscles, to encourage relaxation, to improve posture or provide physical conditioning. Various programmes of stretching–relax regimes are available, including yoga, Alexander technique and Feldenkrais. All have their devotees and the degree of conviction of the therapist is usually an important determinant in the success of the programme. Positive reinforcement has been shown to enhance efficacy of physical therapy.

Manipulation and mobilization – the precise relationship of fibromyalgic or regional pain syndromes to possible spinal abnormality is not known. Various mechanisms have been proposed to link local and referred pain to intervertebral disc, zygapophyseal joints, ligaments and nerve radicals. Such explanations purport to provide an explanation for the undoubted success of various manipulative and mobilizing techniques.

Massage – various types of massage, ranging from effleurage to frictions, have been advocated for management of painful muscle conditions. There are no hard data to demonstrate their effectiveness.

Electrotherapy – radiant heat, microwave, shortwave diathermy, interferential, ultrasound and laser therapy have all been employed in the management of chronic pain. One of the most popular at this time is transcutaneous electrical nerve stimulation, which has the advantage that after satisfactory instruction, the patient can apply the treatment personally, thus taking charge of the treatment. Unfortunately there is little evidence that these forms of treatment produce any lasting benefit and as the provision of treatment of this nature by therapists consumes a substantial amount of health funding, properly constituted clinical trials are urgently required to verify their efficacy.

Acupuncture – this is also commonly employed, providing relief to a proportion of patients without apparently treating the underlying condition.

Infiltration of trigger points – in cases in which there is unusual presistence of symptoms apparently related to clearly defined foci of tenderness and induration in muscles, infiltration with local anaesthetic or local anaesthetic and corticosteroid will provide relief. Unless this procedure is accompanied by a full and effective treatment plan to deal with the whole problem, recurrence of symptoms after a variable interval is likely.

Psychosocial and vocational management
It is essential that the therapeutic team gain full understanding of the problem as it appears to the patient. From the patient's point of view the situation is clouded by concerns relating to diagnosis, prognosis, future employment, financial considerations and the impact of the condition on ability to carry out domestic function and recreational pursuits. The patient requires understanding, explanation and reassurance, together with a supportive attitude at the workplace. Allaying anxiety will reduce tension which may be the cause of perseverance of symptoms.

The use of a small dose of amitriptyline in the evening may improve the sleep pattern and assist elimination of muscle tension. Diazepam may be used for similar purposes, but should only be prescribed in short courses because of the risk of habituation.

6. Progress is monitored by members of the team and discussed at appropriate intervals by the team.

7. A thorough exploration of the work environment is essential. It may be that the tasks performed are almost certain to lead to recurrence of symptoms unless there is some modification of the work scene. Improvements might include the handling technique, the pressure of time constraints, or the organization of the work station with respect to positioning, lighting, etc. The repetitive strain injury epidemic in data-processing personnel in Australia provided many lessons, most especially in the importance of proper workplace organization of a preventative nature and the attitudes of work colleagues, management and unions. These may be crucial factors in a successful rehabilitation after work injury.

Alterations to work stations and work practices where indicated must be carried out or arranged prior to return to work.

Management of return to work

When a person has been unable to work for some months tolerance of the effort required to carry out a full day's activities may well be reduced. For this reason some form of 'work hardening' is appropriate. This might include simulated work at a rehabilitation centre or a graduated increase in hours at the workplace. It is important to ensure that this 'softly, softly' approach is not overdone, lest the client become unduly apprehensive about the possibility of relapse with disproportionate and unrealistic views concerning the fragility of the body system. Ideally the injured person should remain a member of the employment group throughout the rehabilitation process, reporting at the workplace at the usual time in the morning, attending treatment sessions, carrying out alternative duties and signing off in the afternoon. This approach minimizes the risk of the development of the sick person role. A responsive compensation system which provides 'make-up pay' and encourages the employer to collaborate in this way is obviously advantageous.

Conclusions

The key to successful rehabilitation of soft tissue injuries are:

1. Early intervention.
2. Accurate diagnosis of both the anatomical and the functional lesion.
3. Enthusiastic participation in an active exercise programme – move it or lose it!
4. Continuous monitoring to assess progress and adjust the programme accordingly.
5. Awareness of the psychosocial and vocational implications of soft tissue injury.
6. In complicated cases, a team approach characterized by communication, co-ordination and co-operation.

References

Burry HC (1978) Pathogenesis of some traumatic and degenerative disorders of soft tissue. *Australian and New Zealand Journal of Medicine* **8**, (suppl) 163–7.

Cousins MJ, Bridenbaugh PO (eds) (1988) Neural blockade in *Clinical Anaesthesia and Management of Pain*. Philadelphia: JB Lippincott.

Friden J, Sjostrom M, Ekblom B (1983) Myofibrillar damage following intense eccentric exercise in man. *International Journal of Sports Medicine* **4**, 170–6.

Gibson TJ, Burry HC, Poswillo D, Glass J (1976) Effect of intra articular cortico-steroid injections on primate cartilage. *Annals of Rheumatic Disease* **36**, 74–9.

Maitland GD, Corrigan B (1983) *Practical Orthopaedic Medicine*. London: Butterworths.

Moritz V (1979) Evaluation of manipulation and other manual therapy. *Scandinavian Journal of Rehabilitation Medicine* **11**, 173–9.

Nelson DA (1989) Dangers from methyl prednisolone acetate therapy by intraspinal injection. *Archives of Neurology* **45**, 804–6.

Saal JA (1988) Rehabilitation of the injured athlete. In: Delisa JA (ed) Rehabilitation Medicine. Philadelphia: JB Lippincott.

Part III

Sports Injuries

18

Risks and injuries in athletics and running

M. B. Bottomley

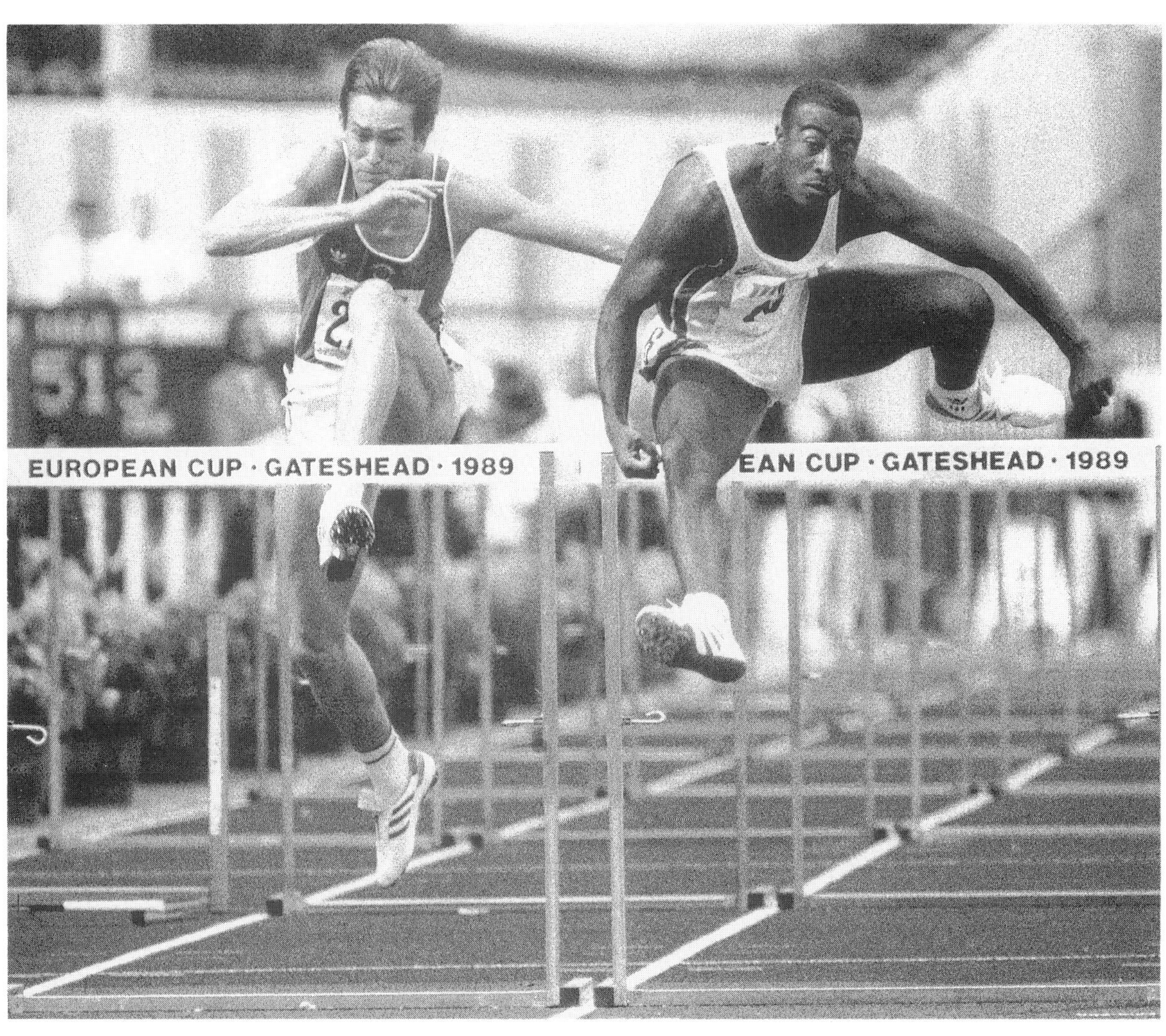

Athletic and running sports cover a wide spectrum of activity. The explosive power of the sprinting events and the tactical manoeuvring of the middle-distance races are familiar to all television viewers. The London and New York Marathons have made endurance running a popular and familiar event, easy to understand and an attainable goal to anyone prepared to spend the necessary time training.

Less well-known are the field events that are part of any athletics competition. Javelin throwers like Tessa Sanderson and Steve Backley have brought some glamour to that event, but only the most dedicated of sports followers can claim to be familiar with contests such as putting the shot, hammer and discus throwing or the pole vault. Whilst everyone has heard of Daley Thompson, few can recite, particularly in the correct order, the 10 events that make up the decathlon and fewer still are aware that a similar competition of seven events is held for women.

Race walking, orienteering, cross-country and fell running attract thousands of competitors each weekend but have little following outside their relatively small band of devotees.

There is more to athletics than merely running. The demands of an oval track put particular stresses on the body. Running long distances on hard and unyielding roads imposes different strains to which the body has to adapt. The highly technical skills of throwing and vaulting involve complicated stresses on the whole body with their own unique implications for injury. Jumping and hurdling events have their own pattern of disabilities. Crossing rough and steep countryside at speed carries the risk of injury unfamiliar to those who run on the track.

Injuries to the ankle

Lateral ligament tear

The lateral ligamentous complex of the ankle is the one which is most frequently injured. This T-shaped arrangement of ligaments runs anteriorly as the anterior talofibular ligament, posteriorly as the posterior talofibular ligament and vertically as the calcaneal ligament.

As the majority of ankle injuries happen with the foot in plantarflexion and therefore with the foot supinated and in adduction, the anterior talofibular ligament is at first risk, being parallel to the axis of the leg and at full stretch from its neutral position at right angles to the leg's axis. With further inversion the ankle becomes more dorsiflexed, thus tightening up the calcaneofibular ligament which is the next most likely to be injured. A calcaneofibular ligament tear is extremely unlikely to be an isolated injury.

The classification of ligamentous injuries depends largely on functional assessment. A type 1 injury has very little bleeding or swelling and minimal functional disability. Type 2 injuries are most commonly presented in the acute stage, with moderate to severe bruising and some functional loss. Type 3 injuries show evidence of joint instability, with the implications of total ligament rupture.

Track and field athletics does not predispose to ankle injuries since most of the activity is regular, well within the normal range of movement of the joint and controlled. Uncontrolled movement, that takes the joint to the limits of its normal range, is always possible; by slipping on the javelin run-up, by an awkward landing in hurdling or steeple chasing; by accidentally stepping on to the curb of the track, quite apart from the obvious risks in fell running or in orienteering.

The symptoms of a lateral ligament tear are immediate pain, usually with some loss of function and swelling, which may be immediate due to bleeding or delayed, caused by inflammatory oedema. There will be tenderness around the lateral aspect of the ankle, maximum over the site of injury, usually the anterior talofibular ligament.

The injured athlete should not continue to compete. Even mild first-degree sprains will have some functional instability which could lead to further damage. For the first 48 hours the basic principles of treatment of a soft tissue injury should apply – cooling, a compression bandage and elevation.

Apart from the history of how the injury happened, with particular emphasis on the loading of the ankle joint at the time and the site of maximum tenderness, it is important to try and make an assessment of the integrity of the ligaments thought to be damaged and to exclude a possible fracture by X-ray.

Tests are probably best carried out with the knee flexed and calf muscles relaxed. For the anterior drawer phenomenon the heel is grasped and drawn forward whilst opposing the movement by backward pressure on the lower leg just above the ankle. In this neutral position of the foot a movement of greater than 2 mm is considered to be suggestive of complete rupture of the anterior talofibular ligament, but an obvious increase on the injured side compared with the normal side would be significant. Increased talar tilt, apparent on forced supination of the foot by grasping the heel, will tend to show rupture of the calcaneofibular ligament if the foot is in the neutral position or of the anterior talofibular ligament if the foot is in plantarflexion. A difference of more than 10° compared with the uninjured side is significant (Lightowler, 1984).

If facilities for stress X-rays are available these tests can be quantified more easily but the amount of spasm due to pain may limit the examination and either a local or general anaesthetic may be necessary for a full evaluation.

Proprioceptive function is important in the ankle and ligamentous injury usually results in a proprioceptive loss. If the athlete is asked to stand on his or her toes, unsteadiness will show up a loss which will be equally demonstrated by a modified Romberg test, standing first with eyes open and then with eyes closed, on the injured leg.

Treatment

Once the diagnosis has been made a treatment plan has to be decided. A recovery time of between 3 and 8 weeks is reasonable: a satisfactory fitness test is essential before return to full activity. Most opinions agree that first- and second- degree tears do well with a positive rehabilitation programme of exercise, following the initial treatment aimed at limiting the extent of injury and reducing oedema. Early mobilization, with or without physiotherapy, offers the most rapid return to functional activity. Patients who have the ankle immobilized in plaster of Paris take longer to recover (Brookes *et al.*, 1981).

With third-degree injuries a similar programme of controlled exercise seems to give satisfactory results. Surgery in the acute stages of ligament rupture gives no better results than late reconstruction (Cass and Morrey, 1984). In more severe cases of ligament rupture, when the two ends of the torn ligament are grossly separated, it is unlikely to heal without surgical intervention. These will be apparent when gross instability persists after conservative treatment and the decision as to when to operate must be a matter of judgement.

The consensus is that these patients should have either plaster of Paris or adhesive strapping support with a gradual return to activity, starting with mobility exercises as soon as possible and gradually introducing weight-bearing and strengthening exercises with regular monitoring of progress. Brostrom (1966) recommends that strapping is the more favourable procedure but, if POP immobilization is used, it should be for 1–2 weeks only, longer periods not improving success.

In the earlier stages of rehabilitation the main aim is to restore a full range of movement. As the ankle improves weight-bearing is reintroduced, with particular emphasis on normal walking patterns. Exercises to strengthen the ankle through its full range of movement, such as standing on the toes and walking barefoot with the feet alternately inverted and everted, may be included as soon as weight-bearing is comfortable. A wobble-board is good exercise, providing that care is taken to avoid an excessive range of movement that may reinjure the healing tissue. The range of movement of the board helps to improve the elasticity of the healing scar and maintaining balance is a stimulus to the proprioceptive function that is vital to satisfactory recovery.

When the athlete can walk with a normal ground push-off and without a limp she or he can start to jog, at first in a straight line on a sympathetic surface like grass. When this is painfree she or he can progress to running slow zig-zags or large figures of eight. As healing progresses the speed can be increased and the angle of turns may become more acute. During this phase side step-ups, placing the injured foot sideways on a step and bringing the normal foot up to it and then reversing the process, can be introduced.

A test of recovery is when the athlete can sustain a series of shuttle runs at full speed and cover a cross-country run without pain.

If possible, rehabilitation should be a daily function. It can be supplemented by physiotherapy modalities. Anti-inflammatory drugs are most useful in the first 24–48 hours after injury, especially if used in adequate dosage, such as 1.8 g ibuprofen daily. These would not be used in athletes with a history suggestive of active inflammatory bowel disease.

Strapping is of benefit. A properly applied zinc oxide strapping can help to avoid not only an inadvertent overstretching of the damaged ligament but also, by its skin contact, it is thought to be a stimulus to proprioception (Freeman, 1965). It also helps minimize swelling.

Preventive strapping is a controversial subject. Whilst functional recovery may allow a return to normal activity, it takes 6 or 7 months for the collagen in the scar to mature fully. Taping to protect the extremes of range of movement may be helpful, particularly in those athletes such as throwers and jumpers whose ankles may be at risk (Fumich *et al.*, 1981).

In those patients who develop persistent pain over the site of the injury, local steroid injections, such as 10–20 mg triamcinolone acetonide, followed by gradual mobilization and rehabilitation as described previously, or local friction massage and mobilization, are helpful.

Plantar fasciitis

Plantar fasciitis is a common condition amongst runners, particularly those on a high weekly mileage. The plantar fascia or aponeurosis is a tough ligamentous band running from the medial tubercle of the calcaneum and branching anteriorly to blend with the ligaments of the metatarsophalangeal joints. Its main function is to stabilize the longitudinal arch of the foot, acting as a springy, rather than elastic, tie rod.

The normal gait cycle of the running foot is that heel strike occurs on the posterolateral aspect of the heel pad, the foot pronating at the subtalar joint through the mid-stance phase, with consequent flattening of the longitudinal arch and stretching of the plantar aponeurosis. Following the stance phase, the foot returns to supination to give a rigid forefoot for the final thrusting off. As the toes are bent, the aponeurosis is tensioned once more.

Pronation is a combination of dorsiflexion, eversion and abduction of the forefoot, supination being the reverse.

The two abnormalities which can cause excessive stresses on the aponeurosis are flat-footedness, which will commonly be associated with a hyperpronated foot, and a high arch, which in an extreme form would be called claw foot. A walking footprint on firm sand or of a wet foot will show the load distribution. A normal print does not show the impression of the medial longitudinal arch, but with excessive pronation the whole sole area is visible. With a high arch the impression of the lateral longitudinal arch is markedly narrowed or absent.

With a flat foot the aponeurosis is stretched to start with and the further flattening in the stance phase will impose added stresses. With a high arch the aponeurosis is short and inelastic, again leading to stresses during the gait cycle. Since, in running at relatively low speeds, when heel strike is still part of the cycle, the loads are greatly increased, an aponeurosis that can cope with walking may well break down as a result of running for endurance training.

Tight calf muscles can also contribute to plantar fascial strain by limiting the amount by which the ankle can dorsiflex, requiring more dorsiflexion of the forefoot, with consequent stretching of the aponeurosis.

The effect of repeated stretching of the plantar aponeurosis is to cause minor tearing of the periosteal insertion. Like many problems of similar cause, the injury is slow to heal, even with appropriate rest. A bony spur may be seen at the site on X-ray. This in itself is not the cause of the pain and may be seen radiologically as a chance finding in patients who have not complained of symptoms.

The symptoms of plantar fasciitis are pain at the calcaneal origin of the aponeurosis, which is worse under load and when getting out of bed, and tenderness on local pressure. The pain can be elicited by standing the athlete on tiptoe.

Treatment

The immediate treatment is rest from the activities that cause pain. Non-steroidal anti-inflammatories may be helpful and physiotherapy by ultrasound or laser is of use. A shock-absorbed heel insert, such as sorbothane, will help and a strapping to reinforce the longitudinal arch will also give relief. Those cases that do not settle with conservative treatment after a month or so may benefit from a local steroid injection, 10–20 mg triamcinolone acetonide, distributed as droplets around the tender area of the ligamentous insertion. The initial reaction will be painful for 2 or 3 days and weight-bearing may not be possible. It is important to reintroduce activities slowly and to include gentle stretching of the fascia, looking for full recovery over 2–3 weeks.

The most important aspects of rehabilitation is to try and identify and correct the possible cause of the injury. Overpronation is a common finding in plantar fasciitis and may be corrected by appropriate orthotic inserts. In view of the expense of permanent orthotics it is worth a trial of a temporary correction, using orthopaedic felt pads on a cork insole, before referring the patient to a specialist, who may be an orthopaedic surgeon or physician but is likely to be a podiatrist.

Tight calf muscles should be improved by appropriate stretching exercises.

Inadequate or inappropriate shoes may be a contributory factor. Modern sports footwear is designed to help the body deal with the immense loads created, particularly by the longer-distance running sports. During heel strike a force of 2.5–3 times the body weight is transmitted through the leg, which in a 150 lb runner can mean some 220 tons of force for every mile on the road. It is essential that the proper shoes are worn and replaced long before they are totally broken down. The efficiency of a running shoe is reduced by 23% after 150 miles and by 45% after 500 miles (McKeag and Dolan, 1989).

Morton's metatarsalgia

Morton's metatarsalgia or neuroma is characterized by a sharp burning pain to the lateral aspect of the forefoot during activity. One of the digital nerves becomes trapped between the heads of adjacent metatarsals, usually the third and fourth, and responds to repeated trauma by local swelling, causing a neuroma.

The pain is relieved by rest and, often, by removing the shoe, suggesting that the shoe is overcompressing the forefoot. There may be some flattening of the normal transverse anterior arch of the forefoot. There may be localized tenderness and the pain may be reproduced by compressing the metatarsal heads.

A small support under the toe to alter the relative alignment of the adjacent metatarsal heads may help. If there is overpronation, correction may help.

Physiotherapy aimed at local relief of inflammation, together with exercises and muscle stimulation to improve the flexors of the foot, may also be of use.

Surgical excision of the neuroma is a last resort, with the risk of resulting scar tissue causing problems postoperatively.

Shin splints

Pains in the lower leg are a frequent complaint amongst runners. Commonly referred to as shin splints, they represent a variety of overuse injuries, including compartment syndromes, stress fractures, musculotendinous and teno-osseus strains and tendinitis (see Chapter 4). Typically the pain is of insidious onset and due to repetitive stress, although it may be made suddenly worse by a particular event that represents the final straw to an overstressed tissue.

A runner takes an average of about 1500 strides to cover 1 mile and, at each heel strike, the leg and foot have to absorb a force of between two and three times the body weight. Simple overuse of body tissues unaccustomed to an activity can precipitate problems and a sudden increase in training load, perhaps to try and catch up with an absence from training due to other causes, is a common feature to the history of the injury. Athletes at the very peak of fitness tread a narrow, and difficult to define, path between peak performance and overuse.

Other causes should be looked for. minor biomechanical abnormalities of gait, for which the body can compensate at lower levels of performance, may decompensate as training loads increase. A change of training surface, perhaps from grass to the much harder road, can vastly increase the load that the soft tissues have to absorb.

Inadequate shoe wear is not always obvious. The loss of stress absorbency has been mentioned, and after 500 miles, which is 2 months' training mileage at the most for a club runner, the sole is reduced to about 55% of its original absorbency.

Medial tibial stress syndrome

The tibialis posterior arises from the upper third of the posterior surface of the fibula and interosseous membrane and the medial border of the lower third of the tibia. It acts as a plantarflexor as well as an adductor and inverter of the foot. The soleus includes the medial border of the upper tibia in its origins, together with the posterior surface of tibia and fibula. It acts, as part of the triceps surae, as an inverter and plantarflexor. Any biomechanical abnormality that either restricts or stresses the full range of plantarflexion and its associated foot inversion and adduction is likely to affect one or more of these muscles.

Medial tibial stress syndrome has been classified into three types:

1. *Type I* is where the pain and tenderness are in the tibia itself and subsequent investigation reveals a stress fracture.
2. *Type II* is where the pain and tenderness are felt along the medial border of the tibia.

   The symptoms are of insidious onset, with the pain developing increasingly earlier during exercise.

   Bone scans of runners presenting with medial tibial pain will often show inflammation along the medial border of the tibia, an area which represents the origin of the soleus. Overpronation, which involves dorsiflexion, inversion and adduction at the subtalar joint of the foot, causes overstretching of the Achilles tendon, of which the soleus tendon forms part. This excessive strain can therefore be transmitted to the origins of the soleus with resulting inflammation at the teno-osseus junction on the medial border of the tibia – a type II medial tibial stress syndrome.
3. *Type III* is the least common and presents with pain and tenderness in the muscle. It is more likely to be an acute muscle tear rather than the insidious-onset pain of types I and II.

The syndrome is common amongst distance runners and is an overuse injury. The pain is typically induced by exercise and tenderness is elicited along the medial border of the tibia. Very localized tenderness in the bone may indicate stress changes within the bone. Application of a vibrating C tuning fork over the site may provoke pain with a stress fracture and the diagnosis is confirmed by a scan.

Treatment

All three types of medial tibial stress syndrome will respond to rest, a reduction of activity to below the pain-producing threshold, and to ice. Types II and III can be treated with physiotherapy and anti-inflammatories. Overpronation will need to be corrected by the appropriate orthotics if a recurrence is to be avoided. Stretching of the posterior muscle groups should be prescribed to encourage a full range of movement.

Most cases will resolve with conservative treatment but resistant problems that have not recovered after 6 weeks or so may benefit from local steroid injection – triamcinolone acetonide 20 mg distributed in droplets in the area of tenderness – followed by total rest for several days, after which rehabilitation exercises and stretching can be started.

Achilles tendon

The Achilles tendon is formed mainly by the conjoined tendons of the gastrocnemius and soleus. The medial head fibres of gastrocnemius wind laterally through 90° as they descend to form the posterior part of the tendon. The fibres of soleus similarly rotate to form the anterior part. This spiral arrangement allows a degree of elongation and elastic recoil which helps the tendon store energy (Shields, 1982).

Gastrocnemius and soleus, together with plantaris, which is largely a redundant muscle, form the triceps surae. This group is not only a powerful plantarflexor, but has a shock-absorbing function in resisting dorsiflexion. The group acts most powerfully with the knee in extension. When the knee is flexed to a right angle, soleus is the main plantarflexor, since gastrocnemius cannot contract further.

The Achilles tendon inserts into the back of the calcaneus. There is a bursa between its deep surface and the bone and a pad of fat at the back of the heel. The tendon has no sheath but it is surrounded by adipose connective tissue from which it receives its blood supply.

A healthy tendon is immensely strong, withstanding forces of up to 2000 lb during fast running (Kulund, 1988), so that rupture is a relatively uncommon event. The tightly packed collagen fibres of the tendon receive their blood supply from vessels entering the paratenon at the teno-osseous junction and the musculotendinous junction. It is therefore the mid-area of the tendon that receives the least blood supply, this is some 2–6 cm above the insertion on the calcaneum. Increasing age does reduce the blood supply to the tendon and, despite its low metabolic rate, degeneration does occur with increasing age. It is widely held that local steroid injections also cause degeneration of the tendon with a high risk of subsequent rupture.

Injury to the Achilles tendon

Rupture therefore usually occurs in the older athlete, during sudden powerful contraction of the triceps surae, often with an audible crack and a sensation of having received a blow on the back of the heel. The definitive test is to squeeze the calf in its middle third with the muscle completely relaxed, either kneeling or prone with the feet jutting beyond the end of the couch. If the ankle fails to dorsiflex, the tendon rupture is complete. The usual rupture site is some 2 cm above the calcaneal insertion and a gap may be palpated at this point, with local swelling.

Surgical repair gives better results than conservative treatment (Shields, 1982).

If conservative treatment is to be successful the two ends, which usually tend to retract on rupture, must be opposed and the leg held in an equinus plaster for 6–10 weeks.

Rehabilitation, to restore mobility and strength, must be carefully monitored and a fitness test must be satisfactory before a complete return to sport.

The tendon can become inflamed for a number of reasons. The change from training shoes to competition spikes without heels produces an increased pull on the tendon. Too rapid an introduction to uphill running may also increase the pull. Direct trauma from too high or too hard a heel tab on the shoes will cause problems. An overpronating foot will stress the medial fibres of the tendon.

Repeated stresses produce various local or diffuse degenerations of the tendon or its surrounding tissues, resulting in adhesions between the paratenon and tendon which may eventually restrict movement (Boni *et al.*, 1985).

Treatment

The treatment of the painful Achilles tendon is in the early stages to rest from activity which provokes pain, icing and physiotherapy aimed at reducing inflammation. Gentle stretching exercises encourage the healing collagen fibres into appropriate alignment. A heel raise of about 0.5 cm will shorten the functional length of the tendon and help to relieve symptoms.

Non-steroidal anti-inflammatory drugs may be of value in the earlier stages, to limit the inflammatory reaction and restrict swelling. Local steroid injections are generally considered inadvisable, being thought to contribute to tendon rupture by their inhibition of collagen synthesis.

As the condition improves a rehabilitation programme of strength and stretching exercises is introduced. Initially, active exercise is through the range of dorsiflexion and plantarflexion without load. This is followed by heel raises and drops whilst standing on the edge of a stair, with the load being increased by holding weights as healing progresses. Most multigyms have apparatus which serves the same purpose. Static stetches will serve to improve the range of movement in muscle and tendon. As improvement progresses the tendon can be exercised on a bicycle and by gentle running with a small stride. The running is accompanied by regular stretching and the heel wedge is discarded. Speed and stride are progressively increased until the athlete can run shuttle sprints without discomfort.

Recovery may take up to 4 weeks. Athletes who do not fully recover and suffer chronic pain may need to be referred for a surgical stripping of the tendon, when areas of degenerate granulation tissue may be removed. This is followed by a full course of rehabilitation exercises.

The knee (see Chapters 5 and 13)

The knee is essentially a hinge joint between the lower end of the femur and the upper surface of the tibia. The anterior surface of the femoral condyles also articulate with the patella. The stability of the knee is maintained by the cruciate ligaments within the joint and the medial and lateral collateral ligaments. The outer border of the medial meniscus is attached to the medial collateral ligament on its deep short fibres. The superficial fibres of the medial ligament are very long and extend down to insert on the tibial shaft. Not only does the ligament resist valgus strains but it also assists the cruciates in resisting rotational movements.

In front, the capsule of the joint is formed by the patella, into the upper and lateral borders of which are inserted the fibres of the three vasti and rectus femoris muscles that make up the quadriceps group. The fibres sweep over the patella and continue as a strong tendon to be inserted into the tibial tubercle. Thin sheets of tissue anchor the sides of the patella to the medial and lateral condyles of the femur, forming the patellar retinaculum.

Posteriorly the knee has a number of overlapping structures. On the medial aspect are semimembranosus and semitendinosus. Between them pass upwards the medial and lateral heads of gastrocnemius, together with plantaris, to their insertion on the lower femur. The semimembranosus muscle gives off an extension to form the oblique popliteal ligament, which extends laterally and proximally to form part of the posterior capsule of the joint. The arcuate popliteal ligament arises from the head of fibula and extends proximally to be inserted into the posterior capsule. It is crossed by the origin of the popliteus muscle arising from the lateral femoral condyle as a tendon that passes distally, deep to the lateral ligament, to be inserted on the tibia. Superficially the biceps femoris tendon is prominent on the lateral aspect of the posterior knee as it passes to its insertion on the head of fibula.

The iliotibial band is the distal attachment of the tensor fascia lata muscle on the thigh, originating at the iliac crest and posterior sacrum. It crosses the lateral side of the knee, anterior to the lateral collateral ligament, to insert in the upper end of the tibia.

There are 13 bursae which surround the knee joint – four anteriorly, four laterally and five anterolaterally.

Knee flexion is part of the shock-absorbing mechanism which includes dorsflexion of the ankle and pronation of the foot, together with a bending moment of tibia and fibula. Abnormality of any one component can set up stresses leading to breakdown somewhere in the chain.

An overpronated foot causes over-rotation of the tibia, leading to valgus strain at the knee, putting at risk the medial capsule. Tight calf muscles limit dorsiflexion of the foot, imposing the need for extra knee flexion which, in turn, adds to loading of the patella, compressing it further into the femoral groove.

Tight hamstrings mean that the quadriceps have to work harder to overcome their resistance, again loading the patella. Any valgus deformity of the knee will increase the angle, called the Q angle, made by the patellar tendon with the pull of the quadriceps in the outer range of knee extension. This increases the tendency to lateral displacement of the patella, resisted by the vastus medialis muscle.

The running surface will affect the biomechanics of the knee. Soft surfaces absorb some of the stresses that are otherwise reflected back up the leg on heel strike. Banked surfaces cause pronation of the uphill leg, giving rise to medial knee pain, whilst the lateral ligaments of the knee suffer in the downhill leg. Downhill running requires powerful eccentric work in the quadriceps, stressing the patellar tendon, whilst popliteus is acting to stabilize the forward movement of the femur, risking a popliteus tenosynovitis.

Pain from the soft tissues around the knee can arise from various sites. Direct trauma to the knee can cause damage not only to the periarticular ligaments, but also to structures within the knee. These are uncommon injuries in track athletes unless arising from an awkward fall. More common are the overuse injuries that cause soreness and inflammation to some of the structures around the knee.

Friction between the iliotibial band and the lateral epicondyle of the knee during flexion and extension occurs in runners. It is a typical overuse problem, arising from continuous repeated stereotyped movements through a relatively short range. It results in either inflammation of the bursa overlying the lateral femoral epicondyle or a direct irritation of the band and adjacent periosteum (Bates Noble *et al.*, 1982). Overpronation of the foot on the affected side may contribute to the syndrome by reason of the internal rotation of the tibia it causes, further pressing the band on to the lateral epicondyle.

The symptoms are those of pain, coming on after starting a run, which increases to the point where activity cannot continue. Running downhill or on heavily cambered surfaces may exacerbate the pain. There is tenderness over the lateral epicondyle of the femur. A specific test can be carried out. With the patient lying supine the knee is flexed to 90° and gradually extended whilst pressing over or just proximal to the lateral epicondyle. The test is positive if pain is felt at about 30° of flexion (Noble, 1979).

Treatment in the acute phase is similar to that for other soft tissue inflammation – rest, ice and anti-inflammatory drugs. Correction of overpronation and regular stretching exercise of the lateral tissues of the thigh will help in preventing recurrences. The athlete stands with the affected leg extended at the hip and adducted so that the affected knee lies in the popliteal fossa of the other leg. The trunk is flexed laterally away from the affected side, the arms stretching down towards the heel of the posterior affected leg. The stretch is held for 10 seconds and repeated three or four times, twice daily. If the condition fails to settle an injection of local steroid into the painful area may be helpful.

Popliteus tendinitis

Popliteus tendinitis may give pain at the lateral side of a runner's knee, particularly when running downhill. It can be confused with pain from a damaged posterior horn of the lateral meniscus, although in the latter case there is usually a clear history of trauma. The popliteus muscle assists the posterior cruciate in controlling forward displacement of the femur on the tibia in the stance phase, as well as being a flexor of the knee joint and medial rotator of the tibia.

The tendon will be over its attachment on the lateral aspect of the femur just anterior to the lateral ligament. This is most easily demonstrated if the patient sits with the injured knee held at 90°, with the foot supported on the opposite knee. This position throws the lateral ligament into prominence and the popliteus tendon may be felt just anterior to the ligament just above the joint line.

Active rest and ice are used in early rehabilitation, together with oral anti-inflammatories. The athlete should avoid pain-provoking situations such as downhill running and cambered roads. In resistant cases a local steroid injection will help to hasten recovery.

Patellar tendinitis

Jumper's knee is the popular term for patellar tendinitis. It is associated more with the mechanical properties of the tendon and bone–tendon junctions than with anatomical or biomechanical derangements of the knee or with trauma (Ferretti, 1986).

Tendons are relatively inelastic structures with enormous strength and capable of transmitting a very high concentration of forces through a small cross-sectional area. The loads in the patellar tendon during running can be extremely high, particularly during the eccentric work that the quadriceps perform as they contract to control the flexion of the knee on landing from a jump. Repeated loading of this kind can eventually cause the cellular structure of the tendon to degenerate, with microtears developing and eventual tendinitis.

Aching and point tenderness occur commonly at the inferior pole of the patella or along the line of the patellar tendon, although it may happen above the patella. Initially the pain is felt after activity, but, as the condition progresses, the pain becomes more persistent until it markedly interferes with normal activity.

Initial treatment is to rest from the activity that causes pain, together with ice and non-steroidal anti-inflammatories. Physiotherapy modalities, such as ultrasound, are useful in helping to promote recovery. As the pain improves, quadriceps exercises can be introduced: straight leg raises to start with, progressing to carefully planned strength training, which will include jumping exercises. Tendons will improve with training but progress must be carefully monitored. Any recurrence of pain should be treated by rest.

In the more long-standing and resistant cases transverse friction massage of the tendon will help to break down adhesions and provoke a healing response, after which rehabilitation can be started.

The really intractable cases, that keep breaking down, may progress to surgery. If ultrasound scanning is available it may confirm areas of tendinitis as well as partial ruptures of the tendon. Areas of granulation and mucoid degeneration can be scraped out; this allows healing to progress, aided by rehabilitation.

In adolescents the stresses in the patellar tendon are transmitted to its attachment at the tibial tubercle – its weakest link, being one of the final epiphyses to fuse at age 16. Inflammation of the epiphysis is called Osgood–Schlatter's disease and has been variously ascribed to avascular necrosis or to minor avulsion fractures (Olympic book of Sports Medicine, 1988). High loading leads to inflammation at the epiphysis with pain, swelling and tenderness. An X-ray may show some fragmentation of the bone. The injury heals spontaneously with rest, although it may be recurrent until the epiphysis finally fuses, when there can be a residual enlargement. Physiotherapy or local steroid injection is not indicated.

The most common cause of anterior knee pain is runner's knee, pain and discomfort around the patellofemoral joint. The purpose of the patella is not only to act as a sesamoid bone to reinforce the tendon but also, by displacing the tendon anteriorly, it increases its leverage on the tibia. The maximum forces in the patellar tendon are in the mid-range of knee movement when the patella is forced firmly into the femoral groove. During the last 15° of extension of the knee there is an apparent lateral displacement of the tibial tubercle resulting in an angle, the Q angle, between the patellar tendon and pull of the quadriceps muscles. Powerful extension of the knee in this outer range induces a bowstring effect to straighten the pull, with a tendency for the patella to move laterally out of the femoral groove. This is resisted by the vastus medialis which attempts to maintain the Q angle

Running, particularly uphill, requires a strong push-off with the extended knee. In the untrained athlete in particular, the vastus medialis will be relatively weak compared with the other components of the quadriceps group, with the result that the patella can displace fractionally, becoming inflamed on its articular surface and showing some of the degenerative changes associated with chondromalacia patellae.

Overpronated feet can lead to rotation of the tibia and an increase in the Q angle, giving a greater risk of runner's knee. Women are said to be more prone to the condition by virtue of their wider pelvis, again leading to a valgus knee with an increased Q angle.

Rest and anti-inflammatories, together with physiotherapy, help in the acute stages. It is important that exercises are prescribed to improve the vastus medialis, which means quadriceps exercises, either with an extended knee or knee-straightening exercise in the outer range of extension. If quadriceps exercises are carried out in the middle and inner range this will only increase the discrepancy between the main bulk and the vastus medialis, which is relatively inactive in these phases.

A firm band around the upper tibia, just below the lower pole of the patella, will help relieve symptoms by pressing the tendon, holding the patella more firmly in the femoral groove. A positive attitude towards rehabilitation exercises should bring relief in 2–3 weeks.

If overpronation is thought to be a contributory factor, temporary correction can be applied by the use of felt pads applied to an insole. If this helps, permanent orthotics should be prescribed by a podiatrist.

The hamstrings

The biceps femoris, semimembranosus and semitendinosus together make up the hamstring muscles. The biceps femoris arises from two heads, the long head from the ischial tuberosity and the short head from the femoral shaft. They unite to insert into the head of the fibula, the tendon being separated from the lateral ligament of the knee by a bursa. The muscle acts as a flexor of the knee joint, the long head also being a hip extensor. Together the heads are a lateral rotator of the flexed lower leg. The semitendinosus and semimembranosus also arise from the ischial tuberosity, to be inserted into the upper tibia. They flex the knee, extend the hip and medially rotate the flexed lower leg.

The hamstrings cross two major joints. Their main action is hip extension and knee flexion, a combination of movements that is rarely used. A delicate control over appropriate relaxation and contraction in the hamstring is therefore necessary in actions such as a sprint start, where both hip and knee extend together.

The hamstrings and quadriceps in their turn act as agonists and antagonists in the various phases of the gait cycle. The hamstrings extend the thigh and flex the knee when the foot is off the ground as well as stabilizing the quadriceps during much of leg extension.

Injury to the hamstrings

Medium-paced running does not require much stretching of the hamstrings but the explosive burst from the sprinter's blocks and a lengthening stride put them on a much fuller stretch, as well as more powerful contractions as the lead leg is pulled down to the ground to increase the rate of striding. It is a regrettably familiar sight to see sprinters or long jumpers suddenly pulling up withing a few strides of their start, clutching at the back of their thigh, due to a muscle pull following this increased demand on range of movement and power of contraction.

In the inexperienced athlete, the commonest cause of this injury is inadequate preparation. Poor hamstring elasticity is a failure to practise a stretch programme. Poor warm-up and a neglect of pre-race stretching invites a muscle tear. In the more experienced athlete an imbalance of strength between hamstrings and quads is usually in favour of the quadriceps, with a consequent risk of tearing in the hamstrings. The relative power requirement between the groups alters from a hamstring output of some 60% of the quads at lower work rates to near equality at maximum work rate. Since hamstrings tend to be relatively neglected in training they come under increasing risk at higher work rates.

Treatment

The immediate treatment is the same as for many soft tissue injuries – rest, ice and a compressing bandage. After 48 hours or so the muscle can be gently exercised through its painfree range of movement. As healing progresses the range of movement will increase and the muscle can be more actively worked under increasing load. With a restored range of movement gentle stretching can be resumed and jogging reintroduced. As the strength of the muscle returns the stride length can be increased, with intervals of high knee lifting and heels kicking towards the buttocks. Once sprinting is possible repetitions, with slow starts and slow finishing, can be introduced and the speed gradually built up. To prevent recurrence, strength training of the hamstring should be included in the training schedules with good warm-up and stretching discipline.

Muscle tears are described as being deep within the muscle bundle or superficial to the bundle, when drainage of oedema fluid is easier along the fascial planes. This will have some effect on the rate of healing and may explain why some muscle injuries are comparatively slow to settle.

The groin

Injury to the groin

Groin pain in athletes commonly arises from overuse of one of the four main muscle groups of the region, but can be from something as simple as lymphadenopathy from minor infection lower down the leg.

Of the adductor group, the adductor longus is the most commonly injured. The muscle origin is on the pubic bone and the insertion is on the posterior aspect of the mid-shaft of the femur. Sprinters are liable to acute adductor strain as they come from the blocks into their first strides. The stance is wide with the feet and legs tending to be externally rotated, putting the adductors under greater tension. Subacute strains arise from unaccustomed running on uneven surfaces, when the adductors are working hard to stabilize the pelvis and legs.

Pain is the presenting symptom. It is typically located at or near the pubic origin of the adductor longus and may radiate down the muscle. Initially the pain may be relieved by exercise but returns afterwards with greater intensity. As the condition develops, functional disability progresses. Although the athlete may not be able to run, other activities, such as cycling, that do not require adductor activity, may be possible.

On examination there may be limitation of range of abduction on the injured side. Resisted adduction will be painful and there is usually local tenderness at the pubic insertion of the muscle. In the more chronic cases – and groin strains are one of the problems that can be resistant to treatment – X-ray of the area may show some calcification of the origin.

The iliopsoas group is a powerful flexor of the hip and assists with lateral rotation. Its origin is from the lumbar vertebrae and the inner aspect of the ilium, running to an insertion on the postero-medial aspect of the femur at the lesser trochanter. Beneath the tendon of the muscle, as it crosses the iliopubic eminence of the pelvis, lies a bursa. The tendon and its bursa can become inflamed from overuse. Training that involves active hip flexion such as uphill running, or the high-stepping drills involved in hurdling, may produce the problem. Pain is again the presenting feature, usually located in the groin. Tenderness may be present, but it is difficult to localize. There is limitation of extension of the hip compared with the uninjured side, but this can be difficult to assess. Resisted hip flexion will cause pain in the groin.

It is not possible to differentiate reliably between a tendinitis and a bursitis. Indeed, the two conditions may exist together. A sensation of tension and swelling in the groin may indicate a bursitis, but for all practical purposes the difference is academic.

The hip flexors

The rectus femoris is one of the four muscles that together make up the quadriceps group. Arising from the anterior inferior spine of the pelvis and the upper margin of the socket of the hip joint, it spans both the hip and knee joint to its common insertion on the tibial tubercle. It acts as a hip flexor, secondary only to the iliposoas, as well as functioning with the rest of the quadriceps group as a knee extensor.

Injury to the hip flexors

Tightness of the hip flexors may lead to problems in sprint training, when the repeated explosive exits from the blocks put the rectus femoris under stress. Strain of the rectus femoris will cause groin pain with discomfort on resisted flexion of the hip and resisted extension of the knee, particularly if the hip is extended. Tenderness will be localized above the anterior to the hip joint.

Pain in the region of the pubic symphysis will be felt with injury to the rectus abdominis, which usually occurs at its insertion on to the pubis. Overuse of the abdominal muscles with repeated sit-ups, or the repeated stretching that happens with the back extension and twisting of the trunk in javelin and other throwing sports, may lead to pain at the muscle insertion. As the condition worsens, functional impairment can progress, causing difficulty in running and walking. The pain has to be differentiated from that of a rupture or even an acute abdominal condition such as appendicitis. Active contraction of the muscle, as with simultaneous head and foot raises when supine, will reproduce the pain.

Treatment

The management of all these conditions is similar, with ice, rest and anti-inflammatory drugs being the treatment of choice in the early stages. This can be followed within a day or two by physiotherapy modalities of heat or ultrasound, together with stretching exercises – gentle at first to discourage muscle spasm, more thorough as healing progresses – to encourage a full range of movement.

These injuries characteristically affect the muscles at or near the teno-osseus junction and they can be disappointingly slow to settle. One reason for this may be the poor blood supply to this area, slowing down healing and encouraging chronicity. In the more resistant cases and those who may have been neglected in the early stages, friction massage may be helpful. Friction across the line of the fibres, with firm localized sweeping movements with the tip of one or possibly two fingertips continued for 10 min or so until the area is numbed, will break down scar tissue and help to stimulate healing once more. Friction massage should be followed by stretching to ensure that the new scar accommodates the full range of movement. As an alternative to frictions, or as a further treatment option should they not be successful, an injection of 10–20 mg triamcinolone acetonide, distributed in droplets in and around the painful area, can be used. This should be followed by at least 24 hours' rest and then followed by the rehabilitation described earlier.

In order to try and prevent a recurrence of what can be an extremely annoying injury, the athlete should be encouraged to include appropriate stretching exercises into the warm-up routine, since it is often a relative tightness in the muscles that leads to the problem.

In the case of iliopsoas pain it is clinically almost impossible to differentiate between tendinous pain and a bursitis. Indeed it is likely that the two conditions may coexist. Aspiration of the bursa is a specialized technique that is best carried out under X-ray control, but it does provide an opportunity to inject a local steroid.

The hip joints

Injury to the hip joints

Soft tissue pains around the hip joint generally arise from either the insertion of the larger muscle groups into the greater trochanter of the femur or from a trochanteric bursitis. There are two bursae that overly the trochanter, a superficial and a deep. The importance of a bursitis is not so much the injury itself, but the underlying cause, which may reflect a biomechanical deficiency.

Prolonged running on banked or cambered surfaces may provoke a bursitis in the higher leg. The pelvic tilt causes greater tension in the overlying muscles and hence more compression of the bursa. For similar reasons leg length discrepancy may cause a bursitis.

The gluteal muscles act as lateral rotators and abductors of the hip. In women runners the comparatively wider pelvis results in medial rotation of the femur, with an increased Q angle at the knee. An overpronated foot will also lead to a compensatory medial rotation of the leg, and therefore the hip. Both of these conditions thus stretch the glutei, with compression of the bursa, leading to a bursitis.

Treatment of the acute condition is rest, ice and anti-inflammatory drugs, followed by physiotherapy. It should settle satisfactorily within 10–14 days. Those cases that do not may benefit from a local injection of triamcinolone acetonide 20 mg into the painful area. It is essential to try and determine a cause for the condition and, if possible, prevent a recurrence by giving advice about training surfaces and appropriate footwear. The overpronated athlete may need referral to a podiatric specialist for a corrective orthotic, but it is always worthwhile testing the effectiveness of a temporary correction, based on a cork insole, before a potentially expensive specialist referral.

If the running sports seem to be biomechanically fairly straightforward, the throwing and vaulting aspects of track and field athletics are, by comparison, highly technical events where technique is vital for optimum performance.

One example is the biomechanical comparison of US javelin throwers and the Olympic finalists after the 1976 Montreal Games. Whilst the US throwers relied on a high running velocity added to the arm thrust at release, the Olympic finalists showed more rotation of the trunk in their throws, which limited their running ability. However, the rapid and severe twisting torque of the body as they unwound gave a higher velocity of the throwing hand at release and therefore longer throws of the javelin.

Similarly, a study of shot-putters demonstrated a steady increase in acceleration of the throwing hand through all the phases of the throw, to give maximum velocity of the throwing hand at release. Less successful athletes were not able to achieve this steady acceleration, slowing down during the middle phases of the throw, adversely affecting the final velocity (Zorins and Andrews, 1985).

Whilst the throwing sports use and need movement of the whole body to achieve maximum velocity of the delivery, the arms and shoulders are very much a part of the delivery process. Both power and flexibility are necessary to perform well and to avoid injury.

Running may be said to be a part of normal everyday activity, but throwing is a rarely used skill, employing muscles and joints in unfamiliar ways. It is important that training is directed towards increasing power and improving range of movement at a rate at which the body can cope.

If throwing is a rarely used skill, pole vaulting is completely unnatural. The vault converts the kinetic energy of the run-up into bending of the glass-fibre pole. The recoil energy of the pole, together with the residual momentum of the athlete, carries the vaulter upwards and forwards whilst he or she uses upper body strength to assume an inverted position on the pole. The final phase is the thrust away from the pole to carry the vaulter over the bar. It is, without doubt, the most technical event and, to its devotees, the most exciting.

The decathlon, the multievent competition for men, includes discus, shot-put and pole vault amongst its 10 events. The womens event, the Heptathlon, also includes discus and shot-put but there is, as yet, no official pole vault competition for women.

The field event athlete is using his or her whole body to gain the necessary power, but the shoulder girdle and elbow come under considerable stress.

The shoulder

There are three bones that make up the shoulder girdle. The ball of the humerus articulates with the glenoid socket of the scapula, the articular fossa of which is increased by the fibrocartilage collar of the glenoid labrum. The blade of the scapula serves as muscle attachment. The shoulder joint is surrounded by a loose capsule that allows for a wide range of movement. The clavicle is firmly bound to the acromion process of the scapula and, medially, to the upper end of the sternum. It acts as a stay or prop, holding the scapula at its proper position on the thorax, which gives the maximum range of movement in the shoulder joint. Other than the prop effect of the clavicle, the stability of the joint depends on the synergistic effect of the many muscles that control movement of the joint.

The action of throwing can be divided into several phases, involving the shoulder and the elbow. In the initial clocking phase the muscles are tensed and wound up, ready for release. The shoulder is abducted and the humerus externally rotated, with the elbow flexed at about 45°.

The following phase of acceleration initially brings forward the shoulder and elbow, leaving the forearm and wrist behind, putting a valgus strain on the elbow. The humerus is then internally rotated and the elbow extends. Finally the forearm rotates into pronation after release of the implement and the shoulder movement decelerates (Zorins and Andrews, 1985).

Not only are there powerful muscle contractions needed to initiate these rapid movements but the antagonistic groups are active in synergistic control.

In the final stage of deceleration, the most violent phase in throwing, the muscles of the rotator cuff together with the latissimus dorsi and pectoralis major act to stabilize the humerus in the glenoid fossa powerfully.

The first half of the arc of elevation of the shoulder takes place at the glenohumeral joint, controlled mainly by supraspinatus and deltoid. The next 60° results from rotation of the scapula, controlled by serratus anterior and the upper part of trapezius. During the final 30° of movement the scapula is again stationary, the humerus being adducted by the pectoralis major. The narrowest space between the tuberosity of the humerus and the arch of the acromion process occurs in mid-abduction, between 80 and 120° (Peginton, 1985).

In examination of the shoulder, active, passive and resisted movements are tested. Any limitation of active elevation is noted, with particular emphasis on a painful arc. Passive movements explore the range of movement of the joint and its end-feel, whether hard, soft or firm. Resisted abduction will test the deltoid, which is rarely affected, and supraspinatus, which is commonly injured. Resisted adduction tests pectoralis major, latissimus dorsi and the teres muscles, although injuries to these are uncommon. Resisted external rotation tests infraspinatus and supraspinatus whilst resisted internal rotation tests mainly the subscapularis.

The shoulder area contains several of the 14 or so trigger sites in the body that have been described in the condition of fibromyalgia or fibrositis. In the throwing sports athletes are particularly conscious of tightness or spasm in their muscles and tenderness can often be elicited at these points. Opinion varies as to whether it is related to exercise, fatigue or stress (Cinque, 1989).

Apart from the tender areas there is usually little to find except some localized muscle tightness. The problem resolves with massage and warmth, or transcutaneous electrical nerve stimulation can be used.

Injury to the shoulder

The most common injury that affects the throwing arm is the *rotator cuff syndrome*. It covers a multitude of pathologies including subacromial bursitis, supraspinatus tendinitis and subscapularis tendinitis. The rotator cuff is composed of four tendons – subscapularis anteriorly, with infraspinatus, supraspinatus and teres that attach to the posterior part of the humerus.

The shoulder joint lies beneath the arch formed by the acromion posteriorly and the coracoacromial ligament anteriorly. Between this arch and the tendons of the rotator cuff lies the subacromial bursa. At the upper extreme of abduction the greater tuberosity moves under the arch and part of the supraspinatus tendon, together with the bursa and the long head of biceps, may become nipped.

The vulnerable part of the supraspinatus tendon is less than 1 cm from its attachment to the humerus. This area has been demonstrated to be relatively avascular when the arm is abducted. A similar area of avascularity lies in that part of the tendon of long head of biceps as it is stretched over the head of the humerus. It is these areas that are easily damaged by impingement and subject to chronic patterns of inflammation (Kulund, 1988). Not only the tendon but also the bursa can become inflamed as a result of repeated entrapment.

If the condition is not adequately treated, and the cycle of inflammation and oedema continues, the tissue of the tendon degenerates and may become the site of calcium deposits. The deposit may enlarge to cause considerable discomfort on abduction of the arm as the calcified area passes under the acromion.

The symptoms are pain of insidious onset that gradually over weeks and months becomes more severe as the overhead stress continues. The pattern may be of intermittent mild soreness, culminating in an acutely painful episode precipitated by a more intensive bout of activity.

Resisted abduction will be painful, perhaps with painful resisted external rotation when the supraspinatus is inflamed. If the lesion lies in the vulnerable area of the tendon a painful arc will be found. The smooth pattern of abduction will be broken as the arm is brought to the horizontal, indicating impingement as the shoulder completes its first 90° of initial elevation. The pain will continue through the next 60° as the scapula rotates and will disappear for the final 30° as the space between the coracoacromial arch and the head of the humerus opens up. There may be weakness of abduction.

If the tendon is inflamed more proximally or at the musculotendinous junction, the painful arc may be absent.

A painful arc in isolation may indicate a subacromial bursitis but, because of their close relationship, the bursa and tendon are often inflamed together.

The supraspinatus tendon can be palpated by medial rotation and slight adduction of the arm. Tenderness will be located over the front of the shoulder joint.

Treatment

Treatment is initially rest, avoiding painful activities, together with anti-inflammatories. Physiotherapy treatment, in the form of ultrasound or other modalities, may be helpful. As the condition improves, mobility and strength training are reintroduced. Improvement will take 2 or 3 weeks and it is better to err on the side of too long a lay-off, especially in younger athletes and those presenting for the first time, to try and avoid recurrences.

Local steroid injection of the supraspinatus tendon subacromial bursa can be highly successful and should certainly be considered if more conservative treatments have not worked. Triamcinolone acetonide (20 mg) into the painful area, when this can be palpated, by droplet distribution around the site will help. Where there is evidence of impingement, but a painful area cannot be found, an injection under the acromion, into the bursa, of 40 mg triacinolone acetonide is effective.

An alternative is a large 20 ml injection of 1% Xylocaine, particularly if the lesion is felt to be primarily a bursitis. The size of the injection is thought to splint the bursa, separating its inflamed surfaces and allowing healing to progress.

In chronic cases, where the inflamed tendon can be palpated, friction massage across the line of the tendon, vertically over the front of the shoulder, is often helpful and should always be followed by mobilizations.

Once the pain is beginning to settle, increasing mobilization and strengthening exercises should be introduced, bearing in mind that weakness of abduction is a feature of the painful arc syndrome. Overuse is the commonest cause of the problem; the athlete's training programme should be looked at and advice given about a slow build-up of training and the need to seek treatment early in the event of a recurrence.

Javelin throwers and shot-putters may suffer problems with the subscapularis tendon. The muscle is a powerful internal rotator of the humerus and is therefore involved in the release and deceleration phase of throwing, when the humerus has a high rate of internal rotation.

Pain is the presenting symptom, particularly when reproducing the action of the muscle. After elevating and internally rotating the humerus, resisting external rotation will cause pain. The tendon runs anteriorly across the shoulder joint to be inserted on to the head of the humerus. It can be palpated with the humerus externally rotated. The bicipital groove is felt anteriorly on the head of the humerus and the subscapularis runs horizontally and medially from the inner edge of the groove.

Bicipital tendinitis is also a common cause of pain on the front of the shoulder. The tendon of long head of biceps runs vertically in the groove, passing over the glenohumeral joint to insert above the glanced fossa. During movement of the shoulder the tendon remains fixed and the humerus slides along the tendon. (Kulund, 1988). In the follow-through phase of throwing, the humerus may leave the socket by as much as 2.5 cm and a tight or roughened bicipital groove may irritate the tendon.

Rest from the painful activity, together with ice and anti-inflammatory tablets, is the treatment for the early stages of these injuries, followed after 24–48 hours by the physiotherapy modalities. Cyriax and Cyriax (1984) were of the opinion that early massage was rapidly successful. For bicipital tendinitis, the physiotherapist's fingers are pressed firmly over the lesion and the humerus is rotated to and fro using the flexed forearm as a lever.

Local steroids are recommended by some; droplet distribution around the tendon without injecting into the substance is the favoured procedure. Like the Achilles tendon, the long head of biceps is prone to rupture, particularly in older athletes where the tendon has become worn and degenerate. As long as cortisone injections are believed to be a contributory factor in tendon rupture it is preferable to avoid them as a standard treatment.

If the long head does rupture, there will be some pain over the anterior aspect of the joint and contraction of the biceps will produce a more prominent swelling of the muscle than normal. About 20% of flexion power is lost as a result of rupture and supination will be affected.

Surgical repair can be considered. If the rupture happens to a younger athlete, operation is to be recommended. In the older athlete it may be appropriate to accept the reduced function and rely on physiotherapy, mobility and strengthening exercises for the appropriate muscle groups to compensate for the loss of biceps function.

Arthroscopy of the shoulder is becoming more widely available. It is an invasive technique which allows the direct visualization of the interior of the glenohumeral joint through a small-diameter operating telescope. The best results are obtained by an experienced operator.

The long head of biceps and the supraspinatus tendon can be inspected, together with the glenoid labrum and the upper border of subscapularis. The arthroscope can be introduced into the subacromial bursa, giving a good view of the supraspinatus tendon.

With arthroscopy it is possible to evaluate more accurately chronic disabilities that have not responded to treatment and to carry out tidying up operations on partial tears of tendons or the glenoid labrum. Loose bodies can be removed.

During the acceleration phase of throwing, the shoulder and elbow are rapidly brought forward. The inertia of the long lever of the forearm means that the wrist and hand tend to be left behind, creating a valgus strain on the elbow, compressing the lateral aspect and opening up the medial side.

As the forearm then accelerates forward the elbow then extends, being resisted by the elbow flexors. The forearm pronates, resisted by the supinates and the olecranon engages with some force into the olecranon fossa.

The elbow

The medial, or ulnar, collateral ligament of the elbow has two main fibre bundles arising from the medial epicondyle of the humerus. The anterior inserts into the anterior surface of the ulna and is a major static stabilizer of the valgus stresses of the joint (McCue, 1988). The weaker posterior bundle inserts into the margin of the olecranon.

The common origin of the wrist flexors on the medial epicondyle is put under strain by the repeated valgus stresses of throwing.

Injury to the elbow

Pain over the medial aspect of the elbow is a common problem with throwers, particularly if their technique is bad. Commonly known as golfer's elbow, the condition is likely to be inflammation of the tendoperiosteal junction. Since the flexors overly the medial ligament it can be difficult to differentiate between a ligamentous and a muscular injury. Apart from localized tenderness, muscle pain will be felt on resisted flexion of the wrist, particularly if the elbow is extended. A sprained ligament will be painful when a valgus stress is applied to the elbow.

Repeated valgus strains of the elbow can lead to stretching and degeneration of the medial ligament, with the possibility of spur formation in the ligament. A degenerate ligament may rupture; this is felt as a sudden snap, leading to valgus instability. To detect instability, the elbow is flexed by about 30° to free the olecranon from its fossa. An assessment is made by comparison with the uninjured elbow.

Treatment

In the acute stages of medial epicondylitis, rest from the activity that causes pain, ice and non-steroidal anti-inflammatories are used. Physiotherapy will be useful after 24–48 hours. As the condition improves, mobilizing and strengthening exercises are introduced and these are always more useful if they approximate to the correct action of the event. Technique is so important in the throwing sports that correction of faults is essential to avoid reinjury. Consultations between coach, athlete, doctor and physiotherapist are the ideal of management – this is not only of benefit to the athlete but also gives the opportunity for each to learn a little more from the others' specialist knowledge.

Injection of the inflamed area is popular; 20 mg triamcinolone acetonide distributed in droplet form in the painful area is a suitable treatment, but it is important for the elbow to be completely rested for 1–2 weeks before rehabilitation is started. There does seem to be a high incidence of recurrence after injection.

In the younger athlete the epiphysis of the medial epicondyle is at risk in throwing. Vigorous pronation is a feature of the release phase and repeated traction on the medial epicondyle can cause inflammation, or even separation of the epiphysis.

The associated pain may be acute or of insidious onset. If it is acute the problem is more likely to be one of avulsion (Booher *et al.*, 1985). X-ray may show separation and displacement of the epiphyseal fragment.

The athlete should rest from the activity that causes pain. Ice applications may be helpful in the acute stage. Non-steroidal anti-inflammatories should be used with caution in adolescents. There is an association with gastrointestinal bleeding and a suggested relationship with a worsening of asthma (*British National Formulary*, 1990).

If an avulsion is not present, local treatment with an anti-inflammatory cream can help. Physiotherapy in the form of the electrical modalities should be used with caution, if at all, since their effect on areas of active growth are uncertain. Mobilization and local massage to encourage organized healing can be used.

It will take some 6–8 weeks for the condition to settle, although longer recovery times up to 12 weeks would not be remarkable. Epiphyseal avulsion will need at least 8 weeks from the pain-provoking activity, followed by careful rehabilitation.

Once the local tenderness has settled, conditioning, mobility and strength-training can be resumed, in consultation with the coach, who should give particular attention to any errors in technique as well as the avoidance of overtraining.

Pain over the medial aspect of the elbow may radiate to the third and fourth fingers, indicating ulnar nerve irritation. Examination may show loss of sensation in the fifth and medial half of the sixth fingers as well as tenderness over the medial epicondyle.

The sensation is a familiar one to most people who have accidentally hit their funnybone, but in throwers the nerve can sublux from its groove, with consequent mechanical irritation.

Rest and anti-inflammatories may help in the early stages but, if the condition is recurrent or if the pain becomes chronic, surgery is helpful. The ulnar nerve is transferred anteriorly so that it is under less tension. (McCue, 1988).

References

Bates Noble H, Hajek MR, Porter M (1982) Diagnosis and treatment of iliotibial band tightness in runners. *Physician and Sports Medicine* **10**, 67–74.

Boni M, Benazzo F, Castelli C (1983) Physiopathology of tendon diseases in sport. Sports medicine in track and field athletics. *Proceedings of the First IAAF Medical Congress*, 1983. International Amateur Athletic Federation and Finnish Amateur Athletic Association, Espoo, Finland.

British National Formulary (1990) No. 19. London: British Medical Association/The Pharmaceutical Press.

Brookes SC, Potter BT, Rainey JB (1981) Treatment for partial tears of the lateral ligament of the ankle; a prospective trial. *British Medical Journal* **282**, 606–7.

Brostrom L (1966) Sprained ankles V. Treatment and prognosis in recent ligament ruptures. *Acta Chirurgica Scandinavica* **132**, 537–55.

Cass JR, Morrey BF (1984) Ankle instability. Current concepts, diagnosis and treatment. *Mayo Clinic Proceedings* **59**, 165–70.

Cinque C (1989) Fibromyalgia. Is exercise the cause or the cure? *Physician and Sports Medicine* **17**, 180–2.

Cyriax JH, Cyriax PJ (1984) *The Illustrated Manual of Orthopaedic Medicine*. London: Bailliere Tyndall.

Ferretti A (1986) The epidemiology of jumper's knee. *Sports Medicine* **3**, 289–95.

Freeman MAR (1965) Treatment of ruptures of the lateral ligament of the ankle. *Journal of Bone and Joint Surgery* **47B**, 661–8.

Fumich RM, Ellison AE, Guerin GJ, Grace PD(1981) The measured effect of taping on the combined foot and ankle motion before and after exercise. *American Journal of Sports Medicine* **9**, 165–70.

Kulund DN (1988) *The Injured Athlete*. Philadelphia: JB Lippincott.

Lightowler CDR (1984) Injury to the lateral ligament of the ankle. *British Medical Journal* **289**, 1249.

McCue FC (1988) The elbow, wrist and hand. In: Kulund DN (ed) *The Injured Athlete*. Philadelphia: JB Lippincott.

McKeag DB, Dolan C (1989) Overuse syndromes of the lower extremity. *Physician and Sports Medicine* **17**, 114.

Noble CA (1979) Iliotibial band friction syndrome. *British Journal of Sports Medicine* **13**, 51–4.

Olympic Book of Sports Medicine (1988) vol 1. Oxford: Blackwell Scientific Publications.

Peginton J (1985) *Clinical Anatomy in Action 1*. Edinburgh: Churchill Livingstone.

Shields C (1982) Achilles tendon injuries and disabling conditions. *Physician and Sports Medicine* **10**, 77–84

Zorins B, Andrews JR, Carson WG (1985) *Injuries to the Throwing Arm*. Philadelphia: WB Saunders.

19

Risks and injuries in rugby football

D. A. D. MacLeod

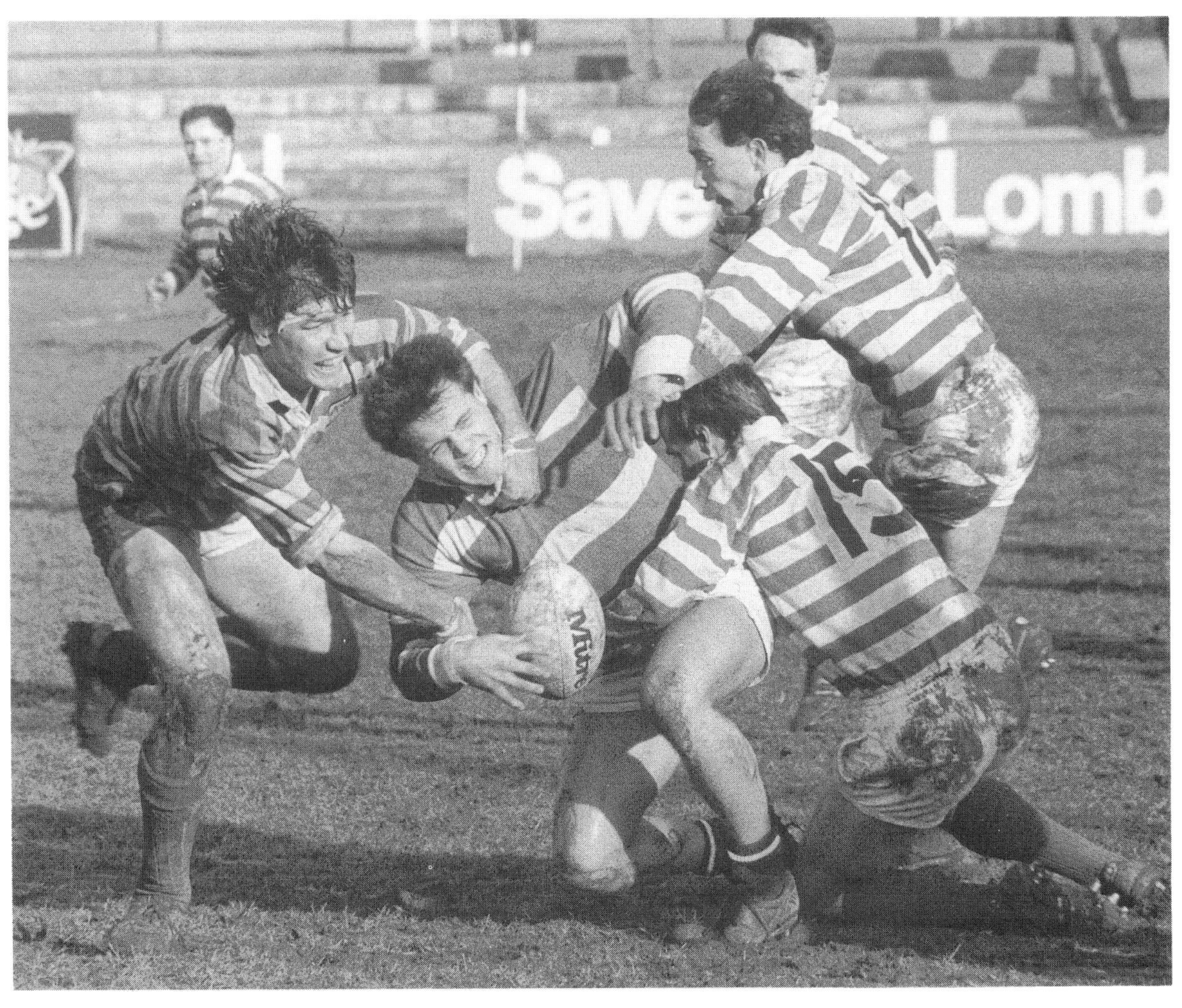

Rugby football is a contact sport which requires a background of aerobic fitness supplemented by the ability to undertake intermittent periods of high-intensity activity in attack or defence, while handling the ball, accelerating into or out of a tackle, rucking, mauling, scrummaging and at the line-out. Rugby caters for a wide range of players with varying physical and psychological characteristics by identifying an appropriate position among the forwards or backs for each individual. Players can be given suitable fitness training programmes in conjunction with developing the basic skills required for the game.

Rugby has proven to be a popular game for all ages, and increasingly among women, because of the player's enjoyment in participation and the good fellowship it promotes. Rugby is played on a worldwide basis in over 100 countries. The game is controlled by the International Rugby Football Board which receives advice on player safety following identification of injury patterns and risk factors by the Medical Advisory Committee which the Board established in 1977. In addition, each country can introduce law modifications into their own domestic game and this is widely done in the interests of player safety and enjoyment, especially for junior or under-age teams and the 'golden oldies'.

The numbers playing rugby on a regular basis have never been accurately documented but estimates include over 200 000 players in England, New Zealand, France, South Africa and 100 000 players in Japan and the USA. Wales has approximately 35 000 regular adult players and Scotland 14 000 players.

Any player participating in a contact sport such as rugby accepts the ordinary risks of injury that occur in the game as the result of collisions between players or falling to the ground. These risks are minimized by ensuring that the laws by which the game is regulated are soundly formulated, are properly supervised by the referee and that the laws, the officials and the opponents are respected by both players and their coaches. The game must be played on a good surface and in a safe environment with padded goal posts, flexible flags to mark the boundaries of the field of play, ground marking lines that have not been painted with lime and an absence of hazards too close to the edge of the pitch.

The individual player must be fit to play and have developed the appropriate skills he needs for the game. Players must also ensure that the equipment they use will not harm an opponent, a point which particularly applies to boots, studs and some of the protective devices used by players to minimize or support injuries they have personally experienced.

Experienced players will always try to protect those parts of their bodies that are particularly vulnerable to injury, such as the ears and shins of forwards or joints that will benefit from adhesive stretch or non-stretch supportive strapping, such as the ankle, fingers or thumbs. All players should use individually fitted mouth-guards, made by a dentist, to reduce the incidence of damage to the teeth, soft tissues of the mouth and concussion.

Many rugby players train and play wearing various different forms of support for previously strained or contused muscles. This protection may range from light-weight Lycra garments to various forms of rubberized material made up as stockings, sleeves or supports and adhesive stretch or non-stretch strappings and other types of compression bandage. There is little or no evidence to suggest that these measures do anything more than minimize heat loss and retain warmth in the affected tissues. They do not provide support to injured muscles.

Additional protection a player may use, that is permitted within the laws of the game, includes a soft pad firmly fixed to the body to protect an injury such as an old subluxation of the acromioclavicular joint. A soft shoulder pad may also be fitted to the player's jersey to protect the acromioclavicular joint. The laws also permit the use of a light-weight soft 'scrum cap' or helmet to protect the player's scalp or ears. Protective supports which incorporate rigid struds or springs, which have been widely recommended to support an injured knee joint, are banned because of the damage such a support might cause an opponent.

The game of rugby football is played in all climates and players should also protect themselves from the elements by ensuring that they are properly equipped to minimize wind-chill and wet or cold climatic conditions in some countries and to allow adequate heat loss and perspiration in others.

The laws of rugby state under the resolutions of the International Rugby Football Board no. 5.5 that:

> the use of drugs by participants in Rugby Football other than for therapeutic reasons in accordance with medical advice is regarded by the board with disapproval and is contrary to the spirit of the game. Any player unable to participate without the administration of drugs or injections to relieve pain or acute illness must be considered unfit to play in a game. The taking of drugs by players to enhance performance is forbidden.

This resolution was written into the regulations whereby the game of rugby football is supervised following advice from the Medical Advisory Committee of the International Rugby Football Board and is designed to protect players from the temptation of requesting or being given medicines or local anaesthetic injections to relieve illness or pain with a view to allowing participation in a game of rugby football.

Local anaesthetic agents such as the short-acting lignocaine or longer-acting Marcain, with or without the addition of adrenaline, have a wide range of pharmacological properties, of which the loss of pain is only one. Their effects include the loss of temperature appreciation, proprioception, touch and pressure sensation. The inability of a player to appreciate pain in conjunction with the loss of proprioception appreciation is particularly dangerous in a contact sport such as rugby football because the underlying injury for which the initial injection was given is liable to a second and much more serious injury following local anaethetic injection. This is particularly important with regard to ligamentous injuries, chest injuries and certain fractures.

The Resolutions of the International Rugby Football Board also specifically identify concussion as an injury requiring special care and attention from rugby players, officials and coaches. Resolution 5.7 states that 'a player who has suffered definite concussion should not participate in any match or training session for a period of at least three weeks from the time of injury, and then only subject to being cleared by a proper neurological examination'.

Implementing the resolutions and recommendations on concussion can be extremely difficult because of the problems encountered with diagnosis, especially with a player who 'engages automatic gear' after a head injury and appears to play perfectly well but has no recall after the match of the injury or any subsequent incidents. Better teaching in the recognition of concussion and the importance of its cumulative effects is required throughout rugby as well as many other sports. The accepted recommendations in modern rugby are that any player having a second concussion in a single season should avoid all contact sport for 3 months; if a third concussion is sustained within the same season he should avoid all contact sport for 6 months.

Skin wounds are relatively common in rugby because of the constant repeated cuts and abrasions of the skin which occur among the ordinary risks of the game. In any activity in which cuts may occur the dangers of tetanus must be acknowledged by ensuring that all players, coaches and officials on the field of play have up-to-date tetanus immunization programmes. The recommendation in a contact sport is that the player should receive tetanus toxoid booster every 5 years after completing a basic immunization programme.

The presence of bleeding must, wherever practical, be controlled before a player continues participating in a match. This can be extremely difficult if the player has a bleeding nose or mouth but most skin wounds can be controlled with Vaseline, the use of topical adrenaline, dressings or sutures. This will be discussed later but on the basis of good hygiene and with the present anxieties about contamination by blood because of the transmission of disease, all players and officials must make every effort to minimize blood loss and ensure that players do not receive external contamination with the blood of other participants in the game.

Skin infections, especially the fungal infections of tinea pedis and tinea cruris, are almost endemic among contact sports players including rugby football. 'Scrumpox' is the most widely recognized skin infection which is particularly related to rugby. During the 1970s, outbreaks due to the Herpes simplex virus were reported among rugby clubs in England (Anonymous, 1974; Shute et al, 1979), and also occasionally affected international touring teams to the British Isles. More recently impetiginous scrumpox affected school rugby teams in Scotland (Sharp and Adam, 1990). The presence of skin 'lesions' along with the abrasive effects of facial stubble, facilitate the spread of infection. The condition also occurs in other combat sports such as judo or wrestling (*herpes gladiatorum*). Scrumpox may be caused by several infectious agents, which can be viral (herpes), bacterial (streptococcal, staphylococcal) or fungal (tinea barbae) in origin.

(i) *Herpes* – This is the most common form of 'scrumpox' and is caused by the Herpes simplex virus type 1, the agent of herpes labialis ('cold sores'). This should not be confused with Herpes simplex virus type 2, the cause of genital herpes. Herpes is highly infectious, spreading directly from person-to-person or indirectly via the sharing of infected towels, clothing or equipment, and on occasion may result in encephalitis. Prevention depends upon the maintenance of high standards of personal hygiene. Treatment requires the use of acyclovir, a specific anti-viral available as a cream or tablets.

(ii) *Impetigo* – this form of 'scrumpox' due to *Streptococcus pyogenes* or *Staphylococcus aureus*, is less common. The use of topical antiseptics may help in minimizing the spread of infection.

(iii) *Erysipelas* – the least common form, caused specifically by *Streptococcus pyogenes*, is potentially the most serious. Treatment requires the use of appropriate antibiotics such as flucloxacillin or erythromycin.

(iv) *Tinea barbae* – a fungal infection which spreads similarly to other forms of 'scrumpox'. Treatment with fungicidal creams or tablets is usually necessary.

An unusual consequence of 'scrumpox', caused by a particularly virulent strain of *Streptococcus pyogenes*, affected several forwards in a hospital rugby team in London in 1984 following a match against a team experiencing an outbreak of impetigo. In addition to being transmitted to front row forwards of yet another team the following week, two girl-friends of affected players in the hospital team were similarly affected one month later, following which salpingitis developed in one girl-friend and acute glomerulonephritis in one player.

Wound Infections

Any wound or abrasion leading to a breaking of the skin surface may become infected by a range of other bacteria (e.g. *Staphylococcus*, *Streptococcus*, *Pseudomonas*), which may be present in the playing or changing room environment, on clothing or equipment, or on the skin or respiratory tract of otherwise healthy carriers. Infection may be localized or may invade other body tissues leading to lymphadenitis, cellulitis or bacteraemia, and in consequence requiring appropriate antibiotic treatment.

Consideration has also to be given to the possibility that infection with hepatitis B virus (HBV) or the human immuno-deficiency virus (HIV) may be transmitted directly from person-to-person via open wounds.

Definition of injury

The ordinary risks of a contact sport such as rugby in which high-speed collisions between players are inevitable, include muscle soreness, contusions and abrasions, sprains and strains. In any study, a practical and clearly described definition of injury is required and this definition must acknowledge but not give undue significance to those injuries that are inevitably associated with what might be described as a good, hard and fast game. In addition the study must clarify whether injuries are being reported on a random basis or whether any attempt is being made to ensure a complete assessment of all injuries meeting the agreed definition.

The definition agreed may cover the occasion when the injury occurs, i.e. playing or training, and the effect of the injury on the player's participation in the event, such as interrupting play, with or without treatment being given, or preventing continuation. The phases of play in which the injury occurred will be a primary consideration – tackling or being tackled, scrummaging, the ruck or maul, the line-out, inadvertent collisions. The acute cause of the injury may be difficult to define; why did one tackle cause injury whereas the previous 50 tackles did not? Was the injury related to poor timing, equipment failure, lack of fitness or skill, fatigue, carelessness or inconsideration shown by an opponent or did an opponent cheat by resorting to the use of violence? The intensity and duration of training will also cause a lot of overuse injuries, such as Achilles tendon strains. After the event, an injury may be defined by whether or not the player seeks medical, chartered physiotherapy or first-aid advice, depending on what is available for minor injuries at a club. If the player has a more significant injury, he will seek advice from his own doctor or by attending the hospital Accident and Emergency department or by visiting his local Sports Injuries clinic.

One of the most common injuries in rugby football potentially requiring medical attention is a simple cut. Many cuts are minor and do not significantly interfere with playing or training but a cut which needs stitching or which may result in permanent scarring must be considered as an injury, although not necessarily of the same significance as a fractured leg.

A practical definition of a significant injury as compared to minor injury in rugby must therefore include lacerations requiring medical attention and/or stitching; admission to hospital, either at the time of the injury or after a period of assessment; injuries which prevent participation of rugby football for a predefined period such as missing 1, 2 or 3 weeks' play, or those injuries which prevent a player following his normal lifestyle outside sport – if he cannot go to work. This type of significant injury may well result in an insurance claim if the player carried an appropriate policy. This gives a very worthwhile and objective definition of a rugby injury and this is the basis of all rugby injury reports from the French Rugby Federation. Over and above this group of significant injuries, there is a separate group of catastrophic injuries resulting in permanent disability or death, such as can occur after a severe head injury, quadriplegia or sudden death as the result of a previously undiagnosed cardiac anomaly or coronary artery disease.

Much discussion has occurred in the past as to whether or not repeated minor or significant injuries will give rise to premature ageing or degenerative osteoarthrosis in a joint. There is increasing evidence that instability and alteration in the biomechanics of a joint such as occurs following total meniscectomy or cruciate ligament injury in the knee will give rise to early osteoarthritis. Players who manage to avoid this type of injury, which significantly disrupts the biomechanics of a joint, do not appear to be at a higher risk of developing osteoarthritis in later life.

Overall patterns of injuries in rugby football

The overall patterns of injuries in rugby football have been widely reported in the medical literature. Series have been based on the 80 injuries experienced in a single club in Ireland (Addley and Faren, 1988), and the 1002 injuries reported by Dalley *et al.* (1982) in Christchurch, New Zealand. A very extensive series has been reported by Dr Sparks (1981) of Rugby School, England, dealing with schoolboy rugby injury patterns.

None of these surveys can be compared directly with each other because of an inconsistency on the definition of injury, in that it can range from a blow requiring a break in play to a cut requiring sutures or an injury preventing play for 3 weeks.

One of the main features identified in all these injury reviews is the high incidence of injury to the head, face and neck, amounting to an average of 30%. Of particular note, the great majority of cuts occur to head and face. In Dr Williams's (1985) survey reporting the incidence of rugby injuries in Wales, she identified 137 lacertation, of which 108 affected the head and face. In her series the definition of an injury was the presence of a cut that required to be sutured or an injury that prevented a player from participating in rugby for 2 weeks or more, of which there were 573.

Injuries to the shoulder girdle and upper limb account for approximately 25% of injuries reported in all surveys. Injuries to the trunk, including the back, account for approximately 10% and the highest incidence of injuries in all series affects the lower limbs – approximately 35%.

Dalley and colleagues, in their survey of injuries in Christchurch (1982), adopted a very useful definition of injury: they suggested that a mild injury was one which required attention but the player was able to participate in rugby football within 1 week. Their definition of a moderate injury was one in which the player missed 1 week and a severe injury was one in which a player missed 2 weeks. Of 1002 injuries, 35.9% were mild, 43.7% moderate and 20.35% severe. In addition 30.23% of their 1002 injuries affected the head and neck, with 18.2% affecting the shoulder and upper limb, 11.7% affecting the trunk and 39.72% affected the lower limbs. This series was based on the review of 5108 players covering training and matches over one season in rugby in New Zealand.

Review of common injuries

The range of minor injuries occurring as a direct result of the contact nature of rugby includes muscle contusion, musculotendonous strains, muscle stiffness with soreness and minor ligamentous injury with associated joint sprain.

The incidence of these minor injuries can be minimized by ensuring that all players are fit and skilful enough to participate in the game or proposed training schedule, wear appropriate protective support and prepare appropriately for the event. This includes adjusting the players' diet on the day of a match and ensuring that they participate in a structured warm-up designed to raise body temperature, enhance flexibility, sharpen skills and ensure a controlled and skilful performance. During the warm-up as well as in the training schedule or match, players should take regular small drinks of water or an appropriate physiological drink such as Dioralyte to help maintain the body fluid and electrolyte balance and replenish glucose levels.

Following the event a structured warm down is invaluable in reducing muscle stiffness. This involves light jogging and muscle stretching followed by a warm bath or shower.

Principles of care

In the event that a minor injury occurs immediate assessment and appropriate management will promote early recovery. The first priorty is to minimize tissue disruption – the relatively minor primary injury tearing muscle, tendon, ligament or joint capsule is aggravated by the size of the subsequent haematoma and degree of tissue oedema. Minimizing the haematoma and tissue oedema will allow an injury to heal by first intention with a minor residual scar.

The steps taken over the initial 36 hours to minimize haematoma formation are rarely carried out well – rest, the application of ice packs, the skilful use of compression and the elevation of the injury all require considerable expertise (see Chapter 4).

1. *Rest.* Rest is designed to ensure that the injured tissues are not subjected to any further damage. During the period of rest the player should be encouraged to undertake gentle, active, minimal movements of the injured tissues within the range of discomfort.
2. *Ice.* Crushed ice packs made up in a damp cloth should be bandaged to the skin at the site of the injury for approximately 20 min starting immediately after the injury and subsequently every 2 or 3 hours during the day for the next 36 hours.
3. *Compression* – Compression is only effective if it is applied following careful assessment of the

objectives to be achieved. Rugby players' limbs are not evenly contoured tubular structures. To apply supportive and compression bandaging to an ankle or knee, for example, requires the use of shaped pieces of thick or medium compressed wool chiropody felt to fill up any hollow around the joint, followed by the application of a non-adhesive, self-adherent stretch bandage. Thereafter additional pressure can be applied to the tissues by the application of intermittent compression three times daily with a Flowtron pump. In addition, the use of a non-adhesive self-adherent bandage facilitates its removal at night.

The use of tapered elasticated tubular bandaging will only maintain pressure on the tissues if it is carefully applied with the use of chiropody felt to enhance its effect.

4. *Elevation* – Elevation of an injury is designed to minimize the development of oedema. This can best be achieved in the lower limb by encouraging the player to rest throughout the day whenever possible with the leg elevated over the back of a chair and to sleep at night with the foot of the bed elevated by approximately 10–15 cm.
5. *Non-steroidal anti-inflammatory drugs.* Non-steroidal anti-inflammatory drugs have been widely recommended to minimize the degree of tissue disruption due to oedema developing following an injury, by inhibiting prostaglandin E_2 release in the tissues. Non-steroidal anti-inflammatory drugs may be most effective in this role if they are given to the player within 48 hours of injury.

Having achieved the immediate priority of minimizing tissue disruption it is then possible to achieve an accurate diagnosis of the degree of injury and recommend an appropriate treatment programme to promote full recovery of the injury, with no increased risk of a second injury or breakdown while maintaining overall fitness. Healing by primary intention is based on the ability to scavenge any haematoma formed by the disrupted tissues, capillary budding and the formation of collagen tissue from fibroblasts. These basic processes cannot by influenced by any medical measures. The maturation of the resultant scar can be assisted by a structured rehabilitation programme designed to ensure rapid alignment of collagen fibres into healthy scar tissue. The duration of the rehabilitation programme will vary with the nature and severity of the original injury and the degree of tissue disruption. At the same time priority must be given to the maintenance of overall fitness.

Throughout the processes of minimizing tissue disruption and promoting recovery it is incumbent upon the doctor and chartered physiotherapist managing the patient's injury to review the diagnosis constantly to ensure that it is accurate, as this will help them provide the player with a reliable prognosis. The injured athlete and coach can become depressed, frustrated and angry with their medical advisory team if they cannot provide them with a structured treatment programme and an accurate outcome.

Summary of management of minor soft tissue injuries

1. Minimize tissue disruption (within 36 hours)
   (a) Rest.
   (b) Ice.
   (c) Compression.
   (d) Elevation.
   (e) Non-steroidal anti-inflammatory drugs.
2. Make an accurate diagnosis.
3. Promote recovery.
   (a) Natural processes.
   (b) Rehabilitation programme.
   (c) Maintain overall fitness.

Catastrophic injuries in rugby football

The incidence of potentially catastrophic and catastrophic injuries in rugby has never been accurately documented.

In an ongoing review undertaken on an annual basis since 1979 by the Scottish Rugby Union attempts have been made to identify clearly all those players admitted to hospital. Among this group the potentially catastrophic injuries that have been identified have included patients with tetanus, haemopneumothorax, ruptured spleen and ruptured kidney. All of these players made a full recovery following appropriate treatment with no residual disability. One player in Scottish rugby has sustained a severe head injury with a cerebral laceration and subdural haematoma requiring specialist neurosurgical care. This player has been left with a permanent disability. Throughout world rugby, there are regular isolated reports of players dying as a result of head injury. These reports are rarely well-documented but at least two players have died following a second head injury occurring within 1 week of an initial concussion.

The catastrophic injury that has been widely recognized to be associated with rugby football is quadriplegia. Considerable effort has been made since the mid 1970s to try and accurately document the incidence of this catastrophic injury but regrettably even in the UK it has not proven possible to obtain comprehensive data.

Quadriplegia

American football has set an example to sports legislators, coaches and doctors by their achievements in dramatically reducing the incidence of catastrophic head and spinal injuries from 1976 onwards. The outstanding contributions made to players' safety without changing the nature of their game are reviewed by Meuller and Blyth in *Clinics in Sports Medicine* January 1987. The key to success was the forward-looking decision made in 1931 by the American Football Coaches Association to collect football fatality data with a view to using the data to make their game safer.

Meuller and Blyth report that lethal head injuries, in spite of the use of protective helmets, have always been and have remained approximately four times more common than lethal cervical injuries – 433 head injury fatalities as against 111 cervical fatalities between 1945 and 1984. During this period, the number of regular participants in American football increased. A dramatic reduction in the number of lethal cervical injuries

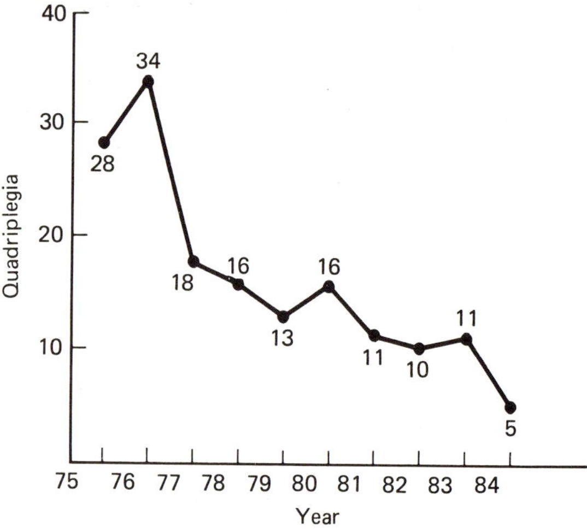

Fig. 19.1 Annual incidence of quadriplegia in American football. From Torg *et al.* (1987), with permission.

(Fig. 19.1) occurred after the law changes made in 1976 which banned initial contact with the helmet or face mask when tackling or blocking. At the same time players started using a helmet which met nationally agreed safety standards.

In rugby football a series of key articles have been published highlighting the problems of fatal and non-fatal quadriplegia in rugby football. Silver and Gill (1988) and Hoskins (1979) from England, the late Humphrey Gowland and his New Zealand colleagues, Burry and Calcinai (Burry and Gowland, 1981; Burry and Calcinai, 1988) Professor AT Scher of South Africa and Professor Brian McKibbin working with JPR Williams and his wife Dr P Williams in Wales (Williams and McKibbin, 1978, 1987) have all contributed to this research. Dr R Vanderfield of Australia, Chairman of the Medical Advisory Committee of the International Rugby Football Board has made a series of presentations to the International Rugby Football Board leading to law changes designed to increasing player safety.

The basic mechanical forces leading to quadriplegia in rugby football are flexion and rotational injuries associated with subluxation, and bilateral or unilateral locking of facet joints at or below the level of the fourth cervical vertebra.

Quadriplegia occurs in rugby in three phases of the game. Approximately one-third of players are injured during the scrum, one-third during the tackle and one-third during the ruck and maul. Recent figures suggest that the overall numbers suffering quadriplegia throughout world rugby – with the possible exception of South Africa – are reducing because of fewer numbers being injured in the scrum and the tackle (Scher, 1990).

Frequency

The overall number of players injured in the scrum in rugby football is low. Regrettably the few injuries that can occur in this controlled phase of the game can be catastrophic in the form of a quadriplegia. The player is usually injured as a result of faulty formation of the scrum due to scrums being unevenly matched, a player being inexperienced or unstable and the front rows charging together. The instability in the front row can then become more manifest by the front row of the scrum collapsing while the second row of both teams continues to exert pressure in the hope of gaining an advantage, and the trapped player, usually a hooker or tighthead prop, has a steady increase in flexion and rotation of his head under his trunk until catastrophic injury results. Occasionally the instability in the front row of the scrum can manifest itself by the tight head prop or hooker riding up or 'popping' with a severe flexion and rotational strain being placed on his neck.

The International Rugby Football Board has recognized and attempted to legislate for all of these problems by trying to control the formation of the scrum and to stop it immediately if there is any sign of significant instability, collapse or a player riding up. As a result, since the mid 1980s, the number of players being injured in the scrum appears to have been reduced.

The tackle in rugby football accounts for approximately one-third of all significant neck injuries, the majority affecting the individual being tackled. Regrettably a badly executed tackle, where the tackling player places his head in front of his opponent's thigh, continues to cause quadriplegia. The majority of tackled players are injured as a result of a multiple tackle in which they are driven to the ground and are rolled over on their head and neck, by the weight of their opponents. It is particularly dangerous if a player has been tackled illegally, above the level of the shoulder.

The overall numbers of players being injured in the tackle appear to be reducing as a result of legislation banning the high tackle and coaches are making a special effort to improve the techniques of tackling.

The remaining third of quadriplegic patients resulting from rugby football arise in the uncontrolled ruck and maul of the game. The overall numbers being injured in this phase of the game do not appear to be reducing. A player can be injured if he charges blindly with his head down into a ruck or maul in much the same way as a player can be hurt poorly executing a tackle. The majority of injuries in the ruck and maul occur when a player is trying to pick up or post a ball while still on his feet and is then driven to the ground in a flexed position while subsequent players pile up on top of him.

These catastrophic injuries have been reviewed by Silver and Gill (1988).

There is no information available with regard to the number of near misses occurring in players who have transient neurological signs with or without significant orthopaedic injury to the neck, which may have required cervical fusion. In addition, the long-term effects of the stresses of rugby football on the cervical spine have yet to be clearly documented but the early onset of traumatic degenerative cervical spondylosis in the neck has been reported.

Concussion

The major problem with the diagnosis of concussion is the lack of a practical assessment of grade I or mild concussion which makes up the vast majority of cases that occur in rugby football.

Concussion is subdivided into three grades:

Grade I – Mild; no loss of consciousness.
Grade II – Moderate; less than 5 min uncon-

sciousness or post-traumatic amnesia of more than 30 min.

Grade III – Severe; unconsciousness for more than 5 min or post-traumatic amensia of more than 24 hours.

The Committee on Head Injury Nomenclature of the Congress of Neurological surgeons has defined concussion as 'a clinical syndrome characterised by the immediate and transient post traumatic impairment of a neural function such as alteration of consciousness, disturbance of vision, equilibrium, etc. due to brain stem injury'. The National Athletic Injury/Illness Reporting System in the USA defines concussion as any disorientation caused by trauma, no matter how momentary the symptoms and no matter what the subsequent disposition of the athlete with regard to further participation in the sport. It is important to note that grade I concussion occurs without the loss of consciousness.

The essential feature with regard to grade I or mild concussion is to recognize that it is associated with brain damage. The player may appear to make a rapid and complete recovery in a very short time but there is a sustained and ill-defined period during which the brain has a reduced ability to process information. In addition the severity and duration of the functional impairment is increased with repeated concussions. The player who has sustained a first concussion is reported to have a four times greater chance of sustaining a second concussion without taking adequate rest. Accordingly, it is of considerable importance that a player suffering a mild as well as a moderate or severe degree of concussion should be removed from the field of play and given an adequate time for recovery. The consensus recommendation is that 3 weeks' rest is appropriate for mild and moderate concussion while severe concussion should be assessed on an individual basis but 6 weeks' rest would be reasonable.

In the incidence of concussion in rugby football it has been reported at approximately 5% of all injuries but these concussional episodes have not been subdivided into Grades I, II or III. There is no doubt that the incidence of grade I concussion is significantly under-reported because of a degree of collusion between players, coaches and medical attendants who are reluctant to make the diagnosis without adequate objective supporting evidence because of the recommendation made by the International Rugby Football Board regarding the 3-week period of rest.

The reported literature suggests that the incidence of concussion in schoolboys may be higher than among adult players. This is certainly the experience identified in studies undertaken in South Africa where Nathan *et al.* (1983) identified a 22% incidence of concussion and Roux *et al.* (1987) identified a 12% incidence of concussion. Roux and his colleagues made specific mention that they felt that of all rugby injuries, concussion was the one most likely to be under-reported. This feature was not confirmed by Sparks (1981) in his review of four seasons of rugby injuries sustained at Rugby School, in which the incidence of concussion was 6%. It is likely that his report gives an accurate reflection of the size of the problem in that he had a captive audience of pupils at a boarding school in England, but the nature of schoolboy rugby in South Africa and England may be widely different.

References

Addley K, Farren J (1988) Irish rugby injury survey: Dungannon Football Club (1986–1987). *British Journal of Sports Medicine* **22**, 22–4.

Burry HC, Calcinai CJ (1988) The need to make rugby safer. *British Medical Journal* **296**, 149–50.

Burry HC, Gowland H (1981) Cervical injury in rugby football: a New Zealand survey. *British Journal of Sports Medicine* **15**, 56–9.

Dalley DR, Lang DR, Rawberry JM, Caird MJ (1982) Rugby injuries: an epidemiological survey, Christchurch 1980. *New Zealand Journal of Sports Medicine* **10**, 5–17.

Hoskins T (1979) Rugby injuries to the cervical spine in English school boys. *Practitioner* **223**, 365–6.

Meuller FD, Blyth CS (1987) Fatalities from head and cervical spine injuries occurring in tackle football: 40 years experience. *Clinics in Sports Medicine* **6**, 185–96.

Nathan M, Goedeke R, Noaken TD (1983) The incidence and nature of rugby injuries experienced at one school during the 1982 rugby season. *South African Medical Journal* **64**, 132–7.

Roux CE, Geodeke R, Visser GR, Van Zyl WA, Noakes TD (1987) The epidemiology of schoolboy rugby injuries. *South African Medical Journal* **71**, 307–13.

Scher AT (1990) Premature degeneration of the cervical spine. *South African Medical Journal* **7**, 557.

Silver J, Gill S (1988) Injuries of the spine sustained during rugby. *Sports Medicine* **5**, 328–34.

Sparks JP (1981) Half a million hours of rugby football. *British Journal of Sports Medicine* **15**, 30–2.

Torg JS, Vegso JJ, Sennet B (1987) *Clinics in Sports Medicine* **6**, 61–72.

Williams P (1985) The epidemiology of rugby injuries Wales 1982–84. The Five Nations Report to the International Rugby Football Board.

Williams JGR, McKibbin B (1978) Cervical spine injuries in Rugby Union Football. *British Medical Journal* **2**, 1747.

Williams P, McKibbin B (1987) Unstable cervical spine injuries in rugby – a 20 year review. *Injury* **18**, 329–32.

20

Risks and injuries in orienteering, fell running and cross-country racing

I. P. McLean
D. A. D. MacLeod

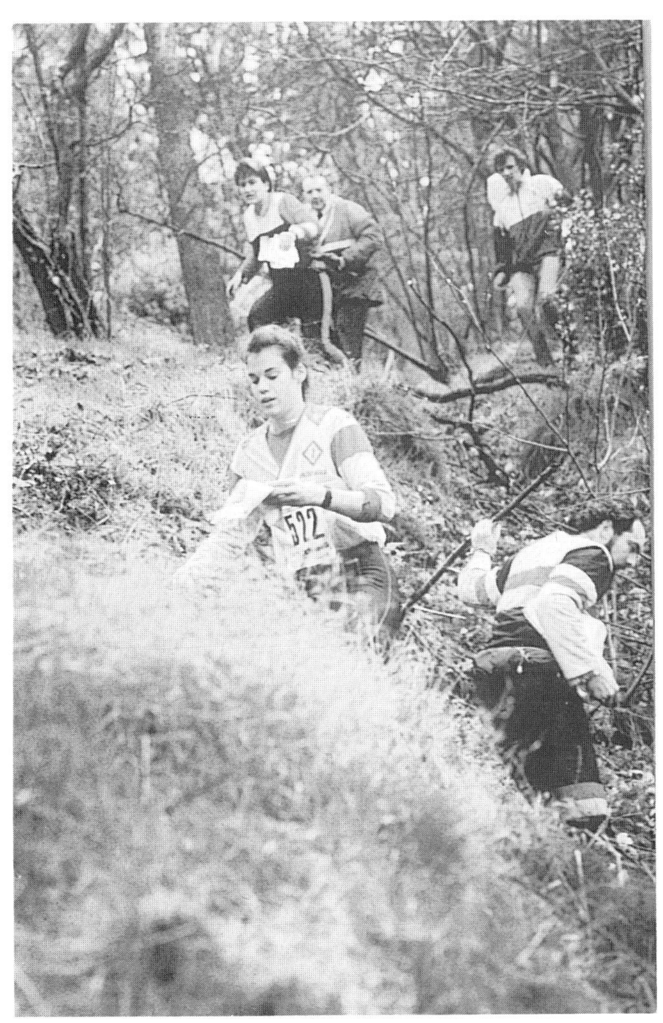

Introduction

All three sports – orienteering, fell running and cross-country racing – evolved from a desire to run in natural surroundings.

Fell racing was born in Scotland in the middle of the 11th century (Smith, 1985). The idea is simple. Competitors start together and run to the summit of one or several nearby hills before finishing, often at the starting point. The route may be fixed or optional, with several checkpoints. The course length may vary from 2 to 35 km or more with 2500 m climbing on the longest races. The Fell Runners' Association, which governs the sport in the UK, categorizes each race according to course length and severity of the terrain, which involves steep, often rocky hills and mountains with numerous other natural hazards. There are some outstanding and versatile athletes who take part in these races who have recently been given the chance to compete internationally. The World Cup races, however, tend to follow the continental European pattern of being mainly uphill, placing less emphasis on the sometimes risky descents.

It was not until the mid 19th century that cross-country running became an established sport in the gentler terrain of southern England (Temple, 1990). Many races still take place over the traditional hilly courses with walls and ploughed fields to cross rather than the racecourses associated with the major events.

The existence of large tracts of unspoiled forest in Sweden meant that navigational aids became necessary before running over the natural terrain could become a popular sport in that country. The first public orienteering event was held near Stockholm in 1919. With advances in map drawing and compass manufacture this has also now become a worldwide sport. Orienteering in the UK experienced a surge in popularity after the World Championships were held in Scotland in 1976. Something similar is expected for North America when the Championships are held there in 1993.

Orienteering is the most complex of the three sports. Each competitor must choose his or her own route between natural features identified on the map as control points set for each race by a course planner. Specially drawn large-scale maps and precision compasses are available as navigational aids.

To reduce the possibility of following each other, competitors start at intervals – 3 min apart for major races. Individuals are timed. The fastest is the winner. The physical demands of orienteering become apparent when one studies the aerobic capacity of top competitors (Saltin, 1981). The aerobic fitness of leading orienteers compares favourably with that of other long-distance runners (Table 20.1).

Table 20.1 A comparison of the maximal oxygen uptake (VO_{2max}) of top male orienteers with competitors in other sports

Sport	VO_{2max} (ml/kg/min)
Cross-country skiing	82
Middle-distance running	79
Orienteering	77
Cyclists	74
Sprinters	67
Untrained	44

Female athletes showed a similar trend.
From Saltin (1981).

Although considerable fitness and running ability are necessary to be successful in orienteering, fell running and cross-country racing, the serious competitors are heavily outnumbered by recreational participants with each of the sports having age-group races. Orienteering, in particular, attracts all ages from toddlers to octogenarians, as the navigational challenge can offset the physical.

Summary of injuries

Although the frequency of injury is greater during competition, a longer time is spent training and so more injuries occur during training. The physical training for each of the three sports is very similar. It is that of any long-distance runner with the addition of appropriate terrain running. This means that the types of injury suffered are very similar in each sport. Those occurring amongst orienteering are the most extensively documented.

Temple (1990) has provided an overview of the injuries suffered by cross-country runners. The occurrence of overuse injuries affecting the lower back and lower limb, such as Achilles tendinitis, anterior knee pain and stress fractures, agrees with that reported by Johansson (1986) and Linde (1986) for orienteers.

Sprains of the lateral ligament complex of the ankle are common problems amongst fell racers (Hodgson, 1986) and are the single most common acute injury affecting élite (Johansson, 1986) and recreational orienteers (McLean, 1990).

A summary of the most common acute and overuse injuries affecting participants in these sports is given in Table 20.2.

Table 20.2 Common injuries in orienteering, fell running and cross-country racing

Acute injuries
Lateral ankle ligament sprain
Lacerations and abrasions (especially to knee, leg, hand and head)
Gastrocnemius strain
Knee ligament injuries
Eye abrasions/foreign bodies
Tick bites

Fractures (e.g. distal fibula, tibia, distal radius) and dislocations (e.g. shoulder and elbow) are rare

Overuse injuries
Medial and anterior tibial syndromes
Iliotibial friction syndrome
Anterior knee pain (chondromalacia patellae)
Blisters
Peroneal tenosynovitis
Low back pain

From Johansson (1986, 1988); Korpi *et al.* (1987); McLean (1990) and Temple (1990).

Among acute injuries, knee problems and lower limb muscle strains are outnumbered by ankle ligament sprains and wounds to various parts of the body.

Stepping in a hole with consequent hyperextension and/or rotation with a fixed foot is one of the mechanisms by which meniscal and ligamentous damage to the knee occurs. Another cause is the steep, uneven descents which are particularly common in fell racing. That such forces can be considerable is demonstrated by Idrissi *et al.* (1985) who report a posterior dislocation of the tibia on the femur with popliteal artery damage in a cross-country runner. Injuries of such severity are, fortunately, unusual in these sports.

A total of 85% of injuries affect the lower limb. Overuse injuries predominate during the winter when training volume is at its greatest and if the transition of high-intensity training is undertaken too abruptly in the spring.

Overuse injuries

The most common overuse injuries can be predicted on anatomical grounds. Orava and Puranen (1979) found a large group of orienteers with medial and anterior tibial syndromes or shin splints in their group of patients with overuse injuries of the leg. Linde (1986) agrees and also found personal tenosynovitis to be a common problem.

These injuries are aggravated by repeated resistance to inversion and eversion at the subtalar and mid-tarsal joints, caused by the uneven ground with consequent tearing of the muscular origins of tibialis anterior and posterior, or swelling within their rigid fascial compartments and friction within the peroneal synovial sheath. Alternatively the peroneal retinacula can be weakened allowing the peroneal tendons to slip over the lateral malleolus.

Stretching and selective strengthening exercises for these muscles may help prevent these injuries.

Pain from the ligament stabilizing the subtalar and midtarsal joints involved in inversion and eversion should be considered in the differential diagnosis of mid-foot pain in these athletes. This may mimic a stress fracture, which is less likely in participants in these sports than in road runners because their usual running surface is softer.

Other overuse injuries are identical to those occurring in other distance runners. Their features and treatment have been extensively reported in previous texts and will not be further considered here.

Ankle ligament sprains

Rough ground explains the frequency of injuries to the lateral ligament of the ankle. Inversion of the foot with internal rotation in relation to the tibia is the usual mechanism of injury. A smaller stress is required to damage the anterior talofibular ligament than the calcaneofibular ligament. The anterior tibiofibular ligament and anterior part of the joint capsule are also damaged but it is unusual for the posterior talofibular ligament to be torn (Cox, 1985).

Although the treatment of ankle sprains is the same irrespective of cause, the nature of the sports requires attention to be paid to certain aspects.

Events are often held in remote areas with difficult access to regular medical facilities. Qualified medical cover is desirable for such events to exert selectivity over which casualties require specialist referral for further treatment. Cox (1985) concludes that surgical repair of the lateral ligaments is inappropriate for most patients. Absolute indications for referral are, therefore, limited to fractures of the distal fibula (King, 1983), talus and fifth metatarsal as well as ruptures of the Achilles tendon and severe sprains to the deltoid ligment on the medial side of the ankle, which are often associated with a fracture to the medial malleolus.

Lateral ligament sprains can be differentiated from fractures by careful attention to clinical detail. The distinction is easier soon after the injury.

The history is important, not only to distinguish sprains from fractures, but also to allow appropriate reduction of displaced fractures by reversing the mechanism of injury. Inability to bear weight suggests a fracture. However, the stoicism of fell runners should not be underestimated. One competitor completed the 80-km élite class at the 2-day Karrimor International Mountain Marathon in 1985 having sustained a fracture to the distal fibula when jumping from a stile shortly after the start!

Careful examination is vital. Inspection will reveal a broadening of the distal tibiofibular joint in significant fractures and often posterior subluxation at the talocrural joint. The site of tenderness should be determined precisely. The surface markings of the three ligaments are shown in Figure 20.1. Tenderness along these lines suggests a sprain. Significant fractures tend to occur about 5 cm proximal to the tip of the lateral malleolus, a distinctly different site.

Examination is also useful in assessing the severity of sprains. The integrity of the anterior talofibular ligament can be determined by the

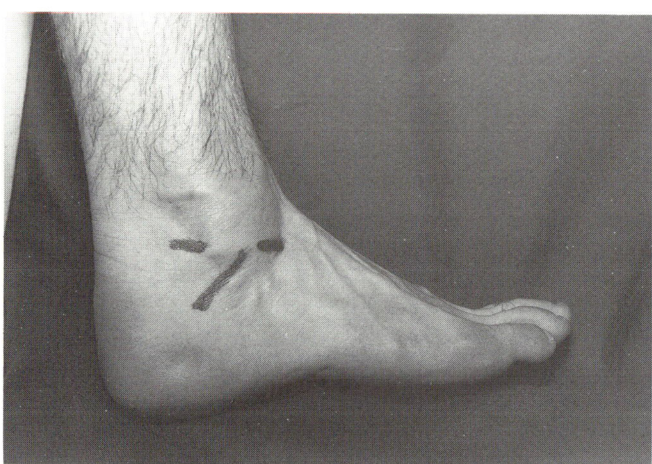

Fig. 20.1 Surface markings of the lateral ligament of the ankle, with the posterior sulcus for the peroneal tendons.

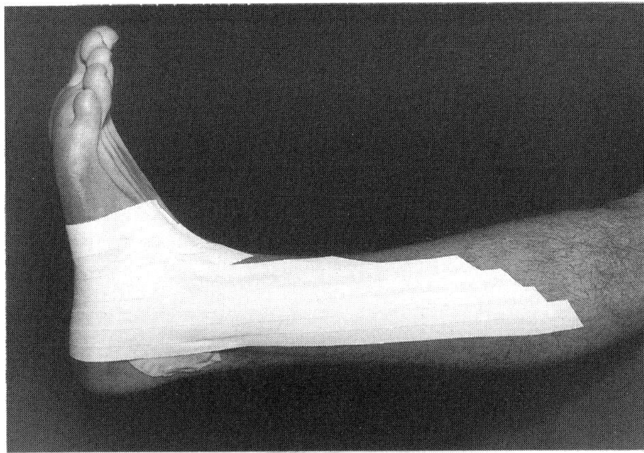

Fig. 20.2 Ankle-supporting technique using shaped chiropody felt and non-stretch tape.

anterior drawer test. In a positive test the foot is drawn straight forwards by one hand behind the heel while the other pushes back on the distal tibia. The patient should be seated to reduce tension in the Achilles tendon.

A slow, sustained inversion stress may reveal instability of the calcaneofibular ligament by opening a gap between the tip of the lateral malleolus and talus at the anterolateral part of the joint (Clain, 1980). Stress radiographs under local or regional anaesthesia may be necessary to demonstrate this, however. The mid-foot should be stabilized during this manoeuvre to prevent the normal inversion at the subtalar and midtarsal joints.

Whatever the severity of the injury, prompt first aid is vital. The affected ankle should be rested and elevated for up to 48 hours with ice applied immediately for 30 min and again at 2-hourly intervals on the day of injury and the following day, and after early attempts at mobilization. A compression bandage should be applied during the daytime.

Of the options available for immobilization, adhesive taping is the most convenient to apply at the race site. McLean (1989) has described a technique which specifically stabilizes the lateral side of the ankle (Fig. 20.2). This peroneal pad and strapping reduce trauma to the skin of the medial side of the leg which will help prevent subsequent irritation and even infection when the competitor returns to muddy terrain. Correctly applied, this taping can give support for 5 days before requiring renewal.

The risk of re-injury is two to three times that of injury to previously healthy ligaments. Taping also has a prophylactic role.

Wounds

Lacerations, grazes and abrasions collectively form the single largest group of traumatic injuries affecting the orienteer in competition. They particularly affect the lower limbs due to collisions with boulders, tree stumps and fallen branches but also affect the scalp, face and eyes because of overhanging branches. Falls frequently cause cuts to the hands.

Wounds are also common problems for fell runners and cross-country runners but the mechanism may differ, such as being struck by falling scree or spiked by running shoes.

It is the exeception for a wound to be severe enough to cause retirement from a race and, as a result, it is usually subjected to mud, streams and undergrowth before receiving attention.

Care of wounds must therefore be meticulous to prevent infection. Paul and Clark (1989) have produced a summary of the micro-organisms commonly found in soil, which should encourage thorough cleaning of any wound! Amongst the common bacteria are *Pseudomonas*, *Bacillus* and

Acitomycetes species as well as *Lactobacillus* and *Enterobacter*. The spore-forming anaerobes of the *Clostridium* genera, *C. tetani* and *C. welchii*, are however those organisms particularly associated with infections in wounds contaminated by soil. Folan (1985) revealed the rather alarming statistic that 27% of a large sample of orienteers could not recall being immunized against tetanus in the previous 10 years. This is particularly sad since 10 years earlier Smith *et al.* (1975) had emphasized the importance of active immunization in tetanus prevention. Competitors need to be educated to improve their cover.

Patients with wounds which are over 6 hours old, dirty, penetrating or with significant tissue damage, and whose immune status is unknown or who last had a course or booster of antitetanus toxoid more than 10 years prior to injury require injection with human tetanus immunoglobulin in addition to active immunization. Additional antibiotic cover may be necessary for penetrating wounds.

Thorough surgical toilet remains the single most important step in preventing tetanus and ensuring that a wound heals without infection. Accordingly patients may require referral to a health centre or hospital Accident and Emergency department.

Hepatitis B

Bacterial infection is not the only complication of wounds in orienteering. From 1957 to 1967 Swedish epidemiologists conducted a classic intervention trial (Ringertz, 1971).

Between December 1957 and May 1960, 169 cases of hepatitis B were reported amongst orienteers in Sweden. Consequently competitors were recommended to wear greater leg protection and not to share soap or towels in the showers after the race. From June 1960 to May 1962 there were 392 more cases. The epidemic had spread to involve people in all parts of the country. Stricter regulations were enforced. All orienteering competitions were cancelled during the spring of 1962, no infected orienteer was allowed to compete until 15 months after the onset of the illness and the 'full-body cover' rule was introduced (Fig. 20.3). In the following year only six cases were reported.

Two years later, however, the preventive measures were relaxed and there were 41 cases in the next 12 months. The 'full-body cover' rule was reintroduced and from 1966 until the present day the risk of contracting hepatitis B at an orienteering event has remained very low.

Other viral illnesses

Commens (1987) and Mobacken and Nordin (1987) report transmission of molluscum contagiosum to orienteers. This common benign poxvirus infection presents as multiple small umbilicated papules. It is transmitted directly from person to person, usually by close bodily contact. In the general population, unlike in orienteers, it is unusual for the lower limbs to be affected (Juel-Jensen, 1987).

A more serious condition to which participants in 'wilderness sports' are exposed is tick-borne viral encephalitis. This disease falls into two groups both geographically and clinically but flaviviruses are responsible for all cases (Simpson, 1987). Far-East Russian encephalitis is a severe paralytic encephalitis transmitted by the tick *Ixodes persulcatus*. Cases occur in the eastern former Soviet Union, around Leningrad and in Czechoslovakia. Central European encephalitis occurs throughout Central Europe extending into Scandinavia. It is transmitted by another ixodid tick, *I. ricinus*. It is generally less severe than the Far-East Russian type.

Prevention of this group of diseases is desirable because of the unfortunate sequelae. Encephalitis following multiple tick bites is associated with a mortality rate in excess of 20% in unvaccinated individuals (Okulova *et al.*, 1989). Single bites to the axilla, upper limb and head seem to be more hazardous than those to the lower limb.

Active immunization offered to the inhabitants of an endemic area consists of a course of three injections at 1- and 6-month intervals. Travellers to these areas are usually only given the first two of these doses but, as orienteers share the predi-

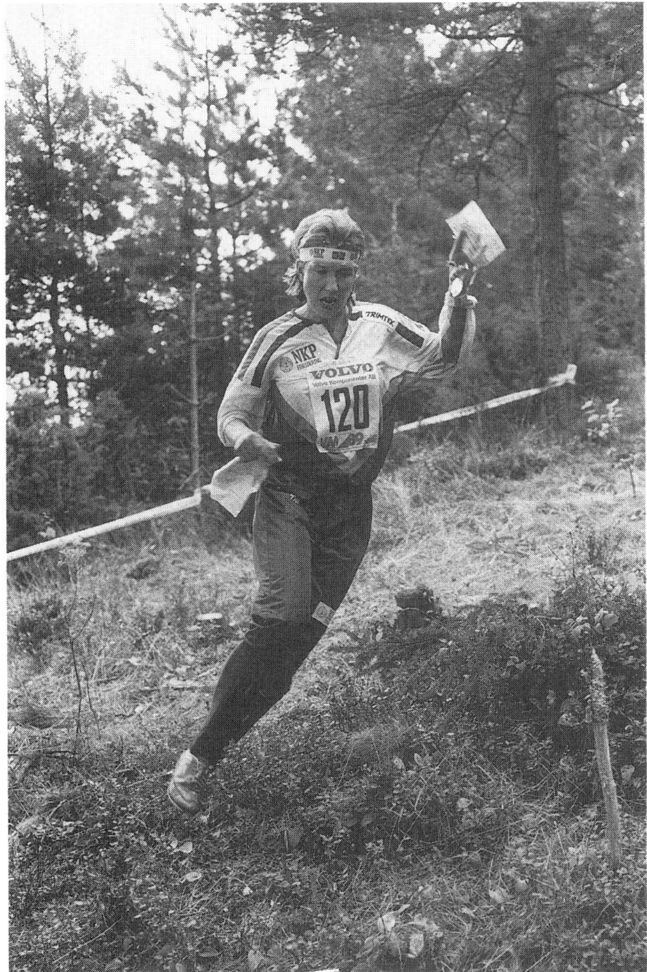

Fig. 20.3 An orienteer demonstrating typical equipment and clothing.

lection of host and vector for forested areas, a sound argument could be put forward for giving the full course to competitive venturing to affected regions.

Lyme Disease

Ixodes ricinus also transmits Lyme disease. First described in Connecticut, USA, in 1975, this is a multi-system disorder caused by the spirochaete, *Borrelia burgdorferi*. Egherman and Rahn (1989) liken the disease to syphilis because of its ability to mimic common illnesses and its staged progression.

Classically it begins with an annular red rash which clears at the centre and is called erythema chronicum migrans. A single lesion starts at the site of a tick-bite within a month after the bite. It spreads and may exceed 50 cm in diameter. If the patient is untreated, similar smaller lesions may develop at other sites over the next week. Both primary and secondary lesions may persist for weeks or months. Haematogenous spread of the causative organism gives rise to a range of non-specific flu-like symptoms.

The second stage of the disease, weeks to

months later, is associated with neurological, cardiac and ophthalmic complications. The neurological ones may be similar to those found in tick-borne viral encephalitis but treatment is entirely different. Other problems at this stage include Bell's palsy, atrioventricular block, conjunctivitis and panophthalmitis with blindness.

Stage III begins months to years after the initial infection. Neurological abnormalities, especially severe fatigue, again occur at this stage but it is arthritis which characterizes this chronic phase of the disease. Indeed the disease first came to light because of an apparent epidemic of juvenile rheumatoid arthritis amongst the inhabitants of Old Lyme and neighbouring communities.

Up to 50% of untreated patients suffer the arthritis which typically affects one or a few large joints, especially the knee, in a series of exacerbations and remissions. Pain is less of a feature than redness and swelling. Some patients, however, suffer a symmetrical polyarthritis, some a chronic, erosive arthritis and others fluctuating, non-arthritic musculoskeletal pain.

The unreliability of the serological investigations to confirm this disease means that diagnosis should be made on clinical grounds. One reason for not relying on such tests is the frequency of asymptomatic infection. Fahrer *et al.* (1988) report a 20% prevalence of immunoglobin G and 4% prevalence of immunoglobulin M antibodies to *Borrelia burgdorferi* amongst a group of 1000 orienteers in Switzerland. Clinical recognition, however, is difficult as the pattern often differs from that described. For example, in one study described by Egherman and Rahn (1989), 80% of patients with Lyme arthritis had no previous history of erythema chronicum migrans.

Early recognition of the disease is important, however, because antibiotic treatment is most effective when given in stage I.

Tetracycline 250 mg q.i.d. or doxycycline 100 mg b.d. orally for 10–21 days is the treatment of choice for stage I disease in adults. The same drugs in the same dose should be given for 2–3 weeks for Bell's palsy or 3 weeks for mild atrioventricular block. Penicillin V or amoxycillin should be substituted in those for whom tetracycline is unsuitable. The later stages and more serious complications require intravenous penicillin G 10–20 Mu q.i.d. or ceftriaxone 2 g q.i.d. for up to 21 days.

Again prevention is desirable. Measures include tick repellents and safe and complete removal of any ticks which do bite. This means a steady, straight pull with blunt forceps held in gloved hands, taking care not to burst the tick. The affected area and the remover's hands should be washed thoroughly afterwards.

Five years after its first description, Lyme disease had been recognized in 19 countries on the three continents of Europe, North America and Australasia (Schmid, 1984). The vectors vary. Mosquitoes have been implicated in Sweden, though most European cases are transmitted by *Ixodes ricinus*. The closely related *I. dammini* and *I. pacificus* are responsible in the USA. The Australian vector is unknown.

Climate and environment

Orienteering, fell running and cross-country racing are all physically demanding sports performed outdoors often in remote, even mountainous countryside. This causes two problems: the effect of extremes of weather and difficulty with access for rescuers in the event of injury or illness. The first of these problems is greater than for many other outdoor sports because of the exposed nature of the terrain. It is most unusual for races to be cancelled because of the weather.

Heat

The American College of Sports Medicine has issued a position statement about prevention of heat injuries during distance running (Strauss, 1979). It advises that water stations should be provided at intervals of 3–4 km in races of 16 km or more. Although primarily intended for road races, these or similar guidelines should be enforced for other distance-running sports. Indeed, even more stringent guidelines may be required. Noakes (1982) reports three cases of heatstroke at the

South African National Cross-Country Running Championships in 1981 at which the longest race was 12 km.

The provision of refreshment during orienteering races is a problem because of the freedom of route choice and the relative inaccessibility of some parts of the course. However, it is a problem which should be addressed because races with recommended winning times of 90 min or more are held in mid-summer.

Fell runners are rarely provided with refreshment on the course. They are expected to carry their own or to drink from streams. Thus, an infection risk is added to that of hyperthermia.

Cold

There are no rules governing the clothing which competitors in any of the three sports should wear to provide protection against hypothermia. Apart from the requirement of cross-country and fell runners to wear club colours and orienteers to be fully clad from neck to feet, clothing is left to the discretion of the individual.

However, it is not always easy to anticipate weather conditions and wind-chill on remote, exposed mountain tops and overdressing has its disadvantages. Head gear is something which tends to be neglected. A considerable amount of heat is lost through the head because of its high surface area to volume ratio and the vascularity of the scalp. This is especially true in children who have proportionately larger heads for their body size. Most hats can be removed and easily carried if weather conditions improve.

Adverse weather conditions at the Ben Nevis fell race in Scotland in September 1988 and the British Orienteering Championship of March 1990 in Yorkshire have stimulated discussion as to the powers of race organizers to force competitors to dress appropriately for the weather. At the former, organizers were thought by some to have been too lenient in allowing inadequately dressed competitors to start. At the latter they were seen to be too officious in disqualifying competitors who did not carry protective clothing! At present the matter remains unresolved but lack of judgement by a competitor can cause an added burden to be placed on first aid and mountain rescue personnel.

Rescue services

In Scotland all medical, first-aid and mountain rescue cover is provided by volunteers. At present the rules of the sports only demand such cover at large events. Most of the casualties are 'walking wounded' and manage to present themselves at the central treatment point. McLean (1990) summarizes the injuries at two Scottish orienteering events. Few required transport from the site of injury. MacGregor (1988) describes the activities of the Scottish Mountain Rescue teams. In the 26 months from 1 January 1985, of 190 accidents reported in his study only one involved a competitor in one of these sports.

Co-operation between organizers and health care workers at the events can improve safety and reduce demands on local medical facilities.

Conclusion

The overall impression of all three sports is of healthy aerobic activity in grand surroundings practised by people of all age groups. The vast majority of the injuries are minor. The unpleasant tick-borne diseases are rare and their possibility does not occur to most competitors.

The medical profession can keep the sports safe by encouraging up-to-date immunization against tetanus for all participants and protection against tick-borne encephalitis for those travelling to or competing in endemic areas. No immunization is available against Lyme disease as yet, but vigilance for the condition in all of its forms will allow the diagnosis to be made earlier with consequent improvement in outcome.

Intervention by the sports' governing bodies in maintaining safety is exemplified by the handling of the hepatitis B outbreak in Sweden. Organizers should be encouraged to enforce dress regulations, not only for protection against wounds but also in extreme weather conditions.

Equipment manufacturers have also contributed to the safety of the sports. Reinforced but light-weight studded or spiked shoes have been developed for each of the sports (Bogdan and Jackson, 1988). Appropriate footwear may reduce the risk of ankle ligament sprains in addition to preventing blisters and many overuse injuries.

In orienteering, the modern, light-weight, snag-resistant nylon suit has evolved (Fig. 20.3). Although the 'full-body cover' rule has been relaxed in some countries to permit short-sleeved tops, it is a requirement of the sport that full leg cover be worn. Many competitors add to the leg protection offered by the orienteering suit by wearing long socks with thin plastic or leather reinforcements to the shins, called 'bramble-bashers', or light-weight padded gaiters. Recent times have seen a growing trend towards wearing stretch tights instead of the conventional trousers and lower leg protection. It will be interesting to see the effect on lower limb trauma in the sport. Reinforcement to the knees of whatever garment is worn may prevent some knee lacerations.

Although the sports are relatively safe, some injuries are inevitable. Prompt and appropriate initial management is the single greatest step to ensuring continued enjoyment for all the participants.

Acknowledgements

We gratefully ackowledge the assistance provided by John Blair-Fish of the Fell Runners' Association, Deeside Orienteering and Leisure Maps, Richard Jones, David McLean, Mrs Margaret Hughes, Dr Philip Henman and the Medical Illustration Department at St John's Hospital.

References

Bogdan RJ, Jackson SJ (1988) Be a step ahead in orienteering. *Australian Orienteer* 6–9.

Clain A (ed.) (1980) The leg and ankle joint. In: *Hamilton Bailey's Demonstration of Physical Signs in Clinical Surgery* 16th edn. Bristol: John Wright, pp 530–3.

Commens CA (1987) Cutaneous transmission of molluscum contagiosum during orienteering competition. *Medical Journal of Australia* **146**, 117.

Cox JS (1985) Surgical and non-surgical treatment of acute ankle sprains. *Clinical Orthopaedics* **198**, 118–26.

Egherman WP, Rahn DW (1989) Lyme disease: unmasking the great masquerader. *Emergency Medicine Reports* **10**, 99–106.

Fahrer H, Sauvain MJ, van den Linden S, Zhioua E, Gern L, Aeschlimann A (1988) Prävalenz der Lyme-Borreliose in einer schweizerischen Risikopopulation. *Schweizerische Medizinische Wochenschrift* **118**, 65–9.

Folan JC (1985) Anti-tentanus immunisation in orienteers. *British Journal of Sports Medicine* **19**, 39–40.

Hodgson S (1986) Ankle injuries. *Fell Runner* 94–5.

Idrissi M, Cardon A, Nicol JB, Kerdiles Y (1985) Complications vasculaires des luxations du genou en pratique sportive (a propos de 3 cas). *Médecine du Sport* **59**, 72–4.

Johansson C (1986) Injuries in elite orienteers. *American Journal of Sports Medicine* **14**, 410–15.

Johansson C (1988) Training, injury and disease in senior and junior elite orienteers. *Scottish Journal of Orienteering* **4**, 3–13.

Juel-Jensen BE (1987) Molluscum contagiosum. In: Weatherall DJ, Ledingham JGG, Warrell DA (eds) *Oxford Textbook of Medicine* 2nd edn. Oxford: Oxford University Press, pp 584–5.

King JB (1983) Fractures: the lower limb – 2. *British Journal of Hospital Medicine* **29**, 267–72.

Korpi J, Haapanen A, Svahn T (1987) Frequency, location and types of orienteering injuries. *Scandinavian Journal of Sports Science* **9**, 53–6.

Linde F (1986) Injuries in orienteering. *British Journal of Sports Medicine* **20**, 125–7.

MacGregor AR (1988) The nature and causes of injuries sustained in 190 Scottish mountain accidents. Research report 1. Edinburgh: The Scottish Sports Council.

McLean DA (1989) Use of adhesive strapping in sport. *British Journal of Sports Medicine* **23**, 147–9.

McLean I (1990) First aid for orienteering in Scotland. *Scottish Journal of Orienteering* **6**, 55–63.

Mobacken H, Nordin P (1987) Molluscum contagiosum among cross-country runners. *Journal of the American Academy of Dermatology* **17**, 519–20.

Noakes TD (1982) Heatstroke during the 1981 national cross-country running championships. *South African Medical Journal* **61**, 145.

Okulova NM, Chunikhin SP, Vavilova VE, Maiorova

AD (1989) The location of the infecting tick bite and the severity of the course of tick-borne encephalitis. *Medinnskaia Parazitologha (Moskua)* 78–85.
Orava S, Puranen J (1979) Athletes' leg pains. *British Journal of Sports Medicine* **13**, 92–7.
Paul EA, Clark FE (1989) Components of the soil biota. In: *Soil Microbiology and Biochemistry*, San Diego: Harcourt Brace Jovanovich, pp 49–73.
Ringertz O (1971) Serum hepatitis in Swedish track-finders. *Scandinavian Journal of Infectious Diseases* **3** (suppl 2), 3–25.
Saltin B (1981) Physical work capacity in orienteering II. IOF Report 9–11.
Schmid GP (1984) The global distribution of Lyme disease. *Yale Journal of Biology and Medicine* **57**, 617–18.
Simpson DIH (1987) Flaviviruses. In: Weatherall DJ, Ledingham JGG, Warrell DA (eds) *Oxford Textbook of Medicine* 2nd edn. Oxford: Oxford University Press, pp 5.122–3.
Smith B (1985) *Stud Marks on the Summits*. Preston: SKG Publications.
Smith JWG, Laurence DR, Evans DG (1975) Prevention of tetanus in the wounded. *British Medical Journal* **3**, 453–5.
Strauss RH (1979) Appendix B: American College of Sports Medicine position statements – prevention of heat injuries during distance running. In: Strauss RH (ed) *Sports Medicine and Physiology*, Philadelphia: WB Saunders, pp 406–8.
Temple C (1990) *Marathon, Cross-country and Road Running*. London: Stanley Paul.

21

Risks and athletic injuries in North American sports

E. C. Percy

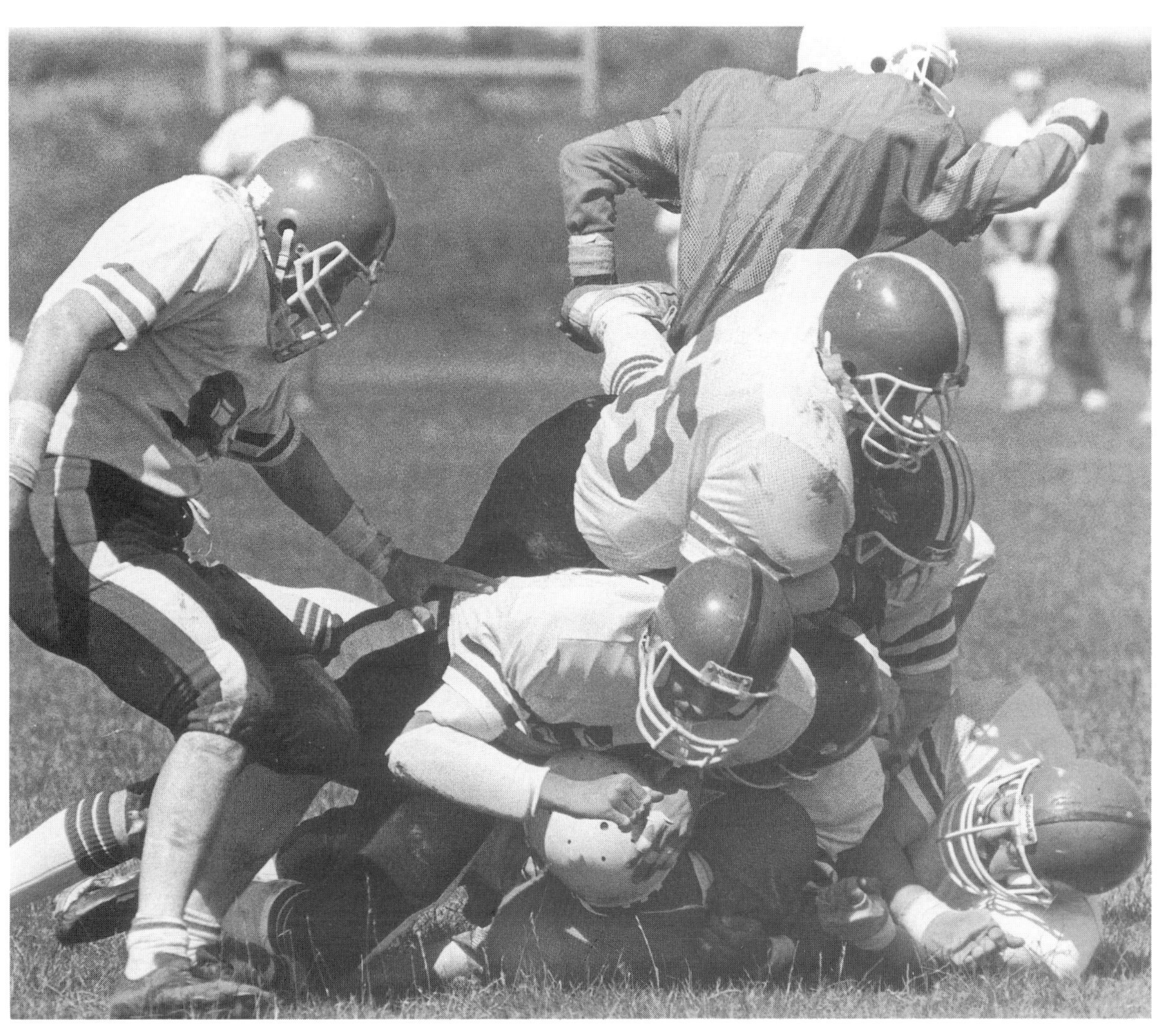

Introduction

It would appear that while the flame of fitness in North America was first kindled in the early 1960s, it was not really until the 1970s that the fitness boom exploded. In this respect North America appears to have lagged far behind the European and Eastern bloc countries during these early days. Certainly in Canada and the USA, while there was some support at governmental levels, we again lagged far behind our eastern-lying neighbours in this area.

Athletic competition at the international level has grown tremendously in both Canada and the USA in the 70s and 80s, largely through the Olympic movement. The national Olympic Committee (NOC) in the USA is funded entirely through private means. In Canada, the funding is largely from the private sector with the Canadian Government's participation amounting to less than 10% of the annual budget. In addition to the Olympics, Canada and the USA compete with the other countries in Central and South America in the Pan American Games. Canada participates also in the Commonwealth Games, composed of those countries who were one time, or who still are, members of the British Commonwealth of Nations. There are many other national and international competitions now being held on the North American continent, Europe and Asia, in which both countries compete.

At the amateur level, at both elementary and high-school levels as well as at the collegiate level, there has been a tremendous growth in the interest and participation in athletics. Indeed, most universities, certainly in the USA, function virtually as farm teams for the professional leagues in the major sports of American football, baseball, basketball and to a lesser degree ice hockey. The majority of professional athletes performing in baseball, basketball and football are university graduates, while in ice hockey the majority of competitors seem to have started on a professional career without the advantage of a college education.

There has been a tremendous growth in interest in physical fitness by recreational athletes. Fitness areobic clubs have sprung up in virtually every city in the USA and Canada. These physical training centres function largely as profit-making corporations and yet obviously perform a valuable function in fitness development. In addition, they act in a sense as a social club or meeting place as a dividend to the health improvement aspects. Associated with this increased involvement in such centres, and in particular with aerobics, a significant number of overuse injuries have resulted.

Industry in North America, following Japan's early lead, was quick to follow suit in developing or sponsoring membership in health clubs for their employees. There is some sound evidence that this effort has reduced tardiness and work loss by their employees in companies so involved (Barnes, 1983). Indeed, many large hotels in North America now include on their property, in addition to swimming pools, fitness centres with standard exercise equipment and even outdoor running tracks for the convenience (and benefit) of their guests.

It is now estimated that in North America upwards of 60 million people are running on a daily or weekly basis and a lesser number are involved in such recreational fitness sports as swimming, cycling, crew (rowing) and cross-country skiing. At the organized level of sporting activities such as team or college sports, cross-over training is now a vital part of the programme regardless of in which sport the participant is partaking. That is to say athletes in training take part in other activities, such as weight-training, as well as their main area of athletic endeavour.

It appears from the current scientific literature that not only has this increased interest in physical fitness resulted in a better lifestyle, but has also possibly contributed to increasing longevity of life and a lessening of morbidity (Bruce, 1984). A dividend that follows along these lines is that most athletes do not generally smoke tobacco products or consume large amounts of alcohol. Athletes in training are more conscious of their diets and proper nutrition nowadays – another factor which should certainly reduce the risk of lung and heart disease. The participation in athletics at the recreational level possibly reduces the drug problem in this particular group of individuals, although it appears that the huge salaries now paid to professional athletes in North America, often out of proportion to the involvement, have led to increasing drug problems at the professional level. We now learn of professional athletes who not only become dependent on drugs such as alcohol, cocaine and anabolic steroids, but also act as purveyors of the same drugs to other athletes. Indeed, it has been jokingly said that the majority of the crime reports in North America are now found on the sports pages due to the large number of athletes involved in drug use and trafficking. Alcohol has become the major problem in American professional athletes, an increasing number seem to have become involved with this major drug problem annually.

The term 'amateur', in essence from the Latin meaning a love of participation, seems no longer to exist in North America other than at the elementary and high-school level. A large number of élite athletes who compete in the USA and Canada at the national and international levels are now being supported to some degree by their NOC or by private funding from major commercial or athletic organizations.

This intense involvement of the North American population in some form or other of physical activity has led to the growing need for health professionals with skills related to the treatment of athletic-incurred injuries. In many of our universities, medical students now ask for sports medicine rotations, as do residents in medicine when applying for hospital training. Because of the demand for expertise in sports medicine an increasing number of physicians lay claim to being experts in the field, without any form of documentation or indeed any specific training. There are a number of professional organizations which offer recognition in the field of sports medicine in this continent, such as the American College of Sports Medicine, the American Orthopedic Society for Sports Medicine, the Canadian Academy of Sports Medicine and the Canadian Association of Sports Sciences, to mention but a few.

The Canadian Academy of Sports Medicine (whose members are all physicians) in 1989 instituted a practical oral and written examination in sports medicine. This test thoroughly covers all areas of sports medicine from clinical to basic science subjects. Successful candidates are granted a certificate of accreditation in sports medicine. There is no 'grandfather clause' and all those physicians who wish to call themselves sports medicine specialists in Canada will undoubtedly seek such accreditation. No such examination board as yet exists in the USA or elsewhere in the world, to the author's knowledge.

There appear weekly dozens of sports medical publications specifically concerned with the treatment and management of athletic injuries. Indeed a large number of standard medical journals often include sports medicine-oriented articles. In addition a large volume of lay periodicals deal with training, performance, diet and injuries: these magazines are available to recreational as well as élite athletes. As a result, athletes in general now have a fairly sophisticated knowledge of proper training methods and some understanding of the injuries that result from participation in sports. They seek out those health professionals who have expertise in the recognition and treatment of athletic injuries.

International teams now travelling the world are accompanied by qualified trainers, physiotherapists and physicians who have a thorough knowledge of injuries caused by athletics. The number of areas of expertise in the athletic health professional field has grown tremendously and there are probably now over 40 interest areas in the field of sports medicine. Family physicians, internists, general surgeons, orthopedic surgeons, exercise physiologists, physiotherapists, trainers, physical educators, nutritionists, psychologists, psychiatrists, osteopaths, neurologists, podiatrists and chiropractors are but a few of these areas.

To orthopaedics seems to have fallen the major involvement of treatment of athletic injuries. This seems to be obvious in that the majority of problems in the health field related to athletics involve the musculoskeletal system. However, many musculoskeletal injuries can well be handled very efficiently by any physician with training in sports medicine and referred on to an orthopaedic surgeon if deemed necessary by the primary care physician.

Biomechanics of injury

While the majority of problems in athletics are related to the musculoskeletal system, fortunately most of these injuries involve the soft tissues and are extra-articular. The articular injuries themselves are of a far more serious nature generally speaking, particularly where joint surfaces are involved or ligaments about the joints are in some way disrupted. Various sports characteristically do have injuries which are more common to that sport than to other forms of athletic endeavour. Sports themselves may be classified in many ways, such as strenuous, moderately strenuous or non-strenuous. Similarly, sports can be broken down into non-contact, limited contact, contact or collision sports. However, some non-contact sports may become collision sports when control is lost, such as in skiing, mountain climbing or hang-gliding.

When a force is exerted on a body its effects are noted in two ways – internally and externally. Take, for example, the bat in baseball striking the ball as it crosses the plate. The external force exerted at the time of contact of the bat with the ball causes the ball to fly through the air. At the same time, an internal force is exerted on the ball itself, leading to mechanical deformation of the ball. Similar effects are noted in the body when a force is applied to part of the musculoskeletal system. When a muscle or a group of muscles is contracted the limb controlled by those muscles moves in response to that contractile force. This results in a stress being applied to the muscles themselves (agonists) or to those opposing this contraction (antagonists) and to the joints over which they have control. Measurable change in the shape of the object being stressed results in a strain to that particular area of the body. This can result in elastic or plastic deformation. If these terms are expressed in the form of a graph we may plot stress in the vertical axis and strain on the horizontal axis. Tissues are able to absorb a limited amount of strain which varies with the structure involved. By stretching, the involved tissue will elongate, depending on the structure involved, and when that stress is removed the tissue will return to its original shape. This is referred to as the elastic strain. When the elastic limit of any particular tissue is exceeded then a plastic phase is entered where partial or complete tearing of the tissues results, and the deformed tissues does not return to its original resting status. This is demonstrated in Fig 21.1 using as an example an adult tendon under stress.

A common problem leading to injuries in the musculoskeletal system is excessive loading of the involved tissues. If any biological system is stressed often and long enough it will break down. These stress effects can be defined as macrotrauma, where there is one excessive uncontrolled force, or microtrauma, where there are multiple repetitive controlled forces. In the former case an example might be the skier who loses control and sustains a fracture of the tibia. In the latter case, a typical example would be the stress or fatigue fracture of a bone.

In general, soft tissue injuries in the body result in either an injury to the musculotendinous unit, which is called a strain, or the injury may lead to damage to the ligamentous structures which support joints and allow motion to various planes – a sprain.

Injuries to the musculotendinous units vary according to the age of the patient and the biomechanical properties of the tissue involved. For example, the adolescent under 16 years of age who receives an injury from excessive stress to the musculotendinous unit will usually suffer from an apophyseal injury because this particular area in the body is the biomechanical weak point in the musculotendinous unit in that age group. A typical example would be an avulsion of the anterior superior iliac spine by excessive force being applied to the sartorius muscle. Another common site of such injury is the tibial apophysis which may be partially avulsed or fractured by an excessive force being applied to the quadriceps. Indeed, it is quite probable that Osgood–Schlatter's disease is in fact a stress fracture of the tibial apophysis. In the adolescent age group the ligaments are far stronger than the epiphyseal line (physis), which is the biomechanical weak point. It is far more common in that age group to sustain an epiphyseal

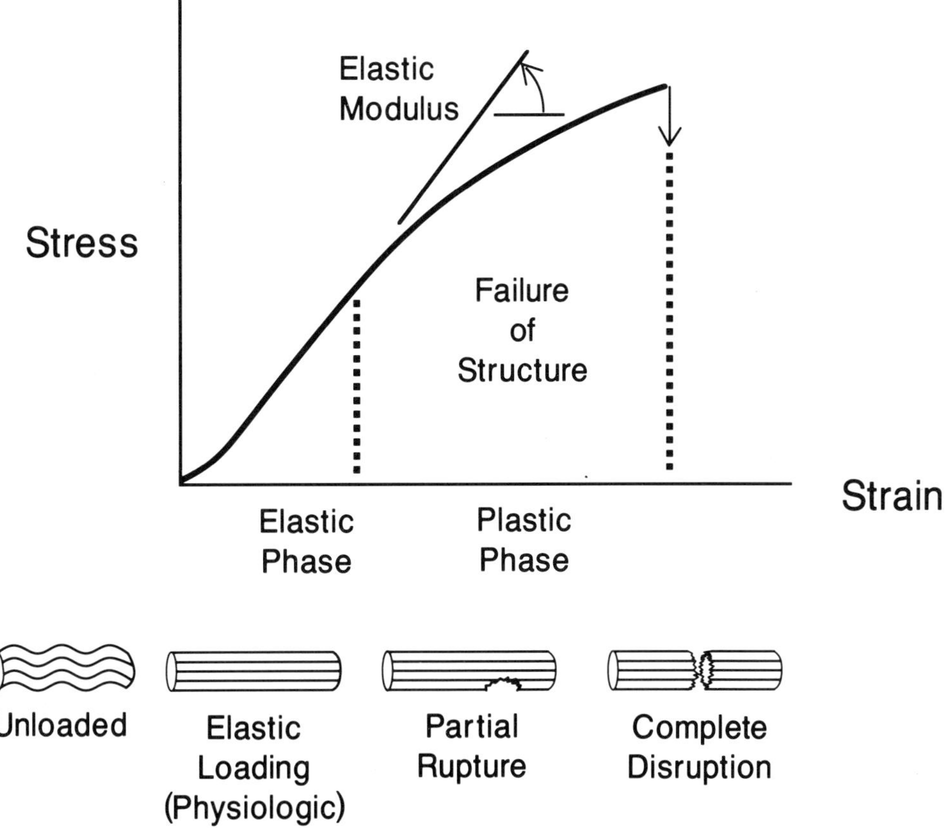

Fig. 21.1 Effect of stress on the tendon and the resultant strain, from resting phase through elastic phase to plastic phase and disruption.

separation of the lower femoral or proximal tibial physis than it is to injure the medial collateral ligament of the knee.

In young adults, from 17 to 40 years of age, the musculotendinous junction is the biomechanical area of weakness other than the tendon of origin or insertion. Usually injuries of this type occur in muscles which cross two joints. Classical examples are a hamstring tear or a partial rupture of the centre slip of the rectus femoris muscle.

Over the age of 40 years the biomechanical weak point is usually the tendon itself. With increasing age degenerative changes occur in the collagen due to the reduction in blood supply and some loss of water content of the tissues so that they lose some of their elastic properties. They become more friable and less resistant to stress. Common examples would be rupture of the long head of the biceps or of the tendo-achilles, although these injuries may also occur in young adults at the level of the musculotendinous junction.

Sprains, in this connotation referring to liagaments about joints, may be divided classically into first, second-or third-degree injuries. First-degree sprains results in partial tear of some of the fibres making up the ligament, but without resultant instability or laxity of that joint. In the second-degree injury, the tearing of the ligamentous structure is more severe, but some fibres remain intact. Thus the joint would show some degree of instability but there would be a check-rein or end-point to testing of the ligament so that the joint does not open widely when a force is applied to that ligament. In the third-degree injury there is complete disruption of the entire ligamentous structure with complete loss of stability in that particular articulation.

General principles of treatment

It is important to realize that the treatment of athletes seeking medical help varies considerably from the treatment offered to health-related problems in the non-athletic population. In the latter group, the emphasis is largely on rest from activity while in the treatment of the injured athlete the emphasis is on altered activities rather than on restriction of activities. The athlete who is told by a well-meaning physician that he or she should stop all physical activities will readily change physician rather than change lifestyle. Hence, the health professional involved in the treatment of athletes must have a thorough knowledge of the make-up of the athlete as well as a general knowledge of the sport in which the athlete was injured.

The mnemonic PRINCER may be used to cover the current principles of treatment which can be applied in general to most of the less serious soft tissue injuries seen in athletics.

Prevention

Many injuries could be prevented or reduced in severity by proper training in the involved sport. The warm-up has been shown to play an important role in the incidence and severity of injuries. Stretching increases the blood supply in soft tissue, making them more viscoelastic, and more resistant to stress. Similarly, the wearing of suitable protective equipment, particularly in North American sports, can prevent or minimize the severity of injuries. Strength training also plays a vital role in prevention of injuries.

Rest

The basic principles of treatment of the athletic injury differ considerably from the treatment of a medical condition of a non-athlete. Absolute rest, the basis of treatment for most non-athletic conditions, is contraindicated in the athletic injury. Rest of the part is the treatment of choice and the athlete should be kept as active as possible so as to maintain general body conditioning.

Icing

Ice should be applied immediately to the injured area and offers many advantages. Its use should not be limited to 24 or 48 hours, but continued as long as the area is painful, even if the pain and swelling last a week or 10 days. The advantages of cryotherapy are that circulation to the area is decreased with a resultant reduced inflammatory response, pain and swelling. It decreases the metabolic demands of the injured cells, resulting in less cellular damage from hypoxia. It decreases pain by depressing sensory nerve conductivity and reduces pain and muscle spasm and as a result lessens disability. A simple method of applying icing locally to the area (which should be done for 8–10 min three or four times a day) is to fill several styrofoam cups with water and place them in the deep-freeze compartment of the refrigerator. When the water is frozen the base of the cup can be torn away circumferentially, exposing the block of ice: the base of the cup can be used as an insulated handle to massage the area.

Heat should be used for the recovery phase to increase circulation of the area and aid in the healing process. Tissues which are warmed have increased elasticity and are less apt to be injured with motion and stretching.

Non-steroidal anti-inflammatory drugs

Non-steriodal anti-inflammatory drugs (NSAIDs) are used commonly in not only acute but chronic injuries. These substances, if used advisedly under a physician's control, act not only as an anti-inflammatory but also as an analgesic. They may also have a function in reducing heterotopic bone formation. There is still argument as to whether or not they increase the risk of articular cartilage damage where joint injuries are involved or whether they have cartilage-sparing effect as in chondromolacia (Casscells, 1986).

Compression

Pressure to the injured area by an elastic stocking or an elastic wrap is an intregal part of the treatment to reduce swelling. It should not be applied too tightly, constricting the circulation in the area distal to its application.

Elevation

As often as possible the injured area should be elevated so as to help reduce the swelling of the injured part.

Rehabilitation

This aspect should really not be considered as a final phase in the treatment but should be started with the initial treatment. In this way not only will inflammation and disability be reduced but joint mobility will be maintained and muscle atrophy prevented. Return to activity should be carried out in a gradually increasing manner depending on the injured athlete's response to treatment.

It is to be emphasized that present-day thinking is mobilization rather than immobilization of the injured athlete. That is to say, the tendency is to use mobile splints and physiotherapy in the treatment even following surgical procedures. Ligamentous and tendons heal more rapidly and with more strength with mobilization rather than immobilization (Tipton *et al.*, 1975; Noyes, 1977). Plaster casting itself has been largely abandoned except for short intervals because of the resultant joint stiffness and tremendous muscle atrophy which occur so rapidly after application of a rigid cast.

While on the subject of treatment in general, injections of a combination of corticosteroid and local anaesthetic can be used under certain circumstances. The very occasional intra-articular use of this combination in the chronic ankle, shoulder (acromioclavicular joint) or knee injury, in the absence of bleeding into the joint, is not to be condemned. Aspiration of joints in general is to be recommended for many reasons. It makes the patient more comfortable by relieving the pressure effects and fluid in a joint, such as in the knee, which can cause reflex quadriceps inhibition. The fluid obtained is often of diagnostic help, blood (haemarthrosis) indicating, for example, a significant soft tissue tear. The pressure of fat which floats freely on the blood (lipohaemarthrosis) indicates a fracture of bone in that joint. Blood itself is a foreign body and eventually on breakdown causes an intense synovitis. Aspiration of the joint aids in the examination/of the joint, increases mobility of that joint and hastens the recovery period. In general, injections into tendons using corticosteroids are not recommended, although it is now recognized that the soluble corticosteroids, as opposed to the insoluble forms, do not lead to collagen breakdown when injected directly into a tendon. It is unlikely that oral corticosteriods play any role in athletic injuries unless given in large doses for a very short time in extenuating circumstances.

Injuries common to the major North American sports

North American football

History relates that the origins of football date back many centuries, the ancient Greeks having played a type of football which was referred to as *harpaston*. (Lechie, 1973). Apparently this sport was played by teams who attempted to pass, kick or run with the ball over the other team's goal line. The early Romans are said to have adopted a similar game which they called *calcio*. This game was brought to Britain by the invading Romans. It became extremely popular in the Middle Ages and eventually became so violent that in many areas it was forbidden by law to play the sport. At that time the ball was generally an inflated bladder or stomach from some animal; later it became more sophisticated and was covered with sewn leather.

The ball was moved by kicking only; running with the ball was forbidden. The players were allowed, however, to keep the ball in play with head shots, resulting in our present-day sport of soccer.

'Football' in Canada and the USA refers to a specific game commonly referred to as American football, while in the rest of the world the term 'football' refers to soccer. Indeed, 'football' is probably an inappropriate term for the North American game because kicking in that sport now plays a relatively minor role compared to soccer or rugby football. It is certainly one of the commonest sports played on the North American continent at all age levels, both amateur and professional. It is classified as a collision sport and as a result produces many significantly serious injuries.

Historically, the North American game evolved from a combination of soccer and rugby football. In 1823 a student at Rugby College School, William Webb Lewis, while playing a type of 'soccer', picked up the ball and ran across the goal line carrying the ball and from that incident the game of rugby football was created (*Sports Encyclopedia*, 1976). In the 19th century a combination of football and rugby was played in North America and at McGill University in Montreal, Canada, a variety of this game was developed with slightly different rules. Harvard University became interested on hearing of this 'McGill game' and invited the Montreal team down to Boston to demonstrate their version of the sport (Pratt and Benagh, 1964). Normally there were 15 players on the team, but McGill University could afford to send only 11 players because of the expense of the train ride. Thus 11 players took part on each side. The game was played in two sections, one using the McGill rules, the other employing the Harvard rules. The McGill game so impressed the Harvard team that they adopted the Canadian game and from it the present North American football game evolved (11 players in the USA and 12 in the Canadian game).

In other than North America the kicking game of football became known as soccer, a derivation of association football, and the ball-carrying variety was labelled rugby football. There are now three varieties played in North America – soccer, rugby football (or rugby) and American football.

Initially, the North American game was played with very little padding or equipment but over the course of 100 years the rules were modified and protective equipment was added so that an enormous amount of expensive equipment is now worn by all players for self-protection.

The most common and most serious injuries encountered in the musculoskeletal system are those involving the knee. Being a heavy contact collision sport, ligamentous injuries about the knee are extremely common. The most debilitating and serious of these injuries are injuries to the anterior or, less commonly, the posterior cruciate ligament. Classically, the player will be supporting the body weight on the flexed knee, which is then struck from the lateral aspect or on which the athlete pivots with the foot fixed on the ground, resulting very often in an audible pop or snap and intense pain in the joint. There is usually very rapidly formed effusion in the joint representing bleeding and aspiration will often reveal fat floating on the the bloody aspirate. There may be an associated torn medial or lateral meniscus in a very high percentage of such injuries involving the cruciate ligament and there may be involvement of a medial (or less commonly, lateral) collateral ligament (DeHaven, 1980; Noyes *et al.*, 1980).

Routine clinical examination reveals a very painful swollen knee with severe pain on attempted ambulation or movement of the joint. There may be instability in the medial or lateral collateral ligament test with the knee flexed at about 30° and there may be a positive anterior cruciate or posterior cruciate ligament drawer test at 30° of flexion (Lachman test). This degree of flexion is the most relaxed position of the cruciates and in this position the hamstrings are also relaxed. The 90° drawer test, which was commonly used in the past, has largely been abandoned as being less accurate, in favour of the Lachman test, because at 90° flexion the posterior horns of the intact menisci may prevent glide of the tibia in the presence of a torn anterior cruciate ligament. There may be joint line tenderness along the line of the meniscus or there may be tenderness along the course of a collateral ligament.

Laxity of the collateral ligaments should be tested at about 30° of flexion. The pivot–shaft test is performed by extending the flexed knee with the leg internally rotated in the abducted position. The knee is then flexed in this position and pressure is applied posteriorly to the proximal fibula on the lateral side; the tibia will be noted to jump back into a posterior position (Galway and MacIntosh, 1980). It is important to realize that with hyperextension in this test the tibia subluxates in an anterolateral position and that with flexion of the knee the tibia relocates to the anatomical position. This test is invalid in the presence of a flexion contracture (i.e. locked knee). A positive test indicates a torn anterior cruciate ligament. Standard X-rays should of course be taken, as well as Merchant patellar views to exclude osteochondral or marginal patellar fractures (Merchant *et al.*, 1974).

If a torn meniscus alone is suspected from the history of physical findings, the role of the arthrograms for confirmation has been abandoned in favour of arthroscopy. This latter procedure allows not only a more accurate assessment of the joint, but also permits the surgeon to deal with the lesion. The state of the art is now most definitely arthroscopic partial meniscectomy or direct suturing of the peripheral tears and salvage of the entire meniscus. The menisci play a vital role in absorption of a larger part of the load across the knee joint (Walker and Erkman, 1975) and their injudicious complete removal is now recognized to be a causative factor in the development of degenerative osteoarthrosis (Fairbank, 1948; Huckell, 1965).

In the presence of a haemarthrosis and a suspected torn cruciate ligament or meniscus, arthroscopy is definitely indicated. If such a procedure is anticipated it is probably unwise to aspirate the joint first in that aspiration can be carried out with the arthroscopy. The recent advent and popularity of magnetic resonance imaging (MRI) is now proving to be a great help in aiding in the diagnosis of torn menisci or cruciates and to a certain degree is taking the place of arthroscopy in that it is non-invasive and less expensive than arthroscopy. Certain ligamentous testing devices are available on the market, such as the KT 1000 and KT 1200 (Medmetric, San Diego, CA); these can be used for testing the stability of the anterior and posterior cruciate ligaments, with objective measurements being obtained clinically at the initial examination.

While certainly the presence of a torn meniscus should be dealt with by arthroscopy, the question of repair of a tear of the collateral ligaments remains debatable. Probably in the élite athlete or someone who intends to pursue an athletic career, third-degree tears of the medial or lateral collateral ligament or capsule, surgical repair should be considered. First- and second-degree tears are best treated by mobile braces which allow healing to take place while at the same time permitting active rehabilitation, preventing muscle atrophy. Salter *et al.* (1980) have demonstrated how the articular cartilage is preserved through joint mobilization rather than immobilization. Tipton *et al.* (1975) have shown how the collagen bundles in healing ligaments are better aligned and strengthened by motion, hence the use of mobile braces to allow early mobilization.

As far as the cruciate ligament is concerned, there is still some debate as to treatment. Certainly, if either cruciate is torn from its origin or insertion it should be reattached surgically. Unfortunately, most of these injuries to the cruciate ligaments occur in their mid-substance and as such they are really not reparable but require reconstructive procedures using biological materials if at all possible. The role of synthetic materials is still uncertain and should probably be reserved for failed biological reconstructions. Allografts are being used in some centres but the fear of AIDS has perhaps limited their general use.

The posterior cruciate ligament injury is one which is most commonly missed at the initial examination due to the fact that it is really extra-articular and may not lead to bleeding within the joint. Furthermore, the secondary restraint of the surrounding capsule and supporting ligaments may mask the true nature of the injury.

The decision to reconstruct cruciate ligaments depends largely on the lifestyle and age of the injured athlete and the future demands to be placed on that knee. Approximately one-third of a group of athletes with a torn anterior cruciate ligament can get by without any treatment other than physical therapy and rehabilitation. A second third can manage by modifying their lifestyle and cutting out strenuous activities which would give rise to symptoms of instability. The final group should probably have reconstruction carried out because of the instability and demands made on that knee. Current general thinking in North America is that all tears of the anterior cruciate ligament in young active athletes should be reconstructed. This allows further participation and also minimizes further joint damage due to instability (McCarroll *et al.*, 1989).

Again, it is important to realize that upwards of 50% of people with severe knee injuries involving torn cruciate ligaments may have an associated tear of the meniscus: in all cases not only are standard X-rays (including Merchant views) necessary but also either MRI or arthroscopy.

As far as rehabilitation is concerned, in North America the plaster cast has essentially been abandoned in the treatment of ligamentous injuries about the knee and the ankle. In the knee it has been replaced by adjustable hinged braces where different degrees of movement can be dialed into the apparatus allowing limited flexion or extension as desired. The emphasis today, as mentioned previously, is on mobilization rather than immobilization of injured or surgically treated joint injuries.

Acute dislocations of the patella are invariably to the lateral aspect of the knee and generally the result of a pre-existing congenitally abnormal patellofemoral relationship (Hughston *et al.*, 1984). There is not infrequently an associated effusion which should be aspirated for diagnostic purposes. A haemarthrosis indicates intra-articular soft tissue tearing involving the synovium and possibly the capsule and insertion of the vastus medialis muscle into the patella. Indeed, with acute dislocation of the patella, the origin of the vastus medialis from the medial intermuscular septum or the muscle belly itself may be disrupted. The disruption of the vastus medialis from its origin is probably, in my opinion, in many cases the cause of the so-called Pelligrini–Stieda's disease rather than the concept of a proximal disruption of the medial collateral ligament as the cause (Houston *et al.*, 1960). With a severe valgus injury to the knee and a resultant tearing of the medial collateral ligament the patella is undoubtedly carried laterally with the lateral displacement of the tibial tubercle, resulting in a possible disruption of the origin of the vastus medialis and a local haemorrhage. This in turn would lead to the formation of heterotopic bone at the region of the adductor tubercle. Free fat and blood indicate the presence of a fracture, which may occur on the margin or undersurface of the patella, or from the lateral femoral condyle as the patella dislocates or relocates (Percy, 1971), as demonstrated in Figure 21.2. In addition to the regular radiographs it is essential to take Merchant views which may demonstrate an osteochondral fracture not otherwise visible.

With lateral patellar dislocation a medial marginal patellar fracture may result at the attachment of the medial capsule to the patella. In such cases, unless grossly displaced, the dislocation can probably be satisfactorily treated by a knee immobilizer for about 4 weeks. A simple knee immobilizer may also be used for the benign dislocation without haemarthrosis (as opposed to a rigid cast) for a few weeks with the immediate institution of quadriceps and hamstring isometric exercises. Recurrent dislocations should generally be treated surgically. If blood, and particularly fat, is present in the aspirate then arthrotomy with lateral release, removal of osteochondral fracture fragments and medial reefing of the vastus medialis should be carried out. Again, a hinged brace may be used in the recovery phase, allowing gradual knee movements after about 3 weeks.

A nagging problem, seen commonly in young athletes and particularly females, is that of maltracking or instability of the patellofemoral complex (Percy and Strother, 1985). Usually physiotherapy modalities will result in amelioration of symptoms but failure to respond to conservative treatment may require lateral patellar release. This author feels that the procedure should be done through a small lateral patellar incision as opposed to arthroscopic release (Dzioba *et al.*, 1985). A more thorough release can be accomplished in this manner and the incidence of postoperative haemarthrosis is reduced. This approach is far less expensive to the patient and arthroscopic assessment should not be necessary prior to the open release unless some other diag-

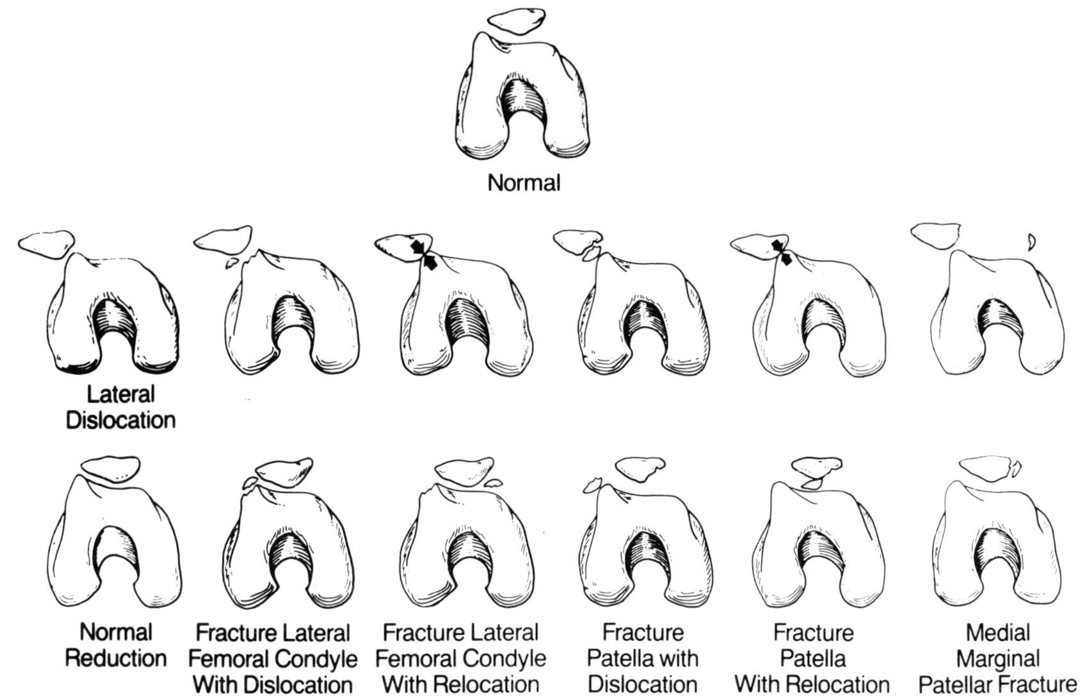

Fig. 21.2 Diagram illustrating acute lateral dislocation of the patella and relocation during dislocation or with reduction. A chondral or an osteochondral fragment can be knapped off the lateral femoral condyle or off the articular surface of the patella or from the medial margin of the patella.

nosis is a possibility or other treatment is required. Should chondromalacia be found which requires surgical treatment, this can easily be carried out through the open lateral approach.

Fortunately, the most severe injury in North American football, that of trauma to the spine, is relatively rare. The medical profession has helped considerably in minimizing this injury by having football management alter its rules and equipment. In spite of this, a total of 105 catastrophic permanent cervical and spinal cord injuries occurred in the USA from 1977 to 1989 (Mueller *et al.*, 1989).

Injuries to other joints are of course common and ankle injuries rank highly in American football statistics. Footballer's ankle (McMurray, 1950), the formation of spurs or osteophytes on the anterior lip of the tibia and the superior aspect of the neck of the talus, is probably more common in soccer but does occur in American football (Vincelette *et al.*, 1972). When present and symptomatic it is probably best treated by surgical excision of the bony protruberances, either by arthrotomy or arthroscopy.

Shoulder injuries involving in particular the acromioclavicular joint or glenohumeral joint are quite common. In the former case, generally speaking, shoulder separations are classified on the grade system: grade 1 and 2 separations are treated conservatively, while in the élite athlete grade 3 separations or dislocations of the acromioclavicular joint should probably be treated surgically (Bannister *et al.*, 1989). Dislocations or subluxations of the glenohumeral joint should certainly be treated conservatively with the first acute episode. While there is generally great pessimism amongst orthopaedic surgeons that acute primary dislocations in the young athlete will go on to recurrent dislocations in the vast majority of cases, MacIntosh *et al.* (1982) have demonstrated that true complete immobilization of the shoulder girdle in the reduced position for 5 uninterrupted weeks will result in a very small percentage of acute primary dislocations going on to recurrent dislocations. Surgery is certainly indicated for the athlete who wishes to compete and who has a history of recurrent dislocations of the shoulder. As well as standard roentgenograms of the shoulder, an axillary view to show the glenohumeral joint should be routine and may demonstrate bony erosion of the anterior lip of the glenoid. The status of the labrum can be assessed by a computed tomography arthrogram or preferably, MRI.

As far as subluxation of the glenohumeral joint is concerned, these may respond to conservative treatment with physiotherapy, as recommended by Jobe and Kvitne (1989), but a significant number will require surgical reconstructive procedures. With the advent of arthroscopy of the shoulder a large number of recurrent dislocations and subluxations of the shoulder are being treated by arthroscopic surgical repair using a staple or screw. Whether or not this approach will replace the conventional open approach remains to be seen. Posterior dislocations of the shoulder, while rare, must be recognized by a clinical awareness of this condition and the mechanism of injury.

The most serious problem in the unstable shoulder ('dead arm syndrome') is that of global instability. Modification of lifestyle and physiotherapy are indicated in this group. Beware of the patient who presents with an atraumatic recurrent subluxation history. These cases do extremely poorly with surgical reconstruction and should in general be treated by physiotherapy.

With the introduction of synthetic turf in North America, a large number of not only professional but also university football games are being played on this artificial surface. This has probably resulted in an increased injury rate as far as minor injuries due to abrasions and impact on this less resilient surface are concerned. The artificial surface has the added disadvantage that it becomes extremely warm on hot days, adding the risk of heat exhaustion. Special football shoes are designed and worn by the athletes who play on these synthetic surfaces. The synthetic surfaces are popular with management because although the initial capital investment is high, the maintenance costs are extremely low. The artificial surface also allows the stadium to be covered for inclement weather conditions. Opinions vary as to whether this artificial surface is responsible for more frequent and more serious injuries than those which result from playing on a natural surface (McCarthy, 1989). Most athletes would certainly prefer to play on natural turf.

A not uncommon injury in American football is that of the contusion with partial rupture of the muscle belly of the quadriceps on the anterior aspect of the thigh. This is usually the result of a direct-impact tackle when an offensive player is running with the football and is struck in the anterior aspect of the thigh by a defensive player's helmet or shoulder both of these areas being protected with a heavy, non-resilient material. While the offensive player is usually wearing a thigh pad, the direct blow to the quadriceps while it is contracting can result in significant tears to the structure. The injury is commonly referred to as a 'Charley horse'. Contrary to lay opinion, a 'Charley horse' is not the result of a spasm of a muscle somewhere in the body, but refers specifically to tearing of the quadriceps from an injury, as described above. The term is interesting historically in that at the turn of the 20th century in an Eastern university (there was of course at that time natural turf on the football field), the university employed a groundskeeper called Charley. The groundskeeper had a horse who pulled the mowing machine to keep the grass cut and trimmed. The unfortunate beast had a rather significant limp and one day, one of the football players, having been struck on the anterior aspect of the thigh (and in those days thigh pads were not worn) limped off the field. One of the other players were heard to remark, 'Oh look, he's limping just like Charley's horse' – hence the true derivation of the rather non-scientific term.

This injury can be quite serious and may keep the player out of action for several months. Treatment is elevation, compressions and icing of the area with immobilization. Gentle active exercises can be started once the pain and swelling have subsided. The use of NSAIDs such as indomethacin is recommended to prevent the formation of myositis ossificans traumatica (heterotopic ossification). Under no circumstances should the area be manipulated or massaged. Attempted aspiration of the haematoma will be unsuccessful for at least 12–14 days following injury due to the clotting of the blood in the area. If myositis ossificans does result from the injury (the ossification does not occur in the muscle cells but rather between the cells) it will usually be diagnosed radiologically within 4–6 weeks of the injury. No attempt should be made to move the resultant calcification and eventual bone formation until the process has become completely arrested, which usually takes about 1 year. Indeed, there is no indication for its removal unless it becomes symptomatic or interferes mechanically with the function of the knee joint. Premature surgery may result in increased formation of bone in the area. A somewhat similar lesion can form in the region of the deltoid insertion in the upper arm of football players due to direct contusion, and is known in this area as 'tackler's exostosis'. A radioactive bone scan may aid in the early diagnosis of this condition: a positive scan will precede definitive radiological evidence. It can also be used to determine when the lesion becomes inactive.

One of the most controversial aspects of the American football game is the ever-changing concept of using prophylactic knee bracing to prevent injuries to this most vulnerable joint in this violent collision sport. The court is still out as regards a final decision as to whether or not such braces will prevent injuries to the knee (Paulos *et al.*, 1986). Certainly it appears that taping of the ankles or the wearing of laced supports on the ankle in the games of basketball, volleyball and football is effective in preventing ankle injuries (Garrick and Requa, 1973). There is some argument that perhaps the wearing of certain types of prophylactic knee braces may increase the risk of injury to the knee (Baker *et al.*, 1989).

Basketball

One of the most popular sports in the USA from the point of view of fan participation is that of basketball. While the game itself is much more popular in the USA than it is in Canada, the credit of its origin must be given to a Canadian, Dr James Naismith from Ontario, and a McGill University graduate, who moved to Springfield, MA, where he developed the sport of basketball in 1891. Naismith used to employ a peach basket affixed to a wall through which the athlete attempted to throw a soccer ball, hence the derivation of the name 'basketball' (Butler, 1985). This game is a particularly fast, exciting contact sport played on a hard surface with no protective padding. The most common injuries incurred are those involving the ankle and foot. The player leaps to make his or her shot and on descending, the involved foot strikes a player's foot or the firm floor, resulting in forced inversion of the ankle and various degrees of sprains up to and including complete disruption of the lateral ligamentous structures or even fractures of the ankle or foot.

Prevention of this disabling and common inversion sprain is very important. Competitors should practise peroneal strengthening exercises: prophylactic strapping with adhesive or a canvas ankle corset, as recommended by Garrick and Requa (1973), has been shown to reduce ankle sprains significantly. Generally, the treatment pendulum for this condition has once again swung to conservatism. The ligaments commonly involved, along with the joint capsule, are the anterior talofibular and the calcaneofibular. The degree of swelling and disability is a clinical index as to the grading of the sprain but the anterior drawer test will aid in assessing the severity and degree of laxity in the acute injury. This is performed by drawing forward on the os calcis with one hand, and pushing backwards on the tibia with the other hand. The patient should be seated with the knee flexed at 90° and the foot hanging free. The degree of laxity present can then be compared with the normal ankle. The author does not rely on the talar-tilt stress test as it is, in my opinion, unreliable and painful so that anaesthesia may be required in the acute injury. Some writers have recommended arthrography to determine the severity of the acute tear but this test is no longer in common use (Percy *et al.*, 1969). Certainly, standard X-rays are mandatory to exclude fractures, particularly those involving the talar dome (transchondral fractures). Fractures of this type have been classified by Berndt and Harty (1959) into types I–IV. Van Beucken *et al.* (1989) recommend early arthroscopic excision of types III and IV if conservative treatments fail. Types I and II are probably best treated conservatively.

Most sprains of all degrees should be treated – with rare exceptions – by the modalities outlined previously. Casting is rarely used now except initially for perhaps 7–10 days in severe sprains, and then merely to control swelling and allow for easier ambulation. Most authorities now prescribe adhesive strapping or the newer plastic removable stirrups splint. This should be followed by early rehabilitation with peroneal strengthening exercises and the use of a tilt board to regain proprioceptive feedback. Surgical repair of the completely disrupted ankle may rarely be required for the élite athlete. In spite of all treatments used, a significant number of acute eversion sprains become chronic and require surgical reconstruction of the lateral ligaments. A rare complications of the inversion sprain injury is that of recurrent dislocation or subluxation of the peroneal tendons requiring surgical reconstruction. Injuries to the medial deltoid ligaments are rare, as are eversion injuries.

Basketball foot injuries are extremely common. The usual common skin conditions such as blisters, calluses and corns are probably more common in this sport than any other athletic activity because of the constant shifting motion on the non-slippery surfaces with starting, stopping and pivoting. Sprains are not uncommon in the smaller joints of the foot and fractures of the metatarsals and tarsal bones can be quite serious if not recognized early. Stress fracture may be the cause of an ill-defined pain in the foot and bone scans may be indicated. Early recognition is important and very often surgery to such a lesion may be indicated primarily. Conservatism in such cases may result in radical procrastination and an inordinate loss of playing time on the part of the athlete. Beware of the simple fracture of the proximal diaphysis of the base of the fifth metacarpal. It requires 6 weeks in a non-weight-bearing below-knee cast. It may go on to non-union, requiring a bone graft and internal fixation (Torg, 1988). Stress fractures can also occur in the tibia and fibula, although are less common in baskeball than in running sports or indeed the most common cause, aerobics.

Ruptures of the Achilles tendon do occur in a younger age group in basketball than in the general population. In younger basketball players the rupture is apt to occur at the musculoskeletal tendinous junction, the point of biomechanical weakness. The diagnosis can be readily missed and one should be aware of the Thompson test to exclude a ruptured tendo-Achilles (Thompson, 1962). A patient with such a condition can often walk on his or her toes because of the power of the other muscles which pass behind the medial and lateral malleoli. To perform the Thompson test, the patient should kneel on a chair facing its back. Compression of the calf muscles with the examiner's hand should result in the foot going into the equinus position by reflex contraction of the triceps surae muscle group. If the tendo-Achilles is ruptured the foot will not go into equinus. While there is still some disagreement as to the advantages of conservative versus surgical treatment, there seems to be little role for conservatism in the treatment of this major tendon injury in the young or élite athlete. Conservative treatment keeps the player immobilized for a much longer time with resultant atrophy, residual permanent weakness and a much higher rate of rerupture (Percy and Conochie, 1978).

Achilles tendinitis is an extremely common condition in all athletes but particularly in those involved in the jumping sports of volleyball or basketball. This represents a stress fracture of the collagen bundles in the tendon itself and would be classified as microtrauma. The patient complains of discomfort in the back of the ankle 5 or 6 cm proximal to the insertion of the tendo-Achilles into the calcaneus. There may be palpable swelling or a lump in this area and/or acute tenderness. The tendo-Achilles is not enclosed in a synovial sheath but a paratenon which brings in its blood supply and this tendon in particular has a minimal blood supply and is prone to partial tears of the fibres. It is not a true tendinitis in the sense that it does not result in an inflammatory response with infiltration of polymorphonuclear leukocytes and would be better labelled as tendonosis. In fact there is very little, if any, cellular response locally to this injury.

Again, prevention is important in this condition by ensuring that the athlete does not have tight tendo-Achilles and when early symptoms present, strengthening and stretching of the triceps surae group is important. A lift in the heel will offload the posterior calf muscles and relieve symptoms during the rehabilitation. Conservative treatment should not, however, be carried on for a prolonged period of time and certainly if there is no relief after 6 months, operation is indicated. If, on the other hand, a palpable tender nodule or lump is present surgery is probably indicated immediately. The surgery consists of gentle dissection of the paratenon and vertical slits are made in the direction of the fibres of the tendo-Achilles in the painful or swollen area. Very often the results are discouragingly negative and yet with closure of the tendon and its sheath and a short period of non-weight-bearing immobilization with active rehabilitation, complete relief will be obtained. If there is a partial rupture demonstrable grossly then that torn portion should be excised and repair carried out. The plantaris tendon, if present, may be used to augment the repair.

Another condition which may confuse the examiner is that of retrocalcaneal bursitis. This may be due to a direct injury or, more commonly, a prominent posterosuperior beak on the os calcis, referred to as a 'pump bump'. Injections of corticosteroid and local anaesthetic into the retrocalcaneal bursa which lies deep to the tendo-Achilles between that structure and the os calcis will often give relief. A lift to the heel may help by altering the tendo-Achilles–calcaneus interface.

NSAID may also give relief to this condition, as well as in Achilles tendonosis. Failure to respond to this conservative treatment should lead the physician to consider excision of the posterosuperior aspect of the os calcis proximal to the insertion of the tendo-Achilles with the bursa.

Another form of tendinitis which may be seen in basketball and/or volleyball is that of 'jumper's knee'. This represents again a so-called tendinitis of the tendon as the result of repeated microtrauma. Again, conservative treatment should be instituted along the lines discussed previously, but surgery may occasionally be indicated. This usually occurs at the origin of the patellar ligament or tendon at the inferior pole of the patella but may also occur at the superior pole of the patella at the insertion of the quadriceps.

Ruptures of both the quadriceps tendon and patella ligament or tendon, while they do occur, are generally rare occurrences. Obviously a surgical repair is indicated in such cases. Strains can occur in the mid-calf in many sports, including basketball, but perhaps more particularly in racket sports. This condition is called 'tennis leg' and refers specifically to that condition in which there is a partial avulsion of the insertion of the medial head of the gastrocnemius into the underlying triceps surae tendon. It seems always to occur at the insertion of the medial gastrocnemius belly, which is larger and lies more distally. It has been mistakenly misdiagnosed over the years as ruptured plantaris, but this diagnosis is no longer tenable. The biomechanical weak point in muscles is at the musculotendinous junction, and this area of the plantaris muscle lies in the popliteal fossa well above the area where the patient complains of discomfort.

Again, the treatment is as mentioned above and the addition of an elastic stocking or an elastic bandage with a lift in the heel and NSAIDs as well as local icing will often give relief in a matter of weeks. The condition is by no means new – it was first reported as 'lawn tennis leg' by Hood in 1884. Knee injuries of course do occur in basketball just as in any other contact or collision sport and should be treated along the lines discussed under American football.

Ice hockey

Although it is difficult to define the origins of ice hockey historically, it seems that while ice skating started in the Netherlands (Vaughan, 1989), the game of hockey originated in Canada. History relates that the true birthplace of this sport was Kingston, Ontario, in 1855, where the present Hockey Hall of Fame is located. Montreal and Halifax have disputed Kingston's claim but apparently the first formal rules for this sport were developed at McGill University 20 years later (Pratt and Benagh, 1964; *Sports Encyclopedia*, 1976). The sport was introduced to the USA in the early 1890s. Its immense popularity today seems to be due entirely to its development as Canada's national sport.

This game is the world's fastest sport and is now played almost universally at the international level. It is unusual in that it is a collision sport played on a slippery surface where the competitors have clubs in their hands, blades on their feet and drive a very heavy missile at speeds of over 150 km/h. Understandably, the majority of injuries in this sport have been lessened considerably with the compulsory use of head gear and facial masks of one type or another. It is surprising that there have not been more major injuries in the past. Each team, although they have six players on the ice, regards the boards circling the hockey arena as a seventh player and use them frequently for checking their opponent (legally or illegally). This accounts for a significant number of injuries. These injuries are generally confined to the shoulder and acromioclavicular separations are a not uncommon injury. In general, shoulder separations can be simplistically classified into three categories – first-, second-, or third-degree. The treatment of these injuries has been discussed under American football and will not be repeated in this section. Shoulder dislocations also are a not uncommon injury, as discussed previously. A trip or a fall on the ice while skating at high speed and then sliding into the boards can result in serious ligamentous injuries to the knee or ankle or the less common fractures of the tibia and fibula. Formerly, a large number of the injuries used to involve the hands and facial area, largely due to fights amongst opposing players. The rules are now being strictly enforced in this area to prevent this unnecessary violence on the ice. Indeed, some unknown humourist in the past made the statement that 'I went to the fights the other night and a hockey game broke out'.

The helmet not only protects the head from serious injuries but also the facial bones and in particular the eyes. Alarming numbers of young hockey players in the past have been rendered legally blind in an eye because of injuries from the stick or the puck. With the use of the helmet alone, sticks which originally would have struck the frontal area of the unprotected facial bones or eyes are now protected by this projecting portion of the helmet. In addition, facial cages or eye shields are often worn although the major complaint here is that the eye shields become fogged up impeding the athlete's vision. In spite of this protective equipment, head and neck injuries can be of a serious nature when the patient moving at high speed is tripped or falls and slides into the board head-first. The addition of the mouth guard has also led to minimizing injuries to the teeth. Years ago, many hockey players in the National Hockey League were missing some or all of their front teeth!

Fractures of the medial or lateral maelleoli have been largely eliminated with the well-fitting and protectively padded boot. It was not uncommon some years ago to see a number of these fractures from defencemen diving in front of the defensive player's slap shot.

In spite of the fact that hockey players do wear a good deal of padding, a not uncommon injury is that of acute bursitis (which may of course become chronic) involving the trochanteric bursa on the lateral aspect of the hip, associated usually with boarding or falling heavily on the ice. Similarly, olecranon bursitis and prepatellar bursitis are commonly seen in this particular sport. In the case of the elbow or the knee, special treatment should be aspiration of the bursa under sterile conditions followed by injection of local anaesthetic with a corticosteroid. This may prevent recurrence but very often these conditions do become recurrent and may require repeated aspirations. Rather than subject the patient to repeated aspirations, the ideal treatment would be excision of the lesion, probably under local anaesthetic as an outpatient procedure at the completion of the season.

In the case of trochanteric bursitis, however, this condition is usually associated with pain and discomfort over the greater trochanteric region of the hip. Again, injections of local anaesthetic and corticosteroids under sterile conditions are recommended. At the same time, stretching of the iliotibial tract should be carried out by a competent therapist so as to reduce the friction of this structure over the greater trochanter. The use of NSAIDs can also be employed in chronic trochanteric bursitis. Occasionally there may be a snapping or clicking associated with problems in that area due to the iliotibial tract snapping over the greater trochanter with flexion and extension of the hip. In addition, an adventitial bursa may be seen lying between the skin and iliotibial tract: this develops due to contusion to the area and haemorrhage. The iliotibial tract may also cause problems distally due to friction as it crosses over the lateral femoral epicondyle, sometimes referred to as 'runner's knee'.

Interestingly enough, while ice hockey and American football are considered very violent sports, they are minor skirmishes compared to the fan violence seen in Europe, the Eastern Bloc countries and South America during and after soccer matches!

Baseball

This sport is the true all-American sport. It is in fact more than just a game – it is an institution just as bull-fighting is in Spain. Its origins are somewhat difficult to trace back in history, but it is possibly a derivation of either cricket or rounders, two sports played in the UK. In 1905 a commission was set up in the USA to determine the origins of baseball; it concluded that in 1839, Abner Doubleday laid out the first diamond-shaped baseball field in Cooperstown, New York. He is credited with having developed the game and its rules as well as the name of the sport (Pratt and Benagh, 1964; *Sports Encyclopedia*, 1976). As a result of this, the present baseball Hall of Fame is located in Cooperstown. There is some dispute about the origins of the game in that the writer Oliver Wendell Holmes claimed to have played baseball at Harvard University in 1829 but the baseball Hall of Fame attributes its origins to Abner Doubleday. The game has grown tremendously in popularity since that time and now is played in many countries throughout the civilized world.

Major injuries can occur in this sport as in any other sport, although baseball by definition is really not a contact or collision sport. However, it is to be remembered that the pitcher is throwing the ball at speeds of up to 170 km/h and unfortunately occasionally the batter is struck directly with the ball. A protective helmet is of course worn but in spite of it serious injuries still occur, particularly to the head and face. At the same time, injuries occur from being struck by the ball which is hit by the batter and the pitcher is in a high-risk position standing on the elevated mound, 60 feet and 6 inches (approximately 18.5 m) from the batter. When the batter does not make direct contact with the ball but the thrown ball is deflected by the bat, the catcher is at risk (in spite of being heavily padded), as is the home plate umpire standing behind the catcher. Occasionally fans in the stands may be injured by an errant batted ball.

This sport is probably the most common of overuse injuries to the shoulder and elbow. These two particular areas are subjected to continued and repeated minor trauma in the throwing mechanism involved in baseball, particularly for the pitcher. Injuries to the shoulder and elbow are so common in pitchers that specific rules have been laid down by the Baseball Commission as far as Little League players are concerned to prevent these repetitive injuries. In pitching, the body acts as a linked system in throwing the ball; energy is developed from the ground up through the body and out through the throwing arm and forearm with release of the ball. As a result, the upper extremity functions much like a snapping whip and tremendous forces are dispersed through the shoulder girdle and elbow joint.

The shoulder joint is the area of the body most subject to wear and tear, no doubt in part due to human's adoption of the upright bipedal posture. With the descent of our ancestors from the role of brachiators (pronograde) in the trees to ambulators (orthograde) on the plains, the shoulder girdle has undergone numerous modifications. The scapula has migrated dorsally, the acromion and coracoid process have increased in size and the biceps groove has moved medially (De Palma, 1983). The glenohumeral joint now depends entirely upon soft tissue support and its stability has been sacrificed for mobility in this joint. Thus the shoulder joint is inherently unstable and subject to overuse problems. It is probably the most commonly dislocated joint in the body. The main humeral head stabilizers are the supraspinatus, infraspinatus, teres minor and subscapularis (rotator cuff) and are placed under continuous stress with global shoulder movements. Similarly, the long head of the biceps, primarily the principal supinator of the forearm, aids in the stabilization and to a lesser degree in shoulder flexion and is subject to tremendous wear and tear. The long head tendon does not move in the intertubercular groove but rather the groove moves in all planes around the tendon. In addition, the rotator cuff and biceps have a rather inadequate blood supply and consequently breakdown of these tissues is common.

Sports which include the throwing motion (baseball, American football, swimming and racket sports) are those in which problems in rotator cuff or biceps tendon are commonly seen due to overuse. In the normal movement of abduction of the arm, 120° occurs at the glenohumeral joint while 60° occurs at the scapulothoracic articulation. For the arm to abduct fully at the glenohumeral joint over 90° of external rotation of the humerus must take place concurrently with the abduction. The acromion, coracoacromial ligament and the coracoid process all form the coracoacromial arch. Lying between these structures and the rotator cuff, the biceps tendon and the tuberosity of the humerus, lies the subdeltoid bursa. If the abduction of the shoulder is not carried out in synchronization with adequate external rotation of the humerus then impingement occurs between these latter structures and the coracoacromial arch. This impingement results in a local breakdown of collagen and an inflammatory response which is reflected in the overlying bursa, resulting in painful abduction and even pain at rest, particularly at night lying in the lateral position. Rathbun and MacNab (1970) have shown that the blood supply to the rotator cuff is further diminished with the upper extremity adducted by the side.

In the early stages the response locally in the rotator cuff is an inflammatory change. This can progress with time to partial and even complete rupture of the rotator cuff and biceps tendon. In addition, new bone may form under the lateral edge of the acromion and degenerative changes occur on the undersurface of the acromioclavicular joint, with new bone formation further abbetting the impingement syndrome. Calcium may be deposited in the degenerative rotator cuff, further increasing the bulk of tissue. This calcium deposit may rupture giving a very painful chemical bursitis.

The same principles of treatment apply in the early phases of the coracoacromial arch syndrome, but surgical decompression of the arch at an early age (i.e. excising the coracoacromial ligament) is now largely done through the arthroscope (Esch, 1989). Decompression and repair of the torn rotator cuff in the older age group may be necessary by open operation. If the biceps tendon rupture occurs proximally in the young adult – a rare occurrence – then repair is indicated, the simplest repair being to suture the proximal end of the tendon to the tip of the coracoid process. In those over 45 years old, repair is usually not necessary, the main function of the biceps being supination of the forearm. On standard X-ray studies (which should include an axillary view) the hallmark of a complete tear of the rotator cuff is elevation of the head of the humerus. The arthrogram may demonstrate a tear in this structure, allowing escape of the contrast medium. This procedure is now being superseded by MRI, which is also taking the place of the computed tomography arthrogram to demonstrate tears or separation of the labrum.

Being an inherently unstable joint (the glenohumeral joint is best described as a golf ball sitting on a tee) stretching of the capsule and soft tissues may result in global glenohumeral stability. This condition is probably best treated with physiotherapy as operation is rarely successful.

'Little Leaguer's shoulder' is in essence an overuse phenomenon which results from young athletes pitching too frequently at too early an age. It is in essence a stress fracture of the Salter–Harris type II through the proximal humeral physis. It should be treated conservatively with rest until there is evidence of healing and relief of symptoms before allowing the athlete to continue.

'Little Leaguer's elbow' was initially a term used

to describe a stress fracture of the medial epicondyle of the throwing arm in pitchers. It is an overuse phenomenon and represents a stress fracture through the physis of the medial epicondyle. It results from valgus strain on the medial side of the elbow caused by the wind-up and cocking motion in pitching. If the displacement is more than 1 cm it probably should be replaced surgically and pinned.

The vast majority of Little Leaguers' problems are, however, associated with damage to the capitular radial head joint. Breakdown of the articular cartilage with separation of chondral or osteochondral fragments into the joint may occur. This results in loose bodies in the joint and as cartilage depends upon its nutrition from the joint fluid, these loose bodies may grow in size. They are a common cause of locking in the elbow joint. If they are of cartilage alone they will not be seen on standard X-rays, but can be seen on an MRI. Changes in the capitelloradial joint result from impingement at that joint with forced abduction of the elbow during the wind-up and cocking phase of the pitching mechanism. Once again, arthroscopy is now taking a dominant role in the treatment of this latter condition.

Injuries to the distal radial epiphysis in children are rare in baseball and more apt to be seen in gymnasts, as are injuries to the spine (Dzioba, 1985).

Neurological problems do occur in sports and baseball is no exception. Entrapment of the suprascapular nerve can result from the throwing mechanism, resulting in paralysis of the supraspinatus and infraspinatus muscle. In addition, injuries to the axillary nerve have been reported in this sport from throwing as well as in volleyball. This nerve is particularly vulnerable to damage with anterior dislocation of the shoulder: adequate neurological as well as vascular assessment should be carried out in the presence of a dislocation. A wise principle is always to take X-rays of an injured area before and after treatment because of the medicolegal problems which exist in today's society.

In sports involving the throwing mechanism, the athlete may be particularly prone to the thoracic outlet syndrome. This can be caused by anatomical variations – malinsertion of the scalenus anticus muscle, a cervical rib or congenital rib abnormalities. It can also occur following malunion of a fractured clavicle. This syndrome can give rise to shoulder and upper extremity symptoms in many forms of athletic endeavours and it should play a part in the differential diagnosis of all upper extremity pain. The examining physician should always be aware of other rare vascular syndromes, such as effort thrombosis or compartment syndromes in both upper and lower extremities. Some athletes may develop the snapping scapula syndrome from overuse or shoulder injury. This is usually the result of postural malalignment of the scapulothoracic articulation and is best treated by physiotherapy and other conservative methods rather than surgery (Percy *et al.*, 1988).

References

Baker BE, Van Hanswyk E, Bogoshian SP et al. (1989) The effect of knee braces on lateral impact loading of the knee. *American Journal of Sports Medicine* **17**, 182–6.

Bannister GC, Wallace WA, Stableforth PG et al. (1989) The management of acute acromioclavicular dislocation. *Journal of Bone and Joint Surgery* **71B**, 848–50.

Barnes I (1983) AAFDBI: Bringing fitness to corporate America. *The Physician and Sportsmedicine* **11**, 127–33.

Berndt AL, Harty M (1959) Transchondral fractures (osteochondritis dissecans of the talus). *Journal of Bone and Joint Surgery* **47A**, 988–1020.

Bruce RA (1984) Exercise, functional aerobic capacity and ageing – another viewpoint. *Medicine and Science in Sports and Exercise* **16**, 8–13.

Butler FT (1985) *The Canadian Encyclopedia* vol 2: Edmonton: Hutrig Publishers, p 1191.

Casscells SW (1986) Are nonsteroidal anti-inflammatory drugs indicated in the treatment of osteoarthritis? *Journal of Arthroscopy and Related Surgery* **2**, 13.

Clancy WG, Narechania RG, Rosenberg TD et al. (1981) Anterior and posterior cruciate ligament reconstruction in rhesus monkeys. *Journal of Bone and Joint Surgery* **63A**, 1270–84.

DeHaven KE (1980) Diagnosis of acute knee injuries with hemarthrosis. *American Journal of Sports Medicine* 9–14.

DePalma AF (1983) *Surgery of the Shoulder*. Philadelphia: JB Lippincott.

Dzioba RB (1985) *Sports Injuries, Mechanism, Prevention and Treatment.* Baltimore: Williams & Wilkins.

Dzioba RB, Strokon A, Mulbry L (1985) Diagnostic arthroscopy and longitudinal open lateral release: a safe and effective treatment for chondromalacia patella. *Journal of Arthroscopic and Related Surgery* **1**, 131–5.

Esch JC (1989) Arthroscopic subacromial decompression. Surgical technique. *Orthopaedic Review* **XVIII**, 733–42.

Fairbank TJ (1948) Knee joint changes after meniscectomy. *Journal of Bone and Joint Surgery* **30B**, 664–70.

Galway HR, MacIntosh DL (1980) The lateral pivot shift. A symptom and sign of anterior cruciate ligament insufficiency. *Clinical Orthopaedics* **147**, 45–50.

Garrick JG, Requa RK (1973) Role of external support in the prevention of ankle sprains. *Medical Science of Sports* **5**, 200–3.

Hood C (1884) On lawn-tennis leg. *Lancet* **1**, 728.

Houston AA, Roy WA, Faust R et al. (1960) Pellegrini-Stieda syndrome: report of 14-cases followed from original injury. *Southern Medical Journal* **53**, 266–72.

Huckell JR (1965) Is meniscectomy a benign procedure? A long term follow-up study. *Canadian Journal of Surgery* **8**, 254–60.

Hughston JC, Walsh WM, Puddu G (1984) *Patellar Subluxation and Dislocation.* Philadelphia: WB Saunders.

Jobe FW, Kvitne RS (1989) Shoulder pain in the overhand or throwing athlete. *Orthopaedic Review* **XVIII**, 963–75.

Leckie R (1973) *The Story of Football.* New York: Random House.

McCarroll JR, Shelbourne KD, Rettig AC (1989) Athletes and their ACL injury. *Surgical Rounds in Orthopaedics* 39–44.

McCarthy P (1989) Artificial turf: does it cause more injuries? *The Physician and Sportsmedicine* **17**, 159–64.

MacIntosh DL, Yoneda B, Welsh RP (1982) Conservative treatment of shoulder dislocations in young males. *Journal of Bone and Joint Surgery* **64B**, 254.

McMurray TP (1950) The footballer's ankle. *Journal of Bone and Joint Surgery* **328**, 68–9.

Merchant AC, Mercer RL, Jacobsen RH, et al. (1974) Roentgenographic analysis of patellofemoral congruence. *Journal of Bone and Joint Surgery* **56A**, 1391.

Mueller FO, Blyth CS, Canter RC (1989) Catastrophic spine injuries in football. *The Physician and Sportsmedicine* **17**, 51–3.

Noyes FR (1977) Functional properties of knee ligaments and alterations induced by immobilization. *Clinical Orthopaedics* **123**, 210–42.

Noyes FR, Bassett RW, Grood ES et al. (1980) Arthroscopy in acute traumatic hemarthrosis of the knee. Incidence of anterior cruciate tears and other injuries. *Journal of Bone and Joint Surgery* **62A**, 687–95.

Paulos LE, Drawbert JP, France P et al. (1986) Lateral knee braces in football: do they prevent injury? *The Physician and Sportsmedicine* **14**, 108–19.

Percy EC (1971) Acute dislocation of the patella. *Canadian Journal* **105**, 1176–8.

Percy EC, Stiother RT (1985) Patellalgia. *The Physician and Sportsmedicine* **13**, 43–59.

Percy EC, Conochie LB (1978) The surgical treatment of ruptured tendoachilles. *American Journal of Sports Medicine* **6**, 132–6.

Percy EC, Hill RO, Callaghan JE (1969) The 'sprained' ankle. *Journal of Trauma* **6**, 972–86.

Percy EC, Birbrager D, Pitt MJ (1988) Snapping scapula: a review of the literature and presentation of 14 patients. *Canadian Journal of Surgery* **31**, 248–50.

Pratt JL, Benagh J (1964) *The Official Encyclopedia of Sports.* New York: Franklin Watts.

Rathbun JB, Macnab I (1970) The microvascular pattern of the rotator cuff. *Journal of Bone and Joint Surgery* **52B**, 540–53.

Salter RB, Simmonds DF, Malcolm BN et al. (1980) The biological effect of continuous passive motion on the healing of full-thickness defects in articular cartilage. *Journal of Bone and Joint Surgery* **62A**, 1232.

Sports Encyclopedia (1976) Ottenheimer Publishers.

Thompson TC (1962) A test for rupture of the tendo-achilles. *Acta Orthopaedica Scandinavinica* **32**, 461.

Tipton CM, Matthes RD, Maynard JA et al. (1975) The influence of physical activity in ligaments and tendons. *Medicine and Science in Sports Exercise* **7**, 165.

Torg JS (1988) Fractures of the base of the fifth metatarsal distal to the tuberosity: a review. *Contemporary Orthopaedics* **19**, 497–505.

Van Beucken K, Barrack RL, Alexander AH et al. (1989) Arthroscopic treatment of transcondylar talar dome fractures. *American Journal of Sports Medicine* **17**, 350–6.

Vaughan CL (1989) *Biomechanics of Sport.* Boca Raton, Florida: CRC Press.

Vincelette P, Laurin CA, Levesque HP (1972) The footballer's ankle and foot. *Canadian Medical Association Journal* **107**, 872–4.

Walker PS, Erkman MJ (1975) The role of the menisci in force transmission across the knee. *Clinical Orthopaedics* **109**, 184–92.

22

Risks and injuries in water sports

M. O'Brien

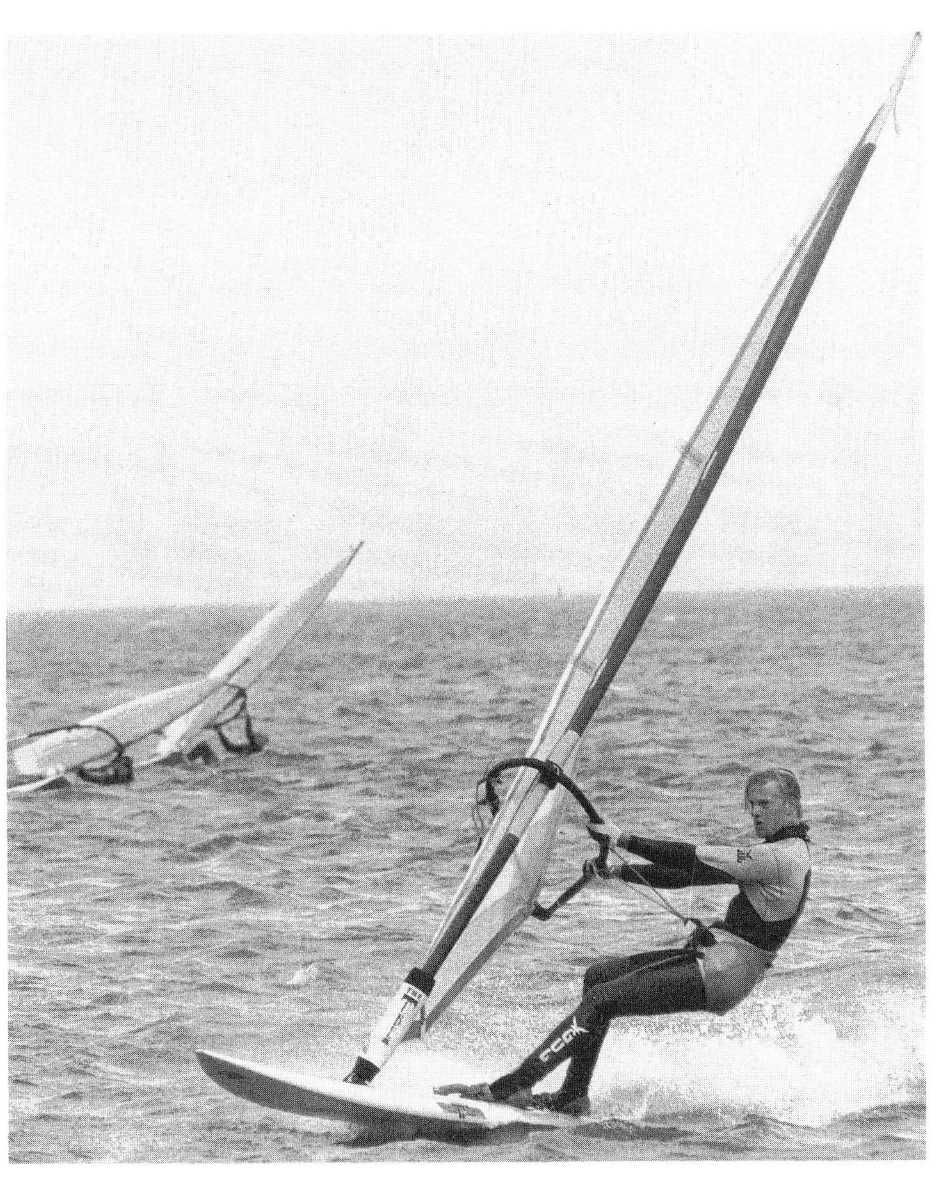

Water-related fatalities are the third leading cause of accidental death in the USA, second in the UK and Australia. The risk of drowning is 2.5 deaths per 100 000 in the USA and 1 per 100 000 in the UK (Metropolitan Life Assurance Company, 1977; Vimpani *et al.*, 1988).

Many factors play a role in drowning. They include ignorance or disregard of danger, an unrealistic idea of swimming ability, lack of knowledge of the area, lack of adequate supervision, inability to cope, the temperature of the water and lack of knowledge of safety procedures and first aid.

There has been a marked increase worldwide in the number of people participating in water sports both at recreational and competitive levels. The risks involved vary greatly depending on the sport, venue, expertise, the temperature of the water and the attention to safety procedures. The one common factor is that drowning may result, even in good swimmers, if safety standards are ignored.

Worldwide the male to female ratio of drowning is 3 : 1. The incidence of drowning has two peaks at 0–4 years and between 15 and 34 years. Females are more at risk below 4 years of age and over 50. In 73% of cases in the 0–4-year age group there was no adult present and swimming ability played a part. In the 0–9-year age group, where this was known, 94% could not swim, but in the 15–24 age group 90% were able to swim (Royal Life Saving Society, 1982). Alcohol was an important contributing cause in 47% of drownings worldwide in the 20–30-year age group (Spyker, 1985).

The highest incidence of drowning in older children and adults occurred in rivers, lakes and in the sea (Orlowski, 1987; Quan *et al.*, 1989). They were usually associated with crafts and boating accidents. Additional causes are cold water, sharp currents and freak waves. Attention to weather reports is essential to prevent accidents on lakes and at sea. On most beaches warning flags are flown to warn the public about strong tides, sharp currents and rough surf and notices are posted warning of hidden rocks and quicksands.

Private swimming pools in some countries are the most common site of drowning, particularly in the younger age group (Rowe *et al.*, 1977; Hassel, 1989; O'Carroll *et al.*, 1988). This may be due to lack of fencing, poor design and poor supervision. In public pools incorrect location of the children's pool close to the deep end of the main pool, or an abrupt change in depth, inadequate or absent depth marks increases the risk of non-swimmers entering the deep water by accident (Royal Society for Prevention of Accidents, 1989/90).

Drowning is death from suffocation by submersion in water, which can be either fresh or salt water (Modell, 1981). There are three forms of drowning: dry, wet and secondary drowning; the latter occurs after an episode of near drowning, which is a term applied to survival after a period of hypnoea due to submersion in water, even if it is only temporary drowning (Modell, 1981).

The most important aspect of drowning is the marked disturbance of gas exchange resulting in hypoxia. The length of time of oxygen lack plays a very important role in the prognosis and clinical sequelae in cases of near drowning.

Dry drowning occurs in approximately 10% of cases; only a small quantity of fluid is aspirated, as severe laryngospasm occurs when fluid is aspirated into the larynx (Modell *et al.*, 1976). The glottis closes and very little water enters the lung. Death is due to apnoea and hypoxia. These patients, if resuscitated before irreversible brain damage has occurred, respond rapidly.

Wet drowning is when hypoxia results, due to the aspiration of fluid into the lungs. When large amounts of fresh water are aspirated, it diffuses rapidly from the alveloi into the circulation, resulting in haemodilution and haemolysis. More than 11 ml per kg body weight of fluid must be aspirated according to studies by Modell and Moya, (1966 and Modell *et al.*, 1967) before this affects the circulation. Fresh water affects the surfactant content of the alveoli and in cases of near drowning may result in atelectasis at a later stage (Giammona and Modell, 1967).

In salt water drowning when large amounts are inhaled there is a shift of fluid from the circulation into the alveoli, with resulting pulmonary oedema, but the surfactant system is not as affected.

In both types of drowning as little as 1.3 ml fluid per kg body weight has a marked effect on the respiratory exchange, as both salt and fresh water affect the alveolar capillary membrane, causing an exudate of fluid and protein (Modell and Moya, 1966; Modell *et al.*, 1967). This effect may not be evident for some hours and should be borne in mind in cases of near drowning.

The differences between fresh and sea water drowning are not as important clinically nowadays. The main factor is the amount of fluid and the temperature of the water.

Secondary drowning is when death occurs after an incident of near drowning. This may occur hours or days after the event, due to pulmonary complications. It may also be due to the effects of hypoxia on the heart, brain or kidney (Sarnaik and Vohra, 1986).

The temperature of the water has a profound effect on survival. A person who has been submerged in water for more than 15 min will usually die, while recovery has occurred after 10–30 min in cold water. This may be due to two factors: firstly, the direct cooling of vital tissues lowers the metabolism and results in decreased oxygen needs, and secondly, the mammalian dive reflex causes peripheral vasoconstriction and shunts blood from the periphery to the brain (Gooden, 1987).

Sudden immersion in cold water may be lethal in a few seconds (Goode *et al.*) 1978. The intense peripheral vasoconstriction and tachycardia from rapid cold immersion may cause vagal arrest (Simpson, 1958) or the marked peripheral vasoconstriction and tachycardia may precipitate a heart attack. Sudden immersion initiates a neurogenic reflex from receptors in the skin to the respiratory centre and results in hyperventilation, with large gasps and an increased respiratory rate, which increases the rate of aspiration and causes a marked fall in arterial carbon dioxide. This may explain the sudden disappearance syndrome (Keatinge 1978).

The drive to breathe on exposure to cold may explain the inability of skin divers to stay under cold water as long as they can under warm water.

If the body is in cold water for some time, despite the vasoconstriction, it is unable to retain the core temperature as it loses heat more rapidly than it can generate it. In water of 10°C, the core temperature starts to cool after 15–20 min. With a core temperature of 34–35°C shivering and tachycardia occur, and there is impairment of mental function. At a core temperature of 30°C unconsciousness results; without the correct flotation device, which keeps the face out of water, drowning will result.

The rate of heat loss depends on the amount of clothing and internal fat insulation. Exercise in water increases heat loss. When the temperature is below 12°C there is a partial failure of vasoconstriction, i.e. a cold paralysis of the peripheral vessels, which results in cold vasodilation. Keatinge (1978) found that fat men had increased heat loss after 40 min in water at 5°C and cooled rapidly despite shivering. A major hazard of cold is ventricular fibrillation. In boating accidents, if there is time, more clothes and a flotation device should be worn, particularly by children, who are more at risk as they lose heat more rapidly. They should get out of the cold water if possible. Movements should be kept to a minimum as swimming increases heat loss which is mainly from the chest wall and groin areas. Use HELP – the heat escape lessening position; curl up the legs and hold the arms close to the body or huddle together if there is more than one person.

Hypothermia is the cause of death in 30% of drownings. If alcohol is involved it will increase heat loss: 52% of all water victims are legally intoxicated at time of death (Royal Life Saving Society, 1982). Alcohol may also affect vision; this may be a factor in boating accidents (MacNeill and Cohen, 1976).

Management

Pull the victim out of the water as soon as possible. Start cardiopulmonary resuscitation (mouth-to-mouth) at once (Spyker, 1985). Ensure clear airways. If the patient is a child, do not hyperextend the neck. If available, oxygen should be given and the patient transferred to hospital as soon as possible. Particular note should be made of cardiac function, ventilation rate and level of consciousness.

In certain sports and situations it is important that the rescuers take adequate precautions or they may become victims:

1. If the water is below 21°C, rescuers should wear wet suits.
2. Safety lines should be used on frozen lakes, in rivers or wild water.

If a head or neck injury is suspected, slide the patient on to a back board and remove him or her quickly from the water. Evaluate the pulse and breathing on dry land or on a boat. Begin cardiopulmonary resuscitation in a pulseless patient if the time of immersion is less than 1 hour (see Chapter 7). The time of submersion and temperature is critical – not dead if cold and pulseless. Cold and dead is not dead.

If hypothermia is present, there should be no attempt at rewarming but the patient should be insulated to prevent further heat loss. Cardiopulmonary and electrocardiogram monitoring should be carried out and the patient should be handled as gently as possible to prevent precipitating ventricular vibrillation. Patients should be transferred to a hospital immediately (Sarnaik and Vohra, 1986). Modell and Conn (1980), in an analysis of near drowning, found that if the patient arrived at a hospital awake there were usually no sequelae. Of those who were comatose when they arrived, 34% died and 18% developed neurological defects.

Breath-holding

There was a vogue some years ago amongst swimmers to hyperventilate before they tried to swim the length of a pool underwater. This resulted in a number of deaths. Craig (1961) found that after hyperventilation breath-holding could be increased from 87 to 146 seconds but the resulting hypoxia due to a low oxygen levels resulted in unconsciousness as the normal increase in levels of carbon dioxide which acts as a stimulus to respiration were delayed.

Injuries

The incidence of injuries in water sports varies considerably. Swimming has a low incidence of injury – 0.03 per 1000 swimming hours (Weightman and Browne 1981). The rate is 0.22 per 100 hours for windsurfing, (sailboard) and is higher in water-skiing and powerboat events. Because swimming is non-weight-bearing, it is frequently used in the rehabilitation of other sports. Running in water is used more frequently in the training phase of some sports to cut down on the injuries which arise due to running on hard surfaces.

Overuse injuries affecting muscles and tendons are common in competitive watersports e.g. bicipital and supraspinatus tendinitis in swimmers and waterpolo players and the extensor tendons of the forearm in rowers. Back problems are common in butterfly swimmers, rowers, sailors and windsurfers. All outdoor participants are liable to become sunburnt and in certain countries may be at risk from jellyfish, coral or even sharks. Competitive swimmers may precipitate a shoulder problem by training errors, such as suddenly increasing both the number of laps and the speed of swimming or by using ill-designed paddles which may produce an impingement syndrome or bicipital tendinitis (Richardson, 1987). Muscle imbalance may result in weakness of the lateral rotators of the shoulder causing posterior subluxation. Scoliosis may develop on the side of the dominant hand (Beker, 1986). There is an increased incidence of low back pain in butterfly swimmers; this is often associated with spondylolisthesis (Mutoh 1976).

Breast-stroke swimmers using the whip kick often complain of medial knee pain (Counsilman 1968). There may be strain and point tenderness of the medial ligament (Kennedy and Hawkins 1974), medial synovial plica, medial synovitis (Keskinen *et al.*, 1980) or patellofemoral syndrome (Fowler and Regan, 1986). A combination of an anatomical variation such as a patella alta and a training error may precipitate the condition. Once the cause has been diagnosed then the appropriate treatment – rest, non-steroidal anti-inflammatories, ice and physiotherapy – can be instituted.

Ankle pain due to excessive kicking (legs only) may occur particularly if flippers or fins have been used.

Fingers may be fractured by hitting them off the

end of the pool in the backstroke or they may be injured by hitting against electronic timing pads or catching a ball when playing water polo.

Water polo combines swimming and throwing and is a contact sport. The eggbeater kick used in waterpolo to keep the player up in the water combines a breast-stroke and freestyle kick. This puts stress on the medial side of the knee, affecting the medial collateral ligament (Dominiquez, 1986) Patella malalignment and wasting of the horizontal fibres of vastus medialis will predispose to patellar subluxation. Shoulder problems are also common.

Lacerations and corneal abrasions may occur, particularly if players have sharp finger or toenails. Blows to the eye may result in a blow-out fracture or hyphaema (see Chapter 15). Muscle contusions may also occur. Trauma to the head may cause rupture of the tympanic membrane of the ear or nasal fracture.

Diving

Accidents occur when people dive into water of unknown depth – they dive without checking the depth of the water. This is more likely to occur in private pools, diving boards on beaches, lakes or into a wave. The design of some pools leads to accidents because the depth is not clearly marked. Competitive diving is relatively safe as there is a minimum depth before a diving board can be erected.

Most injuries in competitive diving occur when the diver is rotating inwards towards the board in reverse or inward dives. This is usually due to faulty technique, i.e. poor take-off, and may result in cervical or head injuries (Carter 1986). Practice on a trampoline with a harness, while learning the correct manoeuvres for a dive, will cut down on injuries. When learning how to dive, a diver may damage the cornea if wearing contact lenses or may lose a lens. It is vital that a diver has no vestibular or auditory problems as this will predispose to injury. Ruptured eardrums and sinusitis are relatively common and divers should not dive unless they are normal. The most serious injuries to the head and cervical spine occur on entry into the water; there should always be a floatable stretcher and trained personnel on the spot to rescue and transport the injured diver to hospital.

Injuries to skin divers are usually due to abrasions on rocks, coral or from jellyfish in the water. They may also be injured by speedboats or wind surfers if they are in areas frequented by these craft.

Scuba diving requires an underwater breathing apparatus, a tank containing compressed air and a regulator that delivers air through a mouthpiece (Fig. 22.1). In cold water a wet suit is required and lead weights are often used to compensate for the air trapped in the suit. These weights are the most common cause of death by drowning when a diver under stress forgets to unbuckle the weight, preventing him or her from rising to the water surface (Strauss, 1979).

Air is composed of 21.6% oxygen and 79% nitrogen. Both these gases are soluble in the blood and diffuse through the tissues. As the depth of water increases the pressure increases and the volume of gas decreases. The pressure increases by 1 atm for every 10 m which the diver descends in the water. The scuba diver breathes compressed air at about the same pressure as the surrounding water. This increased pressure drives more of the gases into the blood and tissues. Normally the compressed air passes via the eustacian tube into the middle ear, equalizing the pressure inside it, but if because of a cold or allergy the mucosa of the tube is blocked and this does not occur, it may cause bleeding into the middle ear and rupture of the tympanic membrane. Cold water will then enter the middle ear, resulting in vertigo, which

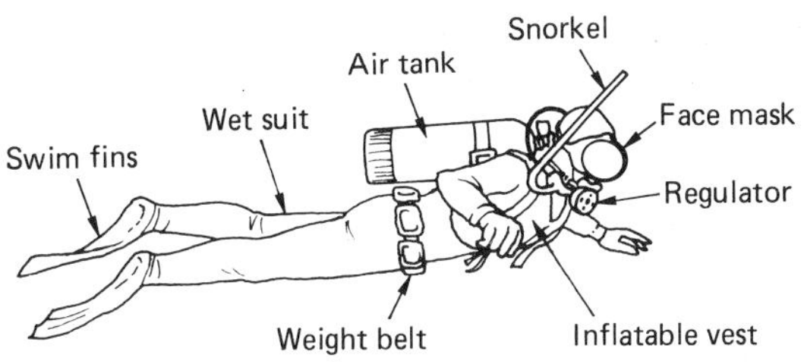

Fig. 22.1 Equipment used in scuba diving.

will cause disorientation – an extremely dangerous situation.

To prevent this occurring, no one with a cold, hayfever or allergy should scuba dive. During descent the diver should equalize the pressure by a manoeuvre such as swallowing. If there is even mild discomfort in the ear, he or she should stop the descent.

It is very important to check the supply of gas – carbon monoxide may occasionally contaminate the air – and to monitor how much has been used. The deeper the dive, the greater the amount of gas required. There is also an increase in the density of the gas, which requires more work to be done by the respiratory muscles. More nitrogen is also dissolved in the blood and tissues at a greater depth; at first this has a euphoric effect and then there is a marked narcotic effect on the central nervous system (Bennett and Elliott, 1975). Therefore 50 m should be the limit for a scuba diver. Professional divers avoid this hazard by replacing part of the nitrogen content with helium (Strauss, 1979).

The most dangerous part of the dive is returning to the surface from a deep dive. There are strict safety guidelines for the time and depth of the dive when it is possible to surface directly – 50 m for 7 min or 20 m for 45 min. If this is exceeded, it is necessary to have a series of stops on the ascent to decompress safely, otherwise the dissolved gases will come out of the solution and air embolism will result. This usually presents as the 'bends', severe joint pain which usually occurs shortly after leaving the water, and is the commonest form of decompression illness. Treatment requires recompression in a decompression chamber.

Sports divers rarely die from decompression sickness, but there may be involvement of the spinal cord and of the brain, resulting in paraplegia or stroke. This may develop over a number of hours and requires immediate recompression at the first sign – usually paraesthesia in the limbs or difficulty with micturition. If the diver holds his or her breath while ascending rapidly to the surface, the volume of gas increases and tends to overinflate the lungs. The lung tissue ruptures. Air enters the pulmonary vessels and emboli may be carried to the heart annd brain, causing a stroke or subcutaneous emphysema. This is most likely to occur if the diver has to ascend rapidly due to a problem with the breathing apparatus.

Women suffering from premenstrual tension are more at risk of developing decompression illness. They are also more accident-prone and should not scuba-dive during this phase of their menstrual cycle. They are also more likely to develop hypothermia (Kizer, 1981).

Diving in a mountain lake also increases the susceptibility to decompression illness, as does flying too soon after a deep dive.

Air embolism can be prevented by breathing normally during the ascent or by exhaling continuously. If a patient has decompression illness or an embolism, place him or her on the left side in the Trendelenburg position, give continuous oxygen and transfer to a hyperbaric chamber as soon as possible.

Stinging jellyfish, sea urchins, sharks or fish with spines may also cause problems. A medical is required for all scuba divers. The minimum age is 15 years. Asthma, eye injury, vertigo and a history of spontaneous pneumothorax are contra-indications. Divers are advised not to dive with hayfever or a perforated ear drum.

Water-skiing

Beginners may injure themselves by falling awkwardly; they may strain leg or arm muscles or injure their shoulder joints. Failure to rise from the starting position may cause forceful retrograde douching, which may cause a haematoma of the vulva or tearing of the vaginal wall. This can be prevented by wearing wet suit pants (Tweedale 1973). The tow rope may also be a cause of friction burns.

Boat drivers should pay careful attention so that boats do not collide or injure fallen skiers. Another boat can cut across the tow rope, causing the skier to be thrown into the air. In one case of this type of accident, the skier injured his brachial plexus, resulting in paralysis of the deltoid and extensor muscles of the forearm (O'Brien *et al.*, 1978).

Rowing

Rowing injuries are often caused by faulty technique or training errors which may result in tenosynovitis of the extensors of the forearm or injury to the back. Correct abdominal strengthening exercises will help prevent back injuries. Blisters on the palms of the hands are very common, and may become infected. Rowers should pay attention to the weather if they are rowing on lakes, particularly in cold weather, as deaths from drowning and hypothermia have occurred.

Canoeing

The risk of injuries in canoeing is greater in wild water events, particularly when negotiating rapids. If the canoeist capsizes and falls against the rocks multiple injuries may result and in some countries there is the added risk of drowning and death from hypothermia.

Windsurfing and yachting

There has been a worldwide increase in windsurfing. The risk of injury is 0.22 per 1000 participant hours and most of the injuries are not significant and may be prevented (McCormick and Davis, 1988). These include abrasions, lacerations, sunburn and muscle strains. It is essential to have good abdominal muscles, otherwise there is an increased risk of back problems; this is especially true of yachting when the crew have to lean out far on a trapeze. In both yachting and windsurfing, injuries may result from the boom, dehydration and sunburn. Cold is the most important factor in increasing the risk of injury.

Speedboat racing

Speedboat or power boat racing is unique in that there is a greater risk of collision. Therefore a seriously injured driver may have to be rescued from the water, possibly with head injuries, multiple fractures and burns. It is essential that there is an adequate number of suitably equipped boats with personnel qualified in first aid and water safety to carry out the rescue. The physician in charge should be competent to treat acute trauma and be able to intubate the injured; if necessary, scuba divers wearing wet suits should be part of the team. Communication is vital to alert the crash boat nearest the accident.

Conclusions

Observing safety precautions, obeying the rules of the sport and having a healthy respect for the water and weather will reduce the incidence of drowing and injuries. Prevention by teaching people to swim and instruction by qualified personnel will allow everybody to enjoy water sports with the minimum of risk.

References

Beker TJ (1986) Scoliosis in swimmers. *Clinics in Sports Medicine* **5**, 149–58.

Bennett PB, Elliott DH (1975) *The Physiology and Medicine of Diving and Compressed Air Work*. Baltimore: Williams & Wilkins.

Carter RL (1986) Prevention of springboard and platform diving injuries. *Clinics in Sports Medicine* **5**, 185–94.

Counsilman JE (1968) *The Science of Swimming*. Englewood Cliffs: Prentice-Hall.

Craig AP (1961) Causes of loss of consciousness diving underwater. *Journal of Applied Physiology* **16**, 583–6.

Dominiquez RH (1986) Water polo injuries. *Clinics in Sports Medicine* **5**, 169–83.

Fowler PJ, Regan WD (1986) Swimming injuries of the knee, foot and ankle and elbow and back. *Clinics in Sports Medicine* **5**, 139–48.

Giammona ST, Modell JH (1967) Drowning by total immersion. Effects on pulmonary surfactant of distilled water, isotonic saline and sea water. *American Journal of Diseases of Childhood* **114**, 612–16.

Goode RC, Romet TT, Duffin J, Beckbache RR, Cunningham DA, O'Hara W (1978) Sudden cold immersion. *Swimming Medicine* **4**, 310–22.

Gooden BA (1987) Drowning and the diving reflex in man. *Medical Journal of Australia* **2**, 583–7.

Hassel IB (1989) Thirty-six consecutive under 5 year old swimming pool drownings. *Australian Paediatric Journal* **25**, 143–6.

Keatinge WR (1978) Cold immersion survival and resuscitation. *Swimming Medicine* **4**, 305–9.

Kennedy JC, Hawkins RJ (1974) Breaststroker's knee. *Sports Medicine* **2**, 33–8.

Keskimen K, Eriksson E, Komi P (1980) Breaststroker's knee. *American Journal of Sports Medicine* **8**, 228.

Kizer K (1981) Women and diving. *Physician and Sports Medicine* **9**, 85–92.

McCormick DP, Davis AL (1988) Injuries in sailboard enthusiasts. *British Journal of Sports Medicine* **22**, 95–7.

MacNeill R, Cohen S (1976) *Recreational Boat Safety. Collision Research Phase 2* vol 2. report no. CG–D23: 11. Springfield, VA: National Technical Information Service.

Metropolitan Life Assurance Company (1977) *Statistical Bulletin*. Metropolitan Life Assurance Company, London, pp 2–3.

Modell JH (1981) Drowning versus near drowning. A discussion of definition. *Critical Care Medicine* **9**, 351–2.

Modell JH, Moya F (1966) The effects of volume of aspirated fluid during chlorinated fresh water drowning. *Anaesthesiology* **27**, 662–72.

Modell JH, Moya F, Newby EJ (1967) The effects of fluid volume in sea water drowning. *Annals of Internal Medicine* **67**, 68–80.

Modell JH, Graves SA, Ketova A (1976) Clinical course of 91 consecutive near drowning victims. *Chest* **70**, 231–8.

Mutoh Y (1978) Low back pain in butterfliers. *Swimming Medicine* **4**, 115–23.

O'Brien M, Bonner FJ, Bonner JF (1978) Echomyographic evaluation of a water skiing injury. *British Journal of Sports Medicine* **12**, 142–4.

O'Carroll PW, Alkon E, Weiss B (1988) Drowning mortality in Los Angeles county. 1976 to 1984. *Journal of the American Medical Association* **19**.

Orlowski JP (1987) Drowning, near-drowning, and ice water submersions. *Paediatric Clinics of North America* **1**, 75–92.

Quan L, Gore EJ, Wentz K, Allen J, Novack AH (1989) Ten years study of pediatric drownings and near-drownings in Kings Country. Washington. **6**, 1035–40.

Richardson AB (1987) Orthopaedic aspects of competitive swimming. *Clinics in Sports Medicine* **6**, 639–45.

Royal Society for the Prevention of Accidents (1989/90) Drowning by design. Winter 6–7.

Royal Life Saving Society 1982. *Drownings in the British Isles*, pp 1–27.

Rowe M, Arango A, Allington G (1977) Profile of paedriatric drowning – victims in a water oriented society. *Journal of Trauma* **17**, 587–91.

Sarnaik P, Vohra MP (1986) Near drowning, fresh, salt and cold water immersion. *Clinics of Sports Medicine* **5**, 33–46.

Simpson CK (1958) *Forensic Medicine*. London: Edward Arnold, p 344.

Spyker DA (1985) Submersion injury. *Paediatric Clinics of North America* **32**, 113–25.

Strauss RH (ed.) (1979) Medical aspects of scuba and breath-hold diving. In: *Sports Medicine and Physiology*. Philadelphia: WB Saunders, pp 344–52.

Tweedale PG (1973) Vaginal lacerations in water skiers. *Canadian Medical Association Journal* 1081; 20.

Vimpani G, Doudle M, Harris R (1988) Child accident mortality in Northern Territory. *Medical Journal of Australia* **148**, 392–5.

Weightman D, Browne RC (1981) Injuries in eleven selected sports. *British Journal of Sports Medicine* **15**, 136–41.

23

Risks and injuries in gymnastics, ballet and dance

J. Howse
S. Hancock

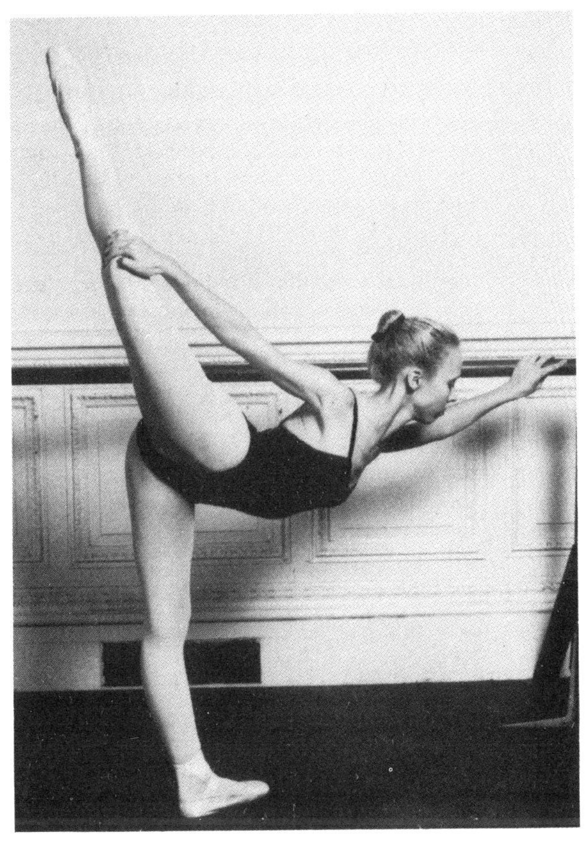

Introduction

Unlike most other athletic activities dance and gymnastics require a large number of different and very varied movements, all of which have to be totally controlled throughout. The necessary precision needs careful and thorough training which can only take place slowly over a period of many years. In the minds of many of the performers injury seems to be accepted as an inevitable consequence of their professional lives. This concept is, however, totally unnecessary and incorrect.

Disregarding the type of accident that can befall any member of the population it is possible to make the dogmatic statement that *all injuries arise from technical faults*. The other concept that must be hammered home into the heads of both performers and teachers is the fact that *injuries are not an act of God*. It is the role of the teacher to make certain that students do not progress faster than they can manage and that they do not attempt techniques of which they are not capable. This latter is particularly important when teaching younger and physically immature students. Children develop at very different rates and there is no doubt that one of the great difficulties teachers have to face is that frequently they have a class of children who are the same chronological age but who are greatly different in maturity and physical development. In these instances it must not be expected that all the children are ready at the same time to progress to the next stage of their training. An excellent example of this is the age that the girl should start pointe work. While 12 years old is given as a rather generalized and blanket age, this must depend entirely upon the physical development of the child as well as the degree of training. Many girls are certainly not strong enough to start pointe work at that age and this may have to be deferred for another year or two, or even more. The strength required is not only in the feet but also in the muscle control of the whole of each lower limb and of the trunk. A very famous ballet dancer was unable to get up on to pointe until she was 16, but this is no way interfered with her career and subsequent success.

In accepting that all dance injuries are due to technical faults it must be understood that these are frequently minor, and it is because they are minor that they are not noticed by the teacher or are ignored with the thought that they can be corrected at a later stage. Unhappily, it is these minor faults which can produce major problems for the dancer.

Technical faults can arise for various reasons. First of all there can be anatomical problems so that the student is physically incapable of achieving the position required or the correct technique. A good example of this is the dancer with a limited turnout who is forced to turn the feet out to 180°. This situation is, of course, brought about by the presence of a teacher who is incapable of accepting the fact that not every student has the flexibility or control required and that forcing the dancer into a position which is physically impossible is only going to cause injury. Anatomical problems therefore cause injury either because a student tries to force something which is unobtainable or an incompetent teacher tries to do the same. Unless corrected, young students will assume that the turnout they see on stage is confined to turning the feet alone out and this correction is the responsibility of the teacher. Before undertaking the training of any child the teacher must accurately assess the degree of flexibility present and this includes any accurate measurement of the amount of external rotation available at each hip. The teacher must realize that the external rotation is not necessarily symmetrical and in these instances the dancer must work symmetrically within the limits of the tighter side. Even established dancers, in whom the technique has been correctly developed, can allow their technique to fall from the ideal from time to time. This happens particularly when the dancer becomes tired. In touring companies one sees the injury rate gradually increase as a tour progresses.

Once performers have sustained a minor injury there will be a great tendency for them to alter technique so that the injury can be accommodated without causing too much pain. Any alteration in technique can only be for the worse and this will frequently lead to the occurrence of further injuries.

The prevention of injury may be thought to be self-evident. Initially children should only be selected if they are physically suitable for the art form required, whether classical ballet, contemporary dance or gymnastics. At this stage the acceptance of someone who is anatomically unsuitable is highly likely to result in injuries at some time in the future. During training, progress and physical demands must be tailored to the development and physical maturity and strength of the student. This must also include the mental ability of the student to learn the technique required. As with academic subjects, so with physical activity requiring special techniques; children will have different learning rates and this must be appreciated by the teachers.

There has to be progress with learning and students must attempt new techniques in order to learn them. A teacher can only prepare students in the best way possible to the point when they should be capable of progressing to something more complicated. However, in any class if several identical injuries occur the teacher *must* ask her- or himself what she or he is doing to the students rather than what the students are doing to themselves.

Once an injury has occurred careful assessment is required. Most injuries when taken individually are relatively easy to treat but unless an accurate assessment is made of the cause of the injury it is highly likely to recur once the student gets back to normal working. It is vital at that stage to assess the presence of any technical faults and to take great care to correct these at the same time as treating the injury. The presence of one technical fault which might have caused the injury does not preclude the presence of others which could be equally or jointly responsible. Only too frequently there are several faults, as the presence of one will fairly rapidly lead to the development of another fault.

During their training, dancers and gymnasts should be educated in the general principles of first-aid treatment and self-help, namely rest, ice and elevation of the injured part. Unless the injury is obviously minor and is settling rapidly with first-aid measures, the injured person should always be encouraged to seek professional advice. Initially this may be from a physiotherapist experienced in the treatment of dancers and gymnasts, or of course the performer may go straight to a physician or surgeon dealing in these types of injuries. It is important that injured performers obtain the best available advice and treatment. There is always great anxiety on their part to return to full work as soon as possible. The risk to the performer and sports player of trying to take the rapid cure cannot be overemphasized. While a quick manipulation, injection or other pain-relieving treatment may appear to have cured the problem, it can only too commonly lead to a recurrence of the same injury or the production of an even more severe injury.

What any athlete, including dancers and gymnasts, requires is:

1. Correct diagnosis.
2. Correct treatment.
3. Full rehabilitation and technical correction.

Rehabilitation is essentially a combination of a suitable exercise programme and thorough technical correction. The exercise programme should be directed at all weak or relatively weak muscle groups. There must be balancing of muscle strength not only between muscle groups but also between the two sides of the body and even within a single group, e.g. quadriceps, lateral versus medial, or hamstrings, lateral versus medial. Imbalance is not uncommon and can be induced by incorrect working. Other treatment modalities, although also important (ultrasound, interferential therapy and ice), are largely an aid to relieving pain and swelling and increasing local blood flow in order to allow the exercise programme and technical correction to proceed. It is essential that the person in charge of a dancer's or gymnast's treatment looks at the patient as a whole, not just treats the injured part. Technical help, it must be remembered, does not only apply to dancers and gymnasts but it also applies to many other sports where the injury is sustained as a result of incorrect performance of that sport, for example throwers of various types, fast bowlers, fencers and golfers, and also surprisingly enough, although not under the heading of sports injuries, musicians.

Sprain of the lateral ligament of the ankle

A survey of dancers carried out over a 10-year period showed that this was the commonest injury and made up 9.4% of the total. A similar figure was found by Dr William Hamilton (personal communication) in a personal survey of dancers he looked after in New York: his patients came from the New York City Ballet, American Ballet Theatre and other small companies and stage shows. It must be admitted though that not all these injuries are sustained during training or performance. Dancers and gymnasts, despite an assumption that they probably have better balance and co-ordination than the average member of the population, appear to be just as liable to fall down the stairs or slip off the pavement kerb as any other member of the population.

In a sprain of the lateral ligament the fibres most commonly affected are those of the anterior talofibular ligament. During performance the injury most often occurs as a result of a bad landing from a jump or the dancer falling off pointe or half-pointe.

Fortunately most of these injuries are relatively minor. A mild sprain consists of the tearing of a few fibres of the ligament accompanied by pain, swelling due to local bleeding and an outpouring of tissue fluid and protective muscle spasm. The severity of the sprain depends upon the degree of tearing of the ligament. It is of vital importance to exclude a complete tear of the ligaments. The initial examination immediately after the injury, before the swelling has developed and before muscle spasm makes examination difficult, may allow clinical confirmation of ankle instability with the talus tilting in the ankle mortice on passive inversion. However, later when there is swelling, protective spasm and much more pain, it may be necessary to carry out stress X-rays under a general anaesthetic. Far more commonly missed and just as important is a complete tear of the anterior talofibular ligament and part of the anterior capsule. This injury allows the talus to slip forwards in the ankle mortice whilst at the same time there is an internal rotational movement of the talus. In this situation the lateral fibres are usually intact and therefore normal stress inversion X-rays will give the impression of stability. This type of damage is best detected on clinical examination and reliance should not be placed on the X-ray examination. Should this damage be missed, chronic problems for the dancer or gymnast will result.

There are many factors which may increase the risk of lateral ligament injury – weak feet (weak intrinsic muscles) and weakness of the muscles controlling the ankle are obvious causes, as there will be insufficient control when landing from jumps and when on half- and full-pointe. However, higher up in the leg, weakness of the muscles controlling the turnout will encourage the foot to be turned out further than the hip, thus altering the line of weight transmission. Weakness around the trunk will also produce faulty jumping. As an extraneous cause, poor floor surfaces, either very slippery or very sticky, can induce technical errors leading to faulty jumping and injury.

At the same time as assessing the degree of ligamentous damage it is essential to exclude bony injury. A fracture of the lateral malleolus is the most common bony injury but a fracture of the base of the fifth metatarsal can occur through a similar mechanism and should also be excluded.

Initial treatment is ice, elevation and rest. The dancer or gymnast must remain non-weight-bearing until fractures have been excluded either on clinical or, if necessary, radiological grounds. Subsequently if the injury is minor, some limited work may be possible with the use of a compression bandage. However, in anything other than a trivial sprain the dancer will have to be off performing and training.

Icing, elevation and rest should continue and a physiotherapist should give ultrasound and interferential therapy. An early start should be made on non-weight-bearing exercises. If these are carried out with the leg in elevation they can be helpful in reducing the swelling more rapidly. An exercise programme must encompass all muscle groups around the ankle. The exercises should be carried out with the foot in full plantar flexion and with the foot at a right angle so as to ensure that all aspects of muscle control are built up.

Specifically at the same time faradic footbaths and intrinsic muscle exercises should be carried out. It may well be that the muscles were weak and at least in part a cause of the sprain, but even if not they tend to waste rapidly after such an injury. As with any other injury the patient can also pay a great deal of attention to doing exercises for all the other groups in the lower limbs and the trunk in order to keep her- or himself in good condition. Part-way through the period of rehabilitation, exercises should be commenced using a balancing board. This can begin when the patient is sitting during the non-weight-bearing phase of treatment. The balancing board can also be used at the barre if some support is required, for example during a partial weight-bearing phase of treatment. The balancing board is an essential tool in the rehabilitation of an ankle injury. When the ligament is sprained there is damage to the nerve endings within the ligament and the joint capsule. The balancing board helps to restore the patient's proprioceptive reflexes which are essential in preventing recurrent sprains of the ankle. Incidentally, the balancing board is also extremely useful in the general rehabilitation of other injuries, whether within the trunk or the lower limb, and indeed in the uninjured performer when trying to build up muscle strength and, in particular, general postural and joint control.

An energetically and conscientiously treated ankle sprain should recover completely and allow the performer to return to full activity without any disability. There is no rule of thumb for the time that rehabilitation should take. This must depend entirely upon the degree of damage. There may be a few days off or even 3 months or more if a ligament has required repair. During recovery the calf muscle may tighten. It is essential that the calf is kept strong and well-stretched during the period of rehabilitation. It is always far more difficult to stretch an area out later than to maintain the flexibility from the beginning.

The complications of ligament injury around the ankle are largely the result of inadequate treatment. Unfortunately ankle sprains tend to be thought of not only by the patient but also by health professionals – who should know better – as a minor injury which will settle spontaneously with little or no treatment and the mere use of a bandage and passage of time. This is far from the case. Inadequate treatment will lead to a chronic condition of recurrent pain, swelling and instability.

Failure to recognize a rupture of a ligament can also lead to chronic problems. For the best results an early surgical repair is essential. Late repairs are far less satisfactory and at an even later date reconstructions are never completely satisfactory.

Sprain of the medial ligament of the ankle

This is not common in gymnasts and dancers. It is, however, important to exclude a fracture of the medial malleolus or a rupture of the ligament as these require immediate orthopaedic treatment. The fracture is best treated by screwing the medial malleolus back into place and a rupture will require early repair. As in injuries of the lateral ligament, damage to the medial aspect of the ankle results commonly from a bad landing from a jump. Treatment is similar to that for the lateral ligament and just as much attention needs to be paid to thorough rehabilitation with correction of any underlying problems.

Chronic sprains of the ankle ligaments

As mentioned above, these may follow inadequate treatment but a chronic injury can also come about by faulty techniques with incorrect weight transmissin through the ankle and foot. This results in repetitive strains being applied to one or other side of the ankle, gradually producing inflammation, thickening and scarring within the ligament. This will usually be accompanied by increasing weakness in some of the muscle groups around the ankle and a steady decrease in the proper control of the ankle and foot. As a result there will be increasingly faulty techniques and even further damage can follow. Recovery will be slow and will probably require a great deal of physiotherapy. It will certainly result in a great deal of time having to be spent on correction of technique. The time spent, however, is well worthwhile as a chronic sprain is an unnecessary and avoidable disability.

Achilles tendon problems

These comprise Achilles tendon bursitis, Achilles tendinitis and peritendinitis and rupture of the Achilles tendon.

The Achilles tendon bursa is situated at the lower end of the tendon and lies between the tendon and the posterior aspect of the calcaneum. It can become inflamed, thickened and swollen if it is irritated. Bursitis may be associated with an Achilles tendinitis or peritendinitis but it may occur as an entity by itself. Most commonly the bursitis is produced by pressure from an ill-fitting shoe or undue prominence of the posterior part of the os calcis or from overuse. In diagnosis it is differentiated from an Achilles tendinitis by its localization. Treatment starts with elimination of the cause. The use of ice, interferential treatment and ultrasound can be helpful. Pulsed microwave is particularly useful in this condition. Once the cause is eliminated the condition usually settles rapidly. Very rarely, an injection of hydrocortisone acetate may be necessary.

Achilles tendinitis is an inflammation of the tendon which may have been precipitated by microtears within the substance of the tendon. A peritendinitis is an inflammation of the tissue immediately surrounding the Achilles tendon. These conditions are most commonly caused by overuse, often precipitated by weakness of various muscle groups, namely the feet, knee and thigh muscles, so that during work extra effort has to be made by the calf muscles, particularly when jumping and landing. A similar result is also produced by extra work when the performer is tired, which is something that can happen during the course of a tour. The situation is aggravated by any factor which causes the weight to be too far back, commonly swayback (hyperextended) knees or a lordosis. Where there is imbalance between the various muscle groups the gastrocnemius may, of necessity, have to overwork because it crosses behind the knee. As a result the soleus may, relative to the gastrocnemius, be underused. This situation can be aggravated in dancers if their pointe is somewhat limited so they cannot work well on three-quarter pointe or if the class work is so structured that there is insufficient three-quarter pointe work to strengthen the calf muscles throughout their range. Three-quarter pointe is essential on all jumps, landings and on *relevés* when rising on to full pointe. Before a dancer starts full-pointe work a considerable amount of time must be spent working in the three-quarter pointe position in order to strengthen the muscles adequately and give full control of the foot and ankle. (In order to avoid any misunderstanding, we must hasten to add that not only do the muscles controlling the feet and ankles have to be strong before starting pointe work but also there must be adequate strength throughout the lower limb and in the trunk. Weakness in any of these areas would make pointe work difficult and perilous.) A tight pointe may also cause overuse as the dancer or gymnast strains to improve the plantar flexion of the foot and ankle. Anything that produces a tight pointe may cause an Achilles tendinitis. The tight pointe may be a general restriction of movement in the ankle and foot or it may be caused by a posterior impingement syndrome due to the presence of an os trigonum or large posterior tubercle of the talus. Inadequately treated calf muscle tears, which are particularly prone to contracture, can lead to an Achilles tendinitis.

Treatment from the physiotherapist will generally be in the form of ice, ultrasound and interferential therapy. The latter should extend to above the knee in order to include the full length of the gastrocnemius. As the symptoms settle the whole calf muscle must be strengthened and this must then be followed by stretching. Incidentally, the stretching should not come first – a weak muscle should never be stretched. Strengthening should take place and following the strengthening should come the stretching. During rehabilitation the causes of the Achilles tendinitis must be eliminated. Any technical correction must be undertaken and there must always be an exercise programme to ensure that all other muscle groups are strengthened. A long-standing Achilles tendinitis can be very slow to resolve. This delay may be associated with a technical fault which has not been noticed and a reassessment of the overall condition of the patient is indicated. Only occasionally will an injection of hydrocortisone acetate or other steroid be necessary. Should it be used, the injection must be given into the peritendinous tissues and not into the tendon itself. An ill-advised injection of steroid may lead to a partial rupture developing into a total rupture as the steroid will interfere with the healing process.

Rupture of the Achilles tendon usually occurs in a dancer or gymnast who has not had any previous Achilles tendon symptoms. The tear is associated with a sudden very powerful calf muscle contraction in a performer who is ill-prepared for such a situation. This lack of preparation occurs in a teacher who is out of training and who suddenly decides to demonstrate a step requiring such a powerful movement or in a performer who has failed to warm up properly before a difficult routine. It can also happen as a result of an uncoordinated muscle contraction in a tired performer. Early diagnosis is vital and if there is any doubt whatsoever, early specialist advice is called for. Initially a gap can frequently be felt in the Achilles tendon but fairly rapidly due to bleeding and local swelling, this gap may be hidden, making the diagnosis more difficult. Pain, local swelling and a flat-footed gait call for urgent expert consultation. With the patient lying face-down with the feet lying over the end of the couch, if there is an Achilles tendon rupture, the affected foot will lie in less plantarflexion than the normal foot because normal muscle tone in the calf will not be transmitted down to the foot. The calf-squeeze test would be positive. In a normal leg if the calf is squeezed the foot goes down into slightly increased plantarflexion. In the presence of an Achilles tendon rupture there is no movement in the foot.

Treatment should be by immediate surgical repair of the rupture. Conservative treatment with a plaster cast gives a less good result, although partial ruptures, if the diagnosis is not in doubt, could certainly be treated successfully in plaster. Unfortunately even following surgical repair dancers or gymnasts may be unable to return to the same high level of performance as before the injury. If they are well on in their career the injury, coupled with their age, may result in the premature ending of their performing life.

Immediately after surgery, as with all other injuries, an exercise programme should be started in order to maintain the muscles in the rest of the body in a high state of training. Once the postoperative plaster has been removed the rehabilitation becomes more intensive as the muscle groups in the affected leg are included in the work programme. During the period of rehabilitation, techniques should be watched to make certain that faults do not develop as a result of any muscle weakness or imbalance which may persist. Usually the rupture will occur out of the blue so there will not necessarily be any technical faults to correct but after any serious injury technical faults can occur during the period when the performer is returning to full activity. The time-scale for full rehabilitation will usually be something in the order of 6 months, although carefully supervised class work can gradually start long before that time.

Tenosynovitis around the ankle and foot

The tendons of tibialis posterior and flexor hallucis longus are those most commonly involved. The extensor hallucis longus tendon not lying in a sheath can, however, develop a peritendinitis or tendinitis.

The common cause is overuse which results in the development of local inflammation. This is often associated with swelling and thickening as well as local tenderness. Frequently, active movements of a tendon can produce a palpable crepitus or creaking. A direct blow may precipitate the condition. This is particularly likely in the case of an extensor hallucis longus tendinitis, which may also be produced by pressure from a shoe or by overuse.

Tibialis posterior tenosynovitis is most commonly caused by an incorrect line of weight-bearing. In the foot that rolls, that is, one where the weight comes on to the medial border of the foot (Fig. 23.1) there can be a great tendency to try and correct the rolling locally at the foot and ankle. This puts considerable strain on both tibialis anterior and tibialis posterior, although it is the latter which more often becomes inflamed. The situation is aggravated by the presence of weak intrinsic muscles. Rolling is usually brought about by allowing the feet to be more turned out than the degree of external rotation which is taking place at the hips. This may be due to limitation of external rotation at the hips or it may be a failure to use the available turnout, either due to a technical error or by weakness of the muscles controlling turnout. If a dancer relaxes when standing in the turned-out position the hips will start to rotate internally but the feet will be held by the friction of the floor and as a result the weight will come on to the medial borders of the feet and the feet will roll.

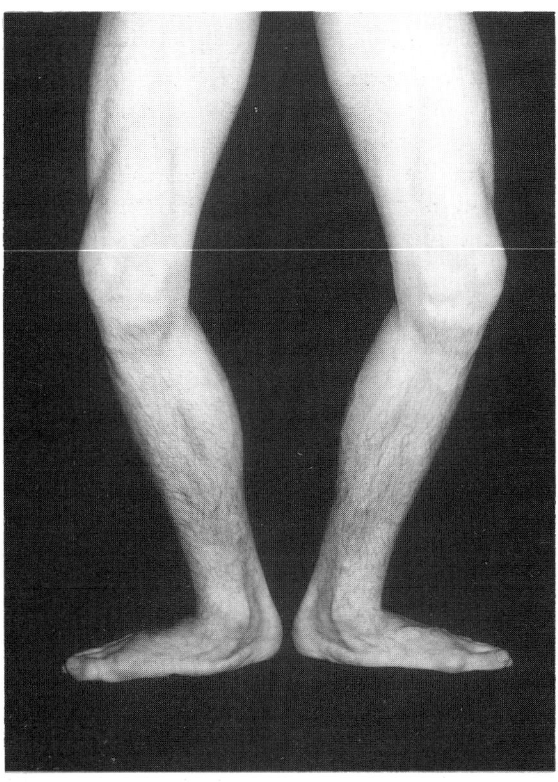

Fig. 23.1 Rolling. The legs are less turned out than the feet so the knees fall inside the feet. The weight comes on to the medial borders of the feet and the longitudinal arches flatten. Strain can be seen over the medial aspects of the ankles. From Howe and Hancock (1988), with permission.

Flexor hallucis longus tenosynovitis is in general caused by incorrect weight-bearing. Additionally, with this tendon, there is another condition associated with the musculotendinous junction. The muscle fibres extend as far as the ankle and the tendon sheath starts immediately distally to this. On full dorsiflexion of the great toe the fleshy musculotendinous junction may be pulled into the tendon sheath. Should this happen repeatedly, it can lead to local swelling which will produce symptoms of persistent pain. The condition is easily relieved surgically by opening the proximal portion of the tendon sheath.

With extensor hallucis longus tendinitis, rolling is an important cause. Tendinitis may also be induced if the weight is back. This will tend to produce clawing of the toes and weakness of the intrinsic muscles. Local pressure from the shoe or an ill-fitting block may also produce a tendinitis.

Tenosynovitis or tendinitis in all three of these tendons is treated with ultrasound, faradic footbaths, intrinsic muscle exercises and technical correction. The latter is particularly important as technical faults are the most common cause of the underlying problems. Unfortunately these conditions can be very slow to settle. The underlying technical faults may be well-established and it may take a long period of help to eliminate them.

In the case of extensor hallucis longus tendinitis a stress fracture of the second metatarsal shaft may give the appearance of pain along the extensor hallucis longus tendon and it certainly needs to be excluded.

Although we are strictly dealing with the soft tissues, stress fractures of the lesser metatarsals, usually the second or third, can occur as a complication of a primary soft tissue problem. For example, weak intrinsic muscles, technical faults, particularly those involving incorrect weight placement (rolling, sickling, overturning or failure to hold the turnout or anything which pushes the weight too far back) can produce stress fractures. Working when the muscle groups are not strong enough or when they have become overtired can cause the performer to land heavily and crash through the foot; if this continues over a period of time then it may result in the development of a stress fracture.

Strains of the capsule of the first metatarsophalangeal joint

This is usually caused by a direct blow, commonly as a result of landing badly, or it is associated with technical faults. Rolling and sickling frequently produce a twisting force on the great toe, straining the capsule. If a hallux valgus deformity is present then in rises a further strain is transmitted to the medial capsule of the joint. The use of worn-out pointe shoes greatly aggravates the situation. As a result of the painful capsular strain there will often be limitation of movements at the joint and this may lead to the faulty diagnosis of a developing hallux rigidus. As it is due to the pain, the limitation of mobility will, of course, regress as the symptoms settle down.

When treating the patient the local use of ultrasound, ice and interferential therapy is helpful. Faradic footbaths and intrinsic muscle exercises are essential in order to strengthen the intrinsics. Passive traction on the toe to stretch gently any tightness that may have occurred in the capsule may be helpful. It is essential to check the shoes and, as ever, to try and correct all the technical faults. Unfortunately long-standing technical faults may have produced permanent rotation of the great toe which no amount of treatment will correct. Therefore full relief of the symptoms may not be obtained. Nevertheless, this does not mean that the condition should be ignored because it will only deteriorate if not treated.

Strain of the plantar fascia

Relatively high longitudinal arches together with weak feet can produce strains of the plantar fascia. The situation is greatly aggravated by wearing shoes that are too short. Boys in particular often tend to wear very short shoes under the misapprehension that it improves the appearance of the foot when they are pointing.

In treating the patient, pulsed microwave, interferential therapy and ultrasound are all helpful and these must be combined with faradic footbaths and intrinsic muscle exercises. Plantar fascia strain can be rather slow to settle unless the symptoms are of a relatively short duration. Obviously shoes must be checked, particularly in boys.

Anterior compartment syndrome

The anterior compartment lies in the front of the leg and is surrounded by non-stretchable fibrous tissue. As a result of the inelasticity of these structures, any swelling that may occur in the anterior compartment will produce symptoms due to the rise in pressure. While a mild degree of anterior compartment syndrome is not uncommon following a return from holiday or an increase in workload, the extreme situation which sometimes occurs in other athletes, when the swelling is so excessive that the rise in pressure obstructs the blood supply, is very rare indeed. A return after a holiday or an increase in work is invariably carried out in a well-structured manner so the build-up in activity is gradual. The causative factor of extra exercise is very much aggravated if the weight is too far back because this increases the tension in the muscle groups in the anterior compartment. It is aggravated yet more by weak feet and by rolling.

Treatment is not usually necessary in very mild cases and the dancer will work through the symptoms, which will gradually settle as muscle condition improves. Should the symptoms be greater then treatment should initially be directed at stimulating the circulation and the venous return. The legs should be elevated, and ice and interferential therapy for the whole lower limb should be used. Exercises must be given to strengthen all the other groups, most of which will certainly be weak. Particular attention must be paid to strengthening the feet and correcting any tendency for the weight to be back.

Surgical decompression of the anterior compartment is necessary if the circulation within the anterior compartment is at risk. If there is any doubt then intracompartmental pressures must be measured. Although a theoretical possibility, the authors have not, in fact, ever seen a case of this severity occurring in a dancer.

A very important differential diagnosis is that of stress fracture of the tibia. In this condition there is warmth, tenderness and thickening in a fairly well-localized area over the tibia as opposed to the anterior compartment itself. X-rays of the tibia will probably not demonstrate a stress fracture until the symptoms have been present for 6–8 weeks and therefore a normal X-ray does not exclude a developing stress fracture. If there is any doubt then an isotope bone scan should be carried out.

Anterior knee pain

Pain over the front of the knee is a very common complaint in both young gymnasts and young dancers. Most frequently it is seen during adolescence but it still continues to be one of the commoner problems in the 20s. Most patients are given the diagnosis of chondromalacia patellae but this diagnosis is usually inaccurate. In anterior knee pain a definitive diagnosis may be difficult and the label of chondromalacia is an easy way of satisfying the patient that the practitioner actually knows the precise diagnosis.

In most patients with anterior knee pain the cause is due to a muscle imbalance within the quadriceps muscle. Careful examination of the knee will show that some degree of lateral tracking of the patella is invariably present. This can range from very mild to very obvious. During an isometric quadriceps contraction the patella can be seen to move both proximally and laterally. The condition is, however, more easily detected by watching the movement of the patella as the quadriceps muscle relaxes after its contraction. In this instance the patella can be seen to relax medially and distally. In patients with anterior knee pain there is retropatellar tenderness and often patellofemoral pain on passive patellar movements and invariably quite severe pain on a resisted isometric quadriceps contraction when the patella is pressed firmly backwards and distally on to the knee and the patient is then asked to do a quadriceps contraction. In most cases this will reproduce the symptomatic pain and most patients will say that the pain is rather worse than they actually experience. Further examination will show that there is increased development of the vastus lateralis and a relative underdevelopment of the vastus medialis. As a result there is always a lateral as well as a proximal pull transmitted during a quadriceps contraction. The importance of the vastus medialis, because of the direction of its muscle fibres, is to counteract the lateral pull and to stabilize the patella so that tracking remains central. Anterior knee pain can happen just as easily when the thigh muscles are well-developed. The vital fact is the imbalance between the medial and lateral sides, not the total strength or development of the thigh muscles as a whole. If the lateral tracking is of long standing there may be some genuine soft tissue and capsular contraction laterally but this lateral tightness only occurs when the lateral/medial imbalance has been present for a long period (the presence of knock-knees, giving an increased Q angle, is most unlikely to present in a dancer or gymnast).

Treatment is directed at correcting the muscle imbalance by active exercise. Considerable strengthening of the vastus medialis is essential and this should be accompanied by strengthening of the adductor muscles. Looking more deeply into the problem it will often be found that there has been incomplete control of the pelvis. This may arise from weakness of the adductors and the hamstrings particularly, but also from the other muscles stabilizing the hip and from weakness of the trunk muscles. Associated with this there is often tightening of the tensor fasciae latae which can in itself prevent a proper adjustment of the pelvis and of weight transference. The physiotherapist's eye therefore has to be cast far further afield and will probably encompass a programme for strengthening the trunk muscles, adjusting the line of weight transmission and stretching out the tensor fasciae latae. In some patients the patellofemoral region is so sensitive that even a simple isometric quadriceps contraction causes pain and therefore inhibition. In these cases the exercise programme will have to start with work on the other muscle groups, particularly the inner side of the thigh, which will allow some overflow into the vastus medialis. This together with very local interferential therapy will usually be sufficient to allow the sensitivity to settle so that work can then proceed more directly on the vastus medialis. One of the important corrections which frequently has to take place is to teach the patient proper control of swayback knees, which are also often present.

Unhappily, only too many patients when first seen have already been subjected to lateral release procedures. The majority of these have been totally unnecessary and a physiotherapy programme correctly carried out would have relieved the situation, although it must be emphasized that this can take a considerable time and the patient must be persuaded not to give up. A lateral release operation will invariably aggravate the situation as there will be an increase in muscle wasting, particularly of the vastus medialis, and therefore an increase in imbalance as a result of the surgical asssault. Should there – extremely rarely – be a true contracture of the lateral capsule, it then becomes even more vital to emphasize to patients the importance of the post-operative physiotherapy and not let them be under any misapprehension that the operative procedure is going to be curative in its own right.

In anterior knee pain probably the most useful feature of an arthroscopy is to exclude for certain the presence of any retropatellar changes which might be contributing to the symptoms.

Patellar tendinitis

This commonly produces pain at the patellotendinous junction rather than in the mid-part of the tendon. It is an inflammatory reaction due to a strain of the tendon fibres where they are inserted into the bone at the inferior pole of the patella.

The commonest cause is lateral tracking of the patella. This produces an unequal pull on the patellar tendon. It is frequently associated with incorrect weight transmission, with the body weight being too far back. This may be accompanied by overturning at the feet and rolling. Swayback knees can cause inadequacy of the quadriceps and this will aggravate any lateral/medial imbalance.

Relative weakness of the feet or calf prevents adequate absorption of the shock in landing from jumps and in these situations the patellar tendon takes the strain and can produce a tightness, especially if there is also some quadriceps inadequacy. During a period of rapid growth all these factors may pertain. There will be relative weakness of muscles. There will be imbalance within the quadriceps and between the quadriceps, calves and feet. The rapid growth may also have produced a temporary tightness at the front of the hip, aggravating the patellar tendinitis.

Growth spurts can pose considerable problems in both gymnasts and dancers. In both these activities training starts very young, when considerable growth is still to be expected. Children grow at different rates and at different ages. In some, growth will be a continuous process but more often it will come in spurts. In class work, which is often structured in age groups, particularly in professional schools where the ballet classes have to be fitted in with academic work, it is difficult to have a mix of ages. As a result the teacher has to cope with a situation where there is a considerable discrepancy in maturity between the various children. During growth spurts the rapid growth tends to take place in the leg followed by the thighs and finally in the trunk, hence the long-legged coltish appearance during these periods. During a spell of rapid growth there are two things in particular which take place which can produce problems in dance and gymnastic teaching. Firstly the muscles become relatively weak and it is this, accompanied by the sudden increase in length, which decreases control and co-ordination. Secondly, there is usually a relative tightening of the soft tissues because bony growth outstrips soft tissue growth. This can lead therefore to obvious tightening of such areas as the hamstrings, the turnout and the front of the hips. The youngsters must be discouraged from injudicious or violent stretching. During this period, provided the class work and training are carried out correctly and in due recognition of the student's temporary difficulties, all the tight areas will gradually settle when the growth spurt creases and the range of movements will return to the pre-growth spurt state. However, this does not mean that the student can just sit back waiting for everything to happen. Usually extra effort is called for in strengthening exercises for the muscle groups in the various weak areas. If this is done the student can just about keep pace with the loss of strength which would otherwise be taking place. Constant reassurance is required to emphasize to students that if they continue working both on their exercises and correctly in class, all will be satisfactory when the growth spurt ceases.

Patellar tendinitis may also be precipitated by direct blows or kneeling routines and it may then be accompanied by an infrapatellar bursitis.

Treatment starts locally with ice, if there is any swelling, together with ultrasound and interferential therapy. Muscle imbalance must be corrected by a suitable exercise programme. This programme usually has to be extended to strengthen any other weak muscle groups which may have been responsible for the onset or potentiation of the patellar tendinitis.

Osgood–Schlatter's disease

Associated with relative quadriceps weakness and also with lateral/medial imbalance of the quadriceps is Osgood–Schlatter's disease (apophysitis of the tibial tubercle). This is common in children who are keen on any form of sport. The weakness and the imbalance in the quadriceps will result in a jerking pull at the insertion of the patellar tendon into the tibial tubercle. If sufficiently painful, there should be a rest from the activity coupled with an exercise programme to strengthen the thigh muscles, quadriceps, adductors, hamstrings and the gluteals. Technical correction is necessary if there are swayback knees as lack of control there will aggravate the situation.

If the child works through the pain the tibial tubercle can undergo a bony enlargement. Girls are upset at the appearance of the enlargement and in both sexes the bony prominence can produce local pain during kneeling routines. It is therefore wise to discourage the student from working through the painful periods. Unfortunately, persistent rapid growth or recurrent growth spurts tend to make this a recurrent condition until growth has ceased and there may be times when the youngster is constantly being on and off work.

Chondromalacia patellae

As has been mentioned, this is a specific entity and not a blanket term and it is really outside the scope of this work on soft tissue injuries. However, it is certainly worth mentioning, if only to underline the importance of the correction of incorrect tracking of the patella, muscle imbalance and muscle weakness. Chondromalacia will most often arise as the sequel to long-standing and uncorrected problems which initially presented as anterior knee pain. Dancers and gymnasts are at risk because there is a very high repetition of particular types of movements. Also both activities, calling as they do for good joint mobility, attract a much higher incidence of swayback knees than is present in the general population. Swayback knees, by increasing the difficulty of thigh muscle control, will be an aggravating factor in the development of a genuine chondromalacia.

Treatment must be directed at strengthening the muscle and correcting any imbalance. It must be emphasized to patients that they must persist with the exercises and keep the muscles really strong if they are going to remain asymptomatic and slow the degenerative processes which have been started by the chondromalacia.

An arthroscopy will confirm the diagnosis. Shaving the retropatellar surface merely causes further damage to the articular cartilage and does nothing to produce a genuine cure. As mentioned earlier, a lateral release operation is contra-indicated unless there is a genuine tightness which persists after a satisfactory programme of strengthening and muscle balancing. A lateral release will aways have to be followed by a long period of further physiotherapy.

Capsular strains of the knee

These usually occur posteriorly and are caused by a forced hyperextension of the knee when the strain may also involve one or both heads of the gastrocnemius. The presence of swayback knees can be a predisoposing factor. Landing from a jump with the weight back can push the knee backwards and cause the injury. Usually these injuries are relatively minor but it is not uncommon for them to be severe enough to produce some bruising and swelling.

Treatment is with ice, ultrasound and interferential therapy. The dancer or gymnast should be off work until the condition has settled. The physiotherapy should include the full range of strenghtening exercises for all muscle groups. As with any knee injury, muscle wasting occurs extremely rapidly. If all the muscle groups controlling the knee are not fully strengthened and the correct balance between groups achieved, then the condition is likely to recur. It is highly likely that more remote muscle groups may be affected, e.g. the gluteals and the adductors. It should be remembered that the gastrocnemius comes behind the knee to take origin from the lower part of the femur and acts as a knee flexor.

Ligamentous injuries of the knee

The ligament most commonly affected is the medial ligament of the knee. As in injuries to other ligaments, these can range from sprains, which are fairly common, to complete tears, which are uncommon. The injury is caused by landing badly from a jump. The degree of force involved will determine the severity of the injury.

Damage to a cruciate ligament, although also coming about from a faulty landing, commonly involves some direct violence and collision with another person or a stage prop.

Lateral ligament injuries are uncommon and usually only occur as a result of a fall. If the rupture is complete the lateral popliteal nerve may also be stretched during the varus strain on the knee and the damage in the nerve is likely to be permanent.

Unless the injury to one of the ligaments is obviously minor an urgent orthopaedic opinion should be sought as a complete tear will require early surgery. The results of late repairs are not particularly satisfactory. Accurate diagnosis is much easier soon after the injury has taken place and before the knee has become swollen and tense. Examination under general anaesthesia, possibily with an arthroscopy, may well be necessary in order to establish an accurate diagnosis. Rehabilitation after repair of a torn ligament is a lengthy process and it will probably be some 4–6 months before the performer can return. In the case of severe cruciate ligament damage the patient may not be able to return to performance.

In sprains the length of time the dancer or gymnast will be off work will depend upon the severity of the sprain. Locally ice, ultrasound and interferential therapy are useful. An exercise programme plays a particularly important part in rehabilitation. The vastus medialis and the adductors tend to be neglected and need special attention; also, unfortunately, the hamstrings are often neglected in knee conditions of all types. Further from the knee, work will also be required with faradic footbaths and intrinsic muscle exercises to strengthen the feet. Attention must be paid to the correct line of weight-bearing. A particular effort should be made to prevent any tendency the dancer has to overturn the feet as overturning always puts an excessive strain on the medial side of the knee joint. As in all situations where rehabilitation tends to be prolonged, great benefit will be obtained from devising a general exercise programme in order to keep all muscle groups strong, not only in the lower limbs but also in the trunk and shoulder girdle.

Medial meniscus injuries

Classically a tear occurs during rotation on a partly flexed knee. This may happen as an acute incident. When working in the turned-out position, particularly if the feet are overturned in relation to the hip, a tear may occur gradually, possibly ending with an acute episode. However, long-standing but lesser symptoms of pain over the medial aspect of the knee, possibly with clicking or a tendency to give way, might lead to an arthroscopy and this can show the presence of a tear even in the absence of any history of an acute episode. Weakness of the adductors makes a tear more likely because the turnout of the hip cannot be controlled properly and the knee will tend to fall inside the line of the foot, giving an appearance of overturning at the foot.

Treatment should start in a conservative fashion unless severe symptoms are occurring, such as locking or marked giving way. The treatment regime will involve correction of the various possible causes together with strengthening exercises, particularly for the adductors and the vastus medialis. If the symptoms are severe, or if they do not subside rapidly with a conservative programme, an arthroscopy is indicated in order to establish a diagnosis and if necessary remove the torn portion of mensicus. Postoperatively the programme of exercises and technical correction will be continued. The exercise programme must encompass all relevant muscle groups. Not infrequently exercises appear to be confined to the quadriceps only but it is always essential to give exercises for the adductors, hamstrings and gluteals. Frequently trunk and foot exercises are also required, as weakness and lack of control in any of these areas may have been a precipitating factor in the original injury.

Lateral meniscus injuries

Tears in the lateral meniscus are most commonly of a chronic type due to repeated minor trauma. They tend to be brought about by a failure to hold the turnout out equally so that on the side which becomes damaged the weight is back and the foot is rolled. The dancer tends to stand with the knees not quite fully extended. Neither the hamstrings nor the quadriceps pull up properly. Due to the passive rotation of the tibia there is a tightening of the soft tissues posteriolaterally and as a result the lateral meniscus becomes chronically compressed and tends to develop a tear of a degenerative nature.

Investigation and treatment are similar to that which was described for the medial meniscus. In the rehabilitation period the technical faults are somewhat different and they need careful assessment and corrections.

Disruption of the extensor mechanism to the knee

This injury can be a rupture of the quadriceps or the patellar tendon or a fracture of the patella. The mechanism is similar in each and is brought about by an explosive contraction of the quadriceps. The patellar fracture is transverse because the patella is snapped back against the femur and breaks and then the two fragments are pulled apart. Normally the injury will occur in someone who is out of training, although occasionally it can be a result of a faulty jump or a technical mishap. Like Achilles tendon ruptures, it may well occur in a teacher who suddenly decides to demonstrate a complex jump.

These are very serious injuries and if they are even suspected, immediate referral for an orthopaedic opinion is necessary. When examined immediately after the injury the gap is easily palpable. However, after a short period the extreme swelling and tension will make a gap difficult to feel. When examined shortly after the accident the patient is unable to carry out a straight leg raise. In most other intra-articular conditions, immediately after the injury the patient is usually able to lift the leg up straight because inhibition of the quadriceps muscle will not by then have occurred. The inhibition will occur some hours later.

A tendon rupture or a patellar fracture requires immediate surgical repair. A delayed repair will almost certainly end a gymnastic or dancing career.

Rehabilitation is lengthy because wasting will become considerable during a period spent in a cast. As always though, even from the beginning, an exercise programme can be devised to keep the rest of the body as strong as possible. Isometric exercises for the affected leg can be used while the cast is on. When it has been removed an intensive exercise programme will be started in order to strengthen the muscle and mobilize the knee. Early bivalving of the plaster for exercises only and then reapplication for the rest of the day will speed recovery.

Technical faults do not in general play any part in the causation of these injuries but care must be taken that faults in technique do not develop when the patient is gradually returning to class work.

Groin strains

The commonest site of a groin strain is the origin of the rectus femoris and of the sartorius, although it is not particularly important to decide which particular muscle is affected.

Groin strains are generally brought about by faulty technique. There may or may not be associated muscle weakness. Occasionally a strain is produced by a sudden overstretching, as when doing the splits. In the main a groin strain is brought about by a failure of the muscles to stabilize the pelvis on the supporting leg, weak adductors and hamstrings are the main cause. The inadequacy of the adductors on the supporting side inhibits those on the working side and this leads to an overuse and strain of the muscles in the groin because the instability results in a tension around the working hip. It is important that the side opposite to that which has been injured is carefully assessed for areas of muscle weakness and imbalance. If the weight is back, particularly on one side with some pelvic rotation, there will be an increased incidence of groin strains. In addition to finding relative weakness within muscle groups in relation from one to another, tightness of the adductors or hamstrings must also be eliminated as a cause and be corrected, as must also any tightness of the tensor fasciae latae. As a result of the lack of stabilization of the pelvis, lumbar spine injuries often occur at the same time as groin injuries.

Commonly, only a limited amount of local treatment is required and this is best in the form of ultrasound and interferential therapy. The exercise programme and technical correction which must be carried on at the same time is the most important part of the rehabilitation. In most instances the symptoms will settle within a week or two but the exercise and technical correction programme will have to continue for very much longer if the injury is not to become recurrent.

Muscle strains

As in other sports, muscle strains and tears usually occur as a result of an uncoordinated muscle contraction associated with failure to warm up properly or by a sudden overstretching. Adductor, hamstring and calf strains and tears are particularly common in dancers and gymnasts. The adductors can be torn by sudden overstretching if the splits are forced. Hamstring injuries often occur during stretching when the dancer is cold or dancing with the weight back and the dancer sitting in the supporting hip when the working leg is being lifted, as in a *grand battement*. With the dancer sitting in the hip and with the weight back the muscle groups around the hip are not working properly and the upper part of the hamstring is then vulnerable to injury. Persistent overturning will lead to weakness of the lateral hamstrings which can then be damaged if subjected to a sudden stretch.

In both hamstring and adductor strains the injury may be at the musculoskeletal attachment and sometimes a piece of bone is avulsed, together with part of the muscle attachment. This can easily be demonstrated on X-ray. In this instance, if stretching is carried out too early, bone cells will be further shed into the haematoma, encouraging the development of myositis ossificans.

Treatment locally will be by ice and rest.

Strengthening exercises should be commenced after the first 2 or 3 days. These may need to be assisted active exercises at first so that further damage is not caused. As in all muscle tears the aim is to obtain healing with the minimum of scar tissue, hence the gradual start to the exercise programme. Once the strengthening programme is underway and there has been restoration of full muscle tone and there is less risk of retearing, the muscle stretching should be gently commenced. Stretching must be at the end of each treatment session when the blood supply is at its maximum. The stretch must be slow and each stretch should last for a minimum of 20 seconds. The stretching programme will have to continue for many months as scar tissue will tend to contract until it is completely mature. It may take 6 or 12 months for the scar tissue finally to mature and settle. The stretching, which must never be violent or forcible, should continue for at least this length of time. Chronic tightening and contracture are almost untreatable and should never have been allowed to occur. In the hamstrings the rehabilitation must also ensure that the strength between the medial and lateral hamstrings is correctly balanced out.

Back injuries

Muscle strains are fairly common and they do not present any particular diagnostic problems. Treatment is as for any other muscle strains. There must be an assessment as to whether there is any trunk muscle weakness and whether there is any imbalance between one side of the trunk and the other. Technical faults may also be present and these must be corrected. Interspinous ligament damage is fairly common. It can be caused by hyperflexion, which causes the ligament to be sprained.

Treatment is with local ultrasound and interferential therapy. If the spine is slightly flexed so as to open up the interspinous area, the treatment can be more effective. In general a great deal of exercise must take place in order to strengthen the trunk muscles.

Of greater interest in the gymnast particularly, but also the dancer, is the hyperextension injury. This can produce an impingment syndrome between adjacent spinous processes when the interspinous ligament becomes squeezed between them. A dancer is taught to 'pull up' with the legs and trunk before starting a backbend and, in doing this, the curve of extension is spread throughout the lumbar spine. Trunk muscle weakness as well as a failure to pull up can cause the hyperextension to take place at one level. From the side this is seen as a sharp kink in the back during the backbend instead of a gentle curve (Fig. 23.2). With most of the hyperextension occurring at one level there is frequently an impingement. Extreme flexibility is required in gymnastics and many gymnasts spend most of their life with a lordotic posture. Any additional hyperextension will then be very liable to produce kinking.

Treatment, as in a hyperflexion sprain, consists of local treatment accompanied by strengthening exercises for the trunk. In the presence of an almost constant lordosis all the trunk muscles, particularly the abdominals, will be extremely weak and rehabilitation, because of the amount of muscle build-up that is required, can be somewhat prolonged. In addition technical help is required to prevent the kinking and hyperextension. The dancer has to learn to get this feeling of pulling up out of the legs and pelvis before going back. Incidentally, although these terms may sound somewhat strange they do portray fairly accurately what the dancer or gymnast feels is happening within the body, although anatomically the expression may sound somewhat nonsensical.

Facet joint strains are not uncommon as the site of injuries in both gymnasts and dancers. These are small synovial joints which are part of the posterior bony arch of adjacent vertebrae. They tend to become injured in sudden uncontrolled movements, particularly when they are carried out in an asymmetrical fashion. This happens most often when jumping. The pain is accompanied by muscle spasm and there is deep tenderness on palpation over the facet joint. The pain is exacerbated on extension, particularly when extension is accompanied by a tilt to one side. Pain can also be produced on flexion and lateral flexion.

Usually some rest from activities is required for at least a few days, together with local treatment in

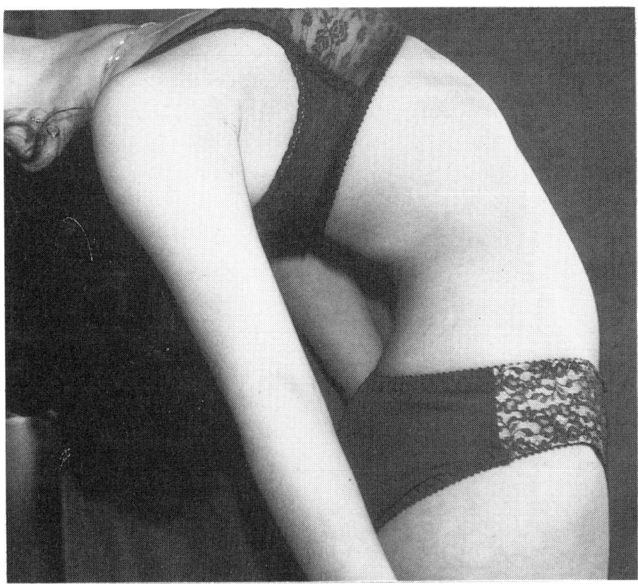

Fig. 23.2 Hyperextension with kinking at one level. In this case there is also a stiff lower lumbar segment which aggravates the situation. From Howe and Hancock (1988), with permission.

the form of ultrasound or interferential therapy to relieve the pain and muscle spasm. An exercise programme will be required as the condition oftens happens in the presence of trunk muscle weakness, particularly if this weakness is asymmetrical. Technical correction is also required if the person has been working in an asymmetrical fashion. Poor control of the turnout can be a factor in precipitation of these injuries and this needs to be investigated. Exercises are required to strengthen the adductors which are the major group controlling the turnout of the hips.

If the condition is resistant, very occasionally an injection of the facet joint with hydrocortisone acetate is helpful. Ideally this should be carried out using an X-ray image intensifier to make certain that the hydrocortisone is injected into the correct place.

A facet joint problem can produce some referred pain because of irritation of the nerve root and may, from the pain distribution, mimic a lumbar disc lesion.

Lumbar disc prolapses are becoming rather more common in dancers, probably as a result of the somewhat bizarre choreography which is sometimes being introduced and also because most dancers have a heavier work load, not only when they are on the stage professionally but also during training. A dancer or gymnast with sciatic pain should be referred for an orthopaedic opinion, particularly if there are any neurological symptoms such as numbness or paraesthesiae. They will have to be off performing until the condition has settled.

Treatment is a routine orthopaedic matter and outside the scope of this chapter. Once the dancer has recovered and has returned for rehabilitation considerable work has to be done in strengthening the trunk, gluteal and lower limb muscles and technical correction of any underlying faults will have to take place.

A gymnast or dancer with persistent well-localized lower lumbar pain which has not responded to adequate physiotherapy or rest should be suspected of having a stress fracture. These are particularly common in cases where there is a lordotic posture. An X-ray may not show the presence of the stress fracture through the pars interarticularis until some 4–8 weeks from the onset of the symptoms and sometimes even longer. If the condition is suspected and X-rays are normal then an isotope bone scan should be carried out.

Early treatment is essential if union of the stress fracture is to take place, allowing the gymnast or dancer to return eventually to full performance.

A lumbar lordosis, although not an injury, is a potent cause of injury in both gymnasts and dancers. It is frequently associated with overturning of the feet either because of limited turnout or because of a failure to hold the available turnout.

Neck injuries

Neck injuries may come about by excessive repetitions of rapid neck movements as in pirouettes or occasionally by direct force. The injuries are all ligamentous. Treatment is by rest if the pain and muscle spasm are marked, possibly using a soft collar, and then by ultrasound, interferential therapy, mobilization and exercises.

An acute torticollis (wry neck) occurs not infrequently in adolescent students. The student will wake with an acute stiff neck, often tilted slightly to one side. This condition is probably identical to that which so frequently happens in any adolescent and is probably unrelated to dance or gymnastics.

Upper limb injuries

In dancers these are not very common. Boys when lifting can sustain muscle and ligament strains but these are usually mild. Treatment is as for similar injuries as described in the lower limb. These injuries may occur either because the girl is inexperienced and fails to hold herself firmly or because the boy does not carry out the lift correctly. In the former case it is much more difficult to lift a floppy ragdoll-type girl than one with strong muscles who can help to support herself. Both the girl and the boy have a very active part to play in a lift.

Of interest in dancers (usually male and therefore probably associated with lifting) as well as in gymnast is a transient nerve palsy affecting the nerve to serratus anterior. It produces the typical winging of the scapula on the affected side. The condition always resolves, usually over a few weeks but sometimes it takes several months. During that time treatment is directed at exercises to strengthen other muscle groups whose weakness may have contributed to the injury and then exercises for the affected serratus anterior as it recovers. There is no treatment which will speed recovery of the nerve palsy itself. The technique must be carefully checked.

Gymnasts have very mobile upper limb joints and it must be remembered that much of their time they are weight-bearing through the upper limbs. They are therefore much more prone to sprains and tears of ligaments and muscles than dancers as a result of this combination of weight-bearing and great flexibility.

In general, treatment is as for other sprains and tears. If there is any doubt at all about joint stability or other serious ligament damage then an urgent orthopaedic referral should be made.

Major tendon rupture may also occur and this requires urgent orthopaedic assessment and possibily repair. Surgery, if indicated, is most effective if carried out very soon after injury rather than as a delayed procedure.

Shoulder injuries in dancers usually affect the boys only and may be associated either with faulty lifting or by injudicious weight-training, especially when using excessively heavy weights. In gymnasts both sexes can be affected. The injury is usually a strain which can produce a capsulitis. This will cause pain around the shoulder with some radiation down the upper arm in the deltoid region. The pain may limit movement and there may also be a painful arc. Treatment is rest together with interferential therapy, pulsed microwave and ultrasound. As the pain settles a well-structured exercise programme should be instituted to replace any unsupervised weight-lifting programme the dancer may have been using. If the condition is not settling over 2–3 weeks and a tear of the rotator cuff can definitely be excluded, then a steroid injection might be considered.

Tears of the rotator cuff at the shoulder should be suspected in any gymnast who cannot fully elevate the arm or when actively lowering a passively elevated arm suddenly cannot sustain the movement and drops the arm. Magnetic resonance imaging or arthrography will be required to confirm the diagnosis and the extent of the injury. Surgical repair is usually indicated. Following the period of postoperative immobilization in abduction rehabilitation will consist of strengthening exercises to all groups and mobilization of the shoulder.

Acromioclavicular joint strain may occur in both gymnasts and dancers. Rest from lifts or weight-bearing on the arms together with local physiotherapy treatments usualy allows resolution but a steroid injection may be required.

In acromioclavicular joint dislocations immediate referral to an orthopaedic surgeon is indicated. Early reduction and fixation in the reduced position using a screw between the acromion and the coracoid is indicated in order to obtain the best possible result. In dancers this is indicated for the cosmetic appearance and in gymnasts to try to obtain the best possible function. Unfortunately when the screw is removed, as has to take place in order to allow movement to take place between the coracoid and the clavicle, some degree of deformity will recur. The injury may prevent a satisfactory return to gymnastics.

General strains around the elbow are common in gymnasts. More specifically they may develop a lateral or medial epicondylitis (tennis or golfer's elbow). These each represent a more acute type of injury than that which is generally seen in other members of the population. Treatment with interferential therapy and ultrasound and an exercise programme to strengthen the extensor/flexor muscle group gently and progressively should be instituted. As damage to the musculotendinous insertion of the bone has taken place the aim is to obtain healing with the minimum of scar tissue and then a gradual build-up of strength to try to avoid re-injury in the future. Steroid injections should be avoided if possible as they will interfere with satisfactory healing. However if the condition has become chronic then a steroid injection may be indicated.

At the wrist in gymnasts there may be various overuse injuries affecting the ligaments and the tendons. In order to weight-bear satisfactorily on the hands the gymnast requires a full 90° of dorsiflexion at the wrist so that the weight-bearing forces can be transmitted through the heel of the hands. If 90° of dorsiflexion is not present then there is a far greater degree of strain transmitted through the tendons and muscles controlling the wrist and hand. Treatment for the tendon and ligamentous injuries is by rest and local ultrasound and interferential therapy. Technical problems should be investigated.

In gymnasts at the ulnar side of the wrist an impingement can occur between the ulnar styloid and the carpus. This is accompanied by local swelling and thickening of the soft tissues that have been crushed between the impinging bones. Treatment is by rest, ice, ultrasound and interferential therapy. This is followed by strengthening exercises to try to make the support around the wrist strong enough to prevent impingement taking place.

Finally, a cautionary word about bone injuries in the upper limbs is necessary. Gymnasts may sustain stress fractures in the upper as well as the lower limbs. The radius is the commonest site (though not nearly as frequent as tibial stress fractures). Always consider a stress fracture when an apparent soft tissue injury is not settling with appropriate treatment and rest. Remember also that a stress fracture may not show up on an X-ray for some weeks after the onset of symptoms. As with stress fractures elsewhere, an isotope bone scan may help with diagnosis. Two other joint conditions which must be considered are an osteochondritis dissecans and an osteochondral fracture. These are not uncommon in the elbow, either in the radial head, which is more common, or in the articular surface of the lower humerus, which is less common.

There are, of course, many technical faults which produce particular types of injuries. Anyone wishing to look after dancers or gymnasts would be well-advised to study technical faults and their consequences.

Acknowledgement

Based on material in *Dance Technique and Injury Prevention* by Justin Howse and Shirley Hancock. Published by A&C Black, London, 1988 and Theatre Arts Books/Routledge, New York, 1988.

24

Risks and injuries in combat sports

G. R. McLatchie

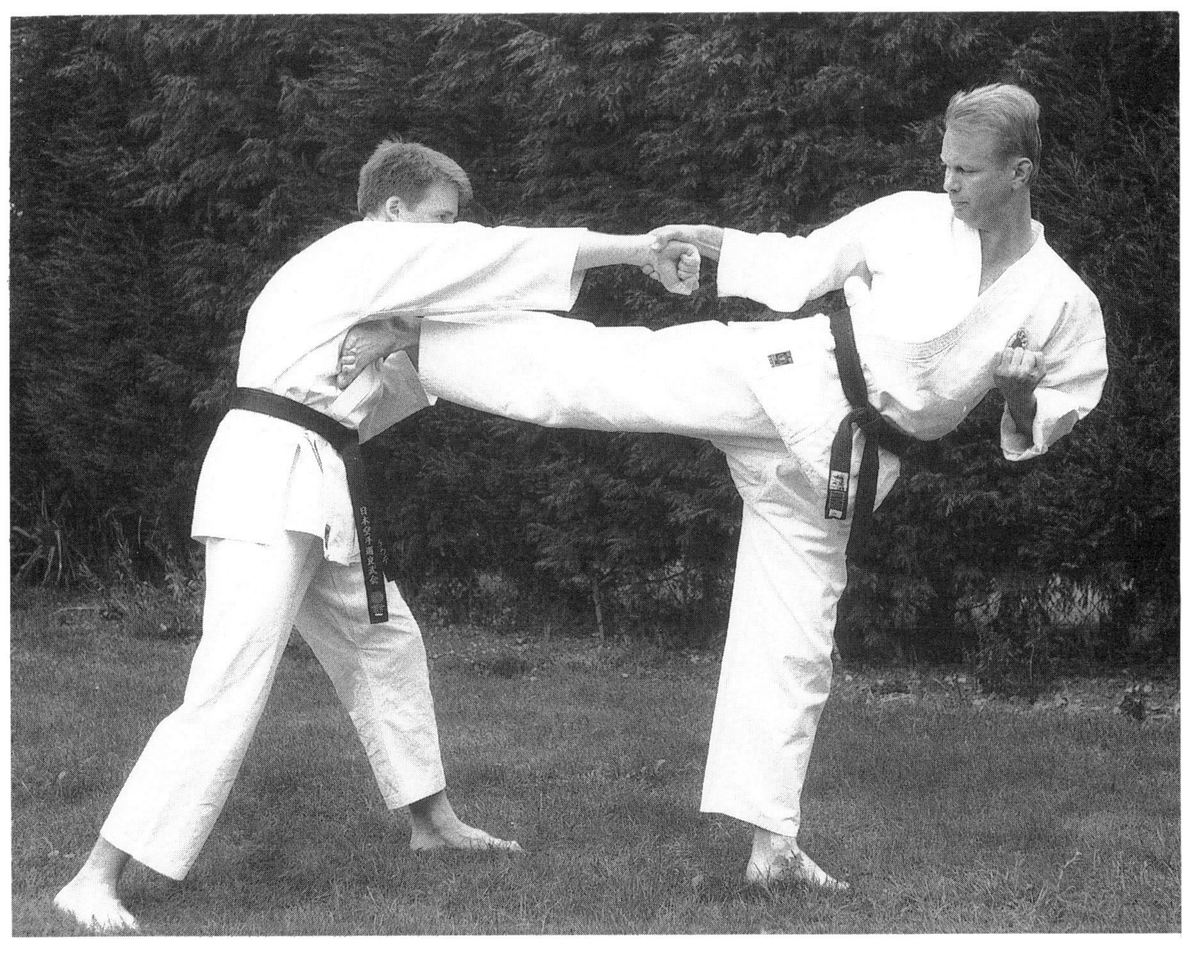

Introduction

Those sports which derived from original combat are three types:

1. Predominantly punching, e.g. boxing, karate.
2. Predominantly grappling and throwing, e.g. aikido, judo, ju-jitsu and wrestling.
3. Weaponry, e.g. kendo, fencing, use of weapons in karate.

The reason for this division is that the injury situations which arise are similar in each group. Sites of injury also tend to conform to each group, although it should be appreciated that an injury can occur to any part of the body from any of the sports.

Punching arts

Boxing

The origins of boxing are ancient with reports as far back as 1100 BC and the fight between Epeus and Euryalus. The purse was a mule and the fighters attacked each other with their fists enclosed in caesti-leather gloves impregnated with metal studs. They had head protection in the form of helmets made of leather but the only rule of note was that the victor should not kill his opponent. Epeus won by a knockout.

Boxing continued to develop through the Roman circuses but after the fall of the Roman empire references to the sport are scant. The first recorded British champion was in the late 17th century when eye-gouging was still legitimate. These contests subsequently gave way to bare-fist fights with rules and then to the modern sport. The first rules of boxing were drawn up in 1743 and lasted until 1838. After several revisions they were superseded by the Queensberry rules in 1866. Further revisions continued until the British Boxing Board of Control produced the current rules.

Boxing has always been a target for criticism by both the lay public and in particular by the medical profession because of the injuries which can occur in the course of a bout or as a result of continued participation in the sport. The very nature of boxing in which two contestants confront each other and attempt to land blows on a particular target must of necessity cause injury. This is compounded by the sport being dominated by the 'no pain – no gain' philosophy, based on the principle that it is impossible to improve unless extreme physical commitment is involved and that injuries can be ignored. While the former is probably true, the latter is certainly false and it is fair to say that this attitude has been eroded in recent years. There is now evidence that injuries can be reduced to a minimum by improvement in equipment and technique. However there will always remain a number of injuries which will require prompt and adequate medical attention by the ring-side doctor whose primary duty is to preserve the health and well-being of his or her patients (the boxers). In philosophical terms, this would mean that a fight should be stopped as soon as a fighter has a bleeding nose or a facial laceration. In practice however only specific injuries will lead to the fight being stopped.

Specific injuries

The main target of attack (the head) and the instrument of attack (the hand) are the commonest sites of injury. Indeed injuries to other parts of the body are rare.

Head injuries

Head injuries are the commonest cause of death and serious disability. For this reason amateur boxing is usually restricted to three rounds as compared to the professional sport where fights last 10–15 rounds because of public demand.

Rules governing a knockout

After a boxer has been knocked out he is not permitted to fight for a 4-week period. Both amateur and professional boxers need to be medically examined before re-entering the ring and in the case of the professional boxer an electro-encephalogram (EEG) is also required. An amateur boxer who sustains more than three knock-outs in a year is suspended indefinitely pending further medical examinations. The professional boxer who has had three knockouts in a year is suspended for at least 3 months and must be certified medically fit before returning to the ring.

Death in the ring

When death occurs from an acute head injury it is nearly always due to intracranial bleeding: sub-dural haemorrhage into one of the middle cranial fossae is the most common post-mortem finding. These haemorrhages are thought to be due to prolonged battering resulting in bleeding from the dural emissary veins (Green, 1978). Traumatic encephalopathy or 'punch drunkenness' was first described in 1928 by Martland. It was commonly seen in the slugging boxer or his sparring partners and has an insidious onset. Clinical signs may be difficult to detect but the deterioration of the boxer can best be observed in the ring. His movements become slowed, he stands on a broad base with impaired reflexes and is less able to avoid punches. At a later stage he appears to be drunk and becomes fatuous, emotionally labile and with slurred speech. The memory and intellect also become impaired and eventually even moral sense is lost. Pathologically there is progressive ventricular dilatation with diffuse cerebellar and cerebral neuronal degeneration. These neuro-logical features have been ascribed to petechial haemorrhages in or near the brainstem and to diffuse cerebral changes particularly affecting the temporal lobes. Recurrent minor head injuries are thought to be the cause (Roberts, 1928).

Almost every year there are reports of fighters either dying in the ring or being left severely disabled. This will continue to happen unless the philosophy of the sport is changed. The stimulus for this will probably come from the public itself, with the regulatory bodies of boxing effecting the change because of public demand. A recent report (Fisher 1991) suggests that the British Medical Association is to step up its campaign against boxing by re-opening its investigation into the medical effects of the sport. This follows the collapse of the boxer Michael Watson in 1991 after a world title fight against Chris Eubank in London. The return of Frank Bruno to the ring following a series of eye operations also adds to the controversy. The British Medical Association has called for boxing to be banned since 1984 and is working with medical organizations in common-wealth countries to get boxing banned from the 1994 Commonweath Games in Canada because 'recent tragedies have made this an area of great public concern' (Fisher, 1991).

In support of boxing there is an argument put forward by coaches and trainers that boxing engenders discipline and well being in working-class boys and this should be examined with respect to assessing risk. There is, for instance, evidence that participating boxers have a very low incidence of cigarette smoking as compared to their peer groups (McLatchie, 1986a). The serious risks attendant upon this habit must be evaluated against the risks of death or injury in the ring.

Injuries to the eye and orbit

Serious eye injuries are rare but cases of retinal detachment, paralytic diplopia and optic atrophy have all been reported (Doggart and Rugg-Gunn, 1965). Following such injuries retirement is mandatory. The commonest injuries, however, are periorbital lacerations and abrasions from punches or head-butting. The gloves themselves can cause abrasions or lacerations of the cornea. The diagnosis of corneal abrasion can be made by instilling a drop of fluorescein into the eye. This stains the lesion and most small abrasions heal in 2 or 3 days; a pad is worn for that period. Periorbital cuts may require suture, thus forcing withdrawal from the bout. Accurate approximation of the skin edges is required to prevent a broad scar and this may best be achieved by a layered closure, other-wise the healed wound is liable to break down again if further traumatized. It is well-known that many boxers have a 'cut problem' – some have even had to undergo specialized surgical techniques to obtain a good repair.

Although serious eye injury is rare, whenever it is suspected or there is visual impairment the patient should be referred promptly to an opthalmic surgeon.

Other injuries

Nose bleeds and nasal fracture with dislocation of the nasal septum are all fairly common and can lead to the typical boxer's nose (Fig. 24.1) with considerable cosmetic deformity. Surprisingly, fractures of the mandible and facial bones are unusual but do occur. Cauliflower ear is a complication of haematoma of the pinna but can be prevented from forming by early aspiration of the haematoma and injection of proteolytic enzymes such as hyaluronidase to allow resolution.

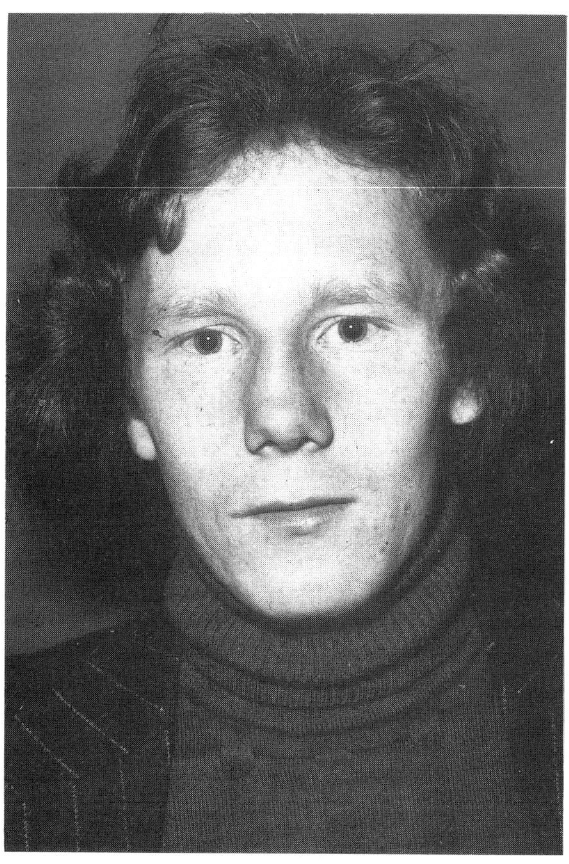

Fig. 24.1 Boxer's nose.

Hand injuries

These are extremely common. More than half of all boxing injuries will occur to the hand. It is obviously important to do all that is possible to avoid injury for a hand injury can keep a fighter out of the ring for months. The most frequent serious injury is fracture or fracture dislocation of the base of the first metacarpal (Montanaro and Francone, 1966). These injuries require manipulative reduction and occasionally surgical fixation because of their instability. The necks of the second and fifth metacarpal bones are also commonly fractured. They should be treated by reduction and immobilization for 3–4 weeks in a dorsal slab.

Changing the glove design would probably make injury to this digit less likely. The most recent designs of gloves have incorporated a flange so that a blow to the thumb will be deflected. However, it is important that the boxer still practises striking correctly. The striking surface of the fist should include the index and middle finger knuckles because they are immobile and the force of any blow passes directly to the radius. Boxers should also try to keep the thumb firmly applied to the rest of the glove when punching.

Gloves

The first gloves were introduced by Broughton in England in the mid 18th century. Their purpose was to protect the face and hands in training. Later gloves were used in championship fights but until the early 1900s they were skin-tight.

Today 6 oz (170 g) gloves are used in fights up to and including welterweight and 8 oz (225 g) gloves from middle-weight onwards and in all amateur contests

Further developments in the form of pneumatic gloves are currently under examination but for light sparring 10 oz (280 g) and 12 oz (335 g) gloves are recommended.

Tapes

Bandages or tapes are permitted for protection of the hands. They must not exceed 9 foot (2.7 m) of 1-inch (2.5 cm) zinc oxide plaster tape or 18 foot (5.4 m) of 2-inch (5 cm) soft bandage for weights up to and including middle-weights. Light heavy and heavy-weights are allowed 11 foot of (3.3 m) of zinc oxide plaster tape. If a fighter uses more than these lengths or applies tape over his knuckles he could seriously injure his opponent. It is important that the referee and/or doctor checks the taping and that an official witnesses its application.

The long-term effects of severe brain damage, both physical and psychological, are now well-recognized but it is not often appreciated that even minor head injuries with brief periods of post-traumatic amnesia or unconsciousness can also be associated with impairment of psychological function. The processing and recall of information are especially impaired (Figs 24.2 and 24.3). The defect can persist for up to 1 month and although in many people no direct symptoms can be attributed to it, in others a post-traumatic syndrome of headaches, irritability and difficulties with concentration and sleeping develops. Such symptoms may take months to resolve.

In any sport where there is the risk of recurrent head injury there is a risk of comulative damage (Fig. 24.3) and further trauma will produce greater psychological impairment (Gronwall and Wrightson 1974, 1975). To date, two sports, boxing and steeple chasing, have been implicated in cases of cumulative brain damage but there have been anecdotal reports of cerebral damage in many other sports in men and women (Corsellis, 1974; Table 24.1). Certainly the incidence of cumulative brain damage in sports such as rugby and American football may be worthy of systematic investigation. Quite recently a high incidence of EEG disturbances, most probably due to neuronal damage as a result of repeated trauma, has been reported in active Norwegian football

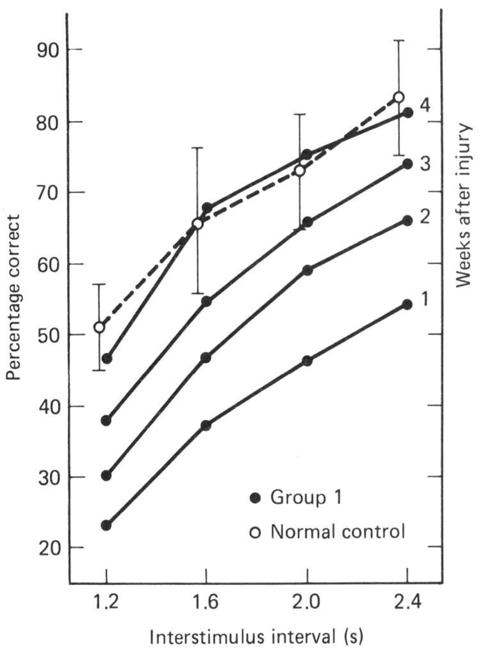

Fig. 24.2 Psychological and intellectual disruption after head injury. Group 1 = Head-injured patients. From Gronwall and Wrightson (1974), with permission.

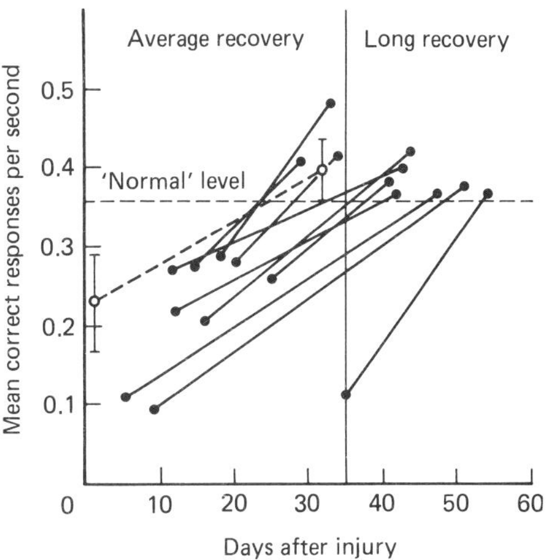

Fig. 24.3 The cumulative effect of concussion. From Gronwall and Wrightson (1975), with permission.

Table 24.1 Head injury in sport causing lasting brain damage: answers to a questionnaire sent to 165 British neurologists: 'Have you ever seen a condition resembling the punch-drunk state in any sportsmen?'

Sport	Number
Professional soccer	5 cases
Rugby football	2 cases
Professional wrestling	2 cases
Parachute jumping	1 case
Steeplechase jockeys	12 cases
Boxing	290 cases

From Corsellis (1974).

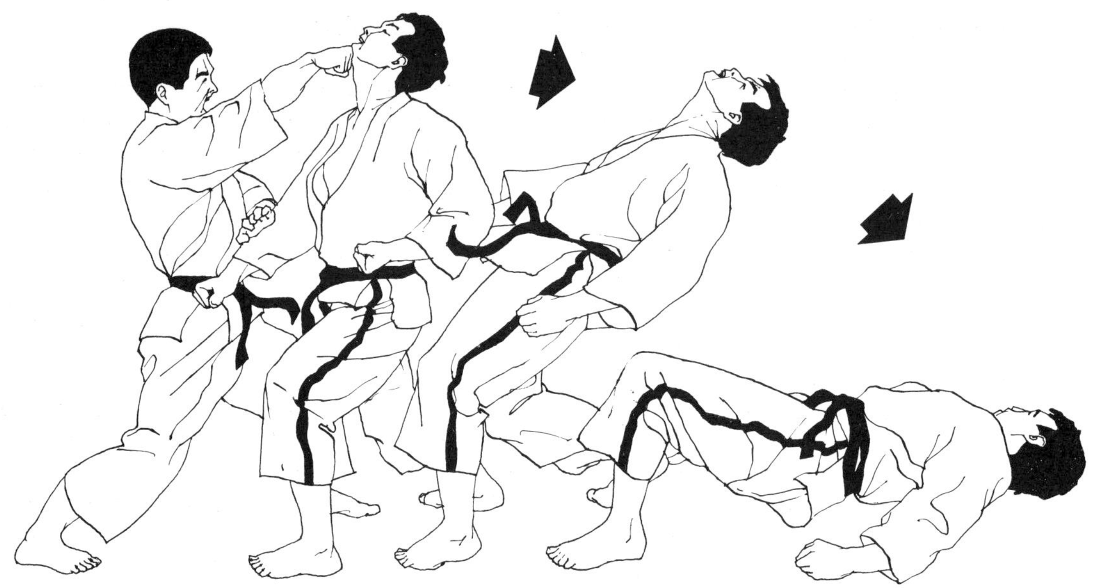

Fig. 24.4 Padded or sprung flooring may reduce the risk of second head injuries after falls.

players and increased EEG abnormalities have also been noted in former football players (Tysvaer and Storli, unpublished observations; Sortland *et al.*, 1989). Although both boxers and steeple-chase jockeys suffer obvious recurrent minor head injuries in their sport it is possible that a centre-half in football, for instance, who may head the ball up to 500 times in each year, or a rugby prop forward sustains similar injuries.

Cumulative damage may be prevented by increasing the awareness of sports officials and participants in sport of the risks of continuing active participation following head injury. In the combat sports such as boxing and karate sprung or padded flooring can reduce the incidence of second head injuries which can occur when a fighter falls to the floor as a result of a blow and then strikes his or her head on the canvas (Fig. 24.4). The use of head gear in boxing has reduced the number of knockouts when studied in Czechoslovakia but paradoxically, whereas a knockout will stop the fight and three knockouts will prevent the boxer fighting for the rest of that year, protective head-gear may simply allow a partically incapacitated fighter to continue the bout sustaining multiple minor traumatic cerebral injuries which can lead to cumulative brain damage.

The evidence for brain damage in professional boxers is conclusive but now there is a strong suggestion that brain damage may also occur in active amateur boxers.

In the search for the most senstive method of detecting abnormal cerebral function and established brain damage, one Finnish study included neuropsychomotry, clinical examinination and EEG and found them all to be equally sensitive (Kaste *et al.*, 1982). The computed tomography (CT) scan was rarely abnormal, but this is not surprising as CT scanning may only detect severe degrees of brain damage. A normal brain scan therefore does not exclude significant brain damage and should not be used as the sole method of detection. Magnetic resonance imaging (MRI) has still to be evaluated in the detection of early cerebral damage in boxers but it may well be of value. Currently the best method of detecting neurological abnormalities and possible brain damage is neuropsychometry. In one study (McLatchie *et al.*, 1987) boxers' neuropsychological performances were compared with a control group and it was noted that in some tests the boxers fared significantly worse than their controls. EEG abnormalities were also twice those of the normal population. Although a single EEG is not the ideal method of diagnosing damage, an abnormal series of EEGs in combination with neuropsychometry and clinical examination carried out by a neurologist is a satisfactory method of detecting early cerebral damage in boxers. In this study, brain damage correlated well with the number of fights. Those boxers who had had more than 40 fights showed a greater incidence of abnormalities than those with less than this number. There is scope here for a change in philosophy in boxing in that fighters who show early changes should be advised either to reduce the number of fights or stop boxing altogether. It may also be possible to plan a boxer's career with, say, a maximum of 40–50 fights in his boxing lifetime to reduce the risk of cumulative damage.

Karate

Historical background

Karate in Japanese means 'empty hand' and in its simplest sense this implies empty-handed combat without the assistance of weapons. In its deepest sense, however, it implies infinity of knowledge, self-discipline and conviction, particularly linked to the Zen philosophy.

Although originally developed in China, modern karate is said to owe its development to the Ryukui islanders who when conquered by the Kyushu in 1609 and subsequently banned from carrying weapons of any kind devised an empty-handed form of combat which was so effective that a trained exponent could punch through the bamboo armour of his oppressors with his hands or fists or dismount a horseman with a jumping kick. In its practice today it still has two distinct forms – one a philosophical way of life linked strongly to the Zen religion; the other a practical martial art concerned with the acquisition of spectacular physical skills and historically linked to the ideology of Bushido (the way of the warrior – the code of conduct for the Samurai).

The concept of Bushido

Bushido was a highly specialized code of honour and conduct which the Samurai warriors of feudal Japan were required and instructed to observe. It loosely related to chivalry and dictated how the fighting nobles should behave in battle and in their daily life. The code was unwritten and had grown out of centuries of military life. For those who diligently adhered to its concept it meant absolute loyalty to one's immediate superior and unquestioning obedience. The Samurai had to be prepared to fight or die without any questions and to be unafraid of pain or death. Obviously such men were daunting adversaries.

The concept of bushido pervaded Japanese thinking and applied to all aspects of life. It was particularly evident during the Second World War. It also applied of course to the teaching and learning of martial arts.

The acceptance of pain as a necessary part of advancement in Japanese karate is one reason why the incidence of injuries was so high in the sport when it originally came to this country. This principle has now gradually been eroded on common-sense grounds, for most people who practise karate in the west are not monks but work for a living. Injuries cause valuable loss of time from work and sometimes, more importantly, sport.

The physics of karate

The most extraordinary feats in karate such as breaking wood or smashing concrete blocks are explicable scientifically. The energy of a karate blow is concentrated in a small area on the target. By taking strobe pictures of punches and kicks this can be calculated. In a straight punch, forces of 300 N/cm^2 are generated by a good standard karateka (black belt and above). More force is required to break wood than concrete because wood is more elastic and absorbs much of the energy applied to it. However, all karate exponents know that wood is easier to break than concrete. When the hand strikes the target only part of the energy is transferred to the target – the remainder is transferred to the puncher and interpreted as pain! Whilst wood absorbs most of the hand's kinetic energy, concrete refuses to absorb at least half of it. This therefore presents a psychological problem for even the most hardened punchers and exaggerates the difficulty of breaking concrete as compared to wood.

Why do the bones of the hands and feet not break in such a collision? Provided the force of collision is directed along the lines of stress in the bone no fracture will occur. This is because bone is tougher than wood or concrete by virtue of its lamellar structure but the striking hand or foot must be held in the correct posture. This aspect of technique is important in the prevention of injury in karate.

Karate competitions

Most competitions are one of three types:

1. Traditional or controlled contact.
2. Semi-contact.
3. Full contact.

Over the period 1974 to 1986 we determined that by careful interpretation of the rules and the strict application of medical recommendations injuries can be reduced in all types (McLatchie, 1986b).

Traditional karate

In this form no actual contact is made although attacks are carried out at full speed, the blows being withdrawn just before they reach the target. Obviously fine judgement is required by the attacker and a basic awareness of human anatomy would permit the easier scoring of competitions. A half-point or a full point is awarded depending on the site of the attack and the force with which it was carried out.

Semi-contact karate

In this sport some areas of the body such as the testicles and face are exempt from attack but full contact is allowed to the head with the feet and to the trunk with the hands and feet. Most injuries in competition occur to the limbs because of persistent low kicks in an attempt to kick an opponent off his or her feet (a fight can be won by a knock-down). At the end of each round a succession of boards must be broken to proceed to the next. This presents inherent dangers and has produced many unnecessary injuries causing loss of time from sport and work. We feel that the application of a points system alone and less emphasis on a knock-down in this style of karate would permit improvements in injury statistics.

Full-contact karate

In this sport blows of unmitigated force are directed against the opponent's target area – the head and trunk.

Full contact increased in popularity during the late 1970s and early 1980s but now seems to be on the decline. Fighters should be well-matched and of equivalent weight. Sparring should be conducted in protective gear and the same rules apply to fighters as to boxers

There are many inherent dangers in this sport. The addition of the feet as weapons compounds the risk of injury. Fights have been mainly well-controlled. The most significant injuries are to the head but injuries to the liver, kidneys and spleen have also occurred. Preventive measures must be directed towards stringent rules with full pre-fight medical examinations, strict refereeing by informed referees and standard recommended lay-off times after specific injuries.

Particular injuries

There are three possible sites of injury (McLatchie 1976, 1990; McLatchie *et al.*, 1980):

1. Head and neck injuries.
2. Injuries to the trunk.
3. Injuries to the limbs.

Head injuries

The potential for knockout always exists, even in non-contact karate. Skull fractures have resulted from falling backwards, striking the head on a solid floor during sweeps or after an uncontrolled punch to the face (Fig. 24.4). Full-contact karate also presents the same injury type of problem as boxing and therefore stringent medical rules regarding fitness to fight should be implemented and all fights should have a doctor in attendance.

Lacerations, abrasions, nosebleeds and black eyes are all common. They do not usually cause withdrawal from a contest unless bleeding is persistent or vision is impaired due to periorbital swelling. Minor lacerations can be treated with Steristrip or sutures; adrenaline packs can be used for serious nosebleeds and may allow the fighter to continue. Nasal fracture is a fairly common injury and karateka can often present with features of boxer's nose. Fracture of the malar bone has also been described; this is recognized by a depression on the affected side, infraorbital paraesthesia due to nerve entrapment and trismus. Fighters with this injury need to withdraw and should be transferred to hospital where after elevation of the malar bone a period of at least 6 weeks should elapse before fighting starts. Cervical injury is not common but cervical dislocation has resulted when attackers have used spinning kicks. Many karate associations have now outlawed these dangerous techniques because of their uncontrollable nature.

If padded or sprung flooring is used at all competitions, this considerably reduces the risk of serious head injury and of soft tissue abrasions and lacerations caused by falls.

Injuries to the trunk

The commonest injury is 'winding', which results from a blow or blows to the region of the solar plexus (the coeliac plexus). The injured person experiences extreme difficulty with inspiration due to transient paralysis of the diaphragm. Fortunately, in most cases the sensation passes off in 30–90 seconds.

Blows to the chest wall have resulted in pneumothorax secondary to rib fracture or rapid decompression of the chest wall caused by the blow. Those injured experience pain and dyspnoea and all have responded well to hospital transfer and chest drainage. No cases of tension pneumothorax have been seen during competition (in the author's experience).

The testes are a recognized target in all self-defence body-charts but are mostly accidentally struck in contest. A blow to the testes can be sickeningly painful and can produce vomiting and unconsciousness and even cardiac arrest, at worst. Usually, however, the pain passes off quickly and most contestants can continue to fight. After such an injury the penis and scrotum should be inspected. If there is extensive bruising the patient should then be transferred to hospital. Testicular injury can be prevented by the wearing of a groin guard and martial arts referees have now been instructed to disqualify a man who is not wearing a groin guard in a competition. This could mean that an opponent could win a fight by accidentally striking a man on the testicles and if he was not wearing a groin guard the injured man would then be disqualified – rough justice indeed!

Injuries to the limbs

As in boxing, the hands and fingers are the commonest sites of injury. Fingers can be dislocated from attempts to parry blows and toes from effectively blocking kicks. Fractures of the bones of the upper and lower limbs are also seen and should be treated as and when they present.

Some injuries are common: both 'gamekeeper's thumb' and 'karate thumb' occur, as well as Bennett's fracture dislocation. In gamekeeper's thumb the ulnar collateral ligament is avulsed from the base of the proximal phalanx with a wedge of bone. This is an unstable injury which requires surgical fixation in most cases. In karate thumb the radial collateral ligament is affected. This can usually be treated conservatively since the injury is stable. In those karate fighters who harden their fists on padded wooden boards or bags, traumatic bursitis over the heads of the second and third metacarpal bones is commonly seen (puncher's knuckle).

Compression syndromes of the leg and quadriceps haematoma are one serious group of injuries caused by low hard kicks to the shins and thighs in some styles of karate. Severe bruising of the large muscles of the thighs can be a source of chronic pain and if there is subsequent calcification with a haematoma, the formation of myositis ossificans occurs. Traumatic anterior tibial compartment syndrome or indeed any fascial compartment compression syndrome of the lower leg can present as a surgical emergency which usually requires fasciotomy. The use of ice packs with elevation and bandaging of the affected limb can considerably relieve the pain and reduce the swelling. Withdrawal from competition in such a situation is mandatory.

Injuries to the knee are fairly common. The method of performing the roundhouse kick is similar to that of kicking a football in that there is a degree of rotation on a fixed tibia which can produce tears of the menisci. Usually the fighter presents with swelling or pain in the affected knee caused by a synovial effusion developing over the first 24 hours. If the swelling develops rapidly after the injury this usually implies blood in the knee joint and more extensive damage, often involving the anterior collateral ligament. Such patients should be seen at hospital on the same day; aspiration of the blood and possible arthroscopy may be indicated. Patients with injured menisci may require subsequent meniscectomy.

Nerve injuries

The peripheral nerves most often injured are:

1. The radial nerve in the upper arm.
2. The ulnar nerve.
3. The superficial peroneal nerve.

The radial nerve in the upper arm

A kick directed to the mid-part of the upper arm can cause neuropraxia of the radial nerve. Injury may also occur following fracture of the humerus. The patient first complains of weakness of the grip and also of tingling over the arm and back of the hand. Most neuropraxias recover spontaneously but a fractured humerus associated with nerve injury may require surgical treatment with repair of the nerve.

Historically kicks (especially mawashi-geri – the roundhouse kick) to the mid-part of the upper arm prevented an armed man from gripping or wielding his sword.

The ulnar nerve

This is most often injured from kicks to the elbow region; the injury produces tingling of the little and ring fingers and half of the hand and weakness of their muscles. A further site of injury to the ulnar nerve is in the hand. It supplies the muscles of the hypothenar eminence and can be damaged by striking firm objects in chop-style over a prolonged period. One such unfortunate student presented to his doctor with wasting of all the muscles of the hypothenar eminence due to traumatic neuropraxia. When he stopped doing breaking techniques his problem resolved.

The superficial peroneal nerve

This nerve is most often injured during sweeping manoevres. The patient complains of tingling and weakness of eversion of the foot. The symptoms usually settle in hours but may persist for several weeks. If the symptoms are associated with a fracture of the neck of the fibula, surgical exploration of the nerve may be necessary. Patients with persistent symptoms may also require nerve conduction studies.

Reduction of injury – example of the Scottish karate injury register

Over a 10-year period (1974–1983) all injuries sustained in traditional karate competitions were recorded (McLatchie, 1986; Tables 24.2–24.5). There were three separate periods of study. After establishing the incidence of injury in the first year of the first 3-year period, preventive measures were introduced, including the use of protective clothing in the form of gumshields, groin guards, knuckle pads, shin guards and floor pads, as well as the introduction of padded flooring; the effects of these changes were audited during the period. In the second 3-year period, following a reduction of injury, a national campaign in the UK was launched to educate referees and participants about the risk of injury, the methods of prevention and the immediate management. Equivalent-weight classes were also introduced during this period (except in the team event) and the banning of dangerous techniques was introduced. The

Table 24.2 Injuries to the head and neck sustained in competition karate from 1974 to 1983

	Numbers of cases		
Injury	1974–76	1977–79	1980–83
Epistaxis	91	17	20
Facial lacerations	110	33	15
Periorbital laceration	51	5	2
Head injury (PTA/ concussion/skull fracture)	170	83	45
Blows to the trachea	23	4	5
Cervical dislocation (C6/7)	1	0	0
Maxillary sinus (rupture with pneumatocele)	2	1	0
Mandibular fracture	7	0	1
Malar fracture	8	2	1
Total	463	145	89

From McLatchie (1986).

Table 24.3 Injuries to the trunk sustained in competition karate from 1974 to 1983

	Numbers of cases		
Injury	1974–76	1977–79	1980–83
Rib fracture	35	22	16
Pneumothroax	15	3	2
Blows to solar plexus	185	115	70
Blows to testes	43	12	15
Splenic rupture	2	2	0
Acute traumatic pancreatitis	0	1	0
Total	280	155	103

From McLatchie (1986).

Table 24.4 Injuries to the limbs sustained in competition karate from 1974 to 1983

	Numbers of cases		
Injury	1974–76	1977–79	1980–83
Fractures	97	13	15
Karate thumb	27	5	4
Gamekeeper's thumb	15	5	3
Traumatic neuropraxia	27	5	7
Anterior tibial compartment syndrome	2	2	1
Retropatellar pain	35	21	13
Meniscus symptoms	80	52	32
Total	283	103	80

From McLatchie (1986).

Table 24.5 Injuries in karate – change in incidence over 10 years (13 566 contests)

	1974–76	1977–79	1980–83
Total injuries	931	403	272
Number of contests	4003	3449	6114
Incidence	1 per 4 contests	1 per 8.5 contests	1 per 22 contests

From McLatchie (1986), with permission.

further recommendation that there should be statutory medical control at all competitions where more than 20 participants take part was supported by the Scottish Karate Board of Control.

The incidence of injury fell from one per four contests in the 1974–1976 period to one per eight contests in 1977–1979 period. The effects of the changes introduced during these 6 years were further emphasized when during the period 1980–1983 the injury rate fell to one per 22 contests.

From this study of over 13 500 karate contests it is apparent that even in a combat sport, where injury may be intended and certainly accepted, the incidence can be considerably reduced by making the environment safer, by avoiding the use of dangerous techniques and by providing adequate medical supervision and attention. There was no evidence from the study that the introduction of preventive measures in the form of protective clothing or coach and participant education adversely affected the fighters' performance. During the 10-year period of the study Scotland won four European championships and the British team won the World Championship on four occasions.

Introduction of safety measures

This has meant that karate fighters could train more regularly and have fewer absences from contests. This has allowed many to train towards their peak and compete more regularly in their chosen sport. The use of padded flooring has been extremely successful in reducing the number of head injuries which occur following sweeps, throws or even accidental contact.

If a fighter sustains a post-traumatic amnesia or a knockout the recommendation is that he or she should not fight again for at least 3 or 4 weeks. The Karate Board of Control introduced a 3-month ban following a knockout on the basis that some participants may feign unconsciousness to win a fight 'lying on his back'. In this way histrionics are avoided.

If a fighter has symptoms of a post-traumatic syndrome the rule is that he or she does not return to the sport until the symptoms have resolved completely. If there has been a head injury severe enough to cause coma or lead to a neurosurgical procedure such fighters should be advised to give up combat sport altogether. In all situations when a serious head injury has been sustained those wishing to return to karate competition should be examined and certified fit by a neurologist.

Forensic aspects of karate

The potential of karate to cause severe injury was illustrated in a case report (Camps, 1959) when a young soldier was murdered. He had a vertical fracture of the thyroid cartilage and in addition several vertical tears of the carotid artery were demonstrated at post-mortem examination. At first it was believed that these injuries were caused by a blunt instrument such as a rod or staff. However when the assailant was apprehended and questioned it became apparent that he had struck the victim several times with the side of his hand using the so-called karate chop, a technique he had learned in the Army. The report emphasized the dangers inherent in the technique and actually popularized the concept of the karate chop, a

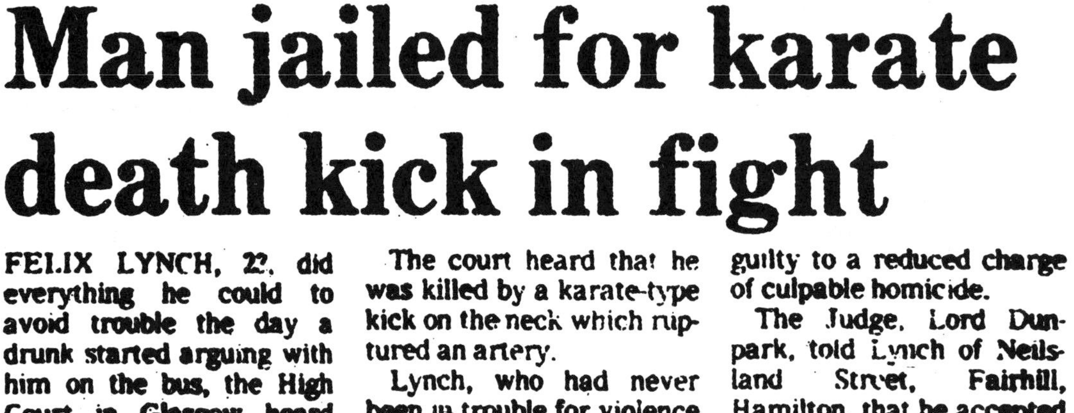

Man jailed for karate death kick in fight

FELIX LYNCH, 22, did everything he could to avoid trouble the day a drunk started arguing with him on the bus, the High Court in Glasgow heard yesterday.

However Peter McCabe, 42, was so abusive that Lynch finally accepted a challenge to get off the bus for a "square go" and the incident ended with McCabe dying on the pavement.

The court heard that he was killed by a karate-type kick on the neck which ruptured an artery.

Lynch, who had never been in trouble for violence before, was charged with murder and was so distressed over what he had done that he developed ulcers and spent his time while awaiting trial in a prison hospital.

Yesterday he was jailed for two years when the Crown accepted his plea of guilty to a reduced charge of culpable homicide.

The Judge, Lord Dunpark, told Lynch of Neilsland Street, Fairhill, Hamilton, that he accepted the deceased had been the aggressor.

Lynch, who hopes to marry when he gets out of jail, admitted punching McCabe, of Woodhead Green, Hamilton, and kicking him on the neck so severely that he died in hospital on August 5.

Fig. 24.5 Newspaper report of a karate kick that killed.

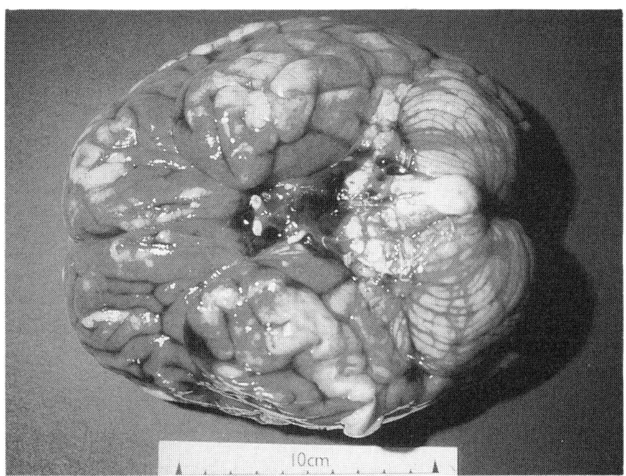

Fig. 24.6 Specimen (brain) showing extensive subarachnoid haemorrhage.

technique rarely used in competition because it is outlawed.

A case of traumatic extracranial subarachnoid haemorrhage was also reported in early 1980. In this situation a young karate fighter was goaded into a fight in the street and defended himself with a high kick to the side of the neck and head of his opponent. Unfortunately, the victim sustained a traumatic rupture of the vertebral artery just as it enters the subarachnoid space and died of traumatic extracranial subarachnoid haemorrhage (Figs 24.5 and 24.6).

A further fatal injury involved a middle-grade karateka at a contest: he was struck with unmitigated force in the chest and died from cardiac arrest due to vagal inhibition.

Other reports are detailed below:

Victim: Young male karateka – contest injury
Experience: International fighter
Injury: Ruptured spleen
Treatment: Splenectomy
Mechanism: Roundhouse kick to the left loin
(McLatchie, 1978)

Victim: Young female karateka
Experience: Second karate lesson
Injury: Ruptured right lobe and dome of liver
Treatment: Partial hepatectomy
Result: Complete recovery
Mechanism: Roundhouse kick to right hypochondrial region
(Cantwell and King, 1973)

Victim: Young male karateka – contest injury
Experience: International fighter
Injury: Acute traumatic pancreatitis (serum amylase greater than 1200 iu)
Result: Complete recovery
Mechanism: Straight punch (gyaku-zuki) to solar plexus
(McLatchie, 1978)

Victim: Middle-aged male tied to chair
Injuries: 1. Several soft tissue bruises to side of neck
2. Fracture of thyroid cartilage into three separate fragments
Mechanism: Karate chop
(Watson, 1978)

Victim: Male university student, blind in right eye
Experience: Low grade at karate lesson
Injury: Orbital blow-out fracture of left eye
Result: Hemi-field defect
Mechanism: Roundhouse kick to left orbit
(McLatchie, 1978)

Victim: Soldier
Injuries: 1. Vertical fracture to thyroid cartilage
2. Several vertical tears of the carotid artery
Mechanism: Knife-hand-strike to the neck (karate chop)
(Camps, 1959)

These case reports are not only of forensic interest, they also demonstrate the destructive power inherent even in minimally trained individuals and should raise suspicion in clinicians involved in the examination of victims of assault – extensive intra-abdominal or intrathoracic organic injury can occur as a result of kicks or punches.

Grappling and throwing sports

Judo

Judo, 'the way of gentleness', has been popular in the UK for more than 40 years. It is an Olympic sport and has become an effective method of self-defence. It is not by definition a martial art: it was invented in the mid 1860s by the Japanese professor, Dr Jigaro Kano, who made a detailed study on the many fighting forms of the Orient and synthesized what he had learned, calling the art *judo*, the gentle way. He argued that the most efficient way of fighting was to use intellect, personal ability and the mistakes of one's opponents so that if an attacker threw a punch he or she could be thrown by the defender as a result of his or her own momentum.

Judo involves rapidly changing one's centre of gravity to perform throws. It also involves the use of ground work and locks against joints to maintain an opponent in a helpless position. Strangles, chokes and locks against the joints are characteristic of ground work and so it is not surprising that injuries may involve many of the joints of the limbs and the neck.

Aikido

This Japanese martial art involves the redirection of an attacker's energy with grappling or striking. On occasions it involves the use of weaponry. Around 1500 people practise the art in the UK.

Ju-jitsu

This Japanese martial art is of uncertain origin and involves locks, throws and holds. Striking techniques are used to weaken or divert the attention of an opponent until a hold can be applied. Several styles exist and there are around 2500 practitioners in the UK.

Particular injuries

Compression of the carotid artery in strangles or chokes can lead to unconsciousness and even death. In all circumstances an episode of unconsciousness should be regarded as if the player has sustained a minor head injury. This involves maintaining the airway, ensuring breathing and circulation are intact and recommending a lay-off period after injury of at least 1 month.

Cervical dislocation resulting in quadriplegia has resulted from the application of strangle holds. Although this is a rare injury it emphasizes the inevitable risks associated with this sport.

Joint injuries in the form of dislocations or sprains are fairly common, especially to the shoulders, elbows and fingers. They should be treated along standard lines.

Mat burns, grazes and bruises are also common but serious abdominal injury is rare.

Injury situations

Participants are most at risk when:

1. A breakfall is poorly executed.
2. A lock was over enthusiastically applied to a joint or not submitted to (Fig. 24.7).
3. A choke or strangle is applied (Fig. 24.8).

The wrist, elbow and head are the most commonly injured after ineffective breakfalls and prevention lies in adequate warm-up and frequent falling practice. It is important to emphasize to players the dangers associated with lockholds applied to a joint and participants and referees should be made aware that a stranglehold applied too vigorously can indeed be fatal.

Injuries to children

Judo is a very popular sport amongst children who commonly suffer from a 'pulled elbow'. In this condition the radial head is actually pulled out of its annular ligament, which leads to immediate pain and tenderness associated with almost complete limitation of pronation and supination.

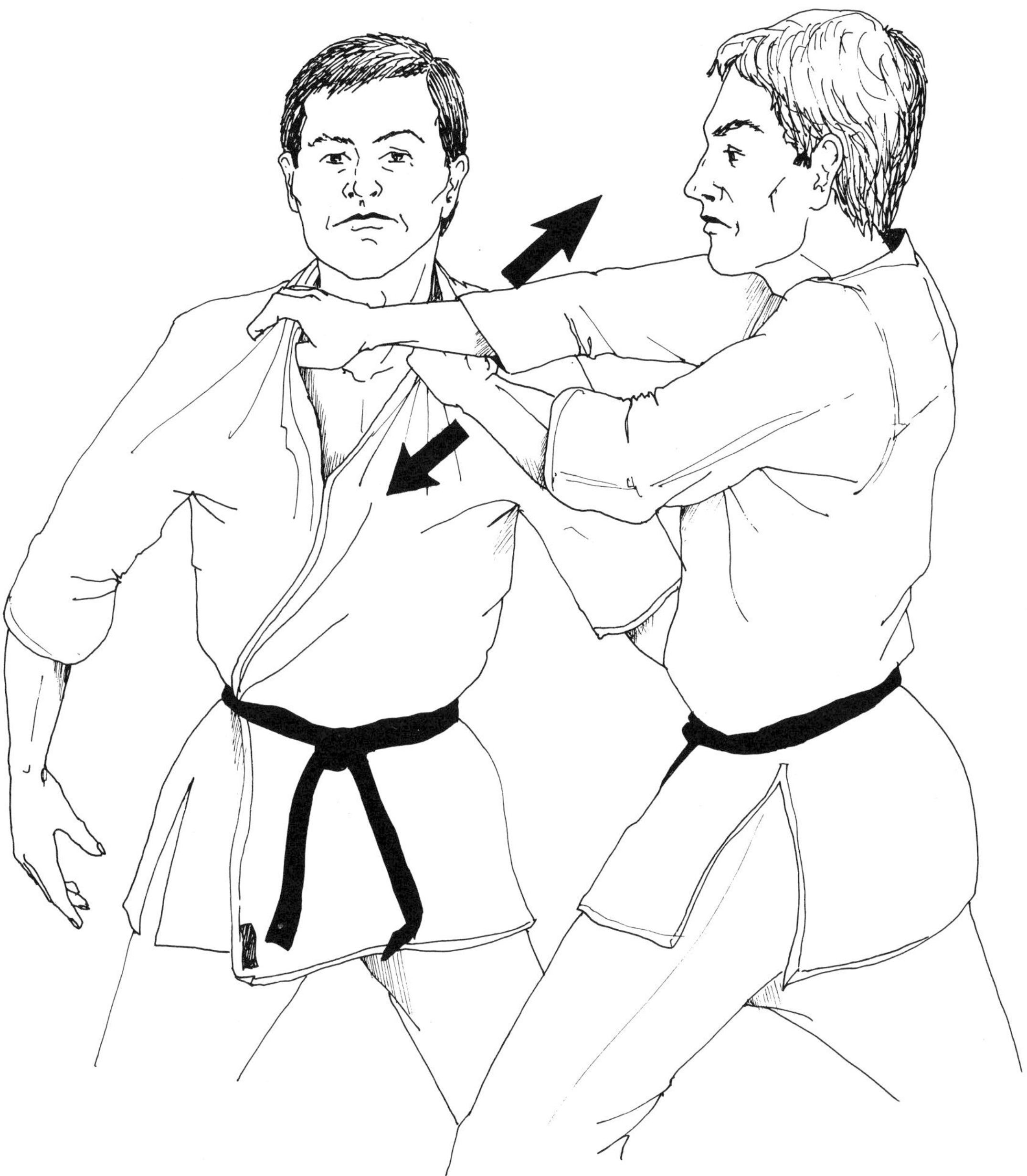

Fig. 24.7 Strangleholds can be applied very rapidly and may lead to unconsciousness in seconds.

Treatment is simple: firm alternate pronation and supination with the elbow held at a right angle allow the radial head to click back into position. Post-traumatic sequelae are rare.

Wrestling

This is one of the oldest sports in the world and probably the most widespread. It was already a highly organized sport in 3000 BC in Egypt and had complicated rules and protocol. Evidence for this

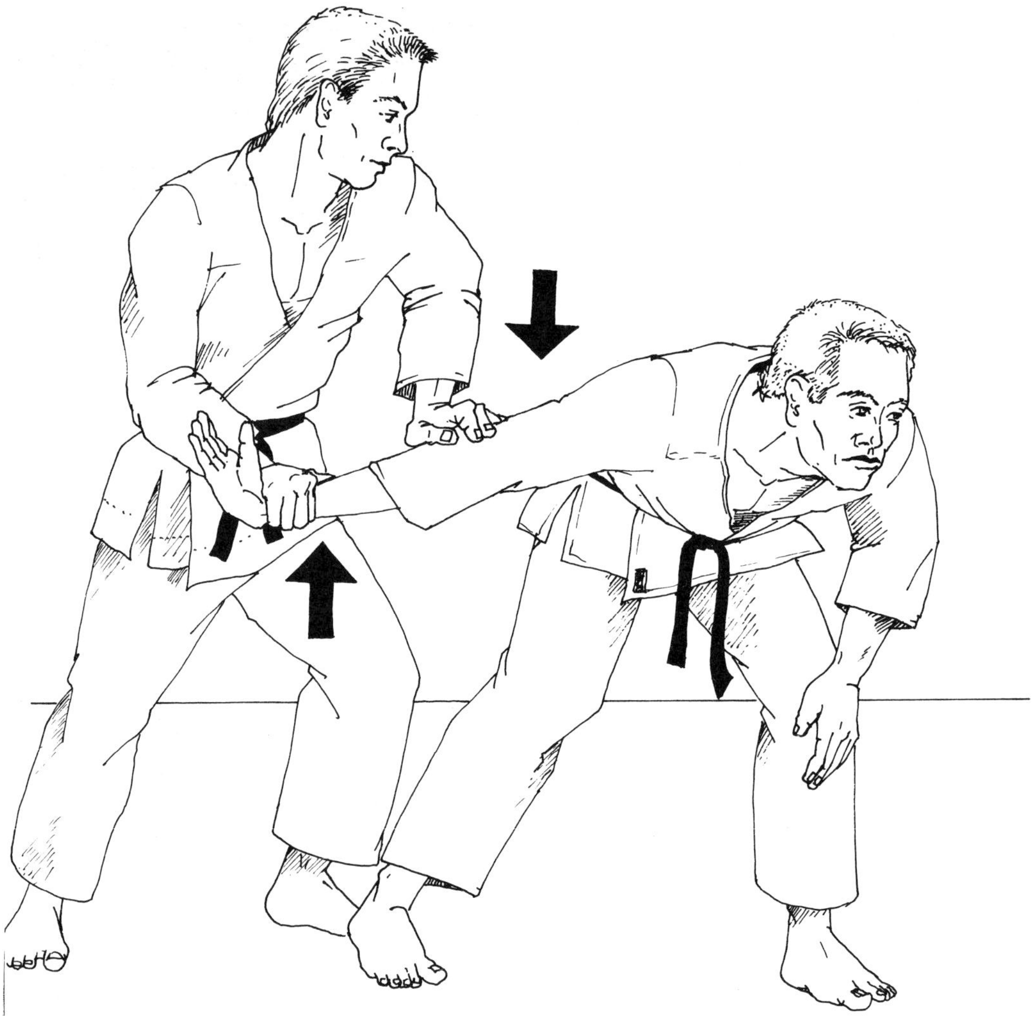

Fig. 24.8 Joint injuries can result from vigorously applied locks.

is found in 4000 or so throws and holds inscribed in the walls of the tomb of Ben-y-Hassam.

There are numerous fabled contents: Ulysses and Ajax wrestled at the funeral games before the walls of Troy; Rustam killed Sohrab, his son, before the King of Afghanistan, and in the 14th century when the Turkish tribes made raids into Europe it is said that two men wrestled for 3 days without decision and then died of exhaustion. In recognition of this contest a 3-day wrestling tournament has been held each year on the site ever since and in Turkish the word for hero and wrestler is the same – *pehlivan*.

In the UK there are three types of wrestling:

1. Olympic or freestyle.
2. Greco-Roman.
3. Professional.

The rules are that the fighters must have well-cut nails and short hair. Their weight should be equivalent and no jewellery is permitted to be worn in a contest. In freestyle wrestling any fair hold is allowed. In the Greco-Roman style, holds below the waist are forbidden and trips or throws using the legs are also illegal.

The spectacular sport of all-in professional wrestling appears to have no holds barred – save direct chokes – and the flat of the hand and forearm (the forearm smash) are permitted as instruments of attack. However, although it is apparently extremely violent, injury and death are indeed rare and due mainly to myocardial ischaemia or head injuries after falling out of the ring. The sport has become increasingly popular with young spectators and is given wide exposure and hype through satellite television networks. There appears to be a high degree of safety for the wrestlers as well as considerable crowd satisfaction for the fans.

Serious injury

Cervical injury used to be common, especially when one contestant could fall heavily on his opponent when he was bridging. A change in the rules has now prevented this type of injury and it is illegal to jump upon a wrestler if he has formed a bridge.

Chronic injuries

The common sites are the knees and the shoulders. They are usually associated with meniscus or ligamentous injuries or innumerable minor muscle strains.

The Sumo wrestlers of Japan, reared from a young age in establishments known as stables, are subject to an interesting range of injuries. They develop stiffness of the metacarpophalangeal joints and proximal phalangeal joints of the fingers and thumbs as a result of the hands being subjected to repeated trauma against padded posts. Anecdotally, they are also said to be at risk of developing a punchdrunk-type syndrome in later life due to the repeated concussions from butting each other in competitions. Described as the fastest athletes in the world over 2 m, they tend to have short lives (usually related to obesity and high fat intake): death is commonly due to ischaemic heart disease.

Prevention of injury

The development of neck strength and skilful bridging techniques is essential to prevent injury.

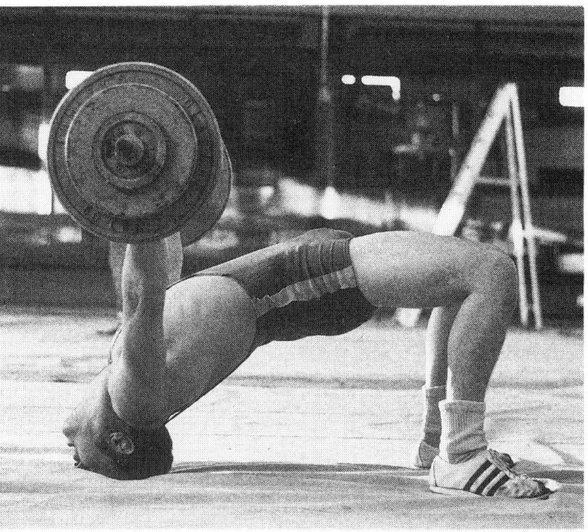

Fig. 24.9 This wrestler could press 250 lb (112 kg) from the position shown. Neck strengthening reduces the risk of injury.

Some wrestlers develop exceptional neck strength and can practise kick-over bridging and bridging with weights (Fig. 24.9). During the souplesse or salto techniques some wrestlers can land on their foreheads in the bridge position. The forehead landing should not be attempted by novices and it may be better for them to 'rotate out' so that their full weight and that of their opponent do not stress the cervical vertebrae.

Neck-strengthening exercises with weights involve shoulder-shrugging and pulling exercises, keeping the weight as close to the body as possible.

Prefight medical examination and rest periods after head injury are mandatory and it is the responsibility of the competition doctor to decide whether a competitor can continue after injury.

Weaponry sports

Fencing

Fencing is a very safe sport and only two fatalities have been reported in the history of British fencing. As in all contact or combat sports, the authorities aim to strike a balance between the safety of the competitors and the essential nature

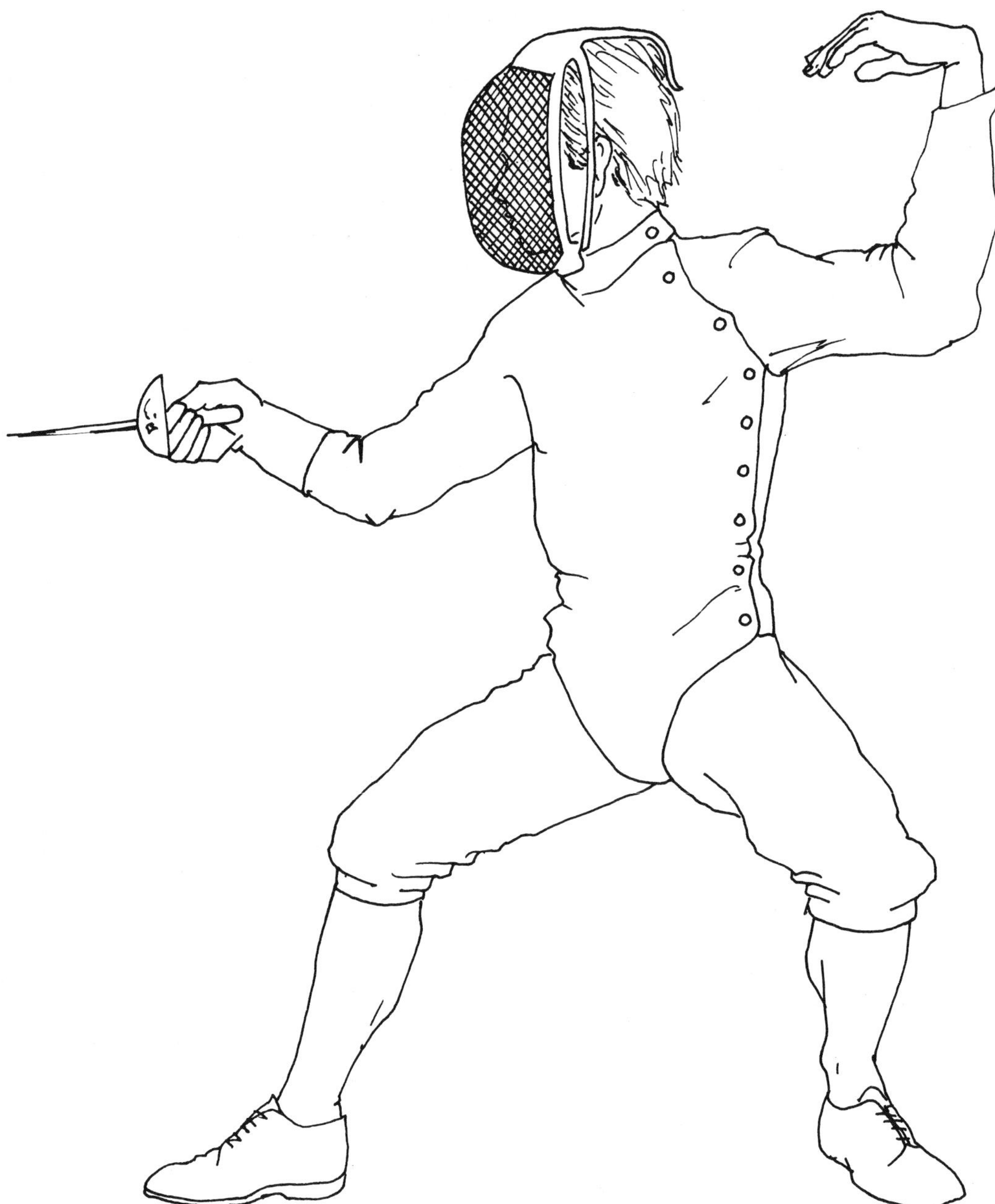

Fig. 24.10 Protective clothing and face guards are an integral part of injury prevention in fencing.

of the sport, which involves two athletes attacking each other with potentially lethal weapons. Currently the move is towards safety and much activity has been devoted to reducing the risks to an ideal minimum. This has involved higher standards of protective clothing (Fig. 24.10) and efforts to make the blade safer by using different types of steel which have been designed to break safely if penetration is a possibility. The theory of a safe blade is probably the most logical step but although initially promising, little success has been recorded in practice.

Blade injuries

Accident statistics in the UK have been kept since 1984 and there have been nine broken blade injuries, including one of the two fatal accidents, and six intact blade injuries. In terms of severity the intact blade injuries were much less serious. Most blade injuries are at foil and the ratio of men to women is 13:2. Accidents are as likely to occur amongst beginners as amongst veterans and club fencers have a similar injury rate to internationals. The neck is particularly vulnerable and modern masks carry heavier protection in this area (Crawford, 1990).

At both fatal accidents a doctor was present in the *salle* but in each case the injury involved penetration of a major vessel (Crawford, 1984).

The initial management of such injuries involves the application of appropriate pressure to the injured area if possible and rapid transfer of the fencer to hospital with the establishment of an intravenous infusion and plasma expander.

The 10-minute rule

When a fencer is injured he or she is allowed a maximum of 10 min recovery to return to the *piste*; failure to do so results in disqualification. This can cause difficulties for the attending doctor who may be summoned from a different part of the competition area to examine a (possibly non-English-speaking) competitor. While it may be possible to strap a sprained ankle or stitch a cut in time for the fencer to return and win the fight, penetrating injuries of the neck, chest and abdomen should be regarded as potentially life-threatening.

There is little evidence of any particular pattern of injury or disease associated with the sport apart possibly from 'fencer's pubalgia', which appears to be associated with shearing forces at the symphysis pubis. There is also anecdotal evidence of an increased risk of osteoarthrosis of the leading hip (the right hip of a right-handed fencer).

In women's fencing the breasts form part of the target area. The protectors leave the lateral aspect of the breasts uncovered and open to injury (usually bruising or superficial lacerations).

Kendo

When death has resulted from an accident in kendo it has been secondary to eye injuries. In the incidents which have happened in *shiai* (kendo sword) shattered and bamboo splinters penetrated the face guard and the orbit. The victim of one such accident died from intracranial bleeding, another from secondary infection. These incidents emphasize the importance of ensuring that protective equipment is in good condition and the need for frequent inspection and care of weapons.

Use of weapons in karate

The use of oriental farming instruments is a popular extension of karate. They also have been increasingly used as weapons of attack in urban violence. Injuries can be avoided in training by using strict control and slow repetitive movements until mastery is achieved. Many inexperienced weapon users find the weapon more dangerous to themselves than to any imaginary opponent.

Recommendations for doctors attending combat sport competitions

The doctor attending such competition should have an interest in sports medicine and be competent in core skills (life-saving techniques). There should also be a good communication system so that injured patients can be transferred quickly to hospital if required. On many occasions it is possible to have representatives from the Red Cross, St John or St Andrew ambulance services in attendance, provided adequate notice is given.

Responsibilities

1. The examination of competitors before the competition, as required by the rules of the sport (particularly boxing, karate, judo, aikido, wrestling and fencing).

2. The inspection of fighting areas to ensure that adequate flooring is in use. In boxing the ring should be sprung and in judo, wrestling and karate padded flooring should be used. If the doctor is unhappy about any of the arrangements for the contest, including inadequate flooring or unsatisfactory medical equipment, the problem should be made known to the officials of the tournament and rectified before the tournament begins (head injury is a common sequel to falls on hard floors).
3. The treatment of minor injuries such as lacerations and sprains.
4. The referral of more seriously injured competitors to hospital after ensuring that the airway, breathing and circulation are adequate.
5. Advising the referees, where requested, as to the fitness of a competitor to continue.
6. Assisting referees with scoring, e.g. in sports such as karate where the potential danger of various techniques may result in a half-point or a full point depending on the potential damage which could be done. It is obvious therefore that the doctor attending such competitions needs to know the sport well.

Injuries which will exclude further participation

1. Fractures.
2. Head injuries which have resulted in disorientation, amnesia or unconsciousness.
3. Ocular injuries, particularly where sight is impaired or there is doubt about the integrity of the globe. This would include periorbital injuries and depends upon clinical examination.
4. Cases of testicular injury where recovery is not rapid and scrotal haematomas are present.

Protective clothing

The governing bodies permit specific types of protective clothing in certain sports. This should be inspected by the officials of the sport concerned and all forms of jewellery, such as earrings in pierced ears, should be removed before any competition takes place.

Fitness to compete

After a knockout a period of at least 4 weeks should elapse before any further competition takes place, although the competitor may be allowed to train but not to spar.

When there is a serious eye or ear injury return to competitive sport should be dictated by expert opinion and the competitor should produce evidence of fitness to compete in the form of a discharge letter from the specialist concerned.

Following bony injuries to the face, nose or hands, time from training and competition will depend on the extent of the injury. Return to competition will be subject to further medical examination.

Guidelines for the management of sportsmen and women with acute head injuries

The most important clinical manifestation of a head injury is alteration of the conscious level. This may present as a knockout, a period of post-traumatic amnesia with automatism, or a fluctuating level of consciousness deteriorating to coma at a variable rate. Where there is a clear-cut loss of consciousness or change in the conscious level, the management is relatively straightforward – the fighter needs to be removed for further examination and possible transfer to hospital.

The difficulty arises when a fighter who has sustained a head injury apparently recovers fully and may be able to speak. On closer examination there may be mild disorientation and post-traumatic amnesia. We believe that all such competitiors should be encouraged to leave the combat area because the mildly concussed individual is more liable to sustain a second head injury and may develop secondary brain damage from an intracranial haematoma.

When there is doubt about the seriousness of a

head injury and there is an altered level of consciousness, even if the fighter is walking and talking, it is essential for a skull X-ray to be performed in order to identify the small number of patients who may have sustained a skull fracture. Lacerations and haematomas must be carefully examined and the possibility of a depressed fracture kept in mind.

The Glasgow Coma Scale (Table 24.6) is a ready means of assessing, recording and displaying the level of consciousness. Its simple terms provide an objective descriptive standard for patients with head injuries and its observations and recordings should be started as soon as possible.

Table 24.6 The Glasgow Coma Scale

Function	Response	Score
Eye opening	Spontaneous	4
	To speech	3
	To pain	2
	None	1
Best verbal response	Oriented	5
	Confused conversation	4
	Inappropriate words	3
	Incomprehensible sounds	2
	None	1
Best motor response	Obeys commands	6
	Localizes	5
	Flexes { normal	4
	Flexes { abnormal	3
	Extends	2
	None	1

(From Teasdale and Jennett, 1974)

If there is prolonged unconsciousness patients should be placed in the coma position and the airway maintained during transport. In less serious cases the advice should be to abstain from eating or drinking for 12 hours and alcohol should be specifically prohibited. After assessment arrangements can be made with relatives, friends or club officials to ensure a safe journey home and adequate subsequent supervision. If there are focal neurological signs or if vomiting or persistent headaches develops further medical aid should be sought and the patient taken to hospital. These instructions can be given to the accompanying person on a printed card (Fig. 24.11).

HEAD INJURY WARNING

Name ....

The above named player has sustained a head injury on

....

1. **He should be seen by an Accident and Emergency Department as soon as possible**
2. **He should not play rugby for 3 weeks but he can, however, attend training sessions (no contact)**
3. **If he develops vomiting, weakness of a limb, any abnormal movement or excess drowsiness or confusion he must be seen by a hospital immediately.**
4. **He must not drink alcohol for 24 hours.**

Fig. 24.11 Head injury warning card.

Treatment of minor injuries

Minor injuries are commonly seen in pugilists and combat sport participants mainly in the form of blisters, friction burns, lacerations or haematomas. Each of these conditions should be treated under as aseptic conditions as possible. If aseptic conditions cannot be guaranteed at the ring side, the patient must be referred to an Accident and Emergency department where this service can be provided.

Blisters caused by shearing forces of the skin, particularly in the hands and feet, are commonly seen in judoka and karateka. The fluid may be aseptically aspirated or drained as often as it accumulates. The roof of the blister should be left intact to act as a biological dressing. This allows healing to occur more rapidly and the areas could be covered with barrier cream or a dressing to prevent further damage.

Mat burns are also generated by friction and are common minor injuries amongst wrestlers and judoka. The affected area should be cooled with tap water or an ice pack and unless extensive, when hospital care is needed, require no further treatment other than simple analgesics.

Lacerations

These are especially common in karate and boxing and usually occur in the periorbital region. The edges of the wound should be carefully approximated with sutures after thoroughly cleaning the area using an aseptic technique and gloved hands, so that infections (particularly AIDS) and excessive scarring can be avoided.

Haematomas often collect following injuries to the soft tissues of the limb, particularly the thighs and around the eye. If the collection is large it may be aspirated, again under aseptic conditions. Haematomas of the lower leg can lead to compartment syndromes unless they are treated promptly by adequate cooling and elevation of the limb.

People taking part in combat sports should be encouraged to have full tetanus immunization.

Conclusions and recommendations

There is considerable potential for preventing injuries in combat sports even further, but this would involve a change in the philosophy of the sport. Referees should be encouraged to stop competitions at early stages to prevent a partially injured competitor becoming more seriously injured and action by the governing bodies is required to alter the rules to ensure that safer practices and equipment are adopted by fighters and officials, both in the competition area and in training.

Audit of injury statistics and the monitoring of potential injury situations are important new developments and should receive further attention in order that the gains in safety already made can be consolidated.

Medical recommendations for reducing injuries

1. A medical certificate of fitness to fight should be presented to the official before a contest.
2. Each fighter should carry a fight record in which previous performances and injuries are recorded.
3. A doctor should be present at all competitions.
4. Following specific injuries (to the eye, ear or head) or heavy contact to the trunk, the competitor should be examined before continuing. A minimum of 4 weeks should elapse after a head injury (knockout, post-traumatic amensia) before fighting again.
5. Equivalent-weight classes should be encouraged and ideally no fighter should outweigh his or her opponent by more than 7lb (3 kg).
6. Referees and instructors should learn first-aid and life-saving techniques.
7. It should be the responsibility of the governing body to issue a summary of the rules of the sport. These should be freely available to all members of the association.
8. If there are any rule changes on the day of a competition, these should be clearly announced beforehand.
9. Protective equipment, as recommended by the governing body in liaison with the medical officer of the sport, should be worn.

References

Camps FE (1959) The case of Emmett Dunne. *Medico-Legal Journal* (Cambridge) **27**, 156.

Cantwell JD, King JT (1973) Karate chops and liver lacerations. *Journal of the American Medical Association* **224**, 1424.

Corsellis JAN (1974) Brain damage in sport. *Lancet* **i**, 401–2.

Crawford AR (1984) Death of a fencer. *British Journal of Sports Medicine* **18**, 220.

Crawford AR (1990) The medical hazards of fencing. In: Payne SD (ed) *Medicine, Sport and the Law*. Oxford: Blackwell, p 360.

Doggart JH, Rugg-Gunn A (1965) Eye injuries. In: Bass AL, Blonstein JL, James RD, Williams JGP (eds) *Medical Aspects of Boxing*. Oxford: Pergamon Press, pp 3–19.

Fisher F (1991). BMA steps-up anti-boxing campaign with new research. *BMA News Review*. November 10.

Green MA (1978) Injury and sudden death in sport. In: Mason JK (ed) *The Pathology of Violent Injury*. London: Edward Arnold, pp 255–77.

Gronwall D, Wrightson P (1974) Delayed recovery of intellectual function after minor head injury. *Lancet* **ii**, 605–9.

Gronwall D, Wrightson P (1975). Cumulative effect of concussion. *Lancet* **ii**, 995–7.

Kaste M, Vilkki J, Sainis K, Kumme T, Katevuo K, Meurala H (1982) Is chronic brain damage in boxing a hazard of the past? *Lancet* **ii**, 1186–8.

McLatchie GR (1976) Analysis of karate injuries sustained in 295 contests. *Injury* **8**, 132–4.

McLatchie GR (1978) Serious injuries in competition karate. Presentation. Glasgow University.

McLatchie GR (1986a) The hard man image of the non-smoker. In: *Proceedings of the 23rd FIMS World Congress of Sports Medicine*. Brisbane. Australia.

McLatchie GR (1986b) Prevention of injuries in combat sports – a 10 year study of competition karate. Brisbane, Australia: World Congress of Sports Medicine.

McLatchie GR (1990) *Skilful Karate*. London: A & C Black, pp 85–9.

McLatchie GR, Davies JE, Caulley J (1980) Injuries in karate – a case for medical control. *American Journal of Trauma* **20**, 956–9.

McLatchie GR, Brooks N, Galbriath S *et al.* (1987) Clinical neurological examination, neuropsychology, electroencephalography and computed tomographic head scanning in active amateur boxers. *Journal of Neurology, Neurosurgery and Psychiatry* **50**, 96–9.

Martland HS (1928) Punch drunk. *Journal of the American Medical Association* **91**, 1103–7.

Montanaro M, Francone A (1966) Roentgencinematographic study of the hand in boxing. In: *Proceedings of the 6th Amateur International Boxing Association Medical Congress, Rome*.

Roberts AH (1928). *Brain damage in boxers*. Tunbridge Wells: Pitman Medical.

Sortland U, Tysvaer AT, Storli OV (1989) Association football injuries to the brain – a neurological and encephalographic study of former football players. *Neuroradiology* **31**, 44.

Teasdale G and Jennett B (1974) Assessment of coma and impaired consciousness. *Lancet* **ii**, 81–4.

Watson AA (1984) Kicking, karate and kung fu. In: Mason JK (ed) *The Pathology of Violent Injury*, London: Edward Arnold, p 286.

25

Risks and injuries in horse-riding sports

J. Lloyd Parry

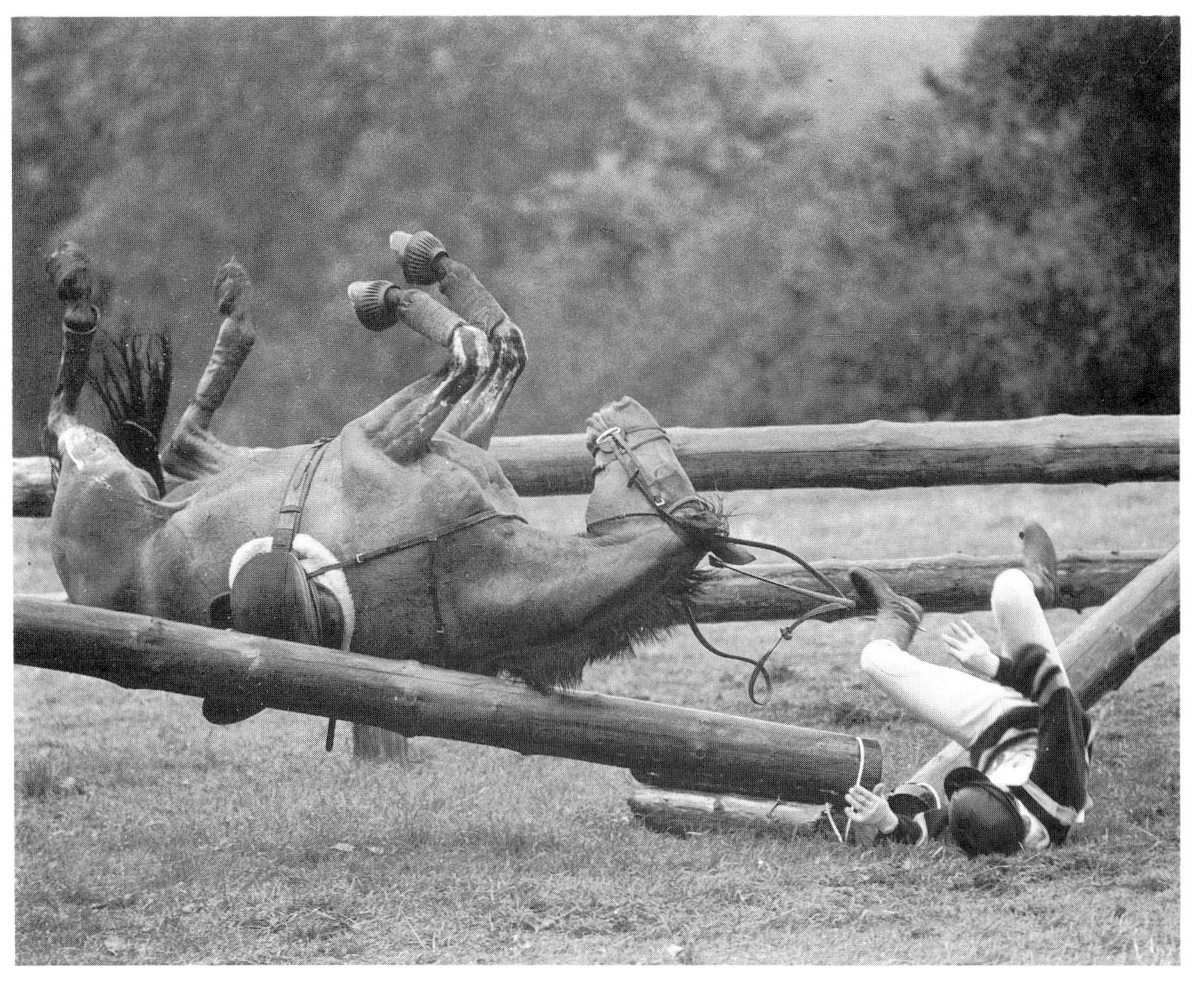

Introduction

The diverse spectrum of horse-riding, which involves as many as 3 million people (British Horse Society Report, 1988), ranges from gymkhanas and Pony Club mounted-games to team-chasing, point-to-point and professional horse-racing. Whilst tent-pegging and vaulting may be considered a minority interest, there is a very large following for show-jumping and eventing (which involves dressage, show-jumping and cross-country fences). Many thousands of spectators annually attend the Badminton and Burghley Horse Trials (Eventing) or the Horse of the Year Show at Wembley (show-jumping), with television coverage producing household names from the most successful competitors. Dressage, polo and carriage-driving command their own enthusiastic and knowledgeable following whilst long-distance riding has continued to advance its appeal. Several types of competition may be seen at horse shows and will include both ridden and unmounted show classes of horse and pony but, undoubtedly, the best-known and most popular of all is horse-racing. The governing body is the Jockey Club which is responsible for all aspects of professional racing both on the flat and over fences. Its influence on the safety of the competitor and public has been considerable and should be emulated by the governing bodies of other high-risk equestrian sports. Unfortunately, hunting is only slowly paying heed to certain aspects of safety and continues to arouse fierce controversy between those who are dedicated to its survival, as a fundamental contribution to rural life, and those who would wish it banned because the manner in which it achieves its objective seems to involve cruelty to the hunted fox or stag. Whilst horse-racing, horse and pony trials and, latterly, show-jumping have seen to it, through their governing bodies, that vulnerable heads are, as far as possible, protected from injury to the brain and its disastrous consequences, a large number of the hunting fraternity remain bound by fashion rather than prudence (Teacher, 1988).

Incidence

The serious nature and severity of horse-riding injuries, most particularly head injury, are alarming and well-documented. It must be remembered

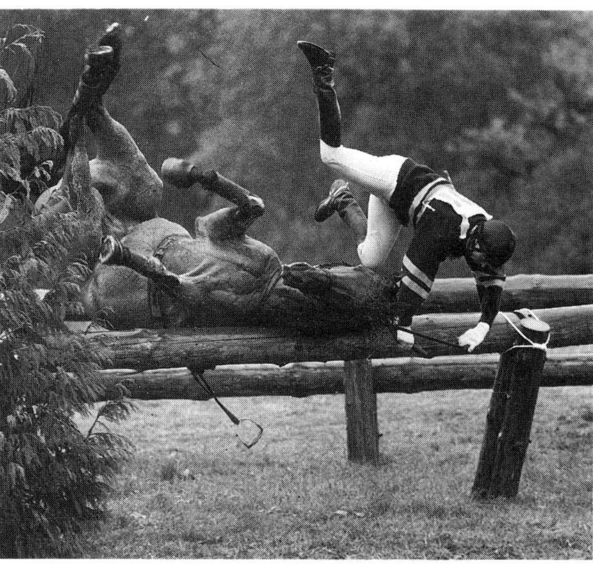

Fig. 25.1 The head leads during many accidents, which explains the high incidence of head and spinal injuries.

that a rider's head may be 3 m from the ground and that a horse can attain a speed of 60 km/h (Miles, 1970). The position adopted is frequently with the head forward and Becker's principle is applicable (Becker, 1959) in that the degree of this position is reflected in the number of head injuries sustained (Fig. 25.1).

In 1980, Lindsay *et al.* from the Neurosurgical Unit in Glasgow noted the link between horse-riding and serious head injury following Barber's earlier work (1973) in Oxford where 67% of 131 admissions to the Radcliffe Infirmary had head injuries. There was a dismal warning from the Department of Neurosurgery of this hospital in 1984 (Ilgren *et al.*, 1984) noting that the six fatalities were either unhelmeted or improperly helmeted and in every instance the individual died of primary brain damage as a consequence of trauma to head and/or neck. Muwanga and Dove at Nottingham in 1985 noted the frequency with which horse-riders with a significant head injury presented to a large Accident and Emergency department and commented that riders warranted the most effective head protection possible; they expressed concern that hats were often not worn or inadequately harnessed. In 1987, McGhee *et al.*

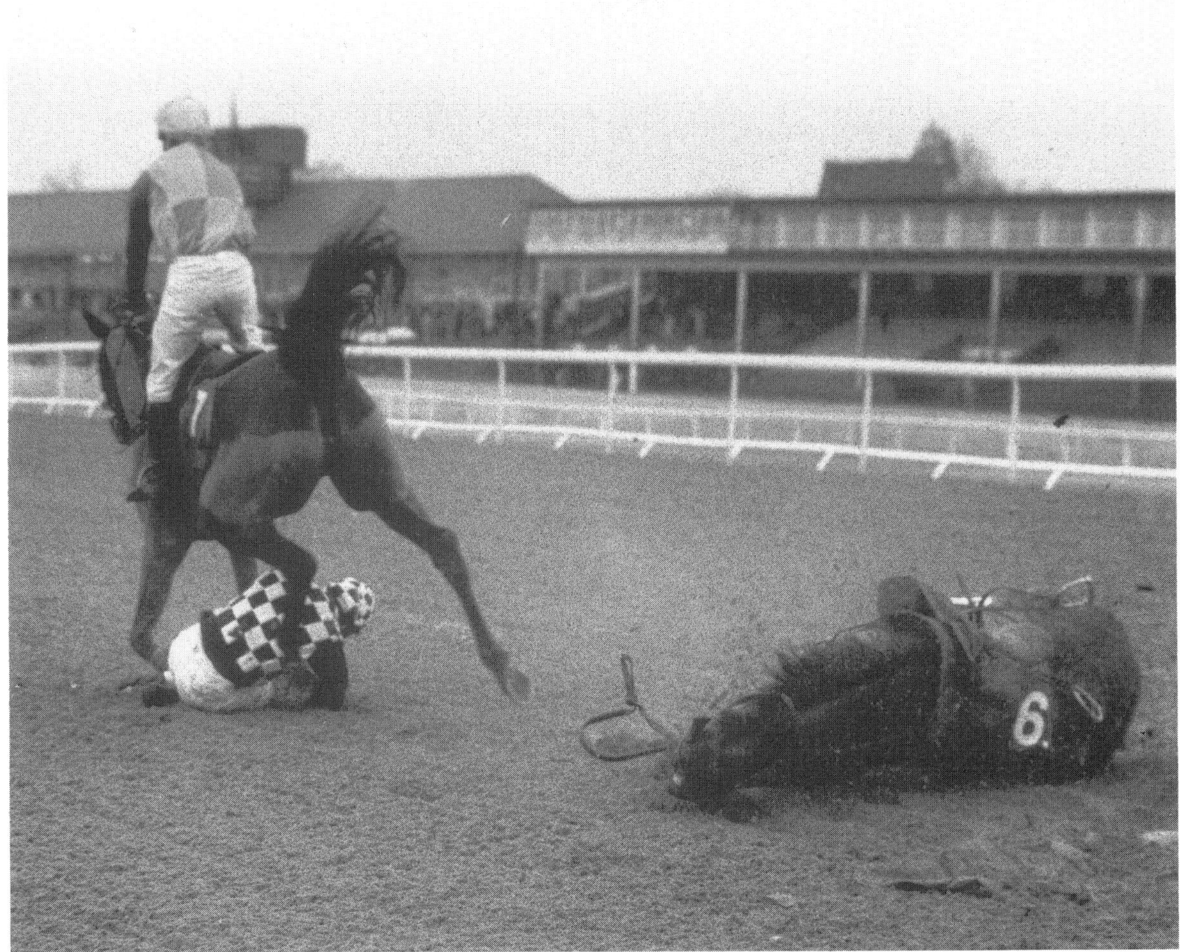

Fig. 25.2 The rider who has survived a fall from one horse may then be seriously injured by being trampled or kicked by another.

Table 25.1 Fatal accidents occurring during sporting and leisure activities

	1981	1982	1983	1984	1985	1986	1987	1988	1989
Horse-riding	10	19	18	23	15	14	12	16	14
Motor sports	8	7	15	23	15	13	10	12	14
Air sports	7	15	8	14	5	18	24	8	9
Ball games	6	14	8	3	9	14	5	3	10

Data from the Office of Population Censuses and Surveys (OPCS 1990).

specifically commented on horse-riding injuries admitted to the University of Edinburgh Royal Infirmary and noted that the usual male predominance of head injury was reversed, with 85% being female, and that in their series there was a predominance of occipital injuries, considered by most neurosurgeons to be a more serious form of head injury.

Where sufficient energy is transferred to the brain to render that individual unconscious, even momentarily, then this should be regarded as a serious head injury (Firth and Galloway, 1990). Whilst unconsciousness or concussion may, therefore, be anticipated it should not be overlooked that other injuries may be serious or even life-threatening. A large study by Whitlock (1988) in the West Midlands found a total of 1554 injuries sustained during the year of 1985, of which over 50% were to those aged 20 years or less, with female dominance (78.8%). Avery (1986) noted that in South Warwickshire in 1980–1984 354 children attended hospital with 67 admissions (61.2% head injuries). One-quarter of the West Midlands injuries occurred during competition whilst of the whole, 10.2% (37 fractures) were to the spine, 5.42% to the chest, including five pneumo-haemothoraces, and 3.73% to the abdomen with 14 visceral ruptures. It was not unexpected that the upper limb (160 fractures) comprised 24.32% but the lower limb also yielded 17.82% (78 fractures). The limb girdles contributed 4.83%, with 41 fractured clavicles and seven fractures of the pelvis. It is very likely that the weight of a horse (500 kg or half a ton) falling on to a rider or a kick from a metal-shod hoof, which can produce a force in excess of 10 kN (Firth, 1985), may demand rapid, skilled care from the attending medical team (Fig. 25.2).

On the other hand, despite this catalogue of potential disasters, it is encouraging to note that the horse-racing scene was transformed by the introduction of compulsory head gear to the required standard and the use of body protectors. Indeed, during the 1989–1990 National Hunt season of 30 000 rides, there were 140 injuries of which 25 were concussion. In the same year flat racing produced only seven cases of such injury (Allen, personal communication). By the same token, the official Horse Trials of the British Horse Society, which enforces similar regulations during the Cross-Country Phase, produced only an average of two injuries to riders during a competition.

In 1990 162 (10 three-day events) Horse Trials took place. The pattern of injury after analysis of accident report forms from a sample of these competitions over the last 3 years (Lloyd Parry, 1990) noted that concussion comprised 13.6% of the injuries sustained. Fractures and dislocations of the upper limb accounted for 21.9%, with injuries to neck and back 19.6%, face 9.67%, chest 7.55% and fractures and dislocations of the lower limb 3.55%.

Unfortunately, fatalities can occur and the Office of Population Censuses and Surveys (OPCS) figures for fatal accidents occurring during sporting and leisure activities may be seen in Table 26.1. It must be observed that these figures are dependent on the details provided by coroners and death certificates and comparison with other organizations shows that the OPCS figures are incomplete to a varying extent (Gloag, 1988).

Prevention and management

The essence of safer riding must lie with a greater awareness of the risks, inherent in the natural unpredictability of the horse's behaviour, and the need for high standards of learning, supervision and training. Whilst care may be taken for the physical adaptation of the horse or pony to its task, the rider's fitness should have equal provision. During a sporting career a tumble seems inevitable, so the art of learning to fall must be acquired in advance of the actual event.

The required protective head gear, suitably harnessed, must be worn at all times when mounted. Indeed, an Act of Parliament (Young Persons Protective Headgear) 1990 came into force on 30 June 1992 to ensure that children under 14 years of age wear suitable head protection when riding. Partly as a consequence of competition rules, the majority of riders now wear BS 4472 (jockey skull cap) adorned by a silk with flexible peak; the alternative riding hat with flexible peak is BS 6473. The harness is attached at four points and often secured by means of a chin-cup. A Duvaxyn RiderCard (Duphar Veterinary Ltd, Southampton) may be carried inside the hat giving details of identity and medical information (Fig. 25.3). It may be obtained free from veterinary surgeons and a caution is given that when information is required, a hat is not to be removed except by those with the necessary skills.

Although it may be forthcoming, body protectors do not have a British Standard. However, recently BETA (British Equestrian Trade Association) have introduced their own blue (standard 5) and red (standard 7) labelled garments. The aim is to prevent or reduce soft tissue injury and possibly minor fractures without restricting the rider's movements.

It is imperative that a foot should not be trapped by the stirrup – dragging injuries can be very severe in nature (Gierup *et al.*, 1976) – and a heeled boot or jodhpur boot (certainly not trainers) must always be worn.

The choice of gloves must be confined to those that do not become slippery. It is perturbing to note that fingers can be avulsed by the unwary who wind a leading rope or reins around their hands (Regan *et al.*, 1991).

The immediate care of injury involves the best standard of airway, breathing and circulation maintenance (ABC; Fig. 25.4) and it is emphasized that the type of fall may predict the severity of the injury. The recognition of concussion will tax the skilled and any evidence of even the briefest loss of consciousness or amnesia will render the rider at risk if remounted.

Spinal injury, so often associated with head injury, requires correct immobilization, lifting and transport. Organizers should be warned of the necessary delay. Assessment of the extent of damage can be facilitated by the use of a Spinex card (Fig. 25.5). Children, with their pliant cervi-

a

Duvaxyn RiderCard

Cardholder:

Allergies:

Medical Conditions:

PTO

b

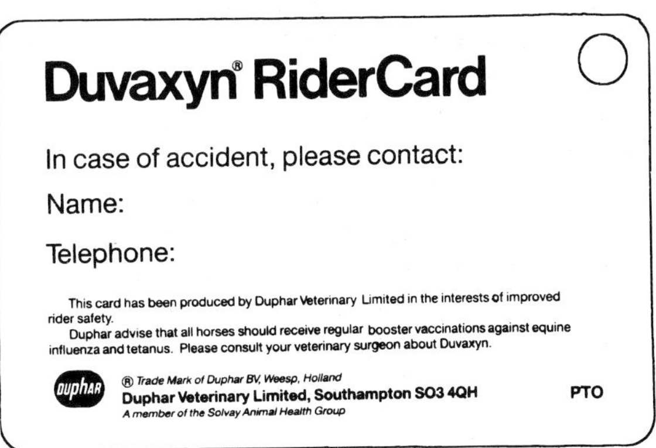

Fig. 25.3 (a) Front and (b) back of the Duvaxyn RiderCard (by kind permission of Solvay–Duphar).

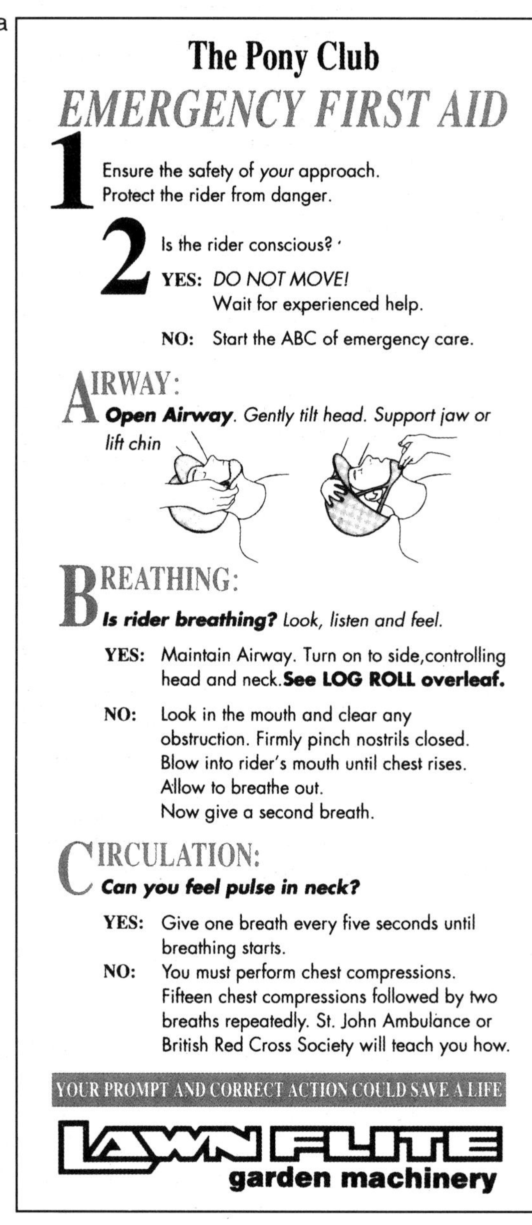

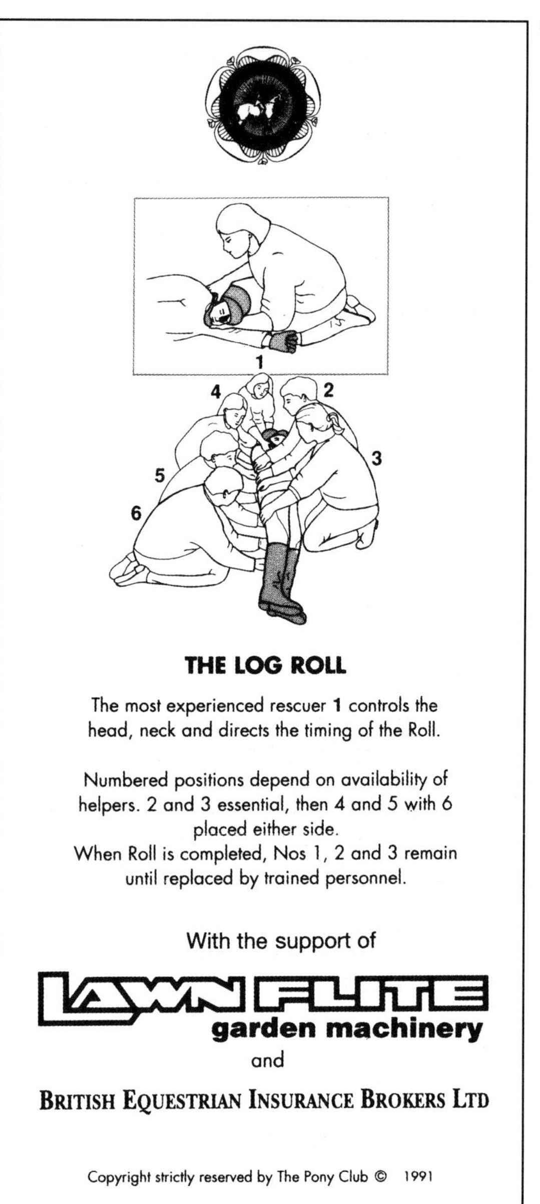

Fig. 25.4 (a) Front and (b) back of the emergency first-aid card, showing the log roll (see also Chapter 12) (by kind permission of the Pony Club).

cal spines, who have transient neurological symptoms must be regarded as having a spinal cord insult with established spinal vasoparesis (Firth and Galloway, 1990).

The prevalence of upper limb injuries has already been noted and damage to the acromioclavicular joint must not be overlooked. However, the greatest emphasis must be on the likelihood of serious pelvic injuries, ruptured viscera or haemo/pneumothorax in the fall of horse on rider.

a

MEDICAL EQUESTRIAN ASSOCIATION
SPINEX CARD
SPINAL CORD INJURY CARD

THE LEVEL AT WHICH SENSATION IS ALTERED OR ABSENT IS THE LEVEL OF INJURY.

IT IS VITAL TO CARRY OUT MOTOR AS WELL AS SENSORY EXAMINATION AS THE PATIENT MAY HAVE MOTOR DAMAGE WITHOUT SENSORY DAMAGE AND VICE VERSA.

SENSORY EXAMINATION
1. EXAMINE BY:
   A. Light touch.
   B. Response to pain.
2. USE:
   The forehead as the guide to what is normal sensation.
3. EXAMINE:
   A. Upper limbs and hands.
   B. Lower limbs and feet.
4. EXAMINE:
   Both sides.
5. T.4 EXAMINATION:
   Must be carried out in the MID–AXILLARY line, NOT the MID-CLAVICULAR line, as C2, C3 and C4 all supply sensation to the nipple line.

C2
C4
T4
C6
T10
T12
C8
S3
L3
L5
S1

IT IS IMPORTANT TO CARRY OUT ALL THE ABOVE AS A VARIETY OF SENSORY CHANGES MAY OCCUR.

The production of this card has been made possible by the financial support of Duphar Veterinary Limited, suppliers of The Duvaxyn RiderCard obtainable from veterinary surgeons.

b

MOTOR EXAMINATION

THE LEVEL AT WHICH WEAKNESS OR ABSENCE OF MOVEMENT IS NOTED IS THE LEVEL OF INJURY.

MOTOR EXAMINATION: EXAMINE BOTH SIDES

UPPER LIMB		LOWER LIMB	
ASK PATIENT TO:		ASK PATIENT TO:	
A. Shrug Shoulders	*C4	A. Flex Hip	*L1 & L2
B. Bend the Elbow	*C5	B. Extend Knee	*L3
C. Push Wrist back	*C6	C. Pull Foot up	*L4
D. Open/Close Hands	*C8	D. Push Foot down	*L5 & S1

THORACIC AND ABDOMINAL MOTOR EXAMINATION : LOOK FOR ACTIVITY OF INTERCOSTAL & ABDOMINAL MUSCLES

DIAGNOSIS OF SPINAL CORD INJURY IN THE UNCONSCIOUS PATIENT

A. Look for paradoxical respiration, as in quadriplegia the loss of use of the intercostal muscles means the diaphragm must be used to breathe.
B. Flaccid limbs.
C. Loss of response to painful stimuli below the level of lesion.
D. Loss of reflexes below the level of lesion.
E. Erection in the unconscious male.
F. Low B.P. (systolic less than 100) associated with a normal pulse or bradycardia indicates patient may be QUADRIPLEGIC.

IF YOU DON'T THINK ABOUT A SPINAL CORD INJURY YOU WILL MISS IT!!!

TREATMENT:
1. A.B.C.
2. Immobilise injured part.
3. Lift patient in one piece in position found.
4. Only move the patient when it is necessary.

We are indebted [illegible] J. Toscano for his original concept and his kind permission to reproduce this card.

Fig. 25.5 (a) front and (b) back of Spinex card. This is an invaluable guide to the rapid assessment of patients with spinal injuries (by kind permission of Solvay–Duphar).

Conclusion

The skill and courage of many equestrian competitors is legendary but they must be prevented from foolhardiness because 'a fall's a hawful thing'; (Surtees, 1843). As to the consequences, the excellent contribution of the Injured Jockey's Fund, The Mark Davies Fund for Injured Riders and The Riding for the Disabled Association command our esteem and support. However, indubitably, we have a responsibility to alert administrators and participants of the possibility of severe injury and the requirement for the management of such accidents (Baker, 1989). There are constraints to the provision of adequate medical care, not least in availability and cost. The new standard that now pertains for medical cover on racecourses is laudable (Jockey Club general Instructions, 1991) but serves to underline the need for doctors with such knowledge to teach all those who will first attend the injured competitor.

References

Avery JG (1986) *Horse Riding Accidents*. Fact Sheets. Child Accident Prevention Trust. Fourth Floor, Clerk's Court, 18–20 Farringdon Lane, London EC1R 3AU.

Baker JHE (1989) The first aid management of spinal cord injury. *Seminars in Orthopaedics* **4**, 2–14.

Barber HM (1973) Horseplay: survey of accidents with horses. *British Medical Journal* **3**, 532–4.

Becker T (1959) Das Stumpfe Schädel Trauma Als Spatunfall. *Mschs. Unfallheidelkunde* **62**, 179.

British Horse Society Report (1988) *The Economic Contribution of the British Equine Industry*. Peak Marwick McLintock.

Firth JL (1985) Equestrian injuries. In: Schneider RC, Kennedy JC, Plant ML, Fowler PJ, Hoff JT, Matthews LS (eds) *Sports Injuries, Mechanisms, Prevention and Treatment*. Baltimore: Williams & Wilkins, pp 431–48.

Firth JL, Galloway NR (1990) Head injuries. In: Hutson MA (ed.) *Sports Injuries*. Oxford: Oxford Medical Publications, p 21.

Gierup J, Larsson M, Lennquist S (1976) Incidence and nature of horse riding injuries. *Acta Chirurgica Scandinavica* **142**, 57–61.

Gloag D (1988) Accidents in sport and leisure activities in: *Strategies for Accident Prevention: A Colloquium*. London: HMSO, p 119.

Ilgren EB, Teddy PJ, Vafadis J, Briggs M, Gardiner NG (1984) Clinical and pathological studies of brain injuries in horse-riding accidents: A description of cases and review with a warning to the unhelmeted. *Clinical Neuropathology* **3**, 253–9.

Jockey Club General Instructions (1991) *Medical Services for Licensed Personnel* N. 11. 1. London: The Jockey Club.

Lindsay KW, McLatchie G, Jennett B (1980) Serious head injuries in sport. *British Medical Journal* **281**, 789–91.

Lloyd Parry JMH (1990) *Official Horse Trials of the British Horse Society*. Accident report forms.

McGhee CNJ, Gullan RW, Miller JD (1987) Horse riding and head injury: admissions to a regional head injury unit. *British Journal of Neurosurgery* **1**, 131–6.

Miles JR (1970) The racecourse medical officer. *Journal of the Royal College of General Practitioners* **19**, 228.

Muwanga LC, Dove AF (1985) Head protection for riders: a cause for concern. *Archives of Emergency Medicine* **2**, 85–7.

OPCS (1990) Fatal accidents occuring during sporting and leisure activities, 1989 registrations. London: Office of Population Censuses and Surveys.

Regan PJ, Roberts JO, Feldberg L, Roberts AHN (1991) Hand injuries from leading horses. *Injury* **22**, 124–6.

Surtees RS (1843) *Jorrocks in Handley Cross*. London: Methuen.

Teacher J (1988) Safety hat appeal after hunting fall. *Horse and Hound*.

Whitlock MR (1988) Horse riding is dangerous for your health. *Australian Guide for Emergency Medicine*, 191.

Index

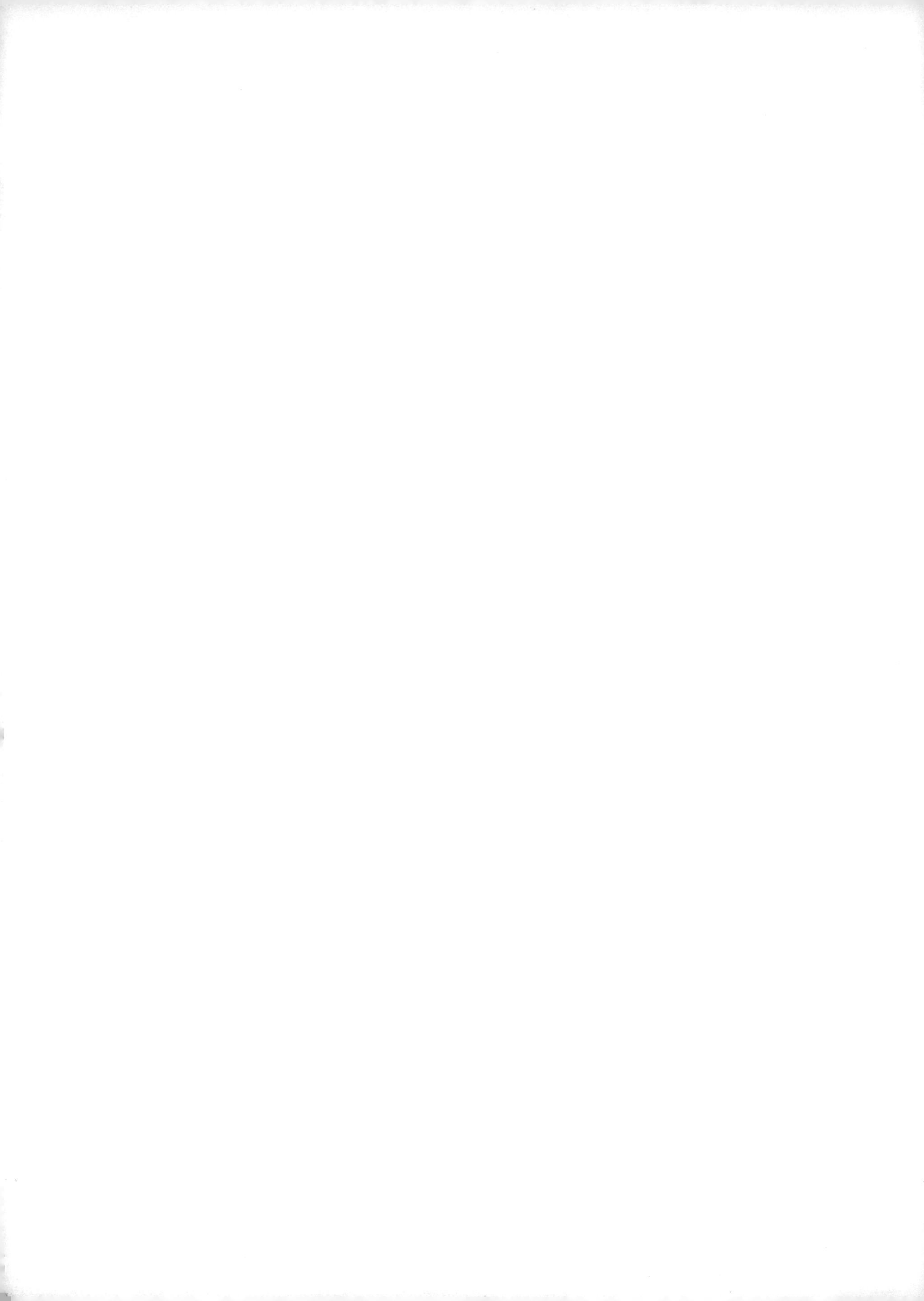

THE SOFT TISSUES

Trauma and Sports Injuries

To our parents and our children